C0-ARI-167

DATE DUE

AUG 28 1990			
DEC 15 1993			

DEMCO 38-297

GYNECOLOGIC CANCER
DIAGNOSIS AND TREATMENT STRATEGIES

The University of Texas
M. D. Anderson Hospital and Tumor Institute at Houston
Twenty-ninth Annual Clinical Conference on Cancer

Published for
The University of Texas
M. D. Anderson Hospital and Tumor Institute at Houston
Houston, Texas, by the University of Texas Press, Austin

The University of Texas
M. D. Anderson Hospital and Tumor Institute at Houston
Twenty-ninth Annual Clinical Conference on Cancer

GYNECOLOGIC CANCER
Diagnosis and Treatment Strategies

Edited by

Felix N. Rutledge, M.D.
Ralph S. Freedman, M.D.
David M. Gershenson, M.D.

University of Texas Press, Austin

Proceedings Editorial Staff

REBECCA TEAFF: Supervising Editor

SUZANNE SIMPSON: Editor

SHERYL BOWEN: Editorial Assistant

Department of Scientific Publications
UT M. D. Anderson Hospital and Tumor Institute

Copyright © 1987
by the University of Texas System Cancer Center
All rights reserved
Printed in the United States of America

First Edition, 1987

Requests for permission to reproduce material from this work should be sent to Permissions, University of Texas Press, Box 7819, Austin, Texas 78713-7819.

Library of Congress Cataloging-in-Publication Data
Clinical Conference on Cancer (29th : 1985 :
M. D. Anderson Hospital and Tumor Institute
at Houston)
Gynecologic cancer.
Held Nov. 13–16, 1985.
Includes bibliographies and index.
1. Generative organs, Female—Cancer—Congresses.
I. Rutledge, Felix N., 1917– . II. Freedman,
Ralph S. III. Gershenson, David M. (David Marc),
1946– . IV. M. D. Anderson Hospital and Tumor
Institute. V. Title. [DNLM: 1. Genital Neoplasms,
Female—diagnosis—congresses. 2. Genital Neoplasms,
Female—therapy—congresses. W3 C162H 29th 1985g /
WP 145 C6405 1985g]
RC280.G5C55 1985 616.99′465 86-30802
ISBN 0-292-72737-2

This volume is a compilation of the proceedings of The University of Texas M. D. Anderson Hospital and Tumor Institute at Houston's 29th Annual Clinical Conference on Cancer, held November 13–16, 1985, in Houston, Texas.

The material contained in this volume was submitted as previously unpublished material, except in instances in which credit has been given to the source from which some of the illustrative material was derived.

Great care has been taken to maintain the accuracy of the information contained in the volume. However, the editorial staff, The University of Texas, and the University of Texas Press cannot be held responsible for errors or for any consequences arising from the use of the information contained herein.

Contents

Rehabilitation

Jeffrey A. Gottlieb Memorial Lecture

Preface

Each year nearly 70,000 new cases of gynecologic cancer are diagnosed, making it the third most common cancer for women. In the past decade, physicians have come to understand more about the risk factors for gynecologic cancer; however, ovarian cancer remains an exception, still claiming more lives than endometrial and cervical cancer combined. It is estimated that one in 70 women will develop carcinoma of the ovary. And most women will present with the disease in an advanced stage, when only palliative treatment is possible.

The purpose of this conference was to provide gynecologists—both specialists and generalists—with information about the latest developments in the detection and treatment of gynecologic cancers. A major emphasis in these proceedings was the trend toward more conservative treatment. Recent clinical investigations have shown, for example, that the traditional treatment for carcinoma of the vulva, which consists of radical vulvectomy and bilateral groin lymphadenectomy, does not protect against local recurrence and may produce high postoperative morbidity. More conservative surgical techniques, such as wide local excision or hemivulvectomy and ipsilateral groin dissection do not increase the recurrence risk and are associated with less infection, shorter hospital stays, and less psychosocial consequences. The adoption of less radical procedures together with new plastic surgery techniques has helped in many cases to restore sexual function.

Innovative treatments combining conventional radiotherapy and chemotherapy with newer modalities for ovarian and other types of gynecologic cancers appear promising. In ovarian cancer treatment, the combined use of biologic response modifiers (BRMs) and chemotherapy is being studied. BRMs, which can increase the resistance of the host to tumor growth, have been shown to have substantial antitumor effects in a variety of animal models. A particularly promising approach to therapy with BRMs involves administering agents in the region of tumor growth.

In the majority of ovarian cancer cases, the tumor remains largely confined to the peritoneal cavity for most of its natural history. Because of this, intraperitoneal administration of chemotherapeutic agents is being thoroughly investigated. It is believed that because the tumor often grows as tiny nodules on the peritoneal surface, the delivery of drug by free-surface diffusion to the tumor might significantly enhance the therapeutic impact of treatment.

The intraarterial infusion of chemotherapeutic agents also appears to be effective in cases of advanced gynecologic cancer, such as FIGO stage III and IV carcinomas of the cervix and vagina. In one study of patients with advanced localized gynecologic malignancies, arterial chemotherapy given prior to radiation treatment produced a 74% response rate.

New uses are being found in gynecologic oncology for other more established therapies. Although it has been applied in the management of gynecologic cancer for 30 years, for example, hormonal therapy has been a topic of renewed interest based on cytosol estrogen and progestin receptors in samples of epithelial ovarian cancer. Hyperthermia is another somewhat established modality, which has recently been effectively combined with chemotherapy and radiotherapy for certain types of metastatic gynecologic cancers. Further clinical investigations are needed, however, to determine whether hyperthermia may be used as primary treatment—development of better deep-heating equipment and noninvasive thermometry are prerequisites to these trials.

Many of the advanced techniques and therapies discussed in these proceedings have been developed only within the last decade. We are confident of the great potential they hold for both basic science and clinical applications in the field of gynecologic oncology. Our judicious use of these therapies combined with the trend toward conservative treatment and the recent emphasis on psychosocial adjustment after radical surgical procedures should help to ensure a better quality of life for our patients.

We would like to extend our appreciation to all those who made possible the 29th Annual Clinical Conference, including members of the program committee, Larry J. Copeland, M.D.; Creighton L. Edwards, M.D.; H. Stephen Gallager, M.D.; John J. Kavanagh, M.D.; Lester J. Peters, M.D.; J. Taylor Wharton, M.D.; and Patton B. Saul, M.D. We also appreciate the contributions of James M. Bowen, Ph.D.; David T. Carr, M.D.; Thomas Gee; Charles A. LeMaistre, M.D.; Bernard Levin, M.D.; Clifton F. Mountain, M.D.; Walter J. Pagel; Jeff Rasco; Steven C. Schultz; and Stephen C. Stuyck.

For their continued support of the U.T. M. D. Anderson Hospital and Tumor Institute at Houston's Clinical Conference on Cancer, we thank the American Cancer Society, Texas Division, Inc. For their generous support, we also thank Abbott Laboratories; Adria Laboratories, Inc.; Bristol Laboratories; Ethicon, Inc.; Lederle Laboratories; Mead Johnson Pharmaceutical Division; Merck, Sharpe & Dohme; Miles Laboratories, Inc.; ONCOR; Roerig-Pfizer; Ross Laboratories; Sandoz, Inc.; Smith Kline & French Laboratories; E. R. Squibb & Sons, Inc., Stuart Pharmaceuticals; Upjohn; and Wyeth Laboratories.

THE EDITORS

GYNECOLOGIC CANCER
DIAGNOSIS AND TREATMENT STRATEGIES

Annual Clinical Conference on Cancer, Vol. 29
Gynecologic Cancer: Diagnosis and Treatment Strategies
© 1987 by The University of Texas System Cancer Center

1. Introduction

Felix N. Rutledge

This recording of the Twenty-ninth Annual Clinical Conference represents the third clinical conference on gynecologic oncology sponsored by The University of Texas M. D. Anderson Hospital and Tumor Institute at Houston. Since our first conference on gynecologic oncology held 25 years ago, we have witnessed growing numbers of highly trained specialists and expansion of clinical experience and research in this field. A comparison of the subjects that we discussed in these proceedings with those of the earlier clinical conferences in 1960 and 1966 is of some historical interest.

In the current proceedings, we have noted an important trend toward conservative treatment of the gynecologic cancer patient when feasible. There is also an emphasis on concern for the psychological and emotional as well as the physical consequences of radical surgical procedures. When major surgery is appropriate, conservation or restoration of sexual function, for example, has become an integral part of the treatment plan.

In recent years, we have abandoned some subjects of controversy and some areas of research, and we have made alterations in our treatment approach to certain types of gynecologic cancer. Because it did not improve cure rates, for example, we no longer perform pelvic lymphadenectomy after full-dose irradiation for cancer of the cervix. Pretreatment laparotomy to stage cancer of the cervix before radiation treatment proved to be intolerable and has also been stopped. Complete vulvectomy for all degrees of intraepithelial carcinoma is no longer routinely applied because less radical resection can be effective. These are lessons we have learned from clinical experience and from forums such as this conference. We have also begun to focus on new discoveries—tumor markers, hormone receptors, nuclear magnetic resonance imaging, immunotherapeutics—that may significantly impact future developments.

Although, as expected, many changes have taken place in this field over the past 25 years, there is still a focus on several specific clinical problems. Among these, ovarian cancer is prominent. We continue to try to define the nature of borderline (low malignant potential) tumors of the ovary, to find the most effective applications of chemotherapy for epithelial ovarian cancer, and to rely on surgical procedures such as second-look laparotomy and pelvic exenteration for control of disease spread.

The publication of our first clinical conference on gynecologic oncology contains the classic article on semimalignant ovarian tumors by Hans-Ludwig Kottmeier (1962). He stressed a need to distinguish patients with these tumors from other patients with cancer of the ovary when determining treatment and assessing survival rates. Many articles, emphasizing both the clinical and pathological aspects of these tumors, have since appeared. Only after many years is Kottmeier's advice being heeded. We have learned that these tumors, which we now call tumors of borderline malignancy, represent a special type of ovarian cancer and thus require accurate clinical evaluation and appropriate treatment.

Also in the first clinical conference volume, S. B. Gusberg and Grace G. Helman (1962) discussed cellular infiltrates in cancer of the cervix that could be used to predict the outcome of radiation treatment. This enduring topic has been researched extensively, but so far no dependable method for predicting radiation sensitivity has been discovered. More sophisticated techniques of DNA determination by flow cytometry and other radiobiological research methods keep this topic interesting.

In 1960, the best treatment for regional nodes along the pelvic wall was being debated by surgeons and radiotherapists. There was a prevalent opinion that irradiation alone was not therapeutically reliable. Early in the 1950s, the staff at U.T. M. D. Anderson Hospital had undertaken to test the success of combined irradiation and surgery. Following full-dose irradiation, pelvic lymphadenectomy was performed. I reported on this experience with a series of 440 patients who had pelvic lymphadenectomy as an adjunct to irradiation for cancer of the cervix (Rutledge 1962b). One of the protocols was designed to determine whether there was improved survival. The negative results of this study led to the decline in the practice of lymphadenectomy in combination with radiation therapy.

The report by Samuels, Howe, and MacDonald (1962), regarding the use of alkylating agents for advanced cancer of the ovary, introduced melphalan as a new agent for this purpose. Our staff utilized this chemotherapy agent and for many years popularized this new treatment. Only after cisplatin became available did melphalan become a secondary drug for this disease.

In the proceedings of the second clinical conference, we reviewed a series of 950 patients with ovarian cancer to illustrate the role of tumor stage and histological type on prognosis (Burns, Underwood, and Rutledge 1969). The importance of grade had not been recognized at that time. Although 239 patients in that series had received chemotherapy, external irradiation remained the preferred treatment. The significance of the size of a residual tumor that could not be resected was recognized. It was noted that residual tumors larger than 3 cm responded poorly to radiation therapy. In the years since that conference in 1966, there has been a decline in the use of external irradiation for stage III and stage IV epithelial tumors. A randomized prospective trial comparing chemotherapy with whole-abdomen irradiation (Smith, Rutledge, and Delclos 1975) was influential in the shift from irradiation to chemotherapy for advanced cancer of the ovary. Second-look laparotomy was practiced extensively during this interim.

Also in the 1966 proceedings, Kottmeier discussed individualized therapy for patients with carcinoma of the endometrium and advocated the role of primary hysterectomy and postoperative radiation therapy, depending upon the extent of the disease (Kottmeier 1969). This philosophy of management was later supported by Morrow, DiSaia, and Townsend (1973), and a new era of individualized therapy has followed. There was a 79% five-year survival rate in Kottmeier's experience with 228 patients with stage I disease who were treated with primary surgery. When the lesions were well differentiated, the five-year survival rate was 91%, but it dropped to 32% when the adenocarcinomas were markedly anaplastic. Kottmeier's views concerning the efficacy of combined surgery and radiation therapy for endometrial carcinoma have been confirmed by observations over the past 20 years and are an important topic in the present conference.

Another emphasis in the care of gynecologic cancer patients at U.T. M. D. Anderson Hospital that deserves mention is the philosophy of treatment, which was outlined in our clinical conference proceedings in 1960 (Rutledge 1962a):

> The first treatment should be the best possible since it has the greatest chance for curing the patient. Every effort should be made to: decide the full extent of the cancer before treatment, raise the level of the patient's general health to achieve the greatest benefit from therapy, give the maximum treatment during the first effort and follow the results closely for possible complication or recurrence.
>
> Should recurrence develop, a cure should again be attempted. This second treatment will be more difficult and more hazardous, and is usually a different method than the first. If a cure is not possible, palliation should be attempted.

We also adhered to the idea that the first physician to prescribe treatment was to consider the initial treatment a serious responsibility that extended until either cure or failure was definite. This indicated a need for a special physician to serve this role. The development in 1970 of the specialty of gynecologic oncology was the solution.

Our staff at U.T. M. D. Anderson Hospital was fortunate in these proceedings to have had the participation of leading authorities from cancer centers throughout the United States and from Canada and England to aid us in covering all the current topics of interest in gynecologic oncology. We hope that this volume will be a useful text for physicians, researchers, and other health professionals involved in the care of gynecologic cancer patients.

References

Burns BC Jr, Underwood PB Jr, Rutledge FN. 1969. A review of carcinoma of the ovary at The University of Texas M. D. Anderson Hospital and Tumor Institute at Houston. In *Cancer of the Uterus and Ovary*, pp. 123–147. Chicago: Year Book Medical.

Gusberg SB, Helman GG. 1962. A radiobiologic contribution to the treatment of patients with cancer of the cervix. In *Carcinoma of the Uterine Cervix, Endometrium and Ovary*, pp. 61–67. Chicago: Year Book Medical.

Kottmeier H-L. 1962. Modern trends in the treatment of patients with semimalignant and malignant ovarian tumors. In *Carcinoma of the Uterine Cervix, Endometrium and Ovary*, pp. 285–298. Chicago: Year Book Medical.

Kottmeier H-L. 1969. Individualization of therapy in carcinoma of the corpus. In *Cancer of the Uterus and Ovary*, pp. 102–108. Chicago: Year Book Medical.

Morrow CP, DiSaia PJ, Townsend DE. 1973. Current management of endometrial carcinoma. *Obstet Gynecol* 42:399–406.

Rutledge FN. 1962a. Cancer of the female genital system: Clinical material and philosophy of treatment. In *Carcinoma of the Uterine Cervix, Endometrium and Ovary*, pp. 13–18. Chicago: Year Book Medical.

Rutledge FN. 1962b. Experience with pelvic lymphadenectomy. In *Carcinoma of the Uterine Cervix, Endometrium and Ovary*, pp. 175–191. Chicago: Year Book Medical.

Samuels ML, Howe CD, MacDonald EJ. 1962. Alkylating agents in the treatment of patients with advanced cancer of ovary. In *Carcinoma of the Uterine Cervix, Endometrium and Ovary*, pp. 329–338. Chicago: Year Book Medical.

Smith JP, Rutledge FN, Delclos L. 1975. Postoperative treatment of early cancer of the ovary: A random trial between postoperative irradiation and chemotherapy. *Natl Cancer Inst Monogr* 42: 149–153.

HEATH MEMORIAL AWARD LECTURE

Annual Clinical Conference on Cancer, Vol. 29
Gynecologic Cancer: Diagnosis and Treatment Strategies
© 1987 by The University of Texas System Cancer Center

2. Pelvic Exenteration: An Update of the U.T. M. D. Anderson Hospital Experience and Review of the Literature

Felix N. Rutledge

Radical pelvic surgical procedures, such as cystectomy combined with vaginectomy and colorectal resection combined with vaginectomy, were performed for several years before Appleby in 1943 combined these operations into what is known today as "pelvic exenteration" (Appleby 1950). Although Appleby, Bricker, and Modlin (1951) were the first physicians to actually perform exenteration, it was Brunschwig (1948) who first reported the procedure in the literature. Brunschwig is also recognized as the originator of exenteration because he established its use in gynecology, particularly in cases of cervical cancer.

Pelvic exenteration is most useful in the treatment of gynecologic cancer when the primary cancer has not been cured by the initial treatment or when new cancer growth has developed locally. Both equipment and techniques for administering radiation have improved greatly in recent years, and chemotherapy has been established as an effective treatment in some cases. Still, some types of cancer are very advanced when discovered, and others simply resist treatment. Therefore, pelvic exenteration is necessary in selected cases.

We recently reviewed 3,793 reported cases of pelvic exenteration (table 2.1), excluding reports from foreign literature. Considering the number of foreign reports and the fact that many other exenteration procedures may not have been reported, we estimate that the total number of cases performed is likely to have been over 6,000. Exenteration, then, is performed infrequently compared with other operations of similar magnitude.

At The University of Texas M. D. Anderson Hospital and Tumor Institute at Houston, this operation is performed as frequently today as it was 10 to 15 years ago. A total of 448 exenteration procedures were done from 1955 to 1984. Although there are variations in the actual number of procedures done each year at this institution, the average frequency has not diminished nor have the ratios of total versus anterior or posterior exenteration changed considerably.

In this type of retrospective review, which focuses on signs of development, improvement, and clinical usefulness of the treatment, the time period of each report must be considered. Since this treatment was introduced, guidelines for patient selection have been amended and technical modifications have been applied for improving patient tolerance and acceptance. One notable improvement has been made in the procedure for urinary diversion. The first patients to undergo this procedure

Table 2.1. *Pelvic Exenteration Cases from 1947 to 1985: Review of the Literature*

Study	Institution	Time Period	No. of Patients
Brunschwig 1970	Memorial Hospital, New York	1947–1965	925
Schmitz et al. 1960	Loyola University, Illinois	1947–1958	75
Parsons 1959	Boston University, Massachusetts	1948–1958	160
Wawro and Howe 1957	Hartford Hospital, Connecticut	1948–1957	44
Douglas and Sweeney 1957	Cornell University, New York	1948–1954	23
Ingersoll and Ulfelder 1966	Harvard University, Massachusetts	1949–1963	116
Turko et al. 1977	University of British Columbia, Canada	1949–1971	22
Thyssen 1956	Finsen Institute, Denmark	1949–1954	14
Bricker 1970	Washington University, Missouri	1950–1965	312
Symmonds, Pratt, and Webb 1975	Mayo Clinic, Minnesota	1950–1971	198
Krieger and Embree 1969	Cleveland Clinic, Ohio	1951–1969	47
Mikuta, Murphy, and Schoenberg 1967	University of Pennsylvania	1952–1965	32
Rutledge 1985 (present study)	U.T. M. D. Anderson Hospital, Texas	1955–1984	448
Ingiulla and Cosmi 1967	University of Florence, Italy	1957–1966	241
Devereux, Sears, and Ketcham 1980	National Cancer Institute, Maryland	1957–1977	245
Karlen and Piver 1975	Roswell Park Hospital, New York	1957–1974	87
Talledo 1985	Medical College of Georgia	1959–1983	42
Boutselis 1973	Ohio State University	1960–1972	17
Galante and Hill 1971	University of California at San Francisco	1961–1969	41
Lifshitz et al. 1981	University of Iowa	1963–1979	58
Onnis et al. 1981	University of Padua, Italy	1963–1977	55
Yu et al. 1976	University of Hong Kong	1964–1975	76
Morley and Lindenauer 1976	University of Michigan	1965–1975	70
Wrigley et al. 1976	University of Minnesota	1965–1974	34
Averette et al. 1984	University of Miami, Florida	1966–1981	92
Bompiani et al. 1985	Catholic University, Italy	1967–1981	44
Orr et al. 1983	University of Alabama	1969–1981	125
Morgan, Daly, and Monif 1980	University of Florida	1970–1978	56
Curry et al. 1981	Pennsylvania State University	1972–1979	37
Berek, Hacker, and Lagasse 1984	University of California at Los Angeles	1976–1982	37
Karlen, Williams, and Summers 1983	Akron Hospital, Ohio	1979–1982	20
		Total	3,793

suffered severely from urinary tract sepsis due to the implantation of the ureter into the colon carrying the fecal stream or from infection of the skin when the ureters opened alongside the colostomy. After the ileal conduit was developed, the risk of urinary infection declined. The early series also contained some patients with hopeless prognoses. In some cases, we now can preoperatively identify patients with cancer that is likely to be found unresectable. At laparotomy, the surgeon may also recognize incurable metastases more effectively before the dissection has progressed to the stage wherein the operation must be completed.

Patient Selection

There was no standard process for patient selection when exenteration was first performed. Overall survival rates from the early years may reflect the number of cases that should have been considered inoperable. In some patients, exenteration was performed to remove pelvic organs destroyed by irradiation treatment. These patients frequently developed severe postoperative complications that often caused early death.

The major factors to be considered in determining a patient's ability to undergo the procedure are physical reserve and the extent of the cancer. Because the lungs, heart, liver, and kidneys are most vulnerable to injury by the operation, each of these vital organs is evaluated preoperatively by a minimal function requirement test. Other general factors to consider are advanced age, chronic hypertension, diabetes, alcoholism, and obesity. In some cases, it is still difficult to adhere rigidly to general criteria of inadequacy and to withhold exenteration—the only remaining treatment likely to be curative. Unless patients have obvious or critical impairments, they may be selected for the procedure.

Illnesses affecting other body organs that are present before the operation have an effect on the postoperative death rate and will determine whether the expected benefits of the operation are realized. Obviously, whether the cancer is curable can never be determined when the patient dies of postoperative complications from vital organ system failure. The therapeutic potential of exenteration cannot be determined when there is a high incidence of early postoperative deaths. The calculated five-year survival rates presently reported are so influenced by early postoperative deaths that the true value of this treatment is yet to be realized.

Universal minimum standards regarding vital organ function in patients requiring exenteration have not been established. In areas such as cardiovascular care, new methods for operative and postoperative cardiac monitoring have added considerable safety for patients at marginal risk; thus, our minimum requirements have been lowered in recent years. Recent literature stresses the role of special care teams to support such vital organ functions both during and following the surgery.

The guidelines that we use to determine location and extent of the cancer as contraindications to exenteration at U.T. M. D. Anderson Hospital also are not universal. We have been able to establish some successful guidelines in areas such as renal obstruction, lymph node metastasis, and special types of cancer. Operability implies that the cancer must be removed; this is dependent on the surgeon's accessibility to the affected organs. Physical factors such as obesity are important considerations in patient selection. Obesity creates technical obstacles, particularly for conduit construction, colostomy formation, and perineal reconstruction. Increased distance imposed by the thick anterior abdominal wall and the crowded space within the pelvis due to excess fat reduces access that the surgeon is ordinarily allowed.

Indications for Treatment with Exenteration

At U.T. M. D. Anderson Hospital, exenteration was the primary treatment in 17.6% of cases and was applied in 82.4% for cancer recurrence (Rutledge 1985, present study). Exenteration was used only infrequently to treat newly diagnosed cancer. Our guidelines for patient selection still exclude those who have not first undergone less radical surgery or irradiation. In earlier years, patients with cancer of the cervix that spread to the bladder were treated with combination radiation therapy and anterior exenteration. We now treat such patients with a full course of radiation and withhold exenteration unless there is a treatment failure. Patients who have had special histological types of cancer that can only be treated appropriately by exenteration are exceptions. In our series, 13 patients—all under the age of 20 — were in this category (table 2.2).

As in most patient series, the most common indication for pelvic exenteration in our patients was recurrent cancer of the cervix or vagina. It was often difficult in such cases to determine the correct site of origin. The majority of our patients had common squamous cell carcinoma (table 2.3); 85.7% originated in the cervix or vagina (table 2.4). The type of exenteration employed was determined by the anatomical site of the cancer. Carcinoma of the cervix or vagina was the diagnosis in 84.4% of patients who had anterior exenterations, in 41.7% of the patients who had posterior exenterations, and in 93.5% of those who had total exenterations. Carcinoma of the vulva was the most common diagnosis in patients requiring posterior exenteration.

Reports of selected groups of patients who underwent exenteration for primary compared with recurrent disease are listed in table 2.5. The National Cancer Insti-

Table 2.2. *Age Incidence for Pelvic Exenteration*

Years	No. of Patients	(%)
0–9	9	(2.0)
10–19	4	(0.9)
20–29	11	(2.5)
30–39	64	(14.3)
40–49	114	(25.4)
50–59	123	(27.4)
60–69	99	(22.1)
70–79	24	(5.4)
Total	448	(100.0)

Table 2.3. *Distribution of Pelvic Exenteration Patients by Histological Types of Cancer*

Histology	No. of Patients	(%)
Squamous	343	(76.6)
Adenocarcinoma	72	(16.1)
Sarcoma botryoides	8	(1.8)
Other sarcomas	7	(1.6)
Clear cell carcinoma	6	(1.3)
Melanoma	4	(0.9)
Cloacogenic	3	(0.7)
Adenocarcinoma (ovary)	2	(0.4)
Granulosa cell carcinoma	1	(0.2)
Endodermal sinus tumor	1	(0.2)
Adenoid cystic carcinoma	1	(0.2)
Total	448	(100.0)

Table 2.4. *Anatomical Site of Cancer Origin in 448 Patients Requiring Pelvic Exenteration*

Site	No. of Patients	(%)
Cervix	329	(73.4)
Vagina	55	(12.3)
Vulva	19	(4.3)
Endometrium	15	(3.3)
Colon/rectum	15	(3.3)
Urethra	7	(1.6)
Ovary	4	(0.9)
Bladder	3	(0.7)
Pelvis	1	(0.2)
Total	448	(100.0)

tute series (Ketcham et al. 1970) shows the highest percentage of primary treatment by exenteration. Most of the patients in that series had cancer of the cervix. Exenteration was undertaken in many of the NCI patients because they were found to be unsuited for planned Wertheim hysterectomies.

Operative Techniques

Urinary Diversion

When we performed the first exenteration procedure at U.T. M. D. Anderson Hospital in 1955, the ileal conduit designed by Bricker was already established as the preferred method for diverting the urine. The rectal pouch (implantation of the ureters into the sigmoid colon with diversion of the sigmoid above with sigmoid colostomy) had been described by Parsons and Taymor (1955) as a means for urinary diversion and maintenance of urinary continence. This procedure would have

Table 2.5. *Pelvic Exenteration for Primary and Recurrent Cancer: Review of the Literature*

Study	Primary Cancer		Recurrent Cancer		Postoperative Deaths	
	No. of Patients	(%)	No. of Patients	(%)	No. of Patients	(%)
Barber and Brunschwig 1966	229/840	(27.3)	611/840	(72.7)	—	—
Parsons 1959	35/120	(29.2)	85/120	(70.8)	27/120	(22.5)
Bricker 1970	105/312	(33.7)	207/312	(66.3)	32/312	(10.3)
Symmonds, Pratt, and Webb 1975	37/198	(18.7)	161/198	(81.3)	16/198	(8.1)
Rutledge et al. 1977	66/296	(22.3)	230/296	(77.7)	40/296	(13.5)
Rutledge 1985 (present study)	79/448	(17.6)	369/448	(82.4)	46/448	(10.3)
Ketcham et al. 1970	68/162	(42.0)	94/162	(58.0)	28/162	(17.3)
Karlen and Piver 1975	18/87	(20.7)	69/87	(79.3)	12/87	(13.8)
Talledo 1985	13/42	(31.0)	29/42	(69.0)	10/42	(23.8)
Morley and Lindenauer 1976	—	—	70/70	(100.0)	1/70	(1.4)
Averette et al. 1984	13/92	(14.1)	79/92	(85.9)	22/92	(23.9)
Orr et al. 1983	21/125	(16.8)	104/125	(83.2)	12/125	(9.6)

been useful in cases of anterior exenteration. It was logically designed so that the colostomy would prevent fecal contamination of the renal units. The problem of recurrent pyelitis with the colon-ureteral implantation was intolerable. Our experience with the rectal pouch procedure was also disappointing. Although we may have eliminated pyelitis, there was a significant fistula incidence, and the rectal sphincter was not continent for urine, especially during sleep.

It was considered feasible to use a segment of sigmoid rather than ileum for a sigmoid conduit before we adopted that technique for frequent use. Our first sigmoid conduit procedure was done in February 1956. Soon the advantages of the procedure were clear, and we began to use the sigmoid conduit as a routine urinary diversion for the total exenteration procedure. Employing a segment of sigmoid was beneficial when the segment could be taken from the proximal end of the severed rectosigmoid as was available when total exenteration was performed. This eliminated the intestinal anastomosis that was necessary for an ileal conduit. Thus, operating time was saved and earlier feeding of the patient was allowed following surgery. Use of the sigmoid conduit also eliminated a source of intestinal fistulization as mentioned above. The sigmoid segment conduit is also advantageous because it evacuates urine well and adapts well without electrolyte reabsorption. Also, the stoma functions satisfactorily for adaption of a prosthesis. Symmonds et al. (1975) of the Mayo Clinic have reported favorable results with the sigmoid conduit, whereas others such as Shingleton (Orr et al. 1982) of Birmingham use it infrequently.

At U.T. M. D. Anderson Hospital, the following types of conduits have been used for urinary diversion in 400 cases of pelvic exenteration: ileal conduit, 227 patients (56.8%); sigmoid conduit, 160 patients (40.0%); transverse colon, 8 patients (2.0%); and rectal pouch, 5 patients (1.2%). Of those patients, 48 underwent posterior exenteration. Of course these numbers do not reflect our preferential use of the sigmoid conduit in recent years. Theoretically, it may be not wise to use the sigmoid conduit because of the possibility of metastatic infiltration of the rectosigmoid, particularly when the intestine has been divided near the specimen. We have never observed any cases of cancer recurrence in the conduit, however, since we began using the sigmoid segment.

Selected representative reports from the literature (table 2.6) show an incidence of postoperative urinary fistula ranging from 4% to 12%. It may be assumed that the

Table 2.6. *Incidence of Urinary Fistula: Review of the Literature*

Study	No. of Patients	(%)
Barber and Brunschwig 1966	43/840	(5.1)
Symmonds, Pratt, and Webb 1975	8/198	(4.0)
Rutledge 1985 (present study)	23/448	(5.1)
Ketcham et al. 1970	9/162	(5.6)
Karlen and Piver 1975	8/87	(9.2)
Talledo 1985	3/42	(7.1)
Morley and Lindenauer 1976	4/70	(5.7)
Averette et al. 1984	11/92	(12.0)
Orr et al. 1982	10/119	(8.4)

primary reason for the postoperative urinary fistula is directly related to the technique for urinary diversion; thus, it is important that this complication be closely monitored and that efforts be made to improve the techniques.

Based on the assumption that the ureter-to-conduit anastomosis was most critical, a more watertight connection was designed. No significant changes have been made in our ureter-to-conduit anastomosis technique since our first report describing exenterative surgery in 1965 (Rutledge and Burns 1965) The semi-soft Silastic tubes are threaded up the ureter, but not coiled, into the renal pelvis. The protruding ends of the catheters are passed through the openings in the intestinal segment and out the stomal end.

The sizes of these catheters are selected to match the maximum calibre of the ureter. Provided urinary antiseptics are used, the catheters induce little tissue reactivity and are well tolerated. To prevent extrusion, the catheter is sutured to the wall of the conduit near the anastomotic site. The small chromic catgut retention sutures dissolve after three weeks, and the catheters are removed by traction upon the ends that protrude outside the abdomen through the stoma.

Good healing of the ureteral anastomosis has been aided by splinting. Our experience with splinting of the ureter has been favorable as demonstrated by a decrease from 17% to 6% in the incidence of urinary fistula in the last 150 patients of our series. One of the most important benefits of splinting is that it helps to achieve a more complete and precise anastomosis of the margins. The walls of the severed ureter and the intestinal mucosa rimming the opening in the side of the conduit are made more distinct by the Silastic tubes. Each suture becomes a purposeful and functional placement. An ample, but not excessive, number of sutures should assure a better anastomotic seal without subsequent stenosis.

Denudation of the Pelvic Cavity

Technical modifications designed to reduce the frequency of intestinal complications associated with denudation of the pelvic cavity have been introduced in recent years. The exenteration procedure that was used at U.T. M. D. Anderson Hospital until the mid 1960s involved filling the pelvic cavity with a gauze pack as Brunschwig (1948) and others recommended. The pack served to control hemorrhage in some patients; in all patients, the pack supported the loops of intestine until they were sufficiently adherent or positioned to support themselves. Because of a high incidence of postoperative intestinal fistula associated with this method, we tested a procedure in which a lid composed of the patient's own tissues was placed across the top of the pelvic cavity. Human tissues were used after synthetic materials had proved to be poorly tolerated. To accomplish the technique, segments of ileum or colon with adjoining mesentery were isolated. The antimesenteric margin of the bowel and the edges of the mesentery were sutured to the edge of the pelvis adjoining the mesentery across the top of the pelvic cavity. This technique excluded the loops of functional intestine and supposedly prevented them from becoming obstructed. The method was eventually abandoned, however, because of severe pelvic sepsis caused by exposure to contamination through the perineal opening.

An alternate method using omental material was then developed to cover the pelvis and to fill the pelvic space. A "pedicle" of omentum was developed by partially separating the omentum along the greater curvature of the stomach and extending the material along the left pericolic gutter of the pelvis to cover the pelvic cavity. The length and strength of omentum varies from one individual to another; in the patient undergoing total exenteration, it is important as a source of blood supply as well as a membrane to separate the intestines and urinary conduit from the pelvic wall. Division of the right gastroepiploic artery and its branches leading to the stomach, after dissection of the omentum from the transverse colon, frees the right three fourths of the omentum to be swung downward. This mobilization of the omentum is simple and can be completed by one surgical team while a second team does the perineal phase of the operation. Detachment of the omentum in our patients was most often from right to left by division of the right gastroepiploic artery. However, in cases of poor development of the left gastroepiploic artery, the right artery could be conserved by creating the pedicle from the left. Successive division of the vessels along the greater curvature of the stomach releases about three fourths of the omentum from the stomach and transverse colon. The remainder, which is attached to the left part of the stomach, the spenic flexure of the colon, and the spleen, contains the blood supply. The mobilized omentum is passed along the lateral pericolic gutter—peripheral to the colostomy exit—over the pelvic brim and into the pelvis. In the pelvis, the edges of the omentum are sutured along the pelvic brim and allowed to drape over the pelvic walls and lie on the pelvic floor. Upon this omental carpet, loops of intestine are allowed to descend and fill the pelvic cavity. The exudate from the pelvic walls that have undergone denudation drains into the pelvic basin beneath and outside the omental covering. This exudate is removed by a drainage tube that penetrates the perineum and is sutured to the fascia in the hollow sacrum. The tube for drainage is maintained for at least five days postoperatively. Although there are disadvantages associated with omental transfer, they are insignificant when we consider the benefits of the procedure.

Vaginal Reconstruction

Several operations designed to restore sexual function after exenteration have been modestly successful. Generally, the vagina and much of the vulva are removed by exenteration; therefore, reconstruction of a functioning vagina is planned for most patients. When the patient can be assured that restoration of vaginal function is feasible, a major obstacle to the patient's acceptance of the exenteration procedure is removed.

Perhaps the most generally employed method of reconstruction of the vagina has been the McIndoe and Banister (1938) procedure in which a split-thickness graft lines a space in the area of the resected vagina. The ectopic skin attaches to the undersurface of the omental pedicle and against the levator muscles and tissues of the perineum. The split-thickness graft may be placed during or after the exenteration procedure. If an obturator is employed to reserve this space by resisting contracture and fibrosis, grafting may be delayed until a bed of granulation tissue is established. Delayed grafting may be advantageous in that the serous and lymph exudate will interfere less with the survival of the graft if applied a week or more after exenteration.

Other methods for vaginal construction have been somewhat successful. A segment of intestine has been used for a neovagina by Pratt (1961) of the Mayo Clinic and by several German surgeons. However, that method has not been popular in recent years.

The Williams procedure (Williams 1964) for vaginal reconstruction was proposed as a simple and safe technique that did not require redissection of the healed perineal defect. We employed the Williams procedure for construction of a neovagina in one series of patients; however, we have since judged it to be unsatisfactory. Although a report from U.T. M. D. Anderson Hospital recommending the technique was published in 1977 (Day and Stanhope 1977), a subsequent patient survey revealed objections to it. Patients claimed that the reconstructed vagina was functionally awkward and that internal hair growth made it esthetically distracting. Some patients judged the procedure to be "useless."

Myocutaneous Gracilis Graft

Currently, the myocutaneous gracilis graft procedure, usually performed at the time of the pelvic exenteration, is the preferred technique for neovaginal construction. The technique, described by McCraw et al. (1976), has been employed with minor changes in the size and method of suspension of the graft. Compared with other techniques, the cosmetic and functional results of using the graft have been superior. The advantage of reconstructing the vagina at the time of exenteration is that it avoids the risk of injury to loops of intestine in areas that have already healed.

Although it is designed for construction of a new vagina, the myocutaneous gracilis graft procedure aids the patient in other ways as well. This mass of gracilis muscle, attached skin, and subcutaneous fat fills the space in the lower pelvic cavity and contributes to the support of the abdominal contents. Like the omental covering, the gracilis graft aids in reducing the serum loss from the pelvic walls after denudation. The graft also adds new vasculature to the pelvic area, which aids in infection control. From a graft that is mobilized from the inner aspect of the thigh, a skin-lined tube is created and inverted into the pelvic cavity as a new vagina. Reduction of the size of the grafts, from approximately 16 cm to 8 cm, as originally recommended by McCraw et al. (1976), allows for easier insertion and better suspension in the pelvic cavity. When the mass of the graft is too large to fit easily into the pelvis, the vascular supply is endangered. Reduction in the size of the graft improves survival and reduces subsequent prolapse. The smaller grafts are ample for construction of the vagina and for filling the pelvic space. Suture attachment of the graft to the cut edges of the pelvic diaphragm and suture fixation of the vagina to the rectus muscle tendon permanently secure the reconstructed vagina.

Complications of the Myocutaneous Graft

Major complications that have followed the construction of a neovagina after pelvic exenteration are listed in table 2.7. Because the viability of the graft depends upon a

Table 2.7. *Complications of Neovagina*

Complication	Early[a] No. of Patients	Early[a] (%)	Late[b] No. of Patients	Late[b] (%)
Prolapse	1	(0.2)	11	(2.5)
Stricture	—	—	2	(0.4)
Necrosis (25%)	4	(0.9)	—	—
Necrosis (50%)	3	(0.7)	—	—
Necrosis (75%)	2	(0.4)	—	—
Necrosis (100%)	1	(0.2)	—	—
Total	11	(2.5)	13	(2.9)

[a] ≤90 days after surgery.
[b] >90 days after surgery.

single blood supply, vascular insufficiency is a major problem. There are several situations in which the blood supply via the vascular pedicle is not optimal. When these are identified, some degree of necrosis of the graft is expected. The more common events are: (1) accidental disruption of the vascular pedicle; (2) constriction of the blood vessel after the graft is moved to the pelvic cavity; and (3) limited blood circulation to the pelvis by division of the vascular pedicle into two or more branches.

Sometimes these situations can be improved by additional dissection to mobilize the artery. If this is not feasible, the vascular pedicle may be sacrificed, but the proximal bony attachment of the gracilis muscle to the pubis must be retained. The blood supply to the graft from this source is usually adequate.

Necrosis is rarely complete when it occurs. Although a portion of the skin may be lost, it will be replaced by new growth from the surviving portion. Major necrosis of the graft that causes sepsis, however, must be removed.

Although there are no anatomical restrictions for sexual readaptation associated with the neovagina, emotional hurdles for recovery from the exenteration may indirectly delay rehabilitation. In addition, other physical changes such as the stoma on the abdominal wall may require major personal adjustment for couples. The degree of sexual rehabilitation that may be achieved after exenteration is not certain.

Modifications of Total Exenteration

Conservation of a continent colon is most desirable if accomplished without jeopardizing the curative potential of a total exenteration. Resection and anastomosis of the rectosigmoid behind the cervix was attempted early in the history of the exenteration, but it was discontinued because of an excessive postoperative incidence of bowel fistula. A recently developed stapling instrument makes a more secure anastomosis, which is particularly useful in the lower part of the pelvis. Because of improved healing, there has been renewed interest in restoring intestinal continuity after total exenteration. The success of this new technique in terms of achieving low incidence of fistula and ample lumen is influenced strongly by the amount of prior radiation treatment. Thus, the procedure may not be appropriate for patients who have received very high doses of radiation. In each case, the surgeon must determine whether the rectosigmoid is involved extensively with cancer, for such a condition would increase the risk of incomplete excision by the modified procedure.

Postoperative Complications

Since the incidence of postoperative complications increases with prior large-dose radiation therapy, the number of patients in this category in any series is important. This factor should be considered when evaluating the incidence of complications and postoperative deaths from various institutions. Indications for pelvic exenteration and operative mortality among various groups of patients and from different time periods are shown in table 2.5. These were selected for comparison with the U.T. M. D. Anderson Hospital series. Among gynecologic oncologists, there is no specific time interval after surgery when a complication or death is attributed to the operation. The "postoperative period" is usually considered to be one to three months after the operation. Most reports stipulate that patients who die after hospital discharge are not to be counted in postoperative death statistics. The higher risk of postoperative death in earlier series gave exenteration a reputation among some gynecologists as being excessively hazardous and prompted editorial comments that condemned the procedure as it was first introduced in the 1940s. Fortunately, today the operative mortality rate is estimated at 3% to 5%.

Intestinal Obstruction and Fistula

The most serious and most common postoperative complications are intestinal obstruction and intestinal fistula. The mechanisms that cause these complications are varied. There may be failure of the anastomosis of the small intestine when an ileal segment is resected for conduit construction. Mechanical intestinal obstruction may be caused by adhesions or constriction when the intestine becomes fixed to the denuded surfaces, and obstruction or fistula may occur when a pelvic abscess erodes the bowel wall. Additional factors, such as prior high-dose external irradiation, contribute to postoperative complications.

The clinical interpretation of intestinal obstruction and intestinal fistula as separate events is imprecise. Although intestinal obstruction usually precedes formation of a fistula, in some patients a fistula is caused by a separate and singular event. The fistula that closes spontaneously is rare; however, it may be that transient ones are not discovered. Intestinal fistula should be suspected when there is excessive drainage of fecal content from the pelvic cavity. The majority of intestinal fistulas discharge through the perineum; others drain from the abdominal wall via the incision. They rarely discharge through the conduit or from one loop of intestine to another. Presence of a fistula may be confirmed by roentgenographic examination or passage of a marker that has been given orally. Intestinal complications prolong hospitalization significantly and increase the risk of postoperative death. Correction of intestinal fistula or obstruction is still considered urgent; however, surgery may be delayed with the aid of hyperalimentation in patients with a serious nutritional or fluid and electrolyte imbalance. Repeat laparotomy for segmental resection or for diverting ostomy is usually necessary.

Imperfect covering of the denuded pelvic surfaces appears to be the major cause of these complications. Although considerable effort has been made to improve the covering of the pelvic area after denudation from surgery, there is still a high incidence of intestinal complications. There are prospects for improvement in that the omental pedicle graft is now used routinely to line the pelvic cavity and there is also stricter selection of the segment of bowel for conduit. When the patient has a history of high-dose irradiation, either a colon conduit or a high ileal segment conduit is preferred.

Urinary Fistula

Failure of healing is a major cause of postoperative complications in cases of exenteration. Urinary leakage from a ureteral anastomosis that fails to heal may cause damage to neighboring structures. However, failure of the ureteral conduit anastomosis is not always a primary event. High pressure within the conduit may cause disruption of the implanted ureter when the anterior abdominal wall compresses the distal end of the ileal segment. It is essential that an ample stoma be created; to accomplish this, the conduit must traverse the layers of the abdominal wall directly. This will avoid compression that can occur when the opening in the fascial layer and muscle are not properly superimposed. Necrosis can occur when there is inadequate blood supply or when the conduit is affected by pelvic abscess, particularly if the abscess is caused by an intestinal fistula that exposes the ileal conduit to the digestive action of intestinal enzymes. Technical omissions, such as failure to attach the bottom of the conduit for support, may lead to evulsion of the ureteral implantation by the weight of the intestine draped across the ureters and conduit. Surgical correction of a failed urinary conduit may be difficult and complex. Occasionally, it is possible to repair the defect, but most often a new conduit is necessary. Like intestinal obstruction and intestinal fistula, postoperative leakage of urine into the abdomen can be a contributing factor in postoperative death. Technical modifications have been instituted at U.T. M. D. Anderson Hospital, and a significant number of modified operations have been performed for an analysis.

Other Postoperative Complications

Additional complications that were noted in the U.T. M. D. Anderson Hospital series are listed in table 2.8. For analysis, we divided these into two categories: early postoperative complications, those occurring within three months, and late complications, those occurring after the three-month period.

Early Complications

Early postoperative complications were seen in 28% of the 448 patients in the U.T. M. D. Anderson Hospital series; the remaining 72% experienced no significant problems. Multiple complications were noted in 5%. As shown in this series and in other patient series, urinary and intestinal complications are the most consistent and

Table 2.8. *Postoperative Complications with Exenteration*

Complication	Early Complications ≤90 days Postoperatively No. of Patients	(%)	Late Complications >90 days Postoperatively No. of Patients	(%)
No complications	325	(72.5)	353	(78.8)
Urinary	37	(8.3)	34	(7.6)
Intestinal	36	(8.0)	30	(6.7)
Cardiovascular	17	(3.8)	3	(0.7)
Hemorrhage	16	(3.6)	1	(0.2)
Sepsis	11	(2.5)	4	(0.9)
Neovagina	11	(2.5)	13	(2.9)
Pulmonary	6	(1.3)	1	(0.2)
Conduit stoma	4	(0.9)	13	(2.9)
Colostomy stoma	3	(0.7)	5	(1.1)
Miscellaneous	4	(0.9)	11	(2.5)
Total	470[a]		468[b]	

[a]Twenty-two patients (5%) had more than one early complication.
[b]Twenty patients (4%) had more than one late complication.

Table 2.9. *Early Postoperative Complications Causing Death*

Complication[a]	No. of Patients	(%)
Intestinal	12	(26.1)
Pelvic hemorrhage	7	(15.2)
Uremia	5	(10.9)
Pneumonia	4	(8.7)
Pulmonary embolus	4	(8.7)
Myocardial infarction	3	(6.5)
Sepsis	3	(6.5)
Liver failure	2	(4.3)
Aspiration	2	(4.3)
Cerebrovascular accident	1	(2.2)
Urinary fistula	1	(2.2)
Arterial thrombosis	1	(2.2)
Failure to thrive	1	(2.2)
Total	46	(100.0)

[a]≤90 days after surgery.

the most serious. The incidence of sepsis is less specific. In the early postoperative period, infection is often the initiating event for other complications, but the subsequent problem deemphasizes the role of infection.

Table 2.9 shows some of the causes other than intestinal and urinary complications that were responsible for early postoperative deaths in our patients. There were incidents of organ failure, including renal failure due to drug toxicity, renal anoxia, or obstructive uropathy. The possibilities of such complications should be considered in the patient selection process. Exposure to anesthesia during the

Table 2.10. *Blood Replacement at Surgery*

No. of Units[a]	No. of Patients[b]
1	4
2	29
3	82
4	81
5	65
6	54
7	38
8	27
9	19
10	14
11	2
12	3
13	5
14	1
15	2
16	3
17	1
18	1
19	1
20	1
21	1
22	1
23	1
25	1

[a] Average blood replacement = 5.6 units.
[b] Eleven patients, 14 years of age or under, were excluded.

lengthy exenteration procedure and the delay of postoperative mobilization imposes a greater risk of pulmonary embolism. The incidence of pulmonary embolism is sufficient to warrant anticoagulation, applying a clamp about the vena cava, or both. Because of excessive blood loss, patients also are at risk of experiencing myocardial infarction, renal failure, or lung and liver failure. The risk of hemorrhage during surgery may be judged from the data given in table 2.10.

In the U.T. M. D. Anderson Hospital series, 261 of 448 (58%) had blood replacement equal to or less than 2,500 ml whereas 152 of 448 (34%) had blood replacement between 3,000 ml and 5,000 ml. The extent of the resection is not the only factor causing blood loss during exenteration. In some situations, an inordinate amount of blood may be lost faster than it can be replaced. This results in hypertensive shock, which increases the risk for all organs to be damaged. Blood volume replacement does not promptly reverse this damage; in fact, blood replacement imposes hazards as well. Patients who experience hypertensive shock while undergoing exenteration will survive only with luck and extraordinary care. In some phases of the procedure, hemorrhage may be unavoidable; therefore, more effort must be directed toward improving the technical aspects of the operation that can cause hemorrhage.

Late Complications

Urinary and intestinal complications dominate the late postoperative stages of exenteration. The renal units continue to be susceptible to damage long after the initial healing period has ended. A common menace is recurrent pyelitis caused by urine stasis or reflux backflow into the renal units. With pyelitis, there is a repeated transport of bacteria into the upper urinary tracts, creating a chronic illness. For some patients, the condition for pyelitis or hydronephrosis existed before exenteration and was not corrected or was perhaps worsened by the surgery. More often, the fault was surgical. Recurrent pyelitis is serious because it causes great suffering and loss of productivity and, worse, destruction of the renal unit. Complications of the stoma are another urinary problem, although they produce more discomfort and inconvenience than illness. Fortunately, enterostomal therapists have made advances in recent years in the reduction of stomal problems by paying greater attention to the location of the stoma, reducing inward traction, and creating a precise approximation of the mucosa to the skin. These precautions help the stomal therapist to create a prosthesis that causes the least burden for the patient.

Survival

Survival statistics from the literature are listed in table 2.11. The high five-year survival of 61.8% reported by Morley and Lindenauer (1976) is exceptional. Improved survival is noted in the more recent reports. For the 448 patients in the U.T. M. D. Anderson Hospital series, the Berkson and Gage (1950) method was used to determine survival (fig. 2.1). As would be expected, during observation periods of more than three years, the survival curve for exposure to all causes of death declines slightly more than the survival curve for death from recurrent cancer only. If we

Table 2.11. *Five-Year Survival Rates after Pelvic Exenteration: Review of the Literature*

Study	No. of Patients	(%)
Brunschwig 1970	760	(19.3)[a]
Parsons 1959	74[c]	(24.3)[a]
Bricker 1970	153[c]	(34.6)[a]
Symmonds et al. 1975	198	(32.0)[b]
Rutledge et al. 1977	269	(42.1)[b]
Rutledge 1985 (present study)	448	(41.0)[b]
Ketcham et al. 1970	162[c]	(38.0)[b]
Karlen and Piver 1975	81	(22.2)[a]
Morley and Lindenauer 1976	34	(61.8)[a]
Averette et al. 1984	33[d]	(58.3)[b]
Orr et al. 1983	104[c]	(45.3)[b]

[a] Absolute survival rate.
[b] Actuarial survival rate.
[c] Cervix only.
[d] Last five-year study period.

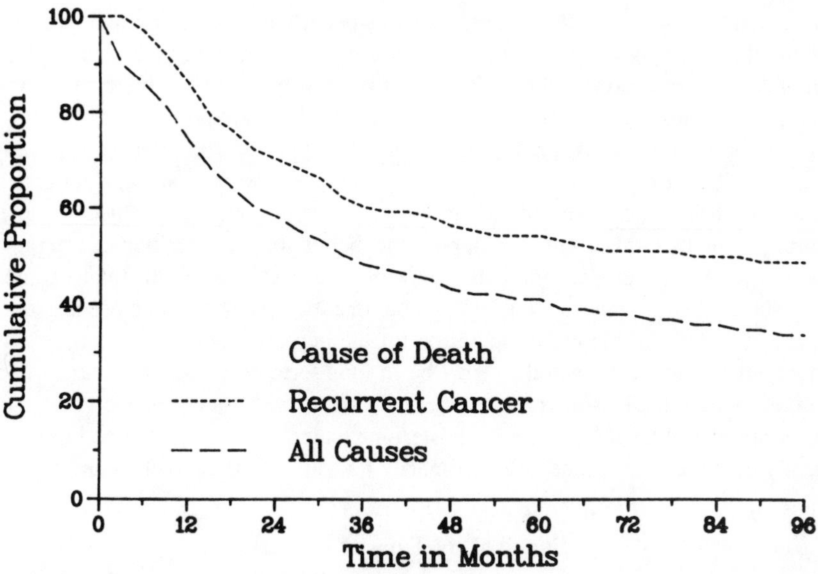

Fig. 2.1 Survival curves are shown for the U.T. M. D. Anderson Hospital series of 448 patients, 1955–1984. The top curve indicates that 53.7% of patients will avoid death from recurrent cancer for five years and that 41% will avoid death from all causes for five years.

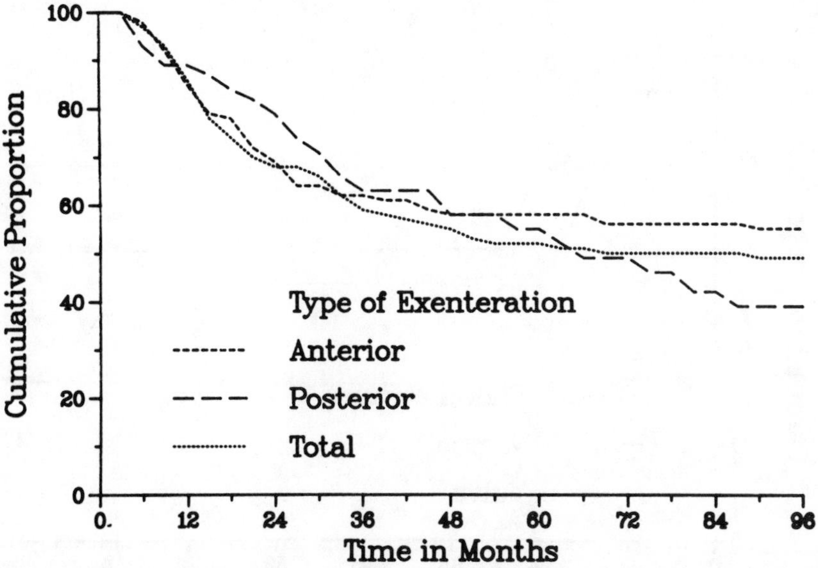

Fig. 2.2 Survival curves are shown comparing the three types of exenterations performed in the U.T. M. D. Anderson Hospital series, 1955–1984. Although the curves are similar, it should be noted that posterior exenteration is performed more frequently than the other procedures for vulvar and anorectal cancer and is associated with more local cancer recurrences.

considered that more life-threatening diseases occur with increasing age, we might assume that both curves would become parallel, showing fewer late deaths due to complications from exenterations. The most significant threat to long-term survival from the operation appears to be failure of the urinary diversion.

A comparison of survival rates among the three types of exenteration is shown in figure 2.2. The similarity of these curves supports the opinion that some patients are suited to a less radical type of exenteration. There may be some objection to the interpretation that these curves support the belief that an anterior exenteration, when properly chosen, accomplishes control of cancer equal with total exenteration. Some types of cancer are more curable than others. Still, the closeness of the curves excludes faulting either operation for the purpose selected. If there is a significant difference to be noted, it may be in long-term outcome of posterior exenteration, which involves a larger number of patients with cancer of the vulva and a higher number of local recurrences. Posterior exenterations are performed more frequently than the other procedures, primarily for vulvar and anorectal cancer.

Survival by Type of Cancer

As shown in our study and reports from other institutions, there is less success with exenteration for cancer of the vulva than with the treatment of recurrent cancer of other sites (fig. 2.3). When there is local recurrence, it is generally assumed that the primary lesion was not completely removed. One of the causes for the low survival

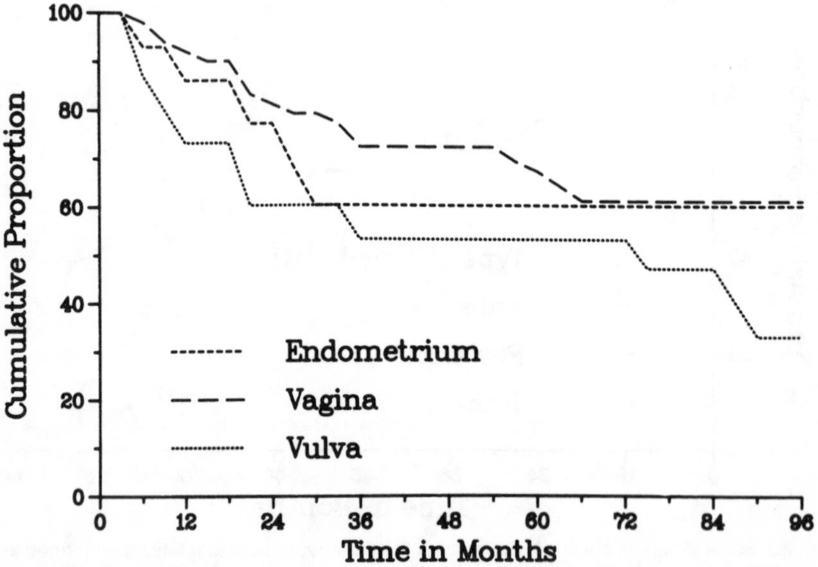

Fig. 2.3 Survival curves are shown comparing three anatomical sites of cancer following pelvic exenteration in the U.T. M. D. Anderson Hospital patient series. The downward curve from 72 to 96 months reflects the high incidence of local recurrence associated with vulvar carcinoma.

curve for patients with vulvar carcinoma has been the incidence of local recurrences; another, perhaps, is the development of new cancer foci. This hypothesis is based on our general knowledge of vulvar cancer treated by other operations and the late recurrences of vulvar cancer compared with recurrences of cancer of the cervix and vagina after exenteration. Local recurrence after radical vulvectomy is the most common treatment failure for carcinoma of the vulva; we assume that reluctance by the surgeon to jeopardize urinary and fecal continence leads to inadequate resection. After vulvectomy, the anogenital tissue that remains may be programmed for a neoplasia. Although these factors may explain the prevalence of local cancer recurrence after radical vulvectomy, they do not explain late local recurrences after exenteration.

Contraindications to Exenteration

More surgical experience, technical improvements, medical advances, and more defined criteria for patient selectivity have all contributed to greater safety in the application of pelvic exenteration. Although vaginal restoration now lessens the crippling consequences of the procedure, patients are still burdened with the care of the stoma. Therefore, exenteration should not be used as a primary treatment if there is reasonable expectation that irradiation or chemotherapy will be equally effective.

There is no consensus about the role of exenteration for patients who have metastases. For example, metastasis to the bladder from cancer of the cervix, in our opinion, is not an indication for immediate exenteration unless the urinary system is irreparably damaged by the cancer. Irradiation therapy could possibly cure this type of stage IV cancer of the cervix or vagina, and if it should fail, radical resection should be as effective as a salvage procedure.

Some gynecologic cancers are radioresistant and are to be treated initially by exenteration. Some of these types of cancer, such as malignant melanoma of the vagina, seem not be influenced, however, by either or both irradiation and resection. Chemotherapy and irradiation have replaced exenteration for sarcoma botryoides of the vagina in the U.T. M. D. Anderson Hospital series. It has rarely been beneficial to perform exenteration for carcinoma of the ovary, although a less radical type of resection is being tested for tumor reduction. Exenteration is not contraindicated for advanced carcinoma of the endometrium and carcinoma of the bladder, but a lower survival than the average can be expected in such cases. These types of cancer also are more likely to be found unresectable at laparotomy.

We concur with opinions expressed in the literature that metastasis to the pelvic wall nodes indicates a poor prognosis with a low cure rate and a short cancer-free interval. However, in our series, exenteration helped to accomplish a 26.3% five-year survival for patients with all types of cancer and a 21.9% five-year survival for patients with lesions of the cervix and vagina associated with lymph node metastases. Therefore, our experience does not support an arbitrary stance to discontinue the procedure upon discovery of lymph node metastasis. The decision to continue should be based on a thorough assessment of the prognostic factors. Positive nodes that have remained after radiation therapy are a more grave finding. Bilateral or multiple nodes and high level node metastases are probably contraindications to the exenteration procedure.

Conclusion

A survey of the recent literature shows that the operative mortality from exenteration has declined. This is also true of the U.T. M. D. Anderson Hospital experience even though we consider death within the first three months after surgery to be a postoperative death. Our postoperative mortality for exenterations performed on 196 patients from 1955 to 1976 was 13.5% (Rutledge et al. 1977) compared with 3.9% for 152 operations performed from 1977 to 1984. Associated with these lower rates are fewer postoperative complications and longer survival.

It is customary to measure the worth of a procedure by the immediate events that may surround it such as intra- and postoperative complications and death. In assessing the risks of exenteration, however, we should remember also the compensation that many patients receive—long-term freedom from recurrent cancer.

References

Appleby LH. 1950. Proctocystectomy: The management of colostomy with ureteral transplants. *Am J Surg* 79:57–60.

Averette HE, Lichtinger M, Sewin BU, Girtanner RE. 1984. Pelvic exenteration: A 15-year experience in a general metropolitan hospital. *Am J Obstet Gynecol* 150:179–184.

Barber HRK, Brunschwig, A. 1966. Urinary tract fistulas following pelvic exenteration. *Obstet Gynecol* 28:754–763.

Berek JS, Hacker NF, Lagasse LD. 1984. Rectosigmoid colectomy and reanastomosis to facilitate resection of primary and recurrent gynecologic cancer. *Obstet Gynecol* 64: 715–720.

Berkson J, Gage RP. 1950. Calculation of survival rates for cancer. *Proc Mayo Clin* 25: 270–286.

Bompiani A, Benedetti Panici P, Greggi S, Margariti PA, Di Roberto P. 1985. Pelvic exenteration in gynaecologic oncology: Analysis of 44 cases. *Eur J Gynaecol Oncol* 6:165–169.

Boutselis JG. 1973. Pelvic exenterations in gynecologic cancer. *Ohio State Med J* 69:266–271.

Bricker EM. 1970. Pelvic exenteration. *Adv Surg* 4:13–72.

Bricker EM, Modlin J. 1951. The role of pelvic evisceration in surgery. *Surgery* 30:76–94.

Brunschwig A. 1948. Complete excision of pelvic viscera for advanced carcinoma: A one-stage abdominoperineal operation with end colostomy and bilateral ureteral implantation into the colon above the colostomy. *Cancer* 1:177–183.

Brunschwig A. 1970. Some reflections on pelvic exenterations after twenty years' experience. *Progress in Gynecology* 5:416–432.

Curry SL, Nahhas WA, Jahshan AE, Whitney CW, Mortel R. 1981. Pelvic exenteration: A 7-year experience. *Gynecol Oncol* 11:119–123.

Day TG Jr, Stanhope R. 1977. Vulvovaginoplasty in gynecologic oncology. *Obstet Gynecol* 50:361–364.

Devereux DF, Sears HF, Ketcham AS. 1980. Intestinal fistula following pelvic exenterative surgery: Predisposing causes and treatment. *J Surg Oncol* 14:227–234.

Douglas RG, Sweeney WJ. 1957. Exenteration operations in the treatment of advanced pelvic cancer. *Am J Obstet Gynecol* 73:1169–1182.

Galante M, Hill EC. 1971. Pelvic exenteration: A critical analysis of a ten-year experience with the use of the team approach. *Am J Obstet Gynecol* 110:180–189.

Ingersoll FM, Ulfelder H. 1966. Pelvic exenteration for carcinoma of the cervix. *N Engl J Med* 274:648–651.

Ingiulla W, Cosmi EV. 1967. Pelvic exenteration for advanced carcinoma of the cervix: Some reflections on 241 cases. *Am J Obstet Gynecol* 99:1083–1086.

Karlen JR, Piver MS. 1975. Reduction of mortality and morbidity associated with pelvic exenteration. *Gynecol Oncol* 3:154–167.

Karlen JR, Williams GB, Summers JL. 1983. The multidisciplinary team approach to exenteration of the pelvis. *Surg Gynecol Obstet* 156:789–794.

Ketcham AS, Deckers PJ, Sugarbaker EV, Hoye RC, Thomas LB, Smith RR. 1970. Pelvic exenteration for carcinoma of the uterine cervix: A 15-year experience. *Cancer* 26:513–521.

Krieger JS, Embree HK. 1969. Pelvic exenteration. *Clev Clin Q* 36:1–8.

Lifshitz S, Johnson R, Roberts JA, Buchsbaum HJ. 1981. Intestinal fistula and obstruction following pelvic exenteration. *Surg Gynecol Obstet* 152:630–632.

McCraw JB, Massey FM, Shanklin KD, Horton CE. 1976. Vaginal reconstruction with gracilis myocutaneous flaps. *Plast Reconstr Surg* 58:176–183.

McIndoe AH, Banister JB. 1938. An operation for the cure of congenital absence of the vagina. *Journal of Obstetrics and Gynaecology of the British Empire* 45:490–494.

Mikuta JJ, Murphy JJ, Schoenberg HW. 1967. Pelvic exenteration for cervical cancer. *Obstet Gynecol* 29:858–861.

Morgan LS, Daly JW, Monif GRG. 1980. Infectious morbidity associated with pelvic exenteration. *Gynecol Oncol* 10:318–328.

Morley GW, Lindenauer SM. 1976. Pelvic exenteration therapy for gynecologic malignancy: An analysis of 70 cases. *Cancer* 38:581–586.

Onnis A, Valente S, Marchetti M, Ozoeze D. 1981. Radical pelvic surgical experience in combined treatment of advanced cervico-carcinomas. *Eur J Gynaecol Oncol* 2:98–101.

Orr JW Jr, Shingleton HM, Hatch KD, Taylor PT, Austin JM Jr, Partridge EE, Soong SJ. 1982. Urinary diversion in patients undergoing pelvic exenteration. *Am J Obstet Gynecol* 142:883–889.

Orr JW Jr, Shingleton HM, Hatch KD, Taylor PT, Partridge EE, Soong SJ. 1983. Gastrointestinal complications associated with pelvic exenteration. *Am J Obstet Gynecol* 145:325–332.

Parsons L. 1959. Pelvic exenteration. *Clin Obstet Gynecol* 2:1151–1170.

Parsons L, Taymor M. 1955. Longevity following pelvic exenteration for carcinoma of the cervix. *Am J Obstet Gynecol* 70:774–785.

Pratt JH. 1961. Sigmoidovaginostomy: A new method of obtaining satisfactory vaginal depth. *Am J Obstet Gynecol* 81:535–545.

Rutledge FN, Burns BC Jr. 1965. Pelvic exenteration. *Am J Obstet Gynecol* 91:692–708.

Rutledge FN, Smith JP, Wharton JT, O'Quinn AG. 1977. Pelvic exenteration: Analysis of 296 patients. *Am J Obstet Gynecol* 128:881–892.

Schmitz RL, Schmitz HE, Smith CJ, Molitor JJ. 1960. Details of pelvic exenteration evolved during an experience with 75 cases. *Am J Obstet Gynecol* 80:43–52.

Symmonds RE, Pratt JH, Webb MJ. 1975. Exenterative operations: Experience with 198 patients. *Am J Obstet Gynecol* 121:907–918.

Talledo OE. 1985. Pelvic exenteration—Medical College of Georgia experience. *Gynecol Oncol* 22:181–188.

Thyssen J. 1956. Preliminary results of attempted radical surgery in recurrent uterine carcinoma. *Acta Obstet Gynecol Scand* 35:1–24.

Turko M, Benedet JL, Boyes DA, Nickerson KG. 1977. Pelvic exenteration: 1949–1971. *Gynecol Oncol* 5:246–250.

Wawro NW, Howe ER. 1957. Experience in a community hospital with multivisceral pelvic resection for advanced pelvic cancer. *Am J Obstet Gynecol* 74:1275–1283.

Williams EA. 1964. Congenital absence of the vagina: A simple operation for its relief. *Journal of Obstetrics and Gynaecology of the British Commonwealth* 71:511–512.

Wrigley JV, Prem KA, Fraley EE. 1976. Pelvic exenteration: Complications of urinary diversion. *J Urol* 116:428–430.

Yu HHY, Leong CH, Ong GB. 1976. Pelvic exenteration for advanced pelvic malignancies. *Aust NZ J Surg* 46:197–201.

OVARIAN CANCER

Annual Clinical Conference on Cancer, Vol. 29
Gynecologic Cancer: Diagnosis and Treatment Strategies
© 1987 by The University of Texas System Cancer Center

3. Surgery for Epithelial Ovarian Carcinoma

J. Taylor Wharton

Surgical therapy for patients with carcinoma of the ovary is utilized in all phases of the management of this complex cancer (Brunschwig and Clark 1962; Munnell, Jacox, and Taylor 1957; Wharton and Herson 1981; Bjorkholm et al. 1982; Hacker et al. 1983). The initial therapy consists of verifying the diagnosis, determining the extent of spread, and removing as much tumor bulk as possible to relieve symptoms and to enhance the therapeutic efficiency of additional therapy. Surgical exploration at specific intervals after chemotherapy provides information concerning drug effectiveness (Copeland, 1985; Copeland et al. 1985; Gershenson et al. 1985; Webb et al. 1982). Frequently, surgical exploration is necessary to relieve bowel obstruction due to advancing disease or to manage a complication induced by prior therapy. The purpose of this paper is to discuss the practices and techniques currently used for prechemotherapy cytoreductive surgery at The University of Texas M. D. Anderson Hospital and Tumor Institute at Houston for patients with advanced cancer.

Surgical exploration of the abdomen and removal of the ovaries and metastatic deposits is universally accepted as the initial therapy in the treatment of epithelial carcinoma of the ovary (Brunschwig and Clark 1962; Munnell, Jacox, and Taylor 1957; Griffiths 1975; Wharton and Edwards 1984). The surgeon has additional responsibilities in the treatment of a patient with carcinoma of the ovary. It is important not only to remove as much tumor as possible but also to determine the extent of the disease (Griffiths, Parker, and Fuller 1979; Griffiths 1975; Wharton and Edwards 1983; Hacker et al. 1983).

Because ovarian cancer is a disease that spreads initially to the abdominal cavity and retroperitoneal lymph nodes, any organ or structure covered by the peritoneum or lymph nodes in the pelvic or aortic areas is at risk and can provide a suitable habitat for implantation of microscopic aggregates of cancer (Feldman and Knapp 1974). The principles of surgical treatment are based on the tenet that when metastases occur, the preferred sites within the abdominal cavity are peritoneal surfaces or retroperitoneal spaces that are surgically accessible through an adequate midline or equivalent laparotomy incision. In surgery for ovarian carcinoma, cutting through cancer masses and leaving small unresectable residuals is an acceptable technical maneuver, although historically, it is considered a poor surgical technique and should be avoided in cancers that are resistant to other forms of therapy. Treatment for ovarian cancers, which are frequently quite sensitive to chemotherapeutic agents and radiation therapy, is never restricted to surgery alone. Therefore, certain technical liberties may be allowed in the surgical management of this group of solid tumors.

Obtaining an accurate histological diagnosis of a primary ovarian tumor is basic in treatment planning. Tissue samples from the uterus, fallopian tubes, and ovaries are usually adequate. It is especially important to have identifiable samples from both ovaries since the diagnosis of the primary tumor is best made when both ovaries can be properly examined. The diagnosis of ovarian tumors of low malignant potential is dependent on histological features exhibited in the ovary and not in the metastatic deposits. The same is true for histological grading (Jolles 1985). Histological grading, utilizing the features found in metastatic foci, is difficult at best and not dependable. Determining the source of the primary tumor when very advanced disease is present is frequently impossible if the pathologist receives only a segment of omentum filled with tumor nodules. Obtaining the correct histological diagnosis is important in planning chemotherapy regimens, which are quite specific for some primary tumors.

The extent of spread to other sites in the abdomen may be documented by performing biopsies of recognizable tumor implants, or from sites selected at random to determine micrometastases. Lavaging the pelvis and upper abdomen with saline is usually done before surgical disturbance of suspected disease sites. The identification of microscopic clusters of adenocarcinoma may provide some information about the spread or biologic potential of the malignancy. This type of thoroughness in surgical examination will allow for proper evaluation of the cancer and determination of the most efficient postoperative therapy. The right hemidiaphragm has received considerable attention as a site in which small metastases implant (Bagley et al. 1973). Evaluation of the diaphragm requires cooperation with the anesthesiologist. A biopsy procedure can be hazardous if the diaphragm is moving; perforation with entry into the pleural space or lung parenchyma is a potentially serious complication. Prognostic factors have been identified and scientific data pertaining to cure of patients with the International Federation of Gynecology and Obstetrics (FIGO) stage III and stage IV disease are expanding. Thus, determining the true extent of the cancer and the extent of surgery needed to achieve a minimal tumor residual, including measurements of the extent of disease remaining, is of critical importance in therapy evaluation and clinical study design (Bjorkholm et al. 1982).

Surgical Strategy

The basic plan of the surgical procedure at U.T. M. D. Anderson Hospital is to leave no residual mass greater than 1 to 2 cm in diameter, if technically possible (Wharton, Edwards, and Rutledge 1984). Convincing data indicate that patients who have a small tumor residual prior to the application of radiation or chemotherapy have a longer disease-free interval than do patients with bulky disease. The important aspect, from the surgical point of view, is the amount of disease left in the abdomen instead of the amount removed. The description of the residual disease, however, is usually based on the greatest diameter of the largest remaining nodule, and it is unrealistic to believe that one 2-cm nodule carries a worse prognosis than many separate and diffuse 0.5-cm nodules or plaques of tumor.

Therefore, the initial responsibilities of the surgeon are as follows: (1) removal of as much tumor as possible with a description of the technical difficulty of the operation, (2) determination of the extent of disease by excision biopsy or adequate sampling of unresectable metastases that have spread beyond the ovaries, and (3) cytoreductive surgery or removal of the ovaries and all clinically recognizable metastatic deposits. Surgical excision of portions of the gastrointestinal and urinary tracts is permissible if all visible disease can be removed.

Patient Preparation

The most favorable results are obtained when an operation is carefully planned. An understanding of the patient's physical, physiological, and psychological strengths and weaknesses is mandatory. Some patients will not accept the psychological trauma of a colostomy, for example, unless a good educational program has been included in the preoperative preparation. There is no substitute for a thorough history and physical examination. The ovaries are a preferential site for metastases from other primaries, and signs and symptoms of these significant other cancers can be missed during the taking of the medical history. The surgeon should be particularly alert for any family history or current signs of malignancies involving the breast or endometrium and should perform the diagnostic tests necessary to rule out an intestinal or pancreatic cancer. Any previous medical or surgical problems involving the urinary system or gastrointestinal tract are of interest. These are particularly important if the patient has a history of diverticular disease and has a left adnexal mass. Diverticular disease with abscess formation easily mimicks ovarian cancer, as do cysts related to endometriosis. Adnexal pathology may mask an occult ovarian cancer, and intraoperative recognition can be difficult. A history of previous abdominal surgical procedures is always important in planning an abdominal operation. Review of what may at first appear to be rather routine pathological material from the previous operation can influence the current plans. For example, prior inflammatory disease of any cause is almost always damaging to the mesothelial cells lining the peritoneum, and adhesions can hamper visualization or impair access to anatomical spaces.

The following laboratory studies are required: blood chemistries, including blood counts and serum electrolyte analysis; coagulation studies; and urinalysis. A bleeding time study may not be routine in many hospitals, and a qualitative platelet abnormality may first express itself as catastrophic intraoperative hemorrhage. Physical examination should also include an electrocardiogram, chest X ray, intravenous pyelogram, and barium enema. Biopsies of the cervix, endocervix, and endometrium may help to detect an unsuspected primary or tumor extension. Special studies such as lymphangiograms, computerized tomography scans, sonograms, and bone and liver scans are ordered only when the surgeon considers them necessary. Cystoscopic examinations and sigmoidoscopies are not routinely done.

Correction of cardiopulmonary, metabolic, or hematologic abnormalities before the operation is axiomatic. Bowel preparation should always include a thorough mechanical cleansing; when gastrointestinal procedures are contemplated, the addition of an antibiotic preparation is indicated. The current preference is neomycin, 1 gram, and erythromycin base, 1 gram, given orally at 3:00, 4:00, and 11:00 the evening before surgery. Patients expected to have extended operations are placed on systemic antibiotics 24 hours before surgery.

Surgical Technique

At U.T. M. D. Anderson Hospital, we prefer to use a midline vertical incision. This incision can be extended to allow access to the upper abdomen, which is necessary if aortic nodes are to be resected or accessible for biopsy. Access to the right hemidiaphragm may require partial mobilization of the liver by division of the right triangular ligament. We do not attempt to strip the peritoneum from the diaphragmatic surface, nor do we attempt to separate the diaphragm from the liver capsule when the subdiaphragmatic space is obliterated by multiple tumor implants. Brisk bleeding can occur during biopsy of the diaphragm since the muscle is richly supplied by branches of the right inferior phrenic artery. With a good light source, these vessels can usually be identified and avoided. Wedge resection of a solitary nodule in the diaphragmatic muscle requires careful closure of the defect and consideration of the placement of a chest tube.

Patients with carcinoma who have extensive replacement of the omentum can have extension high along the greater curvature of the stomach to the level of the phrenocolic ligament and spleen. Removal of the involved omentum, which requires adequate exposure of the left upper quadrant, is an important part of the operative procedure for ovarian cancer. Anatomically, the omentum consists of four folded layers of peritoneum attached to the greater curvature of the stomach and suspended from the transverse colon along an avascular plane. The blood supply comes from the gastroepiploic arch, which arises from the gastroduodenal artery on the right and the terminal branching of the splenic artery on the left. Complete removal of the omentum is justified if it is infiltrated with cancer. Removal of a large portion of omental tissue for biopsy is probably all that is necessary if the omentum clinically appears to be disease-free. A portion attached to the transverse colon should provide the necessary diagnostic information.

The retroperitoneal approach is useful in gaining surgical access to the upper abdominal lymph nodes and is fundamental in the pelvic portion of the operation for removal of the ovaries and uterus. An incision is made through the peritoneum lateral to the ascending or descending colon (fig. 3.1). When a thorough lymphadenectomy is contemplated, the peritoneal incision on the right side is extended around the cecum and along the base of the mesentery of the small bowel to the ligament of Trietz. This maneuver exposes the vena cava and aorta and can be extended to mobilize the duodenum to expose safely the right renal vein and the left ovarian vein. The incisions lateral to the colon allow medial retraction of the colon on both the right and left sides. This allows palpation and inspection of the precaval and aortic nodes. The lymph nodes above the bifurcation of the aorta on the left side are easily removed by reflecting the descending colon medially. This approach is preferred to the transperitoneal midline technique since the inferior mesenteric artery and veins are easier to retract. The ureters are always under direct vision.

The peritoneal incision is extended on both sides; the round ligaments are ligated and the broad ligament opened. Retroperitoneal dissection exposes the ureters, the

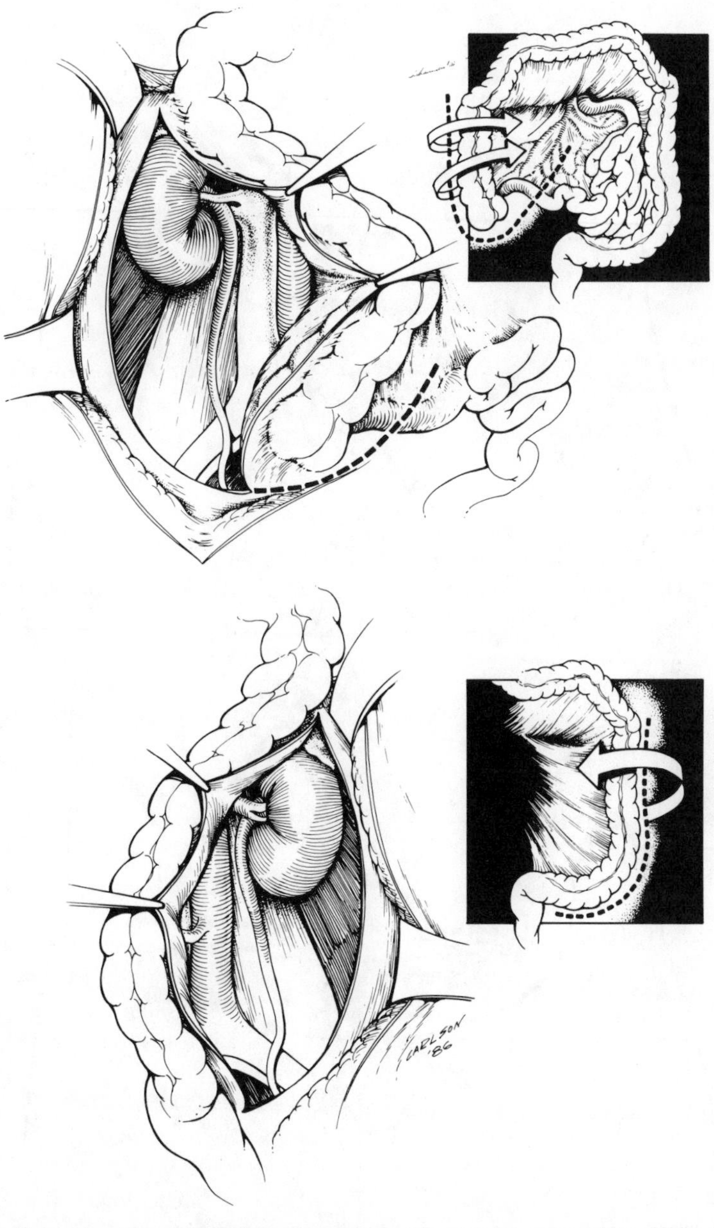

Fig. 3.1. The major retroperitoneal structures and nodes can be exposed by making incisions lateral to the ascending colon or descending colon and reflecting the colon medially. On the right side the incision can be extended along the base of the small bowel mesentery, directly exposing the vena cava and the aortic lymph nodes. Medial retraction of the left colon allows access to the nodes along the lower aspect of the left side of the aorta. Both incisions allow safe identification of the ureters and major blood vessels.

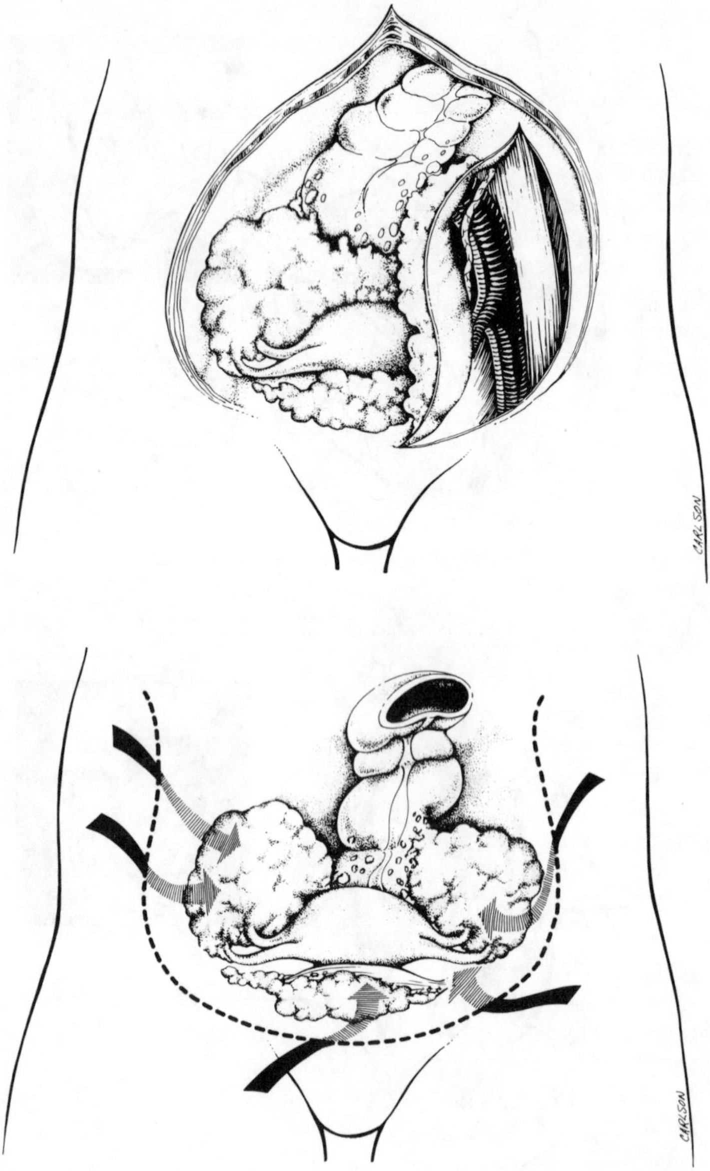

Fig. 3.2. The round ligament is divided and the broad ligament dissected, exposing the ureter and iliac vessels. The infundibulopelvic veins and the pelvic portion of the ureters are easily identified. The hypogastric artery is identified and the perivesical space can be entered by dissection lateral to the superior vesicle artery. The retroperitoneal approach can be employed on either side of the pelvis, as shown in the diagram.

infundibulopelvic vessels at the level of the common iliac artery, the iliac arteries and veins, and the obturator nerve, and establishes boundaries if pelvic lymphadenectomy is indicated. The ureter is then followed in its course to the level of the uterine artery. The external iliac vessels are identified, and the obturator nerve serves as an inferior boundary of the dissected field at this stage of the operation. The perivesical space may be entered by dissection lateral to the superior vesicle artery. Full utilization of this space allows evaluation of bladder involvement (fig. 3.2).

The retroperitoneal spaces are utilized bilaterally, with dissection of the perivesical, pararectal, or retrorectal spaces as required, to gain mobility of the pelvic specimen. Once the surgeon has determined the extent of the cancer, decisions regarding the radicalness of the operation can be made. Persistence in gaining access to these spaces allows mobility and proper exposure of the cancer, major vessels, and ureters, and bulky cancer thought initially to be inoperable can be removed.

Current Standards of Care

The surgeon must develop a systematic, aggressive approach for the patient with advanced disease. Careful documentation in the operative note with diagrams of the sites involved and measurements of the amount of disease remaining after surgery is important. The extent, documented by surgical exploration, is used for FIGO staging purposes and also identifies areas at risk that require biopsy should the patient require a second-look laparotomy (Castaldo et al. 1981; Copeland 1985; Gershenson et al. 1985; Webb et al. 1982).

Cytoreductive surgery, when successful in accomplishing reduction of the cancer masses to a residual of 1 to 2 cm or less, is credited with improvements in survival when these patients are compared with those who have cancers that cannot be removed (figs. 3.3 and 3.4). Data from studies done in the Department of Gynecology at U.T. M. D. Anderson Hospital agree with those of other investigators. Studies of patients with FIGO stage III disease are of particular interest when compared with patients with stage IV disease. Patients with stage III disease may be the best candidates for the extended operation (figs. 3.5 and 3.6). We will accept resection of bowel with anastomosis or colostomy as part of the cytoreduction effort when the remaining residual disease is minimal. Resections of part of the bladder or distal few centimeters of the ureter followed by ureteroneocystostomy are permitted in very select cases. This has also been performed by other investigators (Berek et al. 1982; Castaldo et al. 1981). Exenteration or urinary diversion by ileal or colon conduit or cutaneous bilateral ureterostomy is not recommended.

It would be very difficult to design a prospective randomized study to prove that cytoreductive surgery is of significant value. There is no scientific evidence that the cytoreductive surgery techniques practiced today have an unquestionably favorable impact on survival or on the natural course of the disease. The broad spectrum of surgical procedures required for optimal management of patients with ovarian cancer is the most difficult for the gynecologist to perform. A thorough knowledge of the anatomy of the upper abdomen is a prerequisite to caring for these patients, and experience in performing urological and gastrointestinal procedures is helpful.

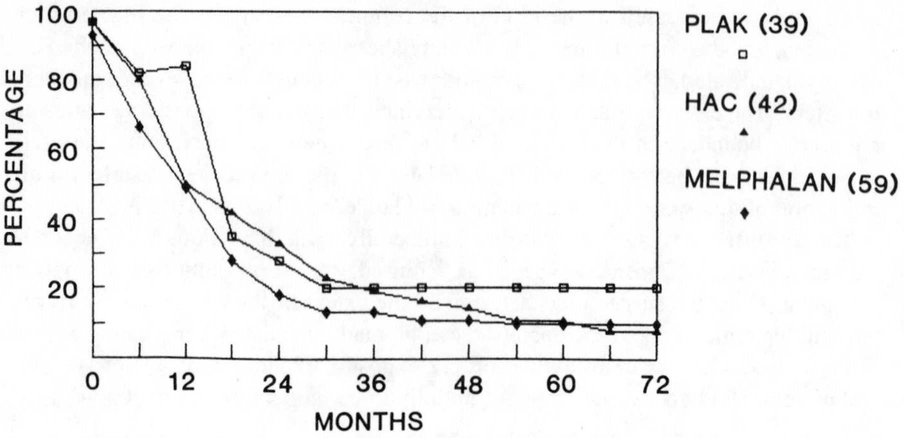

Fig. 3.3 Duration of survival (in months) of 140 patients with FIGO stage III and stage IV ovarian carcinomas is shown. Patients were treated between 1973 and 1980 with single-agent (melphalan) and two combination chemotherapies. All patients had residual tumor masses greater than 2 cm at the initiation of chemotherapy. The survival rate for this group of patients with large residual tumor masses before chemotherapy is lower than the survival rate for patients whose tumors could be resected, leaving a residual of 2 cm or less, as shown in figure 3.4 (*PLAK*: P, *cis*-diamminedichloroplatinum, 20 mg/m^2 i.v., days two, three, and four; LAK, melphalan, 0.66 mg/kg total dose given postoperatively and divided over a five-day period. Repeat every 28 days. *HAC*: H, hexamethylmelamine, 4 mg/kg, days 1–14; A, Adriamycin, 40 mg/m^2 i.v., day 1; C, cyclophosphamide, 400 mg/m^2 i.v., day 1. Repeat every 28 days. *MELPHALAN*: 1 mg/kg given postoperatively and divided over a five-day period. Repeat every 28 days.)

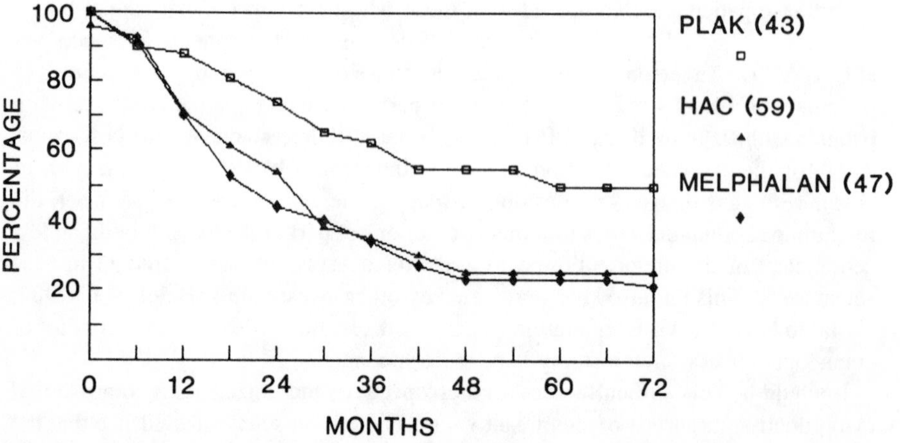

Fig. 3.4. Duration of survival (in months) in 149 patients with FIGO stage III and stage IV ovarian carcinomas is shown. Patients were treated between 1973 and 1980 with chemotherapy. These patients had postoperative residual masses no greater than 2 cm. For a description of chemotherapy regimens, see figure 3.3.

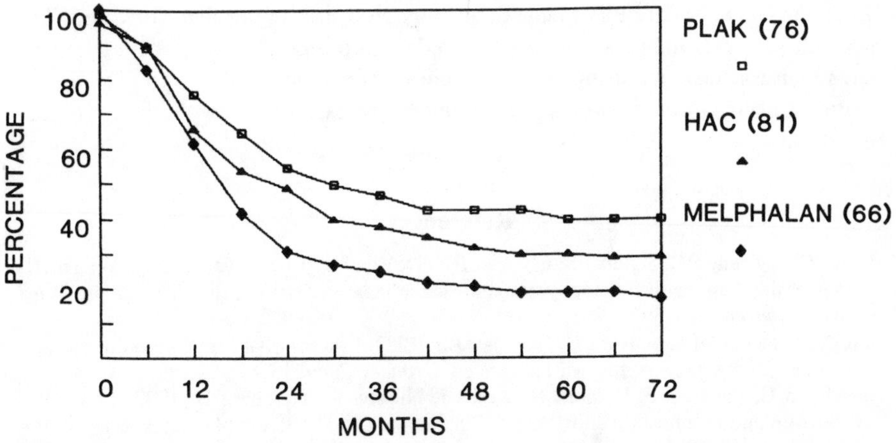

Fig. 3.5. Duration of survival of patients with disease confined to the abdominal peritoneal surfaces and/or retroperitoneal lymph nodes (FIGO stage III) is shown. Patients were treated with chemotherapy between 1973 and 1980. Such patients have potentially resectable tumor masses and probably represent the group most likely to benefit from extended cytoreductive surgery. Comparison of survival times for this group of patients with patients in stage IV disease shows a considerable difference (see fig. 3.6). For a description of chemotherapy regimens, see figure 3.3.

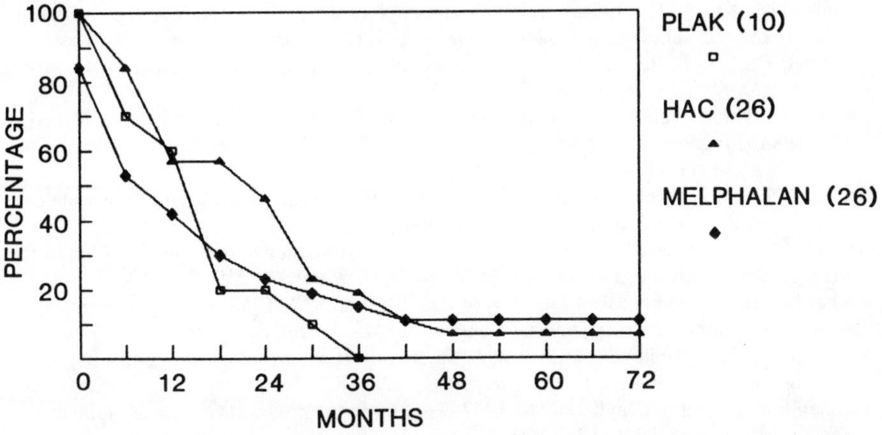

Fig. 3.6. Duration of survival (in months) of 62 patients with FIGO stage IV ovarian carcinomas treated with chemotherapy between 1973 and 1980 is poor. The indications for extended cytoreductive surgery with the accompanying risks are to be carefully considered in therapy planning for such patients. For a description of chemotherapy regimens, see figure 3.3.

Operations must be carefully planned, and any preoperative problem corrected. The medical, surgical, and personal support needs are considerably greater for these patients than for those requiring other gynecologic operations. Major progress in the treatment of this disease will come from intense research and new therapies (Freedman 1985).

References

Bagley CM, Young RC, Schein PS, Chabner BA, DeVita VT. 1973. Ovarian carcinoma metastatic to the diaphragm frequently undiagnosed at laparotomy: A preliminary report. *Am J Obstet Gynecol* 116:397.

Berek JS, Hacker NF, Lagasse LD, Leuchter RS. 1982. Lower urinary tract resections as part of cytoreductive surgery for ovarian cancer. *Gynecol Oncol* 13:87–92.

Bjorkholm E, Peterson F, Einhorn N, Krebs I, Nilsson B, Tjernberg B. 1982. Long-term follow-up and prognostic factors in ovarian carcinoma: The Radiumhemmet series 1958–1973. *Acta Radiol Oncol Radiat Phys Biol* 21:413–419.

Brunschwig A, Clark DCG. 1962. *Intestinal Surgery for Advanced Cancer of the Ovary*. Chicago: Year Book Medical.

Castaldo TW, Petrilli ES, Ballou SC, Lagasse LD. 1981. Intestinal operations in patients with ovarian carcinoma. *Am J Obstet Gynecol* 139:80–84.

Copeland LJ. 1985. Second-look laparotomy for ovarian carcinoma. *Clin Obstet Gynecol* 28: 816–823.

Copeland LJ, Gershenson DM, Wharton JT, Atkinson EN, Sneige N, Edwards CL, Rutledge FN. 1985. Microscopic disease at second-look laparotomy in advanced ovarian cancer. *Cancer* 55:472–478.

Feldman GB, Knapp RC. 1974. Lymphatic drainage of the peritoneal cavity and its significance in ovarian cancer. *Am J Obstet Gynecol* 119:1013–1017.

Freedman RS. 1985. Recent immunologic advances affecting the management of ovarian cancer. *Clin Obstet Gynecol* 28:853–871.

Gershenson DM, Copeland LJ, Wharton JT, Atkinson EN, Sneige N, Edwards CL, Rutledge FN. 1985. Prognosis of surgically determined complete responders in advanced ovarian cancer. *Cancer* 55:1129–1135.

Griffiths CT. 1975. Surgical resection of tumor bulk in the primary treatment of ovarian carcinoma. *Natl Cancer Inst Monogr* 42:101–104.

Griffiths CT, Parker LM, Fuller AF Jr. 1979. Role of cytoreductive surgical treatment in the management of advanced ovarian cancer. *Cancer Treat Rep* 63:225–240.

Hacker NF, Berek JS, Lagasse LD, Niegerg RK, Elashoff RM. 1983. Primary cytoreductive surgery for epithelial cancer. *Obstet Gynecol* 61:413–420.

Jolles CJ. 1985. Ovarian cancer: Histogenetic classification, histologic grading, diagnosis, staging, and epidemiology. *Clin Obstet Gynecol* 28:787–799.

Munnell EW, Jacox HW, Taylor HC Jr. 1957. Treatment and prognosis in cancer of the ovary. *Am J Obstet Gynecol* 74:1187–1200.

Webb MJ, Snyder JA Jr, Williams TJ, Decker DG. 1982. Second-look laparotomy in ovarian cancer. *Gynecol Oncol* 14:285–293.

Wharton JT, Edwards CL. 1983. Cytoreductive surgery for carcinoma of the ovary. In *Management of Advanced Cancer*, ed. P Periman, E Savlov, pp. 221–240. New York: Masson Publishing.

Wharton JT, Edwards CL, Rutledge FN. 1984. Long-term survival after chemotherapy for advanced epithelial ovarian carcinoma. *Am J Obstet Gynecol* 148:997–1005.

Wharton JT, Herson J. 1981. Surgery for common epithelial tumors of the ovary. *Cancer* 48:582–589.

Annual Clinical Conference on Cancer, Vol. 29
Gynecologic Cancer: Diagnosis and Treatment Strategies
© 1987 by The University of Texas System Cancer Center

4. Chemotherapy for Epithelial Ovarian Cancer

David M. Gershenson

Ovarian cancer is the second most common gynecologic malignancy, accounting for approximately 19,000 new cases each year in the United States. The majority of cases are advanced at the time of diagnosis, and this contributes to the fact that ovarian cancer is the most common cause of death from gynecologic malignancy, accounting for approximately 12,000 deaths yearly.

Since the 1950s, chemotherapy has played an increasingly important role in the postoperative treatment of epithelial ovarian cancer. By the early 1970s, single-agent chemotherapy had surpassed radiotherapy as the most popular form of post-operative therapy. The introduction of active drugs other than alkylating agents by the mid-1970s made combination chemotherapy a reality. The use of two or more agents with different mechanisms of action and different toxicities was based on the work of Skipper, Chapman, and Bell (1952).

In this report, I will examine the evolution of chemotherapy from single alkylating agent therapy to modern combination chemotherapy and will attempt to answer some of the important questions concerning the state of chemotherapy for epithelial ovarian cancer in 1985. The comments herein will deal principally with advanced ovarian cancer. A number of clinical trials will be reviewed with regard to two parameters—response and survival. Newer therapies and prospects for the future will also be discussed.

Prognostic Factors

In the last two decades, the influence of several prognostic factors on survival has been elucidated. This information has enabled investigators to better design clinical chemotherapy trials, with the ultimate goal of treatment individualization. In evaluation of chemotherapy trials for advanced ovarian cancer, it is extremely important to analyze carefully the characteristics of the study population with regard to these factors. For example, in randomized studies, it is essential that patients be stratified according to prognostic factors prior to randomization.

Staging by the International Federation of Gynecology and Obstetrics (FIGO) or determination of the extent of disease is a very strong indicator of prognosis. In the reviews by Tobias and Griffiths (1976) and Richardson et al. (1985), statistics compiled from several institutions clearly demonstrate that prognosis worsens as stage increases. In the latter report, five-year survival figures from 76 institutions worldwide, which included 5,254 patients from 1973 to 1975, were as follows: stage I,

66.4%; stage II, 45%; stage III, 13.3%; stage IV, 4.1%. Unfortunately, approximately two thirds of patients will present with either stage III or stage IV disease.

Histological grade is also an extremely important prognostic factor. Several studies (Day, Gallager, and Rutledge 1975; Ozols et al. 1980; Sorbe, Frankendal, and Veress 1981; Sigurdsson, Alm, and Gullberg 1983; Wharton, Edwards, and Rutledge 1984; Malkasian et al. 1984) have firmly documented that patients with poorly differentiated tumors have a worse prognosis than patients with well-differentiated tumors. At The University of Texas M. D. Anderson Hospital and Tumor Institute at Houston, the pattern grading system has been used (Day, Gallager, and Rutledge 1975), whereas the Mayo Clinic experience has been with the Broders' grading system (Broders 1926; Malkasian et al. 1984). Of course, patients with borderline epithelial tumors of the ovary (see Norris, this volume) have the most favorable prognosis of all the ovarian cancer patients.

Residual tumor size also appears to have a great impact on prognosis. Studies of Griffiths (1975, 1979) and Wharton (1981, 1984) have adequately established that patients with minimal residual disease have a better prognosis than patients with bulky residual disease. Those patients who begin chemotherapy with minimal residual disease have a much greater probability of achieving a complete remission than patients who begin chemotherapy with bulky residual disease (Young et al. 1978; Greco et al. 1981; Ehrlich et al. 1979; Edwards et al. 1983). The aforementioned evidence has been used to support the concept of cytoreductive surgery.

Early age at the time of diagnosis is also associated with a favorable prognosis, although it is confounded by the fact that younger patients have a higher proportion of low-grade tumors and less-advanced disease. This factor does not, however, appear to exert as strong an influence on survival as FIGO stage, histological grade, and residual tumor size.

Existing evidence suggests that histological type has minimal influence on prognosis. Several reports (Griffiths 1975; Wharton et al. 1980; Dembo et al. 1982; Deligdisch, Jacobs, and Cohen 1982) have documented that, whenever analyzed within specific stage and grade categories, patients with the common epithelial tumors have similar prognoses.

All of the above-described factors make interpretation of individual, nonrandomized clinical trials extremely difficult. Variations in surgical techniques, patient populations, and patient selection methods exacerbate this confusion. Considering these confounding variables, investigators should be cautious in comparing results of different chemotherapy clinical trials.

Response and Survival

Ovarian cancer is principally an intraabdominal disease, making clinical assessment quite difficult. Thus, response is a very inexact end point. Moreover, in many reports response is not well-defined. It may be evaluated by physical examination (in patients with palpable disease), by surgical procedures (second-look laparotomy), or by radiographic studies (computerized tomography or magnetic resonance imaging).

There are no uniform criteria for definition of response in ovarian cancer patients. The duration required to qualify as a response may vary greatly as well. Surgical evaluation with second-look laparotomy remains the most reliable method of assessing response and continues to be employed in most clinical trials conducted in this country. In Europe, however, it appears to be used less frequently.

Although the category of partial response is important in the search for new active antitumor agents, the only truly meaningful response is a complete response. With rare exception, only those patients who achieve a true complete remission with first-line postoperative therapy have a reasonable probability of cure. Many of these patients, however, will eventually relapse and die of the disease.

Because of the above problems with determination of response, survival is the purest end point for evaluating efficacy of a chemotherapeutic regimen. However, even survival is defined differently in various studies. Some investigators may report absolute survival, others may report corrected survival, and others may report 18- or 24-month survival. Progression-free survival is also commonly analyzed. Most commonly, median survival is analyzed using the life-table methods of Kaplan and Meier (1958) or Berkson and Gage (1952). One problem that adds to the difficulty in evaluating chemotherapy trials is that many studies are published with relatively short follow-up time. In many instances the median survival time has not been reached. Ideally, existing reports should be updated to show five-year survival.

Single-Agent Activity

From the 1950s until the mid-1970s, single alkylating-agent chemotherapy was standard postoperative treatment for patients with advanced epithelial ovarian cancer. Early reports of alkylating agent activity generally were based on poorly controlled studies and retrospective descriptions without definitions of patient populations, previous therapy, or response criteria. Response rates ranged from 35% to 65% when these agents were employed as first-line therapy (Tobias and Griffiths 1976). It also appeared as if the various alkylating agents possessed activity approximately equivalent with other drugs in the same category.

The two most widely used alkylating agents have been melphalan and cyclophosphamide. Melphalan was used as standard postoperative therapy to treat hundreds of patients at U.T. M. D. Anderson Hospital. Cyclophosphamide was mainly popularized by the Mayo Clinic. Table 4.1 shows the response and survival results from some of the larger clinical trials in which melphalan was employed as first-line treatment in advanced ovarian cancer. As noted, the response rates range from 20% to 54%, and median survival is from 12 to 28 months. In table 4.2, similar results are presented from a number of studies employing cyclophosphamide as initial therapy. Although the response rates are similar to those with melphalan, the median survival time of approximately 12 months is shorter. With the use of either agent, approximately 10% to 15% of patients achieved long-term survival.

Beginning in the early 1970s, new nonalkylating agents were introduced into clinical studies involving advanced ovarian cancer. A few studies (De Palo et al.

Table 4.1. *Single-Agent Melphalan*

Study	No. of Patients	Response Rate (%)	Median Survival (Months)
Wharton, Gershenson, and Herson 1983	104	26	18.6 (all)
Piver et al. 1978	111	20	19(CR) 11(PR) 3(NR)
Brodovsky, Temkin, and Sears 1977	114	26	28(CR) 13(PR) 6(NR)
Young et al. 1978	37	54	17 (all)
Omura et al. 1983	64	38	12 (all)
Vogl et al. 1982	119	44	17 (all)
Trope 1981	72	40	16(CR) 15(PR)

Note: CR, complete response; PR, partial response; NR, no response.

Table 4.2. *Single-Agent Cyclophosphamide*

Study	No. of Patients	Response Rate (%)	Median Survival (Months)
Beck and Boyes 1968	126	49	—
Decker et al. 1967	104	37	—
Bolis et al. 1980	33	42	13 (all)
Carmo-Pereira et al. 1981	29	62	11 (all)
Edmonson et al. 1979	35	31	12 (all)
Izbicki et al. 1977	89	45	8 (all)

1975; De Palo, De Lena, and Bonadonna 1977; Wharton et al. 1982) have documented modest first-line activity with doxorubicin HCl. De Palo and coworkers (1975) noted a response rate of 50% in 12 previously untreated patients with ovarian cancer. In a later article (De Palo, De Lena, and Bonadonna 1977), they reported a 42% response rate in 19 patients. In a larger series, Wharton and coworkers (1982) reported a 22% response rate and a median survival of 16 months in 32 previously untreated patients.

In most of the reported studies involving doxorubicin HCl, the agent has primarily been used in second-line treatment after alkylating agent failure. Results from several second-line trials are presented in table 4.3. Response rates in this setting were generally quite low. Nevertheless, doxorubicin HCl assumed a very prominent role in later combination chemotherapy trials.

Hexamethylmelamine also was studied extensively in the 1970s. As in doxorubicin HCl trials, most of the clinical trials with hexamethylmelamine involved patients who had failed alkylating agent therapy. Wharton and coworkers (1979) reported a rare study using hexamethylmelamine as first-line therapy and documented a 32% response rate and median survival of 15 months in 54 patients. Table 4.4 shows results of several second-line studies. As noted, response rates in most of these trials ranged between 20% and 30%, demonstrating some degree of non-cross-resistance with the alkylating agents.

In the early 1970s cisplatin was also entered in phase II trials in ovarian cancer patients. Again, the majority of these studies were performed in patients in whom

Table 4.3. *Single-Agent Doxorubicin HCl: Second-Line Therapy*

Study	No. of Patients	Response Rate (%)	Median Survival (Months)
Bolis et al. 1978	38	8	—
Hubbard, Barkes, and Young 1978	18	0	3
O'Bryan et al. 1973	19	11	—
Stanhope, Smith, and Rutledge 1977	27	0	—
Barlow et al. 1973	4	25	—

Table 4.4. *Single-Agent Hexamethylmelamine: Second-Line Therapy*

Study	No. of Patients	Response Rate (%)	Median Survival (Months)
Johnson et al. 1978	21	28	7
Bolis et al. 1979	34	6	9(CR+PR) 5(NR)
Bonomi et al. 1979	16	25	21(CR+PR) 9(NR)
Omura, Greco, and Birch 1981	39	21	—

Note: CR, complete response; PR, partial response; NR, no response.

Table 4.5. *Single-Agent Cisplatin: First-Line Therapy*

Study	No. of Patients	Response Rate (%)	Median Survival (Months)
Gershenson et al. 1981	22	50	21
Hall, Diasio, and Goplerud 1981	18	50	—
Bruckner et al. 1981	13	31	20
Barlow, Piver, and Lele 1982	12	83	—

therapy had failed with alkylating agents. Table 4.5 presents the results of the few first-line studies in patients with advanced ovarian cancer, with extremely encouraging response and survival data. Results from earlier second-line trials are shown in table 4.6. In those trials, cisplatin unquestionably demonstrated significant activity in previously treated patients and has since assumed a very important role in combination studies.

During this period, other chemotherapeutic agents were also being investigated. These drugs included 5-fluorouracil (Wharton, Gershenson, and Herson 1983; Tobias and Griffiths 1976; Malkasian et al. 1968; Jacobs et al. 1971; Thigpen 1985) and methotrexate (Tobias and Griffiths 1976; Katz et al. 1981; Thigpen 1985). Both agents demonstrated only modest activity against ovarian cancer. Of course, many other agents have been studied in patients with advanced ovarian cancer, but none with the same success as the alkylating agents, cisplatin, hexamethylmelamine, and

Table 4.6. *Single-Agent Cisplatin: Second-Line Therapy*

Study	No. of Patients	Response Rate (%)	Median Survival (Months)
Wiltshaw et al. 1979			
30 mg/m^2	23	28	—
30 mg/m^2 × 3	29	27	—
100 mg/m^2	30	52	12+(CR) 8(PR) 6(NR)
Pesando et al. 1980	32	34	11(CR+PR) 7(NR)
Young et al. 1979	24	29	9(CR+PR) 3(NR)
Bruckner et al. 1978	19	32	6 (all)
Thigpen et al. 1979	34	29	3.5+(CR) 5.5+(PR)
Williams et al. 1979	12	33	5 (all)
Piver et al. 1983	21	43	8 (all)

Note: CR, complete response; PR, partial response; NR, no response.

doxorubicin HCl. Some or all of these agents have therefore been incorporated into most modern combination chemotherapy regimens and will be the principal subject of this discussion.

Combination Chemotherapy

Beginning in the mid-1970s, based on the foundation of proven single-agent activity, a large number of combination chemotherapy trials were undertaken. Investigators were extremely optimistic and hoped that response rates would escalate and that a significantly greater percentage of patients with advanced ovarian cancer would experience long-term survival. Only very recently have we been able to review these studies and put them into proper perspective. The following discussion will address many of the most critical questions concerning combination chemotherapy in 1985.

Single-Agent Versus Combination Chemotherapy

With the advent of combination chemotherapy, the issue of its superiority over single-agent therapy became important. There was little question that the toxicity associated with combination chemotherapy was greater in terms of obvious side effects, i.e., nausea and vomiting and alopecia. Several clinical trials were therefore designed to explore this important issue.

The National Cancer Institute study (Young et al. 1978) comparing hexamethylmelamine, cyclophosphamide, methotrexate, and 5-fluorouracil (Hexa-CAF) with melphalan revealed a statistically superior response rate with the combination (75% vs. 54%) as well as a better median survival (29 months vs. 17 months). Many aspects of this report have been criticized, however, including the relatively young median age of the study population, the relatively high proportion of minimal disease patients in the study, and the fact that survival benefit in the combination arm was observed only in those patients with moderately differentiated tumors. Nevertheless, this study became widely read and often quoted as strong support for combination therapy.

Another major study that underscored the conclusions of the NCI study was that of the Mayo Clinic, comparing the combination of cisplatin and cyclophosphamide with cyclophosphamide alone (Decker et al. 1982). The combination arm was found to be superior in terms of response (76% vs. 26%) as well as median survival (44 months vs. 16.8 months) based on follow-up information. In fact, the single-agent arm was discontinued prematurely because of its obvious inferiority.

Other prospective randomized clinical trials comparing combination with single-agent therapy have not confirmed the above conclusions. In a multicenter study by the Eastern Cooperative Oncology Group, Vogl, Kaplan and Pagano (1982) reported that the combination of cyclophosphamide, hexamethylmelamine, doxorubicin HCl, and cisplatin achieved a significantly better response rate than melphalan (67% vs. 45%) only in those patients who had bulky residual disease or were older than 50. Moreover, there was no difference in median survival between the two arms (18 months each).

In a large randomized clinical trial from Princess Margaret Hospital, Sturgeon et al. (1982) found no differences in survival among patients who received melphalan; a combination of cisplatin, doxorubicin HCl, and cyclophosphamide; or the combination of Hexa-CAF. Toxicity was more severe in those patients receiving combination therapy.

In a recently updated cooperative study from Great Britain, Williams et al. (1985) compared the combination of cisplatin, doxorubicin HCl, and cyclophosphamide with single-agent chlorambucil. Once again, the overall response rate for the combination therapy was higher than that of the single agent (68% vs. 26%), but median survival was not improved (13 months vs. 11 months). The superiority of the combination in terms of response was seen in the patients with bulky residual disease as well as in those patients with minimal residual disease. Furthermore, seven of the eight patients who were continuously disease free (from 30 months to 68 months) received the combination. Since 76% of the patients in this study had bulky disease before undergoing chemotherapy and since there was no superiority in survival with combination therapy, single-agent chemotherapy was recommended for those patients with bulky disease.

Therefore, although early randomized trials suggested a definite benefit of combination therapy over single-agent therapy despite increased toxicity, recent reports cast some doubt on this conclusion. Even in those studies that show a significant survival benefit with combination therapy, there is a question about any long-term advantage, which can only be determined through updated surveys. Although most experts would probably agree that combination chemotherapy represents an improvement in treatment of advanced ovarian cancer over single-agent therapy, there is still no conclusive proof of this.

Cisplatin Versus Non-Cisplatin Combination Activity

Very soon after its introduction into phase II studies, it became evident that cisplatin was an extremely active agent against epithelial ovarian cancer. Its emetic effects, however, have made it very unpopular with patients. Although the recent use of better antiemetic drugs has somewhat alleviated this concern, an important issue is whether cisplatin-containing combination regimens are superior to those that do not contain cisplatin. A number of randomized studies have been undertaken to elucidate this question.

In an early study, Bruckner et al. (1981) compared the combination of triethylenethiophosphoramide and methotrexate with the combination of cisplatin and doxorubicin HCl. The cisplatin-containing combination was superior in terms of both response (68% vs. 29%) and median survival (20 months vs. 11 months). Of course, most investigators would consider the non-cisplatin combination in this study to be an inferior regimen.

In a more realistic comparison by modern standards, Neijt et al. (1984) reported the results of a large multicenter trial comparing Hexa-CAF with the combination of cyclophosphamide, hexamethylmelamine, doxorubicin HCl, and cisplatin. The latter regimen proved superior in terms of response (79% vs. 50%) and median survival (31 months vs. 20 months).

Other randomized trials comparing cisplatin-containing regimens to non-cisplatin-containing regimens have not revealed such differences. In a French cooperative study, Pouillart et al. (1982) found no differences in either response rate or survival in the comparison of the combination of cyclophosphamide, doxorubicin HCl, and 5-fluorouracil with the combination of cyclophosphamide, doxorubicin HCl, 5-fluorouracil, and cisplatin. Likewise, Imholz et al. (1983), comparing the combination of cyclophosphamide, 5-fluorouracil, and doxorubicin HCl with the combination of cisplatin, cyclophosphamide, and doxorubicin HCl, noted no differences in response (65% vs. 57%) or 18-month survival (60% vs. 75%) at the time of analysis.

In a large, prospective randomized trial from U.T. M. D. Anderson Hospital (Edwards et al. 1983), a comparison of the combination of hexamethylmelamine, doxorubicin HCl, and cyclophosphamide with the combination of melphalan and cisplatin produced similar response rates (31% vs. 38%) and median survivals (26 vs. 30 months). Myelosuppression, however, was more severe with the latter combination, and a smaller percentage of patients in this arm received full-dose chemotherapy.

Whether a cisplatin combination regimen is superior to a non-cisplatin combination regimen has not yet been established. Most experts, however, would currently favor a combination that includes cisplatin. Follow-up reports with descriptions of long-term survivors may help to clarify this important issue.

Optimal Combination Regimen

A search for the ideal combination chemotherapy regimen continues. Results of scores of randomized and nonrandomized clinical trials have provided important clues. As noted above, however, comparisons of two or more studies should be made with caution.

Most reports of combination chemotherapy have consisted of two-drug, three-drug, or four-drug regimens. In selecting the optimal combination regimen, both activity and toxicity must be taken into account. Because many clinical investigators have hoped to take advantage of synergistic activity and differing toxicities with the use of multiple agents, the "bigger is better" concept has somewhat pervaded their thinking.

The four most active chemotherapeutic agents in the treatment of advanced epithelial ovarian cancer—cisplatin, an alkylating agent (usually cyclophosphamide), doxorubicin HCl, and hexamethylmelamine—have been studied in combination in several clinical trials. Table 4.7 shows the results of some of these studies. As noted, the response rates are generally quite high, ranging from 67% to 96%, and median survival varies from 18 to 31 months.

Several combination studies with the three-drug regimen of cisplatin, doxorubicin HCl, and cyclophosphamide have produced similar data, as noted in Table 4.8. Response rates range from 44% to 83%, and median survival ranges from 13 to 36 months. Although it is not possible to compare these results with those of four-drug trials because of differences in patient characteristics in study populations (e.g., histological grade, residual disease, and age), the results are not dissimilar.

Likewise, two-drug regimens also have been reported to produce excellent results. The combination of cisplatin and cyclophosphamide, as popularized by the Mayo Clinic, has been used extensively. Table 4.9 presents the results of three

Table 4.7. *Combination Chemotherapy: Cisplatin, Cyclophosphamide, Doxorubicin HCl, and Hexamethylmelamine*

Study	No. of Patients	Response Rate (%)	Median Survival (Months)
Greco et al. 1981	46	96	19+
Vogl, Kaplan, and Pagano 1982	127	67	18
Neijt et al. 1984	92	79	31
Bruckner et al. 1983a	37	83	25
Schulman et al. 1984	28	71	28+

Table 4.8. *Combination Chemotherapy: Cisplatin, Doxorubicin HCl, and Cyclophosphamide*

Study	No. of Patients	Response Rate (%)	Median Survival (Months)
Stehman et al. 1983	56	79	28(V) 24(I)
Belinson et al. 1984	34	—	36
de Konig Gans et al. 1985	57	44	22
Bruckner et al. 1983b	—	52	27
Williams et al. 1985	42	68	13
Budd et al. 1982	36	83	21

Table 4.9. *Combination Chemotherapy: Cisplatin and Cyclophosphamide*

Study	No. of Patients	Response Rate (%)	Median Survival (Months)
Decker et al. 1982	21	76	44
Edmonson et al. 1984	85	—	24
Bell et al. 1982	17	69	17

clinical trials employing this combination. Again, the response rates of up to 76% and median survival times as high as 44 months are not unlike those of regimens using three or four agents.

A number of randomized trials have been conducted to compare two-drug cisplatin regimens with three- and four-drug cisplatin combinations. Bruckner et al. (1983a), based on previous experience with the two-drug combination of cisplatin and doxorubicin HCl (Bruckner et al. 1981; 1983b), compared this regimen with the three-drug regimen of cisplatin, doxorubicin HCl, and cyclophosphamide in a large randomized study involving 130 patients. No differences in either response rate or median survival were observed.

Most of the randomized studies comparing two- and three-drug combinations have employed cisplatin and an alkylating agent in the two-drug arm. Jakobsen et al. (1985), reporting the preliminary results of a large multicenter Danish trial, found that the combination of cisplatin, doxorubicin HCl, and cyclophosphamide produced better results than the combination of cisplatin and cyclophosphamide in terms of a negative second-look laparotomy rate (46% vs. 28%) and three-year survival (48 vs. 20 months). On the other hand, Sertoli et al. (1984), reporting the findings of a randomized study comparing the same two regimens, noted a superior complete response rate with the three-drug combination (55% vs. 21%) but, surprisingly, found a survival advantage for the two-drug regimen at 18 months (75% vs. 49%). The authors concluded that a longer follow-up period was necessary to make definitive assessments.

In a two-arm study comparing the combination of cisplatin and chlorambucil with the combination of cisplatin, chlorambucil, and doxorubicin HCl, Barker and Wiltshaw (1981) reported no differences in either response rate or survival between the two regimens. Moreover, in two separate, large, multicenter randomized trials (Edmonson et al. 1984; Neijt et al. 1985), comparing the four-drug combination of cyclophosphamide, hexamethylmelamine, doxorubicin HCl, and cisplatin with the two-drug regimen of cisplatin and cyclophosphamide, no differences were found in response rate or survival between the two arms. Interestingly, in both studies it was also noted that the four-drug regimen produced significantly more neurotoxicity.

Taking the issue one step further, Mangioni et al. (1985), reporting the preliminary results of a large Italian cooperative three-arm study, compared the efficacy of cisplatin alone with the combination of cisplatin and cyclophosphamide and with the combination of cisplatin, doxorubicin HCl, and cyclophosphamide. Both the two- and three-drug combinations seemed to be more effective than cisplatin alone in inducing a surgically determined complete response. There were, however, no significant differences among the three arms in two-year survival. The authors concluded that longer follow-up was needed.

In summary, the optimal cisplatin-containing combination regimen has not yet been established. Current data suggest, however, that the two-drug combination of cisplatin and cyclophosphamide may indeed be as effective as three- and four-drug regimens without as much toxicity. Resolution of this issue must await maturation of data from ongoing studies.

Optimal Duration of Therapy

The optimal duration of modern postoperative chemotherapy remains unknown. In the early days of single-agent chemotherapy, investigators gradually learned that, to a point, patients who received more cycles of therapy had a greater probability of achieving a complete remission. Eventually, 12 cycles empirically became the standard duration of therapy. Initially, this duration of therapy was transposed to combination chemotherapy. Some investigators (Greco et al. 1981), however, employed only six cycles of combination therapy in selected patients. Currently, most clinical trials appear to include 6 to 12 cycles of treatment.

Presently, there is no information from well-designed prospective randomized trials comparing varying durations of therapy. There is a suggestion from a recently reported study (Stiff, Lanzotti, and Roddick 1983) that patients may achieve maximum benefit from combination chemotherapy after only six cycles. In Stiff's study, 28 patients with advanced epithelial ovarian cancer received six cycles of postoperative chemotherapy consisting of cisplatin, doxorubicin HCl, and cyclophosphamide. Each patient then underwent second-look laparotomy; if persistent disease was noted, the patient received six more cycles of the same chemotherapy and subsequently underwent a third-look laparotomy for assessment of disease status. At the time of the report, eight patients had undergone third-look laparotomy; only one of those patients had negative findings. The other seven had only minimal disease at second-look laparotomy. From the results of this small trial, it appears that more than six cycles of combination chemotherapy carries no additional benefit. Obviously, more information is needed to prove this. Indeed, there may not be an ideal duration of therapy that encompasses all patients with advanced ovarian cancer. Rather, the duration of therapy should be individualized, based on some type of tumor marker. At U.T. M. D. Anderson Hospital, it is our clinical impression that maximum benefit from combination chemotherapy is achieved with six to nine cycles of therapy.

Second-Line Chemotherapy

Historically, second-line chemotherapy for patients with epithelial ovarian cancer who have failed initial therapy has salvaged very few. Stanhope, Smith, and Rutledge (1977) found that only 6.1% of 347 patients responded to second-line therapy for progressive ovarian cancer. The majority of these patients had initially received

Table 4.10. *Cisplatin-Containing Chemotherapy After Alkylating Agent Failure*

Study	Regimen	No. of Patients	Response Rate (%)
Vogl et al. 1979	DDP+ADR+HMM	27	67
Alberts et al. 1979	DDP+HMM+5-FU	74	31
Kane et al. 1979	DDP+CTX+HMM+ADR	35	49
Bernath et al. 1982	DDP+ADR+HMM	27	41
Bruckner et al. 1982	DDP+CTX+ADR+HMM	18	72
Surwit, Alberts, and Crisp 1983	DDP+VBL+BLEO+HMM	35	50

Note: DDP, cisplatin; ADR, doxorubicin HCl; HMM, hexamethylmelamine; 5FU, 5-fluorouracil; CTX, cyclophosphamide; VBL, vinblastine; BLEO, bleomycin.

single-agent chemotherapy. More recent reports involving patients who have previously failed alkylating-agent therapy have documented higher response rates to second-line therapy consisting of hexamethylmelamine (Johnson et al. 1978; Bolis et al. 1979; Bonomi et al. 1979; Omura, Greco, and Birch 1981) and cisplatin (Wiltshaw et al. 1979; Young et al. 1979; Bruckner et al. 1978; Pesando et al. 1980). There are also several reports (table 4.10) of response rates up to 72% with cisplatin-containing combination therapy in patients who previously failed single alkylating-agent therapy. All of these studies were conducted in the late 1970s and early 1980s, an era when it was not uncommon to see many patients with progressive or recurrent ovarian cancer who had previously received only melphalan or cyclophosphamide. Despite the higher response rates, long-term survival nevertheless remained rare. In the last few years, advanced ovarian cancer patients initially treated with single-alkylating agent therapy alone have rarely been encountered because the majority of such patients are initially treated with a cisplatin-containing regimen. It is currently well-appreciated that patients who fail first-line therapy with a cisplatin-containing regimen are rarely salvaged with available second-line treatment, whether it be conventional combination chemotherapy or experimental therapies (Edwards et al. 1983; Sessa et al. 1982; Stehman et al. 1985).

Of those patients with advanced epithelial ovarian cancer who achieve a complete remission with first-line chemotherapy, approximately 25% to 50% will eventually relapse. It has been our observation that many of these patients with true recurrent ovarian cancer will achieve a second response to further chemotherapy, even, in some cases, to the same agents originally administered. Seltzer, Vogl, and Kaplan (1985) also observed this same phenomenon. In their study of 11 patients who relapsed after a complete response to a cisplatin-containing combination, 4 patients had a second complete response and 4 patients had a partial response to repeat administration of a cisplatin-containing combination regimen.

For those patients who achieve a partial response to a cisplatin-containing combination and have persistent minimal disease at second-look laparotomy (microscopic disease or macroscopic disease <1 cm), disappointment with the results achieved with continued systemic chemotherapy has led investigators to study either intraperitoneal chemotherapy or radiotherapy.

For the majority of patients who have bulky residual disease after receiving a cisplatin-containing regimen (which includes some patients who achieve a partial response as well as patients who develop progressive disease on therapy), conventional modalities of therapy appear to be ineffective. These patients are, therefore, candidates for experimental therapies.

Newer Therapies

Because of disappointment in the results achieved with conventional methods of treatment, investigators have turned to innovative types of therapy in an effort to improve survival rates. In the last few years, foremost among these have been alternating, non-cross-resistant chemotherapy; high-dose therapy with either cisplatin or an alkylating agent; and cisplatin analogues.

There is now some evidence that alternating non-cross-resistant chemotherapy may be superior to the use of only one combination regimen in Hodgkin's disease (Bonadonna, Monfardini, and Villa 1977). Similar approaches have been attempted in the treatment of ovarian cancer. Young et al. (1984) treated 39 patients with advanced ovarian cancer, alternating the combination of cisplatin, doxorubicin HCl, and cyclophosphamide with Hexa-CAF. The response rate was 61%, and the median survival was 21 months. These results are not superior to those reported with either combination alone. Hernandez et al. (1983) treated 18 patients with the combination of cisplatin, cyclophosphamide, and hexamethylmelamine, alternating with the combination of doxorubicin HCl, cyclophosphamide, and hexamethylmelamine. The overall response rate was 55%, and the median survival was only 14 months, again not superior to results achieved with only one regimen. Therefore, experience to date with alternating combination chemotherapy does not appear to offer any advantage over conventional methods of administration of a single regimen.

There has also been recent interest in the use of high-dose chemotherapy in an effort to circumvent tumor resistance. Corringham et al. (1983) reported the treatment of two patients with refractory ovarian cancer with high-dose melphalan and autologous bone marrow transplantation. One patient had stable disease for 8 weeks, and the other patient experienced a complete remission for 35 weeks. Maraninchi et al. (1984) also treated two patients with similar therapy. One patient had a complete remission for five weeks, and the other patient failed to respond to therapy. Data concerning this treatment approach is sparse, and more experience will be necessary to clarify its role in the treatment of ovarian cancer.

High-dose cisplatin has also been studied in phase II trials. Ozols et al. (1985b) treated 19 patients with refractory ovarian cancer, including 17 patients who had previously received standard-dose cisplatin regimens, with cisplatin 40 mg/m^2 daily for 5 days with cycles repeated every 28 to 35 days. The overall response rate was 32%, and the median survival was 12 months. Although these data are impressive, the associated toxicity appears to be highly significant. Severe renal toxicity occurred in 32% of patients after the first cycle of therapy, although it appeared to be transient. Neurotoxicity was extremely severe. All patients developed hearing abnormalities in the high-pitch range on audiograms, and one patient required a hearing aid. Peripheral neuropathy occurred in all patients who received more than two cycles of therapy, and it was debilitating in 37% of patients. Two patients became wheelchair dependent. Our assessment of high-dose cisplatin as reported is that the neurotoxicity is prohibitive. More information is needed to evaluate its appropriate status. In the meantime, its use should be restricted to tightly controlled clinical trials.

One of the most promising new chemotherapy agents is carboplatin, an analogue of cisplatin. Evans et al. (1983) reported the use of carboplatin in the treatment of 33 patients who had previously received cisplatin. There were five partial responses and two complete responses noted. Moreover, of the seven responders, four had previously been completely resistant to cisplatin. There were fewer renal, auditory, gastrointestinal, and neurological toxic reactions than would have been expected with cisplatin, but myelosuppression appeared to be more common. Ozols et al. (1985a) noted a 25% response rate in eight patients treated with carboplatin, all of whom had previously received cisplatin. Toxicity data were very similar to those observed by Evans et al. (1983). Therefore, carboplatin not only seems to be associated with much less toxicity than cisplatin, but it also appears to be somewhat non-cross-resistant. This agent will undoubtedly be studied further and may eventually replace cisplatin.

Quality of Life with Chemotherapy

Since the advent of modern combination chemotherapy with its associated side effects, toxicity has been a major issue with patients and medical personnel alike. Some patients have even refused potentially beneficial therapy because of the toxicity. The most devastating effects for the patient with ovarian cancer have been severe nausea and vomiting and alopecia. Of course, other toxicities such as myelosuppression, nephrotoxicity, neurotoxicity, and cardiotoxicity have also had a major effect on some patients, but they are less universal.

Although a thorough discussion of this topic is beyond the scope of this paper, the potential toxic effects of these chemotherapy regimens have made physicians unquestionably more cognizant of and concerned about the quality of life of their patients. Some progress has occurred in the last few years in this area. More effective antiemetic therapy is now available for many patients. Methods of preventing alopecia are also being studied. With meticulous, modern monitoring techniques, severe or life-threatening side effects may become rare. Several prospective studies concerned with quality of life are currently being conducted.

Conclusions

Although much progress has occurred in the last few years in the understanding and treatment of advanced epithelial ovarian cancer, many questions remain unanswered. We have learned a great deal about the influence of prognostic factors. This information should allow investigators to better design clinical trials.

The evidence for superiority of combination chemotherapy over single-agent therapy is confusing. In general, it does appear as if combination chemotherapy produces a somewhat longer median survival in many studies. The crucial issue—its effect on long-term survival—has yet to be answered. Nevertheless, unless a more effective drug is discovered, it is unlikely that we will ever return to single-agent therapy.

Although the evidence for the superiority of a cisplatin-containing combination over a non-cisplatin combination is also equivocal, most experts in this area favor cisplatin combinations. The optimal regimen and duration of therapy remain unclear. Available information suggests that two-drug combinations may be just as efficacious as three- and four-drug regimens. In most cases, the optimal duration of therapy is in the range of six to nine cycles.

Second-line therapy for patients with refractory ovarian cancer remains poor. Multimodality approaches may prove beneficial in patients with minimal disease following chemotherapy. Patients with bulky residual disease following chemotherapy continue to have a dismal prognosis. Future directions include continued study of platinum analogues, a search for new agents, and further trials involving multimodality therapy.

References

Alberts DS, Hilgers RD, Moon TE, Martimbeau PW, Rivkin S. 1979. Combination chemotherapy for alkylator-resistant ovarian carcinoma: A preliminary report of a Southwest Oncology Group trial. *Cancer Treat Rep* 63:301–305.

Barker GH, Wiltshaw E. 1981. Randomized trial comparing low-dose cisplatin and chlorambucil with low-dose cisplatin, chlorambucil, and doxorubicin in advanced ovarian carcinoma. *Lancet* 1:747–750.

Barlow JJ, Piver MS, Chuang JT, Cortes EP, Ohnuma T, Holland JF. 1973. Adriamycin and bleomycin, alone and in combination, in gynecologic cancers. *Cancer* 32:735–743.

Barlow JJ, Piver MS, Lele SB. 1982. Weekly *cis*-platinum remission 'induction' and combination drug consolidation and maintenance in ovarian cancer. *Proceedings of the American Society of Clinical Oncology* 1:119.

Beck RE, Boyes DA. 1968. Treatment of 126 cases of advanced ovarian carcinoma with cyclophosphamide. *Can Med Assoc J* 98:539–541.

Belinson JL, McClure M, Ashikaga T, Krakoff IH. 1984. Treatment of advanced and recurrent ovarian carcinoma with cyclophosphamide, doxorubicin, and cisplatin. *Cancer* 54:1983–1990.

Bell DR, Woods RLK, Levi JA, Fox RM, Tattersall MHN. 1982. Advanced ovarian cancer: A prospective randomized trial of chlorambucil versus combined cyclophosphamide and *cis*-diamminedichloroplatinum. *Aust NZ J Med* 12:245–249.

Berkson J, Gage RP. 1952. Survival for cancer patients following treatment. *Journal of the American Statistical Association* 47:501–515.

Bernath A, Andrews T, Dixon R, Gottlieb R, Judson S, Ellison N, Harvey H, Lipton A. 1982. Long-term follow-up of HAP (hexamethylmelamine, Adriamycin, *cis*-platinum) vs CAP (cyclophosphamide, Adriamycin, *cis*-platinum) in alkylating agent-resistant advanced ovarian carcinoma. *Proceedings of the American Society of Clinical Oncology* 1:110.

Bolis G, Bortolozzi G, Carinelli G, D'Incalci M, Grammellini F, Morasca L, Mangioni C. 1980. Low dose cyclophosphamide in advanced ovarian cancer. *Cancer Chemother Pharmacol* 4:129–132.

Bolis G, D'Incalci M, Grammellini F, Mangioni C. 1978. Adriamycin in ovarian cancer patients resistant to cyclophosphamide. *Eur J Cancer* 14: 1401–1406.

Bolis G, D'Incalci M, Mangioni C, Belloni C. 1979. Hexamethylmelamine in ovarian cancer resistant to cyclophosphamide and Adriamycin. *Cancer Treat Rep* 63:1375–1377.

Bonadonna G, Monfardini S, Villa E. 1977. Non-cross-resistant combinations in stage IV non-Hodgkin's lymphomas. *Cancer Treat Rep* 61:1117–1123.

Bonomi PD, Mladineo J, Morrin B, Wilbanks G, Slayton RE. 1979. Phase II trial of hexamethylmelamine in ovarian cancer resistant to alkylating agents. *Cancer Treat Rep* 63: 137–138.

Broders AC. 1926. Carcinoma: Grading and practical application. *Arch Pathol* 2:376.

Brodovsky HS, Temkin N, Sears M. 1977. Melphalan versus cyclophosphamide, methotrexate and 5-fluorouracil, in women with ovarian cancer. *Proceedings of the American Society of Clinical Oncology* 18:308.

Bruckner HW, Cohen CJ, Deppe G, Sushil B, Zaken D, Storch J, Goldberg J, Holland J. 1982. Ovarian cancer: Schedule modification and dosage intensification of cyclophosphamide, hexamethylmelamine, Adriamycin, cisplatin regimen (CHAP II). *Proceedings of the American Society of Clinical Oncology* 1:107.

Bruckner HW, Cohen CJ, Goldberg JD, Kabakow B, Wallach RC, Deppe G, Greenspan EM, Gusberg SB, Holland JF. 1981. Improved chemotherapy for ovarian cancer with *cis*-diamminedichloroplatinum and Adriamycin. *Cancer* 47:2288–2294.

Bruckner HW, Cohen CJ, Goldberg JD, Kabakow B, Wallach RC, Deppe G, Reisman AZ, Gusberg SB, Holland JF. 1983a. Cisplatin regimens and improved prognosis of patients with poorly differentiated ovarian cancer. *Am J Obstet Gynecol* 145:653–658.

Bruckner HW, Cohen CJ, Goldberg JD, Kabakow B, Wallach RC, Holland JF. 1983b. Ovarian cancer: Comparison of Adriamycin and cisplatin + cyclophosphamide. *Proceedings of the American Society of Clinical Oncology* 2:152.

Bruckner HW, Cohen CJ, Wallach RC, Kabakow B, Deppe G, Greenspan EM, Gusberg SB, Holland JF. 1978. Treatment of advanced ovarian cancer with *cis*-dichlorodiammineplatinum (II): Poor-risk patients with intensive prior therapy. *Cancer Treat Rep* 62: 555–558.

Budd GT, Livingston RB, Webster K, Reimer R, Martimbeau PW, Hewlett JS. 1982. Treatment of advanced ovarian cancer with cisplatin, Adriamycin, and Cytoxan (PAC). *Proceedings of the American Society of Clinical Oncology* 1:117.

Carmo-Pereira J, Oliveira-Costa F, Henriques E, Almeida-Ricardo J. 1981. Advanced ovarian carcinoma: A prospective and randomized clinical trial of cyclophosphamide versus combination cytotoxic therapy (Hexa CAF). *Cancer* 48:1947–1951.

Corringham R, Gilmore M, Prentice HG, Boesen E. 1983. High-dose melphalan with autologous bone marrow transplant. *Cancer* 52:1783–1787.

Day TG Jr, Gallager HS, Rutledge FN. 1975. Epithelial carcinoma of the ovary: Prognostic importance of histologic grade. *Natl Cancer Inst Monogr* 42:15–18.

Decker DG, Fleming TR, Malkasian GD Jr, Webb MJ, Jefferies JA, Edmonson JH. 1982. Cyclophosphamide plus *cis*-platinum in combination: Treatment program for stage III or IV ovarian carcinoma. *Obstet Gynecol* 60:481–487.

Decker DG, Malkasian GD Jr, Mussey E, Johnson CE. 1967. Cyclophosphamide: Evaluation in recurrent and progressive ovarian cancer. *Am J Obstet Gynecol* 97:656–665.

de Konig Gans H, Wils J, Blijham G, Bron H, Eekhout A, van Geuns H, Haest J, Hoogland H, Huiske H, Korman J, Lalisang F, van der Meulen J, Poormann P, Stoot J, Tushuizen P, Vreeswijk J, Wals J. 1985. Combination of surgery and chemotherapy (CAP-1) in stage III–IV epithelial ovarian cancer. A multicenter study. *Proceedings of the American Society of Clinical Oncology* 4:124.

Deligdisch L, Jacobs AJ, Cohen CJ. 1982. Histologic correlates of virulence in ovarian adenocarcinoma. II. Morphologic correlates of host response. *Am J Obstet Gynecol* 144:885.

Dembo AJ, Brown TC, Bush RS, Sturgeon JFG. 1982. Prognostic significance of pathology subtype and differentiation in epithelial carcinoma of ovary (ECO). *Proceedings of the American Society of Clinical Oncology* 1:105.

De Palo GM, De Lena M, Bonadonna G. 1977. Adriamycin versus Adriamycin plus melphalan in advanced ovarian carcinoma. *Cancer Treat Rep* 61:355–357.

De Palo GM, De Lena M, Di Re F, Luciani L, Valagussa P, Bonadonna G. 1975. Melphalan versus Adriamycin in the treatment of advanced carcinoma of the ovary. *Surg Gynecol Obstet* 141:899–902.

Edmonson JH, Fleming TR, Decker DG, Malkasian GD Jr, Jorgensen EO, Jefferies JA, Webb MJ, Kvols LK. 1979. Different chemotherapeutic sensitivities and host factors affecting prognosis in advanced ovarian carcinoma versus minimal residual disease. *Cancer Treat Rep* 63:241–247.

Edmonson JH, McCormack GW, Fleming TR, Cullinan SA, Krook JE, Malkasian GD Jr, Podratz KC, Mailliard JA, Jefferies JA. 1984. Comparison of cyclophosphamide + cisplatin (CP) vs. a combination of hexamethylmelamine, cyclophosphamide, doxorubicin and cisplatin (HCAP) as primary chemotherapy for stage III and IV ovarian carcinoma. *Proceedings of the American Society of Clinical Oncology* 3:169.

Edwards CL, Herson J, Gershenson DM, Copeland LJ, Wharton JT. 1983. A prospective randomized clinical trial of melphalan and *cis*-platinum versus hexamethylmelamine, Adriamycin, and cyclophosphamide in advanced ovarian cancer. *Gynecol Oncol* 15:261–277.

Ehrlich CE, Einhorn L, Williams SD, Morgan J. 1979. Chemotherapy for stage III–IV epithelial ovarian cancer with *cis*-dichlorodiammineplatinum II, Adriamycin, and cyclophosphamide: A preliminary report. *Cancer Treat Rep* 63:281–288.

Evans BD, Raju KS, Calvert AH, Harland SJ, Wiltshaw E. 1983. Phase II study of JM8, a new platinum analog, in advanced ovarian carcinoma. *Cancer Treat Rep* 67:997–1000.

Gershenson DM, Wharton JT, Herson J, Edwards CL, Rutledge FN. 1981. Single-agent *cis*-platinum therapy for advanced ovarian cancer. *Obstet Gynecol* 58:487–495.

Greco FA, Julian CG, Richardson RL, Burnett L, Hande KR, Oldham RK. 1981. Advanced ovarian cancer: Brief intensive combination chemotherapy and second-look operation. *Obstet Gynecol* 58:199–205.

Griffiths CT. 1975. Surgical resection of tumor bulk in the primary treatment of ovarian carcinoma. Seminar on ovarian cancer. *Natl Cancer Inst Monogr* 42:101–104, 113–115.

Griffiths CT, Parker LM, Fuller AF. 1979. Role of cytoreductive surgical treatment in the management of advanced ovarian cancer. *Cancer Treat Rep* 63:235–239.

Hall DJ, Diasio R, Goplerud DR. 1981. *cis*-Platinum in gynecologic cancer. I. Epithelial ovarian cancer. *Am J Obstet Gynecol* 141:299–304.

Hernandez E, Rosenshein NB, Villar J, Dillon B, Ettinger DS, Order SE. 1983. Alternating multiagent chemotherapy for advanced ovarian cancer. *J Surg Oncol* 22: 87–91.

Hubbard SM, Barkes P, Young RC. 1978. Adriamycin therapy for advanced ovarian carcinoma recurrent after chemotherapy. *Cancer Treat Rep* 62:1375–1377.

Imholz G, Mayr AC, Schmoranz W, Gruneisen A, Pschyrembel I, Scholtes G. 1983. Cisplatin, Adriamycin, Cytoxan (PAC) vs. fluorouracil, Adriamycin, Cytoxan (FAC) in ovarian cancer FIGO II B-IV. Preliminary results of a randomized cooperative trial (Abstract). *Proceedings of the American Society of Clinical Oncology* 2:155.

Izbicki RM, Baker RL, Samson MK, McDonald B, Vaitkevicius VK. 1977. 5-Fluorouracil infusion and cyclophosphamide in the treatment of advanced ovarian cancer. *Cancer Treat Rep* 61:1573–1575.

Jacobs EM, Reeves WJ Jr, Wood DA, Pugh R, Braunwald J, Bateman JR. 1971. Treatment of cancer with weekly intravenous 5-fluorouracil: Study by the Western Cooperative Cancer Chemotherapy Group (WCCCG). *Cancer* 27:1302–1305.

Jakobsen A, Bertelsen K, Sell A, Stroyer I, Pedersen M. 1985. Advantage of CAP over CP in terms of survival in advanced ovarian carcinoma. *Proceedings of the American Society of Clinical Oncology* 4:113.

Johnson BL, Fischer RI, Bender RA, DeVita VT, Chabner BA, Young RC. 1978. Hexamethylmelamine in alkylating agent-resistant ovarian carcinoma. *Cancer* 42:2157–2161.

Kane R, Harvey H, Andrews T, Bernath A, Curry S, Dixon R, Gottlieb R, Kukrika M, Lipton A, Mortel R, Ricci J, White D. 1979. Phase II trial of cyclophosphamide, hexamethylmelamine, Adriamycin, and *cis*-dichlorodiammineplatinum (II) combination chemotherapy in advanced ovarian carcinoma. *Cancer Treat Rep* 63:307–309.

Kaplan EL, Meier P. Nonparametric estimation from incomplete observations. 1958. *Journal of the American Statistical Association* 53:457–481.

Katz ME, Schwartz PE, Kapp DS, Luikart S. 1981. Epithelial carcinoma of the ovary: Current strategies. *Ann Intern Med* 95:98–111.

Malkasian GD Jr, Decker DG, Mussey E, Johnson CE. 1968. Observations on gynecologic malignancy treated with 5-fluorouracil. *Am J Obstet Gynecol* 100:1012–1017.

Malkasian GD Jr, Melton LJ III, O'Brien PC, Greene MH. 1984. Prognostic significance of histologic classification and grading of epithelial malignancies of the ovary. *Am J Obstet Gynecol* 149:274.

Mangioni C, Bianchi UA, Bolis G, Bortolozzi G, Colombo N, Epis A, Valsecchi MG, Sanpaolo P, Pecorelli S. 1985. Randomized trial comparing two platinum (P) combinations to P alone in advanced ovarian carcinoma (OC). *Proceedings of the American Society of Clinical Oncology* 4:117.

Maraninchi D, Abecasis M, Gastaut JA, Herve P, Sebanhoun G, Flesch M, Blanc AP, Carcassone Y. 1984. High-dose melphalan with autologous bone marrow rescue for the treatment of advanced adult solid tumors. *Cancer Treat Rep* 68: 471–474.

Neijt JP, ten Bokkel Huinink WW, van der Burg MEL, van Oosterom AT, Vriesendorp R, Heintz APM, van Lent M, Bouma J, van Houwelingen JC, Pinedo HM. 1985. Combination chemotherapy with CHAP-5 and CP in advanced ovarian carcinoma: A randomized trial of the Netherlands Joint Study Group for ovarian cancer. *Proceedings of the American Society of Clinical Oncology* 4:114.

Neijt JP, ten Bokkel Huinink WW, van der Burg MEL, van Oosterom AT, Vriesendorp R, Kooyman CD, van Lindert ACM, Hamerlynck JVTH, van Lent M, van Houwelingen JC. 1984. Randomized trial comparing two combination chemotherapy regimens (HEXA-CAF vs. CHAP-5) in advanced ovarian carcinoma. *Lancet* 2:594–600.

O'Bryan RM, Luce JK, Talley RW, Gottlieb JA, Baker LH, Bonadonna G. 1973. Phase II evaluation of Adriamycin in human neoplasia. *Cancer* 32:1–8.

Omura GA, Greco FA, Birch R. 1981. Hexamethylmelamine in mustard-resistant ovarian adenocarcinoma. *Cancer Treat Rep* 65:530–531.

Omura GA, Morrow CP, Blessing JA, Miller A, Buchsbaum HJ, Homesley HD, Leone L. 1983. A randomized comparison of melphalan versus melphalan plus hexamethylmelamine versus Adriamycin plus cyclophosphamide in ovarian carcinoma. *Cancer* 51:783–789.

Ozols RF, Garvin J, Costa J, Simon RM, Young RC. 1980. Correlation of histologic grade with response to therapy and survival. *Cancer* 45:572–581.

Ozols RF, Ostchega Y, Curt G, Myers C, Young RC. 1985a. High dose (HD) cisplatin (P) [40 mg/m^2 qd x 5] and HD carboplatinum (CBDCA) [400 mg/m^2 qd x 2] in refractory ovarian cancer: Active salvage drugs with different toxicities. *Proceedings of the American Society of Clinical Oncology* 4:119.

Ozols RF, Ostchega Y, Myers CE, Young RC. 1985b. High-dose cisplatin in hypertonic saline in refractory ovarian cancer. *J Clin Oncol* 3:1246–1250.

Pesando JM, Come SE, Stark J, Parker LM, Griffiths CT, Canellos GP. 1980. *Cis*-diamminedichloroplatinum (II) therapy for advanced ovarian cancer. *Cancer Treat Rep* 64:1147–1148.

Piver MS, Barlow JJ, Lele SB, Malfetano JH, McPhee ME. 1983. *Cis*-diamminedichloroplatinum (II): Second line induction chemotherapy in advanced ovarian adenocarcinoma. *J Surg Oncol* 24: 329–331.

Piver MS, Barlow JJ, Yazigi R, Blumenson LE. 1978. Melphalan chemotherapy in advanced ovarian carcinoma. *Obstet Gynecol* 51:352–356.

Pouillart P, Bretaudeau B, Palangil T, Jouve M, Garcia-Giralt E, Asselain B. 1982. Adenocarcinoma of the ovary (stage III and IV) treated with a combination of Adriamycin, cyclophosphamide, 5-fluorouracil and *cis*-DDP: A study of the therapeutic role of *cis*-DDP in combination. *Bull Cancer* (Paris) 69:434–442.

Richardson GS, Sculley RE, Nikrui N, Nelson JH Jr. 1985. Common epithelial cancer of the ovary. *N Engl J Med* 312: 415–424, 474–483.

Schulman P, Kleinbaum Z, Budman D, Weiselberg L, Vinciguerra V, Lovecchio J, Allen S, Degnan TJ. 1984. Long term follow up of patients with epithelial carcinoma of the ovary on Cytoxan, Adriamycin, cisplatin and hexamethylmelamine (HEXA-CAP). *Proceedings of the American Society of Clinical Oncology* 3:165.

Seltzer V, Vogl S, Kaplan B. 1985. Recurrent ovarian carcinoma: Retreatment utilizing combination chemotherapy including *cis*-diamminedichloroplatinum in patients previously responding to this agent. *Gynecol Oncol* 21:167–176.

Sertoli MR, Conte PF, Rosso R, Bruzzone M, Rubagotti A, Carnino F, Mossett C, Guercio E, Siliquini PN, Relato ML, Durando C, Cottini M, Giaccone G, Calciati A, Bentivoglio G, Pescetto G. 1984. A randomized study to evaluate the addition of Adriamycin (A) to cisplatin (P) + Cytoxan (C) combination chemotherapy in advanced ovarian cancer. *Proceedings of the American Society of Clinical Oncology* 3:176.

Sessa C, D'Incalci M, Valente I, Bolis G, Colombo N, Mangioni C. 1982. Hexamethylmelamine-CAF (cyclophosphamide, methotrexate, and 5-FU) and cisplatin-CAF in refractory ovarian cancer. *Cancer Treat Rep* 66:1233–1234.

Sigurdsson K, Alm P, Gullberg B. 1983. Prognostic factors in malignant epithelial ovarian tumors. *Gynecol Oncol* 15:370–380.

Skipper HC, Chapman JB, Bell M. 1952. The anti-leukemic action of combinations of certain known anti-leukemia agents. *Cancer Res* 11:109–114.

Sorbe B, Frankendal B, Veress B. 1981. Importance of histologic grading in the prognosis of epithelial ovarian carcinoma. *Obstet Gynecol* 59:576–583.

Stanhope CR, Smith JP, Rutledge FN. 1977. Second trial drugs in ovarian cancer. *Gynecol Oncol* 5:52–58.

Stehman FB, Ehrlich CE, Einhorn LH, Williams SD, Roth LM. 1983. Long-term follow-up and survival in stage III–IV epithelial ovarian cancer treated with *cis*-dichlorodiammineplatinum, Adriamycin, and cyclophosphamide (PAC). *Proceedings of the American Society of Clinical Oncology* 3:147.

Stehman FB, Ehrlich CE, Williams SD, Einhorn LH. 1985. Cisplatin, vinblastine, and bleomycin as second-trial therapy in ovarian carcinoma. A pilot study of the Gynecologic Oncology Group. *Am J Clin Oncol* 3:27–31.

Stiff PJ, Lanzotti VJ, Roddick JW. 1983. Prolonged combination chemotherapy for ovarian carcinoma does not increase the rate of surgical complete remissions. *Proceedings of the American Society of Clinical Oncology* 2:156.

Sturgeon JFG, Fine S, Gospodarowicz MK, Dembo AJ, Bean HA, Bush RS, Beale FA, Pringle JF, Thomas GM, Herman JG. 1982. A randomized trial of melphalan alone versus combination chemotherapy in advanced ovarian cancer. *Proceedings of the American Society of Clinical Oncology* 1:108.

Surwit EA, Alberts DS, Crisp W. 1983. Multiagent chemotherapy in relapsing ovarian cancer. *Am J Obstet Gynecol* 146:613–616.

Thigpen JT. 1985. Single agent chemotherapy in the management of ovarian carcinoma. In *Ovarian Cancer*, ed. DS Alberts, EA Surwit, pp. 115–146. Boston: Martinus Nijhoff.

Thigpen T, Shingleton H, Homesley H, Lagasse L, Blessing J. 1979. *cis*-dichlorodiammineplatinum (II) therapy for advanced ovarian cancer. *Cancer Treat Rep* 63:1549–1555.

Tobias JS, Griffiths CT. 1976. Management in ovarian carcinoma: Current concepts and future prospects. *N Engl J Med* 294:818–823, 877–882.

Trope C. 1981. A prospective and randomized trial comparison of melphalan vs. Adriamycin-melphalan in advanced ovarian carcinoma by the Swedish Cooperative Ovarian Cancer Study Group. *Proceedings of the American Society of Clinical Oncology* 22:469.

Vogl SE, Greenwald E, Kaplan BH, Moukhtar M, Wollner D. 1979. Ovarian cancer: Effective treatment after alkylating-agent failure. *JAMA* 241:1908–1911.

Vogl SE, Kaplan B, Pagano M. 1982. Diamminedichloroplatinum (D)-based combination chemotherapy (CT) is superior to melphalan (M) for advanced ovarian cancer (OvCa) when age is >50 & tumor diameter is >2 cm. *Proceedings of the American Society of Clinical Oncology* 1:119.

Wharton JT, Edwards CL, Rutledge FN. 1984. Long-term survival after chemotherapy for advanced epithelial ovarian carcinoma. *Am J Obstet Gynecol* 148:997–1005.

Wharton JT, Gershenson DM, Herson J. 1983. Chemotherapy of ovarian malignancies at M. D. Anderson. In *Carcinoma of the Ovary*, ed. HG Bender, L Beck, pp. 151–159. New York and Stuttgart: Gustav Fischer Verlag.

Wharton JT, Herson J. 1981. Surgery for common epithelial tumors of the ovary. *Cancer* 48:582–589.

Wharton JT, Herson J, Edwards CL, Griffith AB. 1982. Single-agent Adriamycin followed by combination hexamethylmelamine-cyclophosphamide for advanced ovarian carcinoma. *Gynecol Oncol* 14:262–270.

Wharton JT, Herson J, Edwards CL, Seski J, Hodge MD. 1980. Long-term survival following chemotherapy for advanced epithelial ovarian carcinoma. In *Therapeutic Progress in Ovarian Cancer, Testicular Cancer and the Sarcomas*. ed. AT van Oosterom, FM Muggia, FJ Cleton, pp. 96–112. The Hague: Martinus Nijhoff.

Wharton JT, Rutledge FN, Smith JP, Herson J, Hodge MP. 1979. Hexamethylmelamine: An evaluation of its role in the treatment of ovarian cancer. *Am J Obstet Gynecol* 133:833–844.

Williams CJ, Mead GM, Macbeth FR, Thompson J, Whitehouse JMA, MacDonald H, Harvey VJ, Slevin ML, Lister TA, Shepherd JH, Golding P. 1985. Cisplatin combination chemotherapy versus chlorambucil in advanced ovarian carcinoma: Mature results of a randomized trial. *J Clin Oncol* 3:1455–1462.

Williams CJ, Stevenson KE, Buchanan RB, Whitehouse JMA. 1979. Advanced ovarian carcinoma: A pilot study of *cis*-dichlorodiammineplatinum (II) in combination with Adriamycin and cyclophosphamide in previously untreated patients and as a single agent in previously treated patients. *Cancer Treat Rep* 63:1745–1753.

Wiltshaw E, Subramarian S, Alexopoulos C, Barker GH. 1979. Cancer of the ovary: A summary of experience with *cis*-dichlorodiammineplatinum (II) at the Royal Marsden Hospital. *Cancer Treat Rep* 63:1545–1548.

Young JA, Johnson A, Kroener J, Koziol JA, Saltzstein S, Yon JL, Campbell TN, Lucas W, Green MR. 1984. Alternating combination chemotherapy for stages III and IV ovarian carcinoma. *J Clin Oncol* 2:1317–1320.

Young RC, Chabner BA, Hubbard SP, Fisher RI, Bender RA, Anderson T, Simon RM, Canellos GP, DeVita VT Jr. 1978. Advanced ovarian adenocarcinoma: A prospective clinical trial of melphalan (L-Pam) versus combination chemotherapy. *N Engl J Med* 299:1261–1266.

Young RC, Von Hoff DD, Gormley P, Makuch R, Cassidy J, Howser D, Bull JM. 1979. *Cis*-dichlorodiammineplatinum (II) for the treatment of advanced ovarian cancer. *Cancer Treat Rep* 63:1539–1544.

Annual Clinical Conference on Cancer, Vol. 29
Gynecologic Cancer: Diagnosis and Treatment Strategies
© 1987 by The University of Texas System Cancer Center

5. Intraperitoneal Chemotherapy for Epithelial Ovarian Cancer

Maurie Markman

Epithelial ovarian carcinoma is one of the most chemotherapy-sensitive nonhematopoietic malignancies. Response rates exceeding 60% have been reported with a cisplatin-based combination chemotherapy regimen (Richardson et al. 1985). Unfortunately, the vast majority of patients with advanced (stage III or IV) ovarian carcinoma eventually die of the disease. Thus, it is not surprising that there has been great interest in innovative approaches to treating this malignancy.

There are several reasons why the intraperitoneal administration of chemotherapeutic agents in ovarian carcinoma has significant theoretical appeal. First, in most patients the tumor remains largely confined to the peritoneal cavity for most of its natural history. Second, there are several agents with known activity against ovarian carcinoma that might be investigated for delivery by the intraperitoneal route. Finally, the tumor often grows as tiny nodules on the peritoneal surface, and it is possible that the delivery of drug by free-surface diffusion to the tumor might significantly enhance the therapeutic impact of treatment.

Although the intraperitoneal delivery of chemotherapeutic agents has a long history in the treatment of ovarian carcinoma (Green 1959; Kottmeier 1968), only recently has this technique been thoroughly investigated (Markman 1985b). Mathematical modeling studies based on anatomic and physiological considerations as well as known characteristics of chemotherapeutic agents have suggested a major pharmacokinetic advantage for exposure of the peritoneal cavity to certain drugs compared with treatment by systemic circulation (Dedrick et al. 1978). In addition, although drugs placed into the peritoneal cavity can theoretically exit the cavity by one of three routes (portal circulation, direct entry into systemic circulation, uptake into lymphatics), experimental data would suggest that the principal means of exit is through the portal circulation (Kraft, Tompkins, and Jesseph 1968; Lukas, Brindle, and Greengard 1971). Thus, a chemotherapeutic agent metabolized (into a nontoxic form) in the liver might demonstrate a significant pharmacokinetic advantage when delivered by direct intraperitoneal instillation. Examples of such agents include 5-fluorouracil and cytarabine.

An additional potential advantage of intraperitoneal chemotherapy would be the opportunity to deliver neutralizing agents (for the cytotoxic drugs) into the systemic circulation simultaneously with or subsequent to intraperitoneal drug instillation. In this way, systemic toxicity might be reduced while allowing further escalation of dosage of the cytotoxic drug or drugs. Unfortunately, it is not possible to keep the neutralizing agent completely out of the peritoneal cavity, and the effectiveness of treatment might be influenced by inhibition of cytotoxicity. An obvious cytotoxic agent–neutralizing agent pair to investigate would be methotrexate and folinic acid (Leucovorin). A second combination examined at the University of California, San Diego (UCSD) Cancer Center is that of cisplatin and sodium thiosulfate.

Intraperitoneal administration of certain chemotherapeutic agents in ovarian carcinoma may result in a pharmacokinetic advantage, but such a treatment strategy does not ensure delivery of drug-containing fluid to all sections of the peritoneal cavity. The difficulty of achieving adequate distribution of radioactive material placed into the peritoneal cavity in small volumes in ovarian carcinoma has been demonstrated (Tully, Goldberg, and Locken 1974; Taylor et al. 1975; Vider, Deland, and Maruyama 1976). There are several reasons for this problem, including tumor masses that can prevent access to large portions of the abdominal cavity and significant intraabdominal adhesions produced by prior surgeries or induced by the tumor itself that further compromise drug distribution. The ability of large treatment volumes to overcome this problem of inadequate distribution has been demonstrated both experimentally in an animal model (Rosenshein et al. 1978) and in patients with advanced intraabdominal malignancies (including ovarian carcinoma) undergoing intraperitoneal chemotherapy (Dunnick et al. 1979; Howell et al. 1982). Most clinical trials of intraperitoneal chemotherapy now employ at least a 2-L treatment volume, which appears to result in adequate drug distribution in 70% to 80% of patients, even those with advanced intraabdominal malignancies.

A second major practical issue in intraperitoneal chemotherapy is that of establishing a safe and effective treatment delivery system. Although it is possible to administer the treatment volume by the percutaneous placement of a temporary peritoneal dialysis or paracentesis catheter with each treatment course, there is concern that patients with adhesions will be at considerable risk of bowel perforation (Kaplan et al. 1985). In addition, because the location of the catheter will be different with each placement, it would be necessary to evaluate the adequacy of distribution before each treatment course.

As an alternative to percutaneous catheter placement, patients can have semipermanent indwelling catheters surgically implanted prior to the institution of the treatment program (Myers 1984; Jenkins et al. 1982; Lucas 1984; Pfeifle et al. 1984). These catheters can be brought out through the skin (Tenckhoff type), and they can also be attached to subcutaneously placed portal systems. This latter approach has the advantage of providing an added barrier to the introduction of infection and appears to be more easily accepted by patients undergoing intraperitoneal therapy.

Infection remains a major concern with the surgically implanted catheters. Not surprisingly, the most common organisms implicated are *Staphylococcus epidermidis* and *Staphylococcus aureus* (Kaplan et al. 1985). An attempt can be made to treat established infections medically, but persistence of fever, positive cultures, or an obvious tunnel infection requires catheter removal.

A final important issue in intraperitoneal chemotherapy is that of the unique toxicities associated with this approach (Alberts et al. 1980). A major concern is the possible production of a chemical peritonitis leading to fibrosis and bowel obstruction. In a recent review of the experience of UCSD with chronic complications of intraperitoneal chemotherapy, seven episodes of partial small bowel obstruction had developed in a population of 115 patients followed 1,103 patient-months (Markman et al. in press[a]). Although several of these episodes were likely due to the tumor itself, at least two were definitely caused by the therapy because no tumor was found at laparotomy. Further follow-up of these and other patients treated with intraperitoneal chemotherapy will be necessary to determine the incidence and seriousness of the chronic complications of this treatment technique.

The acute side effects of intraperitoneal chemotherapy can be principally systemic or local (Markman 1984). If dose-limiting toxicity is not local, then the concentration of drug delivered into the peritoneal cavity can be escalated to the point that as much drug is reaching the plasma as when the drug is administered systemically (Markman and Howell 1985). Thus, all the side effects encountered with intravenous therapy will be observed with intraperitoneal drug delivery. For example, when cisplatin is administered intraperitoneally, dose-limiting toxicity is nephrotoxicity and emesis (Howell et al. 1982). However, for other agents, such as mitomycin and doxorubicin HCl, the dose-limiting side effect is the production of a chemical peritonitis and abdominal pain, and significant systemic toxicity is not encountered because the concentration of the drug cannot be safely increased to allow for major systemic exposure (Gyves et al. 1982; Ozols et al. 1982).

Intraperitoneal Chemotherapy Trials

Researchers have conducted intraperitoneal chemotherapy trials with melphalan, cisplatin, 5-fluorouracil, methotrexate, cytarabine, doxorubicin HCl (table 5.1), and combinations of drugs.

Melphalan

Melphalan is one of the most active drugs in ovarian carcinoma when delivered systemically (Tobias and Griffiths 1976). Unfortunately, the extent of absorption can be

Table 5.1. *Pharmacokinetic Advantage of Chemotherapeutic Agents Administered Intraperitoneally in Ovarian Carcinoma*

	Peritoneum/Plasma		
Agent	Mean Peak Concentration Ratio	Mean AUC Ratio[a]	Study
Melphalan	93	65	Howell, Pfeifle, and Olshen 1984
Cisplatin	20	12	Howell et al. 1982
5-Fluorouracil	298	367	Speyer et al. 1980
Methotrexate	92	—	Howell et al. 1981
Cytarabine	664	474	King, Pfeifle, and Howell 1984
Doxorubicin HCl	474	—	Ozols et al. 1982

[a] AUC, area under the curve.

unpredictable when the drug is administered orally. The intraperitoneal delivery of melphalan in ovarian carcinoma has been investigated in two phase I trials (Holcenberg et al. 1983; Howell, Pfeifle, and Olshen 1984). Although very limited efficacy was observed in a group of patients with advanced refractory disease, local toxicity was not excessive and a major pharmacokinetic advantage for peritoneal cavity exposure to the agent compared with exposure through the plasma was demonstrated. In fact, in one trial, the dose of intraperitoneally administered melphalan was safely escalated to the point at which dose-limiting toxicity was systemic (myelosuppression), suggesting that as much active drug was reaching the tumor by capillary flow as it would have if the drug had been given orally or intravenously (Howell, Pfeifle, and Olshen 1984). On the basis of this experience, it could reasonably be questioned whether the intraperitoneal delivery of melphalan might be the optimal method of this drug's administration in ovarian carcinoma. Further evaluation of this issue in phase II and eventually randomized controlled clinical trials appears indicated.

Cisplatin

Intraperitoneal delivery of cisplatin in ovarian carcinoma has been investigated by several groups (Casper et al 1983; Pretorius et al. 1983; Howell et al. 1982). At the University of California, Los Angeles (UCLA) Medical Center, patients with refractory ovarian carcinoma were given cisplatin by the intraperitoneal route with the treatment volume being removed 20 minutes following drug instillation (Pretorius et al. 1983). In this way, 75% of the administered dose was recovered and systemic exposure to the agent was minimized. Several objective responses were observed, but kidney damage was not totally avoided.

A systemically administered neutralizing agent (sodium thiosulfate) for cisplatin has been employed in several intraperitoneal trials at UCSD Medical Center (Howell et al. 1982; Markman et al. 1984, 1985b). Thiosulfate has been demonstrated experimentally to protect against cisplatin-induced renal dysfunction (Howell and Taetle 1980; Howell et al. 1983). In a phase I trial, it was shown that the dose of cisplatin delivered intraperitoneally could be escalated to 270 mg/m^2 with minimal nephrotoxicity and limited interference with active cisplatin delivery to the tumor by capillary flow (Howell et al. 1982). In a series of cisplatin-based intraperitoneal chemotherapy trials conducted at the UCSD Medical Center using thiosulfate protection, the incidence of clinically relevant (elevation of serum creatinine level out of the normal range) nephrotoxicity has been $< 3\%$ (Markman, Cleary, and Howell in press). Similarly, and somewhat unexpectedly, the incidence of neurotoxicity in this patient population heavily pretreated with intravenous cisplatin has been quite low (Markman et al. in press[b]).

A phase II trial of intraperitoneal cisplatin in patients with minimal residual ovarian carcinoma following initial cisplatin-based intravenous chemotherapy has been conducted by the Netherlands Cancer Center (McVie et al. 1985). Approximately 30% of patients with positive second-look laparotomies were found to be disease free at third-look surgery following treatment with intraperitoneal cisplatin.

Several of these complete responders have relapsed, but others remain disease free more than two years following treatment.

5-Fluorouracil

Metabolized in the liver, 5-fluorouracil has demonstrated a major pharmacokinetic advantage in intraperitoneal drug delivery (Speyer et al. 1980). The route of exit of 5-fluorouracil from the peritoneal cavity has been investigated in a limited but detailed study in human beings, and it has been estimated that from 29% to 100% of the drug is taken up into the portal circulation (Speyer et al. 1981). In a phase I clinical trial, dose-limiting toxicity appeared to be both systemic (mucositis, myelosuppression) and local (abdominal pain) (Speyer et al. 1980). In a phase II trial in refractory ovarian carcinoma, a response rate of only 7% was observed (Ozols et al. 1984). However, most of the patients treated in this trial had previously received intravenous 5-fluorouracil, and the one responding patient had a surgically defined complete remission.

Methotrexate

The intraperitoneal delivery of methotrexate in ovarian carcinoma has major appeal because of the availability of a known effective antidote (Leucovorin) for the cytotoxic drug. The Leucovorin can be used either in a rescue mode (following methotrexate administration) or in a neutralizing mode (administered intravenously simultaneously with intraperitoneal methotrexate). The former approach has been investigated at the National Cancer Institute (Jones et al. 1981), and the latter has been examined at UCSD Medical Center (Howell et al. 1981). In both situations, a significant pharmacokinetic advantage for cavity exposure to the methotrexate has been demonstrated, but limited clinical efficacy was observed in refractory ovarian carcinoma in the UCSD trial. When the Leucovorin was used in the rescue mode, the duration of cavity exposure had to be limited because of the production of systemic toxicity. When the Leucovorin was used simultaneously with the intraperitoneally delivered methotrexate, researchers were able to extend exposure to 120 hours; however, it is not known how much of the methotrexate was inactivated by Leucovorin entering the peritoneal cavity. With longer cavity exposure times there was evidence of a chemical serositis.

Cytarabine

Cytarabine would not normally be considered to be a drug with activity against ovarian carcinoma (Wasserman et al. 1975; Markman 1985a); however, because of the tremendous pharmacokinetic advantage achieved for peritoneal cavity exposure to the agent compared with the effects of systemic administration (because of rapid deamination in the liver), it is possible that the extremely high concentrations present in the cavity will be cytotoxic to ovarian carcinoma. In fact, in a clonogenic assay, it has been demonstrated that ovarian carcinoma from some patients with refractory disease is sensitive to this agent in a concentration-dependent manner (King, Pfeifle, and Howell 1984). In a phase II trial in patients with refractory ovarian carcinoma treated with cytarabine by dialysis exchange for five days each month, two patients with minimal residual disease achieved a clinically defined complete remission that has persisted for longer than two years (King, Pfeifle, and Howell 1984).

Doxorubicin HCl

Doxorubicin HCl was one of the first drugs to be examined for its usefulness as an intraperitoneally delivered agent in ovarian carcinoma (Ozols et al. 1982), both because of its known activity in this disease when delivered systemically (Tobias and Griffiths 1976) and experimental data that suggested major efficacy when the agent was administered by the intraperitoneal route (Ozols et al. 1979a). Unfortunately, though definite clinical activity has been observed, the dose-limiting side effect is abdominal pain, which can be quite severe (Ozols et al. 1982; Demicheli et al. 1985; Roboz et al. 1981). Thus, the dose of this agent that can be delivered by the intraperitoneal route is limited. In initial clinical evaluation, mitoxantrone (a closely related, nonsclerosing anthracycline) appears to be equally active when administered by the intraperitoneal route in ovarian carcinoma without producing a chemical peritonitis (Alberts, Mackel, and Peng 1985). Further investigation of this agent in ovarian carcinoma when delivered by the intraperitoneal route appears indicated.

Combination Intraperitoneal Chemotherapy

As systemically delivered combination chemotherapy has improved the response rate and possibly survival rate in ovarian carcinoma, it is reasonable to consider a combination intraperitoneal chemotherapy regimen in this disease (Richardson et al. 1985; Young et al. 1978). One must be cautious about combining several drugs for delivery into the peritoneal cavity because alterations in individual components may produce excessive toxicity.

One major theoretical advantage of intraperitoneal administration over systemic delivery of a combination chemotherapy regimen is the opportunity to examine the clinical relevance of concentration-dependent synergy demonstrated experimentally in vitro (Markman 1985b). It is possible that synergy may be important at the concentrations achievable with intraperitoneal drug delivery but not safely attainable when the drugs are administered systemically. An example of this is the observation of marked synergy in vitro between cisplatin and cytarabine against a colon carcinoma cell line (LoVo), which is highly concentration dependent, the most dramatic synergy being demonstrated at concentrations of cytarabine not achievable following intravenous administration but at least approachable when the drug is given by the intraperitoneal route (Bergerat et al. 1981). Whether such in vitro observations are clinically important or relevant in the case of ovarian carcinoma is unknown.

Several cisplatin-based combination intraperitoneal trials have been conducted at UCSD Medical Center (Markman et al. 1984, 1985a, 1985b). In addition to cisplatin, all patients received cytarabine, and some were given doxorubicin HCl or bleomycin. The local toxicity of the regimens that included either doxorubicin HCl or bleomycin has been greater than that seen with cisplatin plus cytarabine alone. As expected, the observed response rate and survival of patients with bulky residual ovarian carcinoma (disease > 2 cm in diameter) has been poor. However, surgically defined complete remissions in patients with minimal residual disease following cisplatin-based intravenous chemotherapy have been noted, and several patients remain disease free more than three years following the institution of intraperitoneal therapy.

Conclusion

Although there is great theoretical appeal in the intraperitoneal delivery of chemotherapeutic agents in ovarian carcinoma, much work remains to be done in this area before it can be determined what role (if any) this treatment technique should play in the management of this disease. It is clear that surgically defined complete remissions can result from the intraperitoneal administration of cisplatin in patients with minimal residual ovarian carcinoma. What is not known, however, is how the efficacy of this approach compares with that of other treatment techniques, including whole-abdominal radiotherapy (Hacker et al. 1985) and intraperitoneal immunotherapy (Berek et al. 1985). Eventually, randomized controlled clinical trials will be required to answer this question. Because the penetration of chemotherapeutic agents into tumor in vitro or in vivo is quite limited (West, Weichselbau, and Little 1980; Durand 1981; Ozols et al. 1979b), the greatest potential impact of this innovative treatment approach in ovarian carcinoma will be in those individuals with the smallest quantities of residual tumor following debulking surgery or systemically administered chemotherapy.

References

Alberts DS, Chen HSG, Chang SY, Peng YM. 1980. The disposition of intraperitoneal bleomycin, melphalan, and vinblastine in cancer patients. *Recent Results Cancer Res* 74:293–299.

Alberts DS, Mackel C, Peng YM. 1985. Comparative activity of anticancer drugs used in high dose by the intraperitoneal route for the treatment of advanced ovarian cancer (abstract). *Proceedings of the American Society of Clinical Oncology* 4:36.

Berek JS, Hacker NF, Lichtenstein A, Jung T, Spina C, Knox RM, Brady J, Greene T, Ettinger LM, Lagasse L, Bonnem EM, Spiegel RJ, Zighelboim J. 1985. Intraperitoneal recombinant alpha-interferon for "salvage" immunotherapy in stage III epithelial ovarian cancer: A gynecologic oncology group study. *Cancer Res* 45:4447–4453.

Bergerat JP, Drewinko B, Corry P, Barlogie B, Ho DH. 1981. Synergistic lethal effect of *cis*-dichlorodiammineplatinum and 1-beta-D-arabinofuranosylcytosine. *Cancer Res* 41:25–30.

Casper ES, Kelsen DP, Alcock NW, Lewis JL Jr. 1983. Ip cisplatin in patients with malignant ascites: Pharmacokinetic evaluation and comparison with the iv route. *Cancer Treat Rep* 67:235–238.

Dedrick RL, Myers CE, Bungay PM, DeVita VT Jr. 1978. Pharmacokinetic rationale for peritoneal drug administration in the treatment of ovarian cancer. *Cancer Treat Rep* 62:1–9.

Demicheli R, Bonciarelli G, Jirillo A, Foroni R, Petrosino L, Targa L, Garusi G. 1985. Pharmacologic data and technical feasibility of intraperitoneal doxorubicin administration. *Tumori* 71:63–68.

Dunnick NR, Jones RB, Doppmen JL, Speyer J, Myers CE. 1979. Intraperitoneal contrast infusion for assessment of intraperitoneal fluid dynamics. *AJR* 133:221–223.

Durand RE. 1981. Flow cytometry studies of intracellular Adriamycin in multicell spheroids in vitro. *Cancer Res* 41:3495–3498.

Green TH. 1959. Hemisulfur mustard in the palliation of patients with metastatic ovarian carcinoma. *Obstet Gynecol* 13:383–393.

Gyves J, Ensminger W, Niederhuber J, Manuzak P, Van Harken D, Janis MA, Stetson P, Knutsen C, Doan K. 1982. Phase I study of intraperitoneal 5 day continuous 5-FU infusion and bolus mitomycin C (abstract). *Proceedings of the American Society of Clinical Oncology* 1:15.

Hacker NF, Berek JS, Burnison CM, Heintz PM, Juillard GJF, Lagasse LD. 1985. Whole abdominal radiation as salvage therapy for epithelial ovarian cancer. *Obstet Gynecol* 65:60–66.

Holcenberg J, Anderson T, Ritch P, Skibba J, Howser D, Ring B, Adams S, Helmsworth M. 1983. Intraperitoneal chemotherapy with melphalan plus glutaminase. *Cancer Res* 43: 1381–1388.

Howell SB, Chu BCF, Wung WE, Metha BM, Mendelsohn J. 1981. Long-duration intracavitary infusion of methotrexate with systemic Leucovorin protection in patients with malignant effusions. *J Clin Invest* 67:1161–1170.

Howell SB, Pfeifle CE, Olshen RA. 1984. Intraperitoneal chemotherapy with melphalan. *Ann Intern Med* 101:14–18.

Howell SB, Pfeifle CE, Wung WE, Olshen RA. 1983. Intraperitoneal cisplatin with systemic thiosulfate protection. *Cancer Res* 43:1426–1431.

Howell SB, Pfeifle CE, Wung WE, Olshen RA, Lucas WE, Yon JL, Green M. 1982. Intraperitoneal cisplatin with systemic thiosulfate protection. *Ann Intern Med* 97:845–851.

Howell SB, Taetle R. 1980. Effect of sodium thiosulfate on cisdichlorodiammineplatinum (II) toxicity and antitumor activity in L1210 leukemia. *Cancer Treat Rep* 64:611–616.

Jenkins J, Sugarbaker PH, Gianola FJ, Myers CE. 1982. Technical considerations in the use of intraperitoneal chemotherapy administered by Tenckhoff catheter. *Surg Gynecol Obstet* 154:858–864.

Jones RB, Collins JM, Myers CE, Brooks AE, Hubbard S, Balow JE, Brennan MR, Dedrick RL, DeVita VT. 1981. High-volume intraperitoneal chemotherapy with methotrexate in patients with cancer. *Cancer Res* 41:55–59.

Kaplan RA, Markman M, Lucas WE, Pfeifle C, Howell SB. 1985. Infectious peritonitis in patients receiving intraperitoneal chemotherapy. *Am J Med* 78:49–53.

King ME, Pfeifle CE, Howell SB. 1984. Intraperitoneal cytosine arabinoside in ovarian carcinoma. *J Clin Oncol* 2:662–669.

Kottmeier HL. 1968. Treatment of ovarian cancer with thiotepa. *Clin Obstet Gynecol* 11: 447–448.

Kraft AR, Tompkins RK, Jesseph JE. 1968. Peritoneal electrolyte absorption: Analysis of portal, systemic venous and lymphatic transport. *Surgery* 64:148–153.

Lucas WE. 1984. Surgical principles of intraperitoneal access and therapy. In *Intra-arterial and Intracavitary Chemotherapy*, ed. SB Howell, pp. 53–60. Boston: Martinus Nijhoff.

Lukas G, Brindle S, Greengard P. 1971. The route of absorption of intraperitoneally administered compounds. *J Pharmacol Exp Ther* 178:562–566.

McVie JG, ten Bokkel Huinink WW, Aartsen E, Simonetti G, Dubbelman R, Franklin H. 1985. Intraperitoneal chemotherapy in minimal residual ovarian cancer with cisplatin and iv sodium thiosulfate protection (abstract). *Proceedings of the American Society of Clinical Oncology* 4:125.

Markman M. 1984. Medical principles of intraperitoneal and intrapleural chemotherapy. In *Intra-arterial and Intracavitary Chemotherapy*, ed. SB Howell, pp. 61–69. Boston: Martinus Nijhoff.

Markman M. 1985a. The intracavitary administration of cytarabine to patients with nonhematopoietic malignancies: Pharmacologic rationale and results of clinical trials. *Semin Oncol* 12(Suppl 3):177–183.

Markman M. 1985b. Intracavitary chemotherapy for malignant disease confined to body cavities. *West J Med* 142:364–368.

Markman M, Cleary S, Howell SB. In press. Nephrotoxicity of high-dose intracavitary cisplatin with intravenous thiosulfate protection. *Eur J Cancer Clin Oncol.*

Markman M, Cleary S, Howell SB, Lucas WE. In press(a). Complications of extensive adhesion formation following intraperitoneal chemotherapy. *Surg Gynecol Oncol.*

Markman M, Cleary S, Lucas WE, Howell SB. 1985a. Combination intraperitoneal chemotherapy with cisplatin, cytarabine, and bleomycin (abstract). *Proceedings of the American Society of Clinical Oncology* 4:112.

Markman M, Cleary S, Pfeifle CE, Howell SB. In press(b). High-dose intracavitary cisplatin with intravenous thiosulfate: Low incidence of serious neurotoxicity. *Cancer.*

Markman M, Howell SB. 1985. Intraperitoneal chemotherapy for ovarian carcinoma. In *Gyn Oncology*, ed. D Albert, E Surwitt, pp. 179–212. Boston: Martinus Nijhoff.

Markman M, Howell SB, Cleary S, Lucas WE. 1985b. Intraperitoneal chemotherapy with high dose cisplatin and cytarabine for refractory ovarian carcinoma and other malignancies principally involving the peritoneal cavity. *J Clin Oncol* 3:925–931.

Markman M, Howell SB, Lucas WE, Pfeifle CE, Green MR. 1984. Combination intraperitoneal chemotherapy with cisplatin, cytarabine, and doxorubicin for refractory ovarian carcinoma and other malignancies principally confined to the peritoneal cavity. *J Clin Oncol* 2:1321–1326.

Myers C. 1984. The use of intraperitoneal chemotherapy in the treatment of ovarian cancer. *Semin Oncol* 11:275–284.

Ozols RF, Grotzinger KR, Fisher RI, Myers CE, Young RC. 1979a. Kinetic characterization and response to chemotherapy in a transplantable murine ovarian cancer. *Cancer Res* 39:3202–3208.

Ozols RF, Locker GY, Doroshow JH, Grotzinger KR, Myers CE, Young RC. 1979b. Pharmacokinetics of Adriamycin and tissue penetration in murine ovarian cancer. *Cancer Res* 39:3209–3214.

Ozols RF, Speyer JL, Jenkins J, Myers CE. 1984. Phase II trial of 5-FU administered Ip to patients with refractory ovarian cancer. *Cancer Treat Rep* 68:1229–1232.

Ozols RF, Young RC, Speyer JL, Sugarbaker PH, Green R, Jenkins J, Myers CE. 1982. Phase 1 and pharmacological studies of Adriamycin administered intraperitoneally to patients with ovarian cancer. *Cancer Res* 42:4265–4269.

Pfeifle CE, Howell SB, Markman M, Lucas WE. 1984. Totally implantable system for peritoneal access. *J Clin Oncol* 2:1277–1280.

Pretorius RG, Hacker NF, Berek JS, Ford LC, Hoeschele JD, Butler TA, Lagasse LD. 1983. Pharmacokinetics of Ip cisplatin in refractory ovarian carcinoma. *Cancer Treat Rep* 67: 1085–1092.

Richardson GS, Scully RE, Nikrui N, Nelson JH. 1985. Common epithelial cancer of the ovary. *N Engl J Med* 312:415–424, 474–483.

Roboz J, Jacobs AJ, Holland JF, Deppe G, Cohen CJ. 1981. Intraperitoneal infusion of doxorubicin in the treatment of gynecologic carcinomas. *Med Pediatr Oncol* 9:245–250.

Rosenshein N, Blake D, McIntyre PA, Parmley T, Natarajan TK, Dvornicky J, Nickoloff E. 1978. The effect of volume on the distribution of substances instilled into the peritoneal cavity. *Gynecol Oncol* 6:106–110.

Speyer JL, Collins JM, Dedrick RL, Brennan MF, Buckpitt AR, Londer H, DeVita VT, Myers CE. 1980. Phase I pharmacological studies of 5-fluorouracil administered intraperitoneally. *Cancer Res* 40:567.

Speyer JL, Sugarbaker PH, Collins JM, Dedrick RL, Klecker RW, Myers CE. 1981. Portal levels and hepatic clearance of 5-fluorouracil after intraperitoneal administration in humans. *Cancer Res* 41:1916–1922.

Taylor A, Baily NA, Halpern SE, Ashburn WL. 1975. Loculation as a contraindication to intracavitary ^{32}P chromic phosphate therapy. *J Nucl Med* 16:318–319.

Tobias JS, Griffiths CT. 1976. Management of ovarian carcinoma: Current concept and future prospects. *N Engl J Med* 294:877–882.

Tully TE, Goldberg ME, Locken MK. 1974. The use of 99 Tc-sulfur colloid to assess the distribution of ^{32}P chromic phosphate. *J Nucl Med* 15:190–191.

Vider M, Deland FM, Maruyama Y. 1976. Loculation as a contraindication to intracavitary ^{32}P chromic phosphate therapy. *J Nucl Med* 17:150–151.

Wasserman TH, Comis RL, Goldsmith M, Handelsman H, Penta JS, Slavik M, Soper WT, Carter SK. 1975. Tabular analysis of the clinical chemotherapy of solid tumors. *Cancer Chemother Rep* 6:399–419.

West GW, Weichselbau R, Little JB. 1980. Limited penetration of methotrexate into human osteosarcoma spheroids as a proposed model for solid tumor resistance to adjuvant chemotherapy. *Cancer Res* 40:3665–3668.

Young RC, Chabner BA, Hubbard SP, Fisher RI, Bender RA, Anderson T, Simon RM, Cancellos GP, DeVita VT. 1978. Advanced ovarian adenocarcinoma: A prospective clinical trial of melphalan (L-PAM) versus combination chemotherapy. *N Engl J Med* 299:1261–1266.

Annual Clinical Conference on Cancer, Vol. 29
Gynecologic Cancer: Diagnosis and Treatment Strategies
© 1987 by The University of Texas System Cancer Center

6. Radiation Therapy for Epithelial Ovarian Cancer

Alon J. Dembo

Several principles governing the cure of patients with ovarian cancer by radiotherapy were established during the last decade. I shall review some of the studies at The Princess Margaret Hospital (PMH), which led to the establishment of the following principles:

1. The entire peritoneal cavity should be encompassed by the treatment field, because once the disease has spread beyond the ovary, the entire peritoneal cavity is at risk for recurrent cancer.
2. The moving-strip and open-field techniques are equally effective in tumor control.
3. Late complications can be kept to a minimum (< 5% bowel surgery, < 1% radiation hepatitis, < 1% treatment mortality), but their frequency increases with increasing total radiation dosage, increasing fraction size, and possibly the extent of the previous surgical procedures (Dembo 1985a).
4. Optimal selection of patients for radiotherapy compared with other forms of treatment is based on grouping of patients according to prognostic factors, including presenting stage of disease, amount and site of residual tumor, and histopathologic features.
5. The potential exists for abdominopelvic radiation to be applied curatively as consolidation or as salvage therapy for patients whose disease has not been completely eradicated by chemotherapy; however, further study is needed to clarify the magnitude of this benefit, the situations in which radiotherapy is indicated, and factors that determine the toxicity of the combined-modality treatment.

Study in Stage IA

Between 1971 and 1977 a randomized study was conducted with 54 patients whose invasive ovarian cancer was confined to one ovary at presentation (Bush et al. 1977; Dembo et al. 1979a, Dembo 1982). After patient stratification by age, grade, and pathology, postoperative treatment was randomized, with 27 patients being observed and 27 patients receiving 4500 rad pelvic irradiation in 20 fractions. The nine patients who experienced relapse were almost evenly distributed between the two study arms, indicating no curative benefit for pelvic irradiation. Relapsing tumors occurred throughout the abdominal cavity, suggesting that even in stage IA the entire peritoneal cavity is at risk for relapse. Although it reduced the frequency of pelvic recurrence, pelvic irradiation did not reduce the overall risk of relapse (Dembo 1982). The study was terminated when we realized that control of pelvic disease is an inadequate objective of treatment.

No relapses occurred in patients with well-differentiated carcinomas, even though nine patients (33%) had experienced cyst rupture, and four patients (15%) had ascites. All relapses occurred in patients with poorly and moderately differentiated tumors (p,0.008, Fisher two-tail). Even in these patients, rupture, ascites, and capsular penetration did not predict relapse. Although stage IB ovarian cancer is less common than stage IA, in our experience the disease behavior is similar, so that since 1978 we have treated patients with stage IA and stage IB disease in a similar manner. For well-differentiated stage I cancers, we recommend no postoperative treatment (except for the occasional patient with positive peritoneal cytology).

For stage I patients with poorly or moderately differentiated tumors, we direct therapy at the whole peritoneal cavity using pelvic and abdominopelvic irradiation. To date, however, no study in stage I has demonstrated that postoperative treatment improves cure rates over those obtainable with operation alone. Treatment recommendations, including our own, are extrapolated from therapeutic experiences in patients with more advanced lesions.

Studies in Stages IB, II, and III

Another study, conducted between 1971 and 1975, involved 190 patients who had presentations of stages IB, II, and III ovarian cancer. The patients in stage III were asymptomatic, that is, they had no tumor-related symptoms or ascites four to six weeks postoperatively (Bush et al. 1977; Dembo 1982; Dembo et al. 1979b, 1979c). Before randomization, we stratified patients by age, stage, pathology, grade, and whether or not bilateral salpingo-oophorectomy and hysterectomy (BSOH) was complete. For patients in stages IB and II, 4500 rad pelvic irradiation midplane in 20 fractions was administered as the standard postoperative therapy. The objective was to determine whether survival could be improved by adding either 6 mg/day of chlorambucil for two years or irradiation of the upper abdomen. Stage III patients were randomized only between the last two treatment methods.

The essential features of the abdominopelvic irradiation technique were that it began with 2250 rad pelvic irradiation midplane in 10 fractions and was followed immediately by a downward-moving strip that encompassed the entire abdomen and pelvis. The moving-strip dose was 2250 rad midplane in 10 fractions. The upper border was radiologically verified to be at least 1 cm above the diaphragm in expiration. No liver shielding was used, but posterior renal shielding (5 half-value layers, HVL) was used throughout. Patients were treated prone, two fields per day with an isocentric technique (Dembo et al. 1979c). The survival rate of the 76 patients treated with pelvic plus abdominopelvic irradiation was significantly superior to that of the 71 patients treated with pelvic irradiation and chlorambucil (58% vs. 40%, $P < 0.05$) (Dembo et al. 1979b). However, the survival benefit applied only to patients in whom BSOH had been performed, that is, patients with small or no macroscopic residual disease (Bush et al. 1977; Dembo et al. 1979a, 1979b).

Patients with large residual tumor lesions (incomplete BSOH) were rarely cured, and all three treatment methods yielded similar survival and relapse-free rates. Among patients with small or no macroscopic residual tumor, however, the survival rate of those treated with abdominopelvic irradiation was increased by about 25% to 30% over that observed with the other two treatment methods, because this type of irradiation achieved significantly better control of occult upper abdominal disease (Bush et al. 1977; Dembo et al. 1979b). In the complete BSOH group of patients, the greatest benefit of abdominopelvic irradiation was observed in those with completely resected disease (i.e., no macroscopic residual disease).

Subsequent to this study, a randomized study was conducted between 1976 and 1982 to compare two techniques of abdominopelvic irradiation: the moving-strip (2250 rad in 10 fractions) and the open-field (2250 rad in 22 fractions) (Dembo et al. 1983). In the latter, the whole abdomen is treated in one parallel opposed treatment portal with no liver shielding but with posterior kidney shielding after 1500 rad. A pelvic boost dose (2250 rad in 10 fractions) was given in each case before the whole abdomen was irradiated. Survival, relapse-free rates, and tumor failure patterns were identical for both techniques. Significant late toxicity occurred infrequently with either technique but was less common with the open-field technique. The other principal advantages of the open-field technique are its simplicity and shorter duration (6–7 weeks vs. 11–13 weeks). Because of these results, we have adopted the open-field as our standard radiation technique.

The therapeutic principles derived from these two studies are briefly summarized:

1. When external beam radiotherapy is indicated, a technique that encompasses the contents of the entire peritoneal cavity is superior to pelvic or partial abdominal

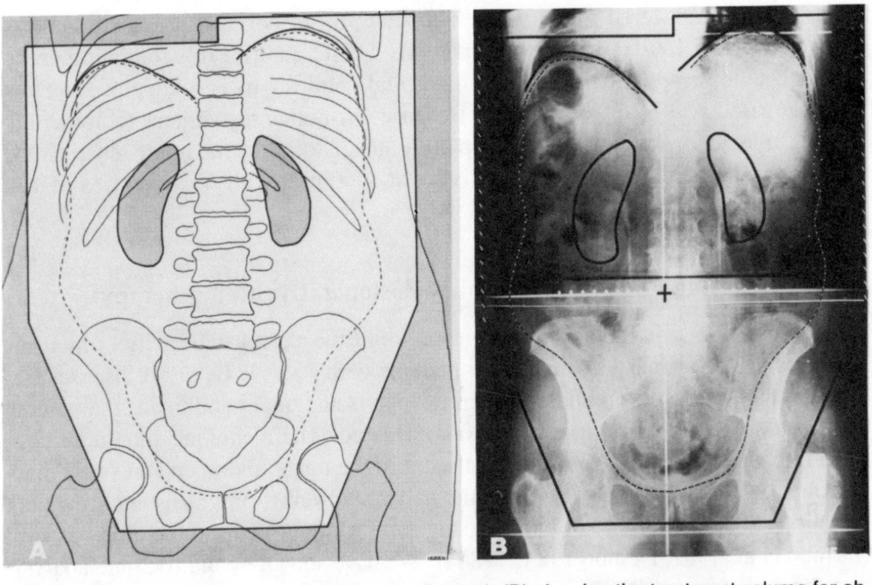

Fig. 6.1. Line drawing (A) from a simulator radiograph (B) showing the treatment volume for abdominopelvic radiotherapy. A generous margin is allowed between the treatment field edges (solid line) and the peritoneum (dotted line). Note that the field extends outside the iliac crests. Kidney shielding is from the posterior to keep the renal dose between 1800 and 2000 rad. The pelvic boost field is not shown. This is the posterior (prone) projection.

irradiation. Radiological verification of the treatment volume is essential, and no liver shielding should be used (fig. 6.1).

2. The moving-strip and open-field techniques are equally effective.
3. Patients with large residual tumors or metastatic spread beyond the abdomen or to liver parenchyma should not be treated primarily with pelvic plus abdominopelvic irradiation because they are rarely cured. (The same applies to patients with small residual macroscopic lesions in the abdomen, with the possible exception of serous grade 1 lesions.)
4. The radiation dosage to the abdomen should be within liver tolerance, and the irradiation dosage to the pelvis should be within bowel tolerance levels to irradiation.
5. In patients deemed suitable for primary postoperative treatment with abdominopelvic radiotherapy, the risk of pelvic and paraaortic lymph node involvement is small (5% is probably a realistic estimate). A boost dose to the paraaortic region therefore is not warranted, nor, probably, is lymph node sampling of impalpable nodes at the time of surgery justified, if radiotherapy is planned. The yield of these procedures is very low, and they may carry an increased risk of bowel toxicity. Unfortunately, the toxicity will be borne by the node-negative patients, who did not require the sampling procedure. Furthermore, it is uncertain whether patients presenting with paraaortic nodal metastases can be cured by radiotherapy. When abdominopelvic radiotherapy is administered after chemotherapy, a boost dose is usually given to the nodes if they were known to be involved before chemotherapy, and if the blood counts permit. In this situation, after 2500 rad has been administered to the whole abdomen, the pelvic and paraaortic field is given a further 1500 rad in 150-rad fractions. Until a curative role for radiotherapy after chemotherapy can be shown, our hospital's philosophy is not to place patients at increased risk of major toxicity. Because chemotherapy-surgery-radiotherapy toxic interactions are still not completely understood, a maximum dose to the extended field boost area currently is set at 4000 rad, with fraction sizes of 150 rad or less.

Selecting Patients for Primary Postoperative Radiotherapy

Abdominopelvic radiotherapy encompasses only the peritoneal cavity, which restricts its use as primary treatment for patients with stage I, II, or III disease. Because of the dosage differential between the pelvis and upper abdomen, the volume and location of residual tumor are also considered. The technique should be confined to patients with no macroscopic disease in the upper abdomen and small macroscopic (2–3 cm) residual disease in the pelvis. However, prognosis and treatment selection should be based not only on stage and residuum but on histology as well (Dembo et al. 1982; Dembo 1984, 1985a). We have shown by multivariate analysis that the major prognostic factors in ovarian cancer are histopathologic characteristics, size of residual tumor, and presenting stage. Each of these factors gives prognostic information independent of the other two, and the prognostic effects of all

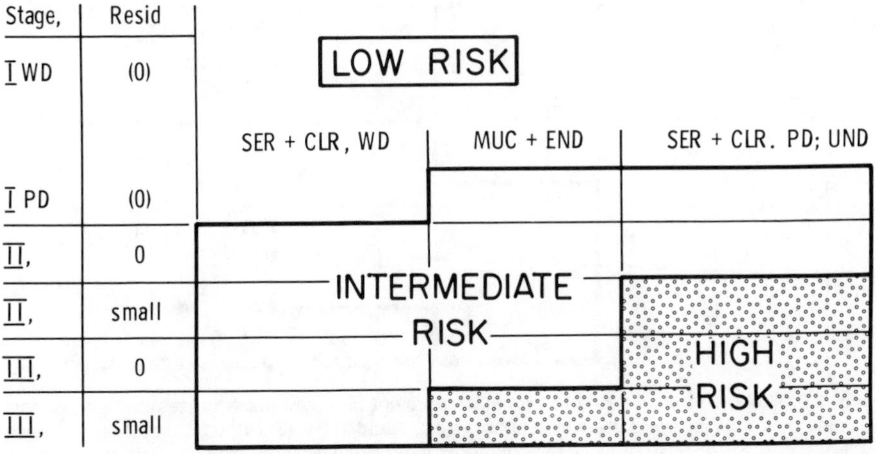

Fig. 6.2. Definition of three patient subgroups according to stage, residuum, and pathological category in stage I, II, and III, with small and no residuum. Patients treated by abdominopelvic irradiation had significantly fewer relapses than those treated by other methods in the intermediate-risk subgroup but not in the high-risk subgroup. (Resid, residuum; SER, serous; CLR, clear cell; WD, well-differentiated, grade 1; PD, poorly differentiated, grades 2 & 3; MUC, mucinous; END, endometrioid; UND, undifferentiated or unclassified.)

three are therefore additive. With respect to histopathologic features, patients may be classified by grade alone, but we have found in our patients that the discriminant function of histopathology is enhanced if histological subtype is considered in addition to tumor grade, according to these three groupings (Dembo et al. 1982): (1) serous (SER) grade 1 and clear cell (CLR) grade 1; (2) mucinous (MUC) and endometrioid (END), all grades; (3) grades 2 and 3 SER and CLR, and all unclassified/undifferentiated (UND) tumors.

From the phase III studies described above, we concluded that abdominopelvic irradiation is indicated for all patients with small or no residuum in stages I, II, and III (55% of the total), with the exception of patients with stage I grade 1 tumors, for whom we recommend no postoperative treatment. Patients with stage I well-differentiated tumors are a low-risk group (fig. 6.2) who compose 6% of our total patient population and whose five-year survival approaches 95% when treated with surgery alone.

By combining the prognostic effects of stage, residuum, and histopathology, we were able to subdivide further the remaining zero- or small-residuum, stage I–III patients into two subgroups. In Figure 6.3, these data are shown in a matrix of the proportion of relapses by stage, residuum, and histology. In two subgroups of patients indicated, the first (unshaded) had an average risk of relapse of about 30% when treated by abdominopelvic irradiation (intermediate risk), and the second (shaded) had approximately an 80% risk of relapse (high risk). If a similar table were constructed using grades 1, 2, and 3 instead of the three histological categories shown, the partitioning of patients would be very similar to that of figure 6.3,

STAGE	RESID	GRD 1 SER + CLR	ALL MUC + ENDO	GRD II/III SER + CLR; UND
I	0	N/A	.21 (29)	.29 (31)
II	0/?	.06 (17)	.22 (45)	.46 (41)
II	YES	.11 (9)	.27 (11)	.73 (22)
III	0/?	.14 (7)	.42 (12)	.75 (24)
III	YES	.22 (9)	.78 (27)	.83 (41)

Fig. 6.3. Proportion of relapses (decimal) and patient numbers (parentheses) in 325 patients treated by abdominopelvic irradiation between 1971 and 1981. (Excluded were 12 patients with stage I, grade 1 disease, and 17 patients for whom grades 2 and 3 disease were not reported separately.) The Princess Margaret Hospital histological grouping is used. (RESID, residuum; GRD, grade; SER, serous; CLR, clear cell; MUC, mucinous; END, endometrioid; UND, undifferentiated or unclassified.)

though not quite as finely tuned (Dembo 1985a). In both situations, the addition of histopathologic information substantially enhances prognostic grouping compared with that using only stage and residuum.

Figure 6.2 shows how we divide patients with small or no macroscopic residuum into low-, intermediate-, and high-risk subgroups. Patients in the intermediate-risk group, about one third of all patients referred to our institution, have a five-year survival rate of 75% when treated with abdominopelvic irradiation (Dembo 1985a). These results are significantly better in this subgroup of patients than those of the other treatment methods we have studied; abdominopelvic irradiation remains our treatment of choice for intermediate-risk patients.

By contrast, the high-risk patients, about 15% of our total population, have a five-year survival rate of 30% with abdominopelvic irradiation. Since 1981 we no longer treat the high-risk patients with irradiation alone but are studying a combined-modality approach, which consists of six courses of chemotherapy with cyclophosphamide-Adriamycin-cisplatin (CAP) followed by abdominopelvic irradiation. With this approach we are attempting to improve long-term survival rates in these patients by chemically "debulking" the disease before irradiation. Preliminary results suggest a significantly improved three-year relapse-free rate.

Radiation Dose-Control Considerations

The therapeutic effectiveness of 2250 to 2750 rad has been questioned, usually on the basis of dose-control data for squamous cell carcinoma of the head and neck. A dosage of 5000 rad in 200-rad daily fractions is believed necessary to control 90% or more of the subclinical metastases in neck nodes (Fletcher 1972). These dose-control factors may not apply to patients with ovarian cancer for several reasons. First, in summarizing the head and neck data from ten publications, Cummings found that the 90% control point for subclinical disease was reached at about 4000 rad and not at 5000 rad (Cummings in press). Second, control of *subclinical* neck-node disease should be distinguished from *microscopic* peritoneal disease, in which tumor volumes may be lower. The former applies to impalpable lesions that could be as large as 5 mm; the latter to lesions invisible to the eye and perhaps smaller than 0.1 mm. Even if the radiation sensitivity of ovarian adenocarcinoma were the same as that of head and neck squamous cancer, 2250 rad might be reasonably expected to control 25% to 50% of microscopic ovarian lesions because they represent a smaller tumor volume. Although the clinically observed radiation responses of high-grade ovarian cancer may be similar to those of squamous cancer of the head and neck, low and intermediate grade 1 ovarian lesions have a slower doubling time. This suggests that a given volume of low-grade tumor contains fewer critical target cells that determine cure by radiation than does a high-grade lesion, and so the low-grade tumor might be more frequently controlled by a lower radiation dosage. For example, considering the patients in stage III with no or questionable macroscopic residuum (fig. 6.3), 18 of 24 (75%) with the least favorable histological types relapsed, whereas tumor control rates were more than twice as high for patients with tumors of the two more favorable pathology types (6/19=32% relapsed). This marked difference in tumor control, according to histological differentiation, has not been observed in squamous cancers of the head and neck, which suggests that the dose-control factors for squamous cancer of the head and neck might not apply to ovarian carcinoma.

Combined Modality Therapy

Both chemotherapy and radiotherapy are active treatments for ovarian cancer, yet a way of combining the two modalities to obtain an additive effect on survival has been elusive. The simultaneous use of large-field irradiation and chemotherapy is limited by myelosuppression, although the possibilities of low-dose systemic cisplatin or intraperitoneal administration of chemotherapy during a course of whole-abdomen irradiation are innovative approaches being studied by others. A detailed discussion of the theoretical considerations pertaining to the sequential multiple modality treatment of ovarian cancer has been presented elsewhere (Dembo 1985b). The limited information available from uncontrolled studies (Dembo 1985b) suggests that the use of abdominopelvic radiotherapy after chemotherapy should be restricted to patients with a negative second-look laparotomy but a high risk of relapse, patients with a microscopic positive second-look, and possibly those with macroscopic residuum of less than 5 mm (though one would be quite skeptical of the curative potential of radiotherapy in patients with *any* macroscopic disease after chemotherapy).

Because ovarian cancer is such a complex disease, and the outcome after negative or microscopically-positive second-look laparotomy can vary so greatly, it is unlikely that the magnitude of the curative potential (if any) of abdominopelvic radiotherapy after chemotherapy will be made clear except by a randomized study. The need to perform this study is twofold. Patients in many centers are now receiving radiotherapy, and physicians need to learn whether and under what circumstances such an approach is of value. In addition, very few alternative, potentially curative treatment options are available at present for patients whose tumors have not responded completely to systemic therapy.

References

Bush RS, Allt WEC, Beale FA, Jenkin RDT, Bean HA, Dembo AJ, Pringle JF. 1977. Treatment of epithelial carcinoma of the ovary: Operation, irradiation and chemotherapy. *Am J Obstet Gynecol* 127:692–704.

Cummings BJ. In press. Radiation therapy and the treatment of cervical lymph nodes. In *Otolaryngology–Head and Neck Surgery*, ed. CW Cummings, JM Fredrickson, LA Harker, CJ Krause, DE Schuller. St. Louis: C. V. Mosby.

Dembo AJ. 1982. The role of radiotherapy in ovarian cancer. *Bull Cancer (Paris)* 69:275–284.

Dembo AJ. 1984. Radiotherapeutic management of ovarian cancer. *Semin Oncol* 11:238–250.

Dembo AJ. 1985a. Abdominopelvic radiotherapy in ovarian cancer: A 10-year experience. *Cancer* 55:2285–2290.

Dembo AJ. 1985b. The sequential multiple modality treatment of ovarian cancer (Editorial). *Radiother Oncol* 3:187–192.

Dembo AJ, Bush RS, Beale FA, Bean HA, Fine S, Gospodarowicz M, Herman J, Pringle JF, Sturgeon J, Thomas GM. 1983. A randomized clinical trial of moving strip versus open field whole abdominal irradiation in patients with invasive epithelial cancer of ovary. *Proceedings of the American Society of Clinical Oncologists* (Abstract C571).

Dembo AJ, Bush RS, Beale FA, Bean HA, Pringle JF, Sturgeon J. 1979a. The Princess Margaret study of ovarian cancer: Stages I, II and asymptomatic III presentations. *Cancer Treat Rep* 63:249–254.

Dembo AJ, Bush RS, Beale FA, Bean HA, Pringle JF, Sturgeon J, Reid JG. 1979b. Ovarian carcinoma: Improved survival following abdominopelvic irradiation in patients with a completed pelvic operation. *Am J Obstet Gynecol* 134:793–800.

Dembo AJ, Bush RS, Brown TC. 1982. Clinicopathological correlates in ovarian cancer. *Bull Cancer (Paris)* 69:292–298.

Dembo AJ, Van Dyk J, Japp B, Bean HA, Beale FA, Pringle JF, Bush RS. 1979c. Whole abdominal irradiation by a moving-strip technique for patients with ovarian cancer. *Int J Radiat Oncol Biol Phys* 5:1933–1942.

Fletcher GH. 1972. Elective irradiation of subclinical disease in cancers of the head and neck. *Cancer* 29:1450.

Annual Clinical Conference on Cancer, Vol. 29
Gynecologic Cancer: Diagnosis and Treatment Strategies
© 1987 by The University of Texas System Cancer Center

7. Second-Look Laparotomy in Epithelial Ovarian Cancer

Larry J. Copeland

The popularity of surgical reexamination after treatment in ovarian cancer patients (Rutledge and Burns 1966) gained momentum in the 1970s (Wallach and Blinick 1970; Smith, Delgado, and Rutledge 1976). In the years that followed, as the treatment of ovarian cancer became less dependent on radiotherapy and more dependent on chemotherapy, second-look laparotomy became part of the standard care for these patients (Copeland 1985; Decker et al. 1982; Ehrlich et al. 1983; Edwards et al. 1983; Greco et al. 1981; G.V. Krepart, M.D., personal communication, March 1985; Lewis, Cain, and Pierce 1983; Podratz et al. 1985). The application of second-look laparotomy, according to its intended purpose, has not been consistent. When first introduced in the management of colon cancer, the intent of the surgery was to monitor tumor growth and debulk tumor tissue at intermittent intervals (Wangensteen, Lewis, and Tongen 1951). Subsequently, the procedure has been applied in restaging or upstaging laparotomy prior to initiating chemotherapy (Webster and Ballard 1981). Also included in some reports are second-look procedures on patients with persistent clinical evidence of disease after chemotherapy (Jones, Khoo, and Whitaker 1981; Luesley et al. 1984; Mangioni, Mattioli, and Natale 1975; Phibbs, Smith, and Stanhope 1983; Phillips, Buchsbaum, and Lifshitz 1979; Smith, Delgado, and Rutledge 1976; Stuart et al. 1982; Misset et al. 1980). In addition, when a patient is reexplored for progressive disease or complications of progressive disease (Stuart et al. 1982; Jacobs et al. 1983), this should not be referred to as a second-look laparotomy. As noted by many recent authors, the term *second look* should be restricted to a laparotomy in a patient clinically disease-free after a treatment program (Ballon et al. 1984; Barnhill et al. 1984; Berek et al. 1984; Curry et al. 1981; Smirz et al. 1985; Webb et al. 1982). With current treatment programs of 10 to 12 cycles of chemotherapy, it is estimated that 50% to 60% of patients with advanced ovarian cancer will be candidates for a second-look operation (Edwards et al. 1983; Decker et al. 1982). With fewer cycles, this percentage could be higher. When performing a second-look laparotomy, one must be as thorough as possible in order to define accurately the disease status. Occasionally, extensive adhesions will render it impossible or highly impractical to perform a satisfactory exploration. Such patients should be categorized as having an inadequate second-look procedure.

Review of the Literature

The second-look laparotomy technique has been adequately described in prior publications and thus will not be reiterated here (Greer, Rutledge, and Gallager 1980; Phibbs, Smith, and Stanhope 1983). The general acceptance of the procedure in the management of patients with ovarian cancer is reflected by the large number of recent reports in the literature. Reports of second-look laparotomies in 20 or more patients are summarized in table 7.1. Because of overlapping time intervals, a few reports are not included in this table (Greco et al. 1981; Schwartz and Smith 1980; Rutledge and Burns 1966; Wiltshaw, Raju, and Dawson 1985). Most reports include patients with all stages of disease. Including patients with early stage disease, the likelihood of having negative second-look findings exceeds 45%. However, if the analysis is limited to patients with advanced disease (stages III and IV), the percentage of patients with negative findings is approximately 33% (Berek et al. 1984; Gershenson et al. 1985; Podratz et al. 1985; Roberts et al. 1982; Smirz et al. 1985; G.V. Krepart, M.D., personal communication, March 1985; Webb et al. 1982). In contrast, the fraction of patients with microscopically positive findings (no gross tumor but tumor identified in biopsy or cytology tissue specimens) is approximately one in five (Copeland et al. 1985; Podratz et al. 1985; Smirz et al. 1985; G.V. Krepart, M.D., personal communication, March 1985).

In many reports, the discouraging problem of tumor recurrence after a complete surgical response (i.e., a negative second look), although described, is not identified as a major concern (table 7.2). This is because many reports concerned patients with early stage tumors, and the length of follow-up was short (Ballon et al. 1984; Coleman, Pasmantier, and Silver 1985; Curry et al. 1981; Schwartz and Smith 1980; Rocereto et al. 1984). Also, the recurrence rates after negative second-look findings were not as high as those now recognized (Barnhill et al. 1984; Roberts et al. 1982).

Second-look laparotomy has been accepted as an excellent method for defining tumor response to chemotherapy, but whether the information gained at second-look surgery can be acted upon to extend patient survival has not been adequately evaluated. Wiltshaw and colleagues (1985), in attempting such an evaluation, found no significant influence of second-look laparotomy on survival. However, their study design was flawed in that patients were randomized to second-look laparotomy only if a hysterectomy had not been done at the initial surgery. Since patients with more aggressive or infiltrative disease are more likely not to have a hysterectomy, the method of randomization imposed a negative bias on the group of patients undergoing the second-look procedure.

Currently, a number of tumor markers are under evaluation for their reliability in detecting the presence of epithelial ovarian carcinoma (Dembo, Chang, and Urbach 1985; Bast et al. 1983). Although preliminary studies suggest a low rate of false-positive results, the rate of false-negatives is of concern, and the accurate identification of small-volume disease poses a significant problem (Atack et al. 1986). Nonetheless, these tumor markers should continue to be correlated to second-look findings, since sufficient information may be accumulated to permit the use of such tumor markers in directing therapy in selected cases (Podratz et al. 1985; Atack et al. 1986).

Alternate Methods of Evaluation

When gross or macroscopic disease is present at the second-look laparotomy, the value of the surgery is limited. For this reason, it has been suggested that patients have less invasive procedures such as laparoscopy performed to identify macroscopic disease and thereby avert a second-look laparotomy. Although noninvasive procedures may play a role, there are associated limitations. Laparoscopy can be used to identify small-volume disease in evaluable areas, but some important areas, such as retroperitoneal lymph nodes and bowel mesentery, will not be accessible with this procedure. Because of these limitations, as well as increased operating time and associated complications, laparoscopy has not gained widespread acceptance (Averette and Sevin 1982). Computerized tomography (CT) cannot be relied upon to identify tumor nodules less than 2 cm in diameter (Brenner et al. 1985; Clarke-Pearson et al. 1986; Stern et al. 1981; Whitley et al. 1981; Goldhirsch et al. 1983). On occasion, nodules up to 4 cm in size have been overlooked with CT scanning (Clarke-Pearson et al. 1986). Also, because of the risk of obtaining a false-positive CT scan, treatment alterations should be based on histological (needle biopsy) or cytological (fine-needle aspiration) confirmation that the abnormality is persistent neoplasm. However, tomography is excellent for the identification of occult disease in the liver parenchyma. Approximately 20% of patients may avoid a second-look procedure if CT scanning is routinely used prior to second-look laparotomy (Brenner et al. 1985; Clarke-Pearson et al. 1986).

Macroscopic Positive Findings at Second-Look Laparotomy

At the time of second-look laparotomy, grossly suspicious areas should be resected or generously sampled. Since fibrosis, necrotic tumor, and suture granulomas can be difficult to distinguish from viable tumor, it is best to confirm the presence of tumor by frozen-section analysis prior to abbreviating the random sampling technique. Otherwise, an inappropriate abbreviation of random sampling may result in negative findings but an incomplete sampling procedure.

When confronted with gross or macroscopic tumor, the question of tumor debulking arises. Although the value of debulking gross tumor at second-look surgery has not been proved (Raju et al. 1982), it is appropriate to individualize the degree of aggressiveness. Factors that discourage extensive tumor debulking at second-look surgery include (1) parenchymal tumor, (2) progressive tumor growth during treatment, and (3) extensive previous treatment that may preclude effective postoperative treatment. In contrast, factors that may encourage an aggressive approach to macroscopic disease at second look include (1) inadequate prior treatment (surgery or chemotherapy), (2) good tumor response to treatment, (3) well-differentiated or slow-growing tumor, (4) absence of parenchymal or unresectable tumor, and (5) op-

Table 7.1. *Second-Look Laparotomy: Reports of 20 or More Patients*

Study	No. of Patients	Stage	Second-Look Findings		
			Negative	Microscopic Positive	Macroscopic Positive
Mangioni, Mattioli, and Natale 1975	26[a]	I-III[b]	10	5	11
Smith, Delgado, and Rutledge 1976	103[c]	IC-IV	23	11	69
Phillips, Buchsbaum, and Lifshitz 1979	24[d]	I-IV	21	1	2
Misset et al. 1980	40[c]	I-IV	11	—[e]	29[e]
Curry et al. 1981	27[a]	I-IV[b]	17	3	7
Jones et al. 1981	25[a]	I-III	19	3	3
Webster and Ballard 1981	20	II-IV	14	3	3
Raju et al. 1982	65[c]	III-IV	12	4	49
Roberts et al. 1982	63[a]	I-IV[b]	36	—[e]	27[e]
Stuart et al. 1982	21	I-IV	15	—[e]	6[e]
Webb et al. 1982	59[a]	I-IV	32	—[e]	27[e]
Cohen et al. 1983	116	III-IV	50	16	37
Varia et al. 1983	38	I-III	26	—[e]	12[e]
Lewis, Cain, and Pierce 1983	118	I-IV	82	—[e]	36[e]
Maggino et al. 1983	48	III-IV	25	—[e]	23[e]
Phibbs, Smith, and Stanhope 1983	42[c,d]	I-IV	17	3	22

Rorat and Wallach 1983	31	I-III	6	1	24
Ballon et al. 1984	25	I-IV	11	6	8
Barnhill et al. 1984	96[a]	I-IV	48	—[e]	48[e]
Rocereto et al. 1984	36[a]	I-IV	23	8	5
Berek et al. 1984	56	III	18	8	30
Mead et al. 1984	20[c,f]	III-IV	8	—[e]	12[e]
Luesley et al. 1984	50	II-IV	12	12	26
Brenner et al. 1985	52	IC-IV	17	10	25
Coffin, Adcock, and Dehner 1985	76	I-III	55	—[e]	21[e]
Gershenson et al. 1985, and Copeland et al. 1985	246	III-IV	85	50	111
Krepart 1985 (personal communication)	141	I-IV	71	23	47
Podratz et al. 1985	135[a]	I-IV	77	24	34
Smirz et al. 1985	79	I-IV[b]	30	14	35

Unless noted otherwise, all patients had epithelial tumors (treated with chemotherapy) and had no clinical evidence of disease prior to second-look laparotomy.

[a] Includes patients treated with radiotherapy.
[b] Also includes patients with recurrence.
[c] Not all patients were clinically without disease.
[d] Includes nonepithelial ovarian tumors.
[e] Microscopic positive findings not identified.
[f] Includes inadequate explorations.

Table 7.2. *Recurrence of Epithelial Ovarian Carcinoma after Negative Second-Look Laparotomy: Reports of 10 or More Patients*

Study	Negative Second Look No. of Patients	Stage	Follow-Up	Disease Recurrence No. of Patients	Median Time to Recurrence (Mo.)	Recurrence Rate (%)
Mangioni et al. 1975	10	I-III[a]	13–72(32[b])	0	—	0
Smith et al. 1976	23	I-IV	?	4	?	17
Phillips et al. 1979	21	I-IV	7–119[c]	1	18	4.8
Missett et al. 1980	11	I-IV	10–57	3		27
Curry et al. 1981	17	I-IV[a]	8–48	3	15	18
Jones et al. 1981	25	I-III	6–40	1	17	4
Webster and Ballard 1981	14	II-IV	3–14	1	11	7
Webb et al. 1982	32	I-IV	?	4	?	13
Stuart et al. 1982	15	I-IV	32[cd]	2	?	13
Roberts et al. 1982	36	I-IV[a]	2–108	6	?	17
	8	III-IV		4	?	50
Raju et al. 1982	12	III-IV	18–74[c]	1	4	13
Varia et al. 1983	26[d]	I-III	40[b]	2	?	7.7
Jacobs et al. 1983	10	I-IV		1	?	10
Lewis et al. 1983	82	I-IV	24(?)–144(?)[c]	7	?	8.5
Ballon et al. 1984	11	I-IV	4–25	1	3	9
	9	III-IV		1	3	11
Barnhill et al. 1984	48	I-IV	13–108[c]	6	22	13
	18	III-IV		5	?	28(64[e])
Berek et al. 1984	18	III	6–68	4	16	22
Rocereto et al. 1984	23	I-III	10–83	1	?	4.3
Luesley et al. 1984	12[d]	II-IV	22	4	<12	33
Podratz et al. 1985	77	I-IV	21–94[c]	12	>12,<24[c]	16
	30	III-IV		8		27
Smirz et al. 1985	30	I-IV[a]	2–100(24[b])	8	21	27
Krepart 1985 (personal communication)	71	I-IV	15–96[c]	10	19[c]	14
Gershenson et al. 1985	85	III-IV	23–138	20	18.5	24(27[e])

[a] Includes patients treated for recurrences.
[b] Median follow-up.
[c] Extrapolated from other information.
[d] Some patients treated after second-look.
[e] Recurrence rate when well-differentiated lesions are excluded.

portunity to convert the tumor status into a clinical situation that will be amenable to an alternate therapy. When tumor debulking is not appropriate, the surgeon should consider generous tumor sampling for research purposes, such as hormone receptor analysis, stem cell assays, cell kinetics, and karyotype analysis.

Macroscopic Negative Findings at Second-Look Laparotomy

At second-look laparotomy, approximately 50% of the patients will have no gross evidence of tumor (macroscopically negative). Over half of these, 30% to 35% of the total, will have no pathological evidence of tumor (negative second look). The others, 20% of the total, will have evidence of tumor on random biopsies or cytology (microscopically positive second look). An analysis of patients with stages III and IV epithelial ovarian cancer who underwent second-look laparotomy at The University of Texas M. D. Anderson Hospital and Tumor Institute at Houston from January 1971 to December 1981 was the subject of two reports (Gershenson et al. 1985; Copeland et al. 1985). The survival rates of the patients with microscopically positive findings were not significantly different from those of the patients with negative findings. Although the time intervals and methods of analysis were identical, there were recognizable biases in favor of the group of patients with microscopically positive findings. Most of the patients with microscopically positive findings (90%) received additional chemotherapy, whereas a minority (9%) of patients with negative second-look findings received additional treatment. Also, the proportion of well-differentiated lesions was higher in the positive group (26%) than in the negative group (13%). Another aspect, currently under detailed analysis, is the nature of the tumor described as being microscopically positive. It appears that müllerian rests (benign glandular inclusions), with or without atypia, were occasionally interpreted as persistent tumor. Treatment of these atypical findings is probably inappropriate (Coffin, Adcock, and Dehner 1985; Donnell, Greco, and Julian 1980). Although it was not reported in the journal *Cancer* until early 1985, analysis of survival for the two aforementioned studies from U.T. M. D. Anderson Hospital was performed in September 1982. Therefore, these two groups of patients were subjected to an updated analysis as of November 1, 1985. The survival update for the negative second-look patients (fig. 7.1) shows a drop in five-year survival from 85% to 69%. In contrast, there was minimal change in the survival curve (five-year survival, 72%) of the patients with microscopically positive findings (fig. 7.2). There continued to be no significant difference shown between the populations with negative and those with microscopically positive findings.

If no macroscopic disease is identified at second-look surgery, patients with low-grade tumors (borderline and grade 1) have an excellent prognosis. However, if the analysis of recurrence is limited to patients with grades 2 and 3 disease, the predicted long-term recurrence rate is approximately 50% (table 7.3). This recurrence rate is expected both in patients with negative second-look findings who receive no additional treatment and in patients with microscopically positive second-look findings who receive additional chemotherapy. Serious consideration must be given to the additional treatment of patients with moderate or poorly differentiated tumors

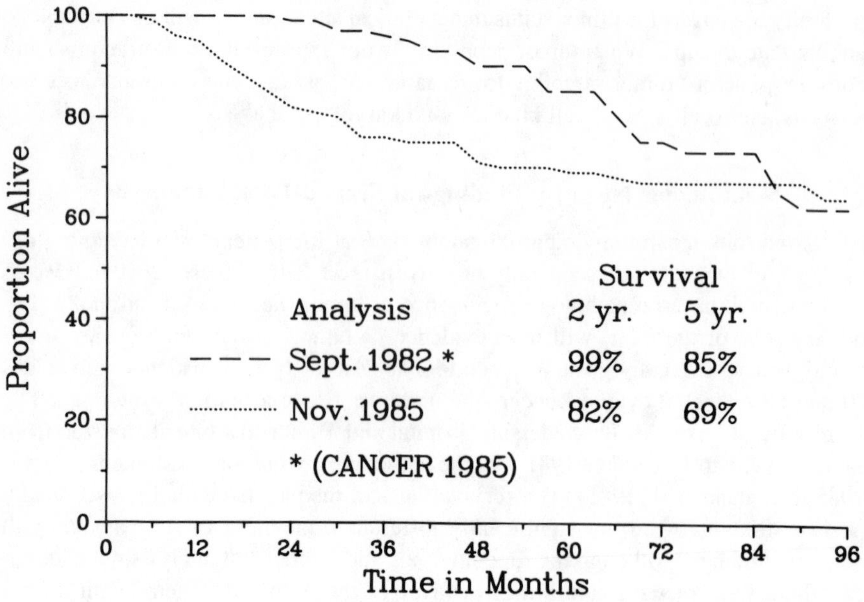

Fig. 7.1. Updated survival of patients with negative findings at second-look laparotomy.

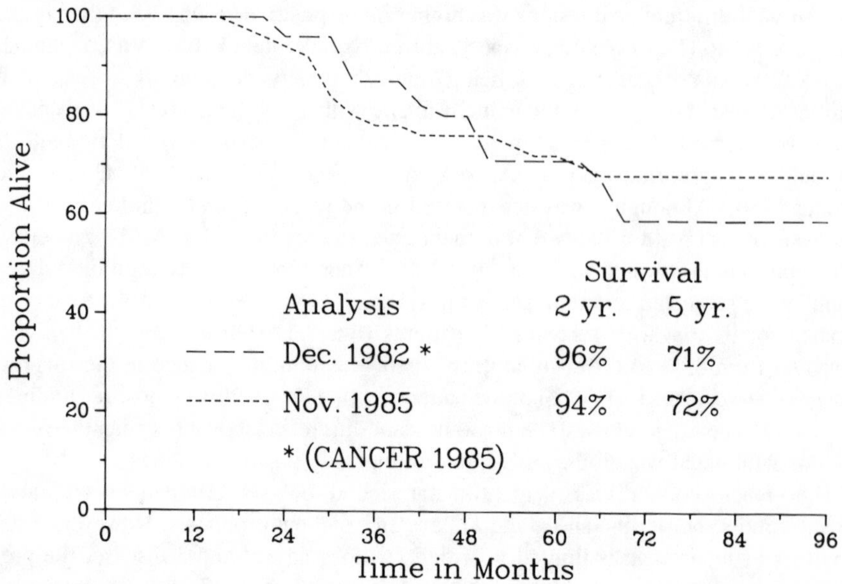

Fig. 7.2. Updated survival of patients with microscopically positive findings at second-look laparotomy.

Table 7.3. *Analysis of Recurrences in Patients with Grade 2 or 3 Ovarian Carcinomas with No Macroscopic Tumor at Second-Look Laparotomy*

	Second-Look Findings	
	Negative	Microscopic Positive
No. of patients	74	37
No. of recurrences	28 (38%)	17 (46%)
Minimum follow-up	48 mo.	48 mo.
Percentage of recurrences after 48 months	14%	12%
Additional recurrences expected	6	2
Predicted long-term recurrence rate	46%	51%

who have negative or microscopically positive second-look findings. In terms of tumor volume, these patients represent an optimal treatment population. Current treatment programs include immunotherapy, radiotherapy, intraperitoneal chemotherapy or radiocolloids (Smirz et al. 1985; Pezner et al. 1978; Varia et al. 1983), and systemic chemotherapy. Previous discouraging reports of radiation therapy following chemotherapy may have resulted from the interruption or delay of the radiation treatment because of myelosuppression (Hainsworth et al. 1983). Adjustments in the type and length of preceding chemotherapy may provide a better tolerance to curative radiation doses. Although it is hoped that new treatment programs will reduce the recurrence rates to a more acceptable level, it should be remembered that 50% of these patients are long-term survivors, and any serious treatment toxicity will be difficult to accept. If effective treatment is developed for this "no macroscopic disease" population, the role of the second-look laparotomy will be more clearly justified.

Clinical Impressions

Review of the experience with second-look procedures reveals many clinical impressions regarding the natural history of epithelial ovarian cancer and the relative role of second-look surgery in various circumstances. However, the following clinical impressions are not firmly substantiated by currently available data.

1. Overall, it is unknown whether the second-look laparotomy contributes to an improvement in patient survival.
2. Patients with borderline tumors probably do not benefit from a second-look procedure.
3. Patients with grade 1 disease who have had all gross tumor removed are not likely to benefit from a second-look procedure if they are clinically disease-free (including noninvasive evaluation, e.g., CT).
4. Patients with grade 1 tumor or very slowly progressive disease but persistent clinical disease may benefit from a second operation, better stated as a repeat tumor reduction rather than a second-look laparotomy.
5. Patients with grade 2 or 3 disease and persistent macroscopic disease are unlikely to benefit from extensive tumor reduction at second-look laparotomy. The pos-

sible exception to this is if previous therapy, surgery or chemotherapy, has been inadequate. Even in these patients, reports of successful outcomes from secondary tumor reduction may be anecdotal, with the majority of attempts unrewarding or possibly harmful.

6. In patients with advanced ovarian carcinoma (stages III and IV, grade 2 or 3), recurrence after negative second-look laparotomy is a significant problem. Many reports do not identify this problem because they have included patients with early stage disease and the follow-up has been short.
7. Patients with negative and those with microscopically positive second-look findings are potentially curable, and both groups of patients may benefit from experimental therapy of a nontoxic nature.

In the treatment of epithelial ovarian cancer, second-look laparotomy will continue to be subjected to critical analysis and may evolve into a procedure limited to more specific clinical applications than those currently used.

References

Atack DB, Nisker JA, Allen HH, Tustanoff ER, Levin L. 1986. CA 125 surveillance and second-look laparotomy in ovarian carcinoma. *Am J Obstet Gynecol* 154:287–289.

Averette HE, Sevin BU. 1982. Debulking surgery and second-look operation. *Int J Radiat Oncol Biol Phys* 8:891–892.

Ballon SC, Portnuff JC, Sikic BI, Turbow MM, Teng NNH, Soriero OM. 1984. Second-look laparotomy in epithelial ovarian carcinoma: Precise definition, sensitivity, and specificity of the operative procedure. *Gynecol Oncol* 17:154–160.

Barnhill DR, Hoskins WJ, Heller PB, Park RC. 1984. The second-look surgical reassessment for epithelial ovarian carcinoma. *Gynecol Oncol* 19:148–154.

Bast RC Jr, Klug TL, St. John E, Jenison E, Nilhoff JM, Lazarus H, Berkowitz RS, Leavitt T, Griffiths CT, Parker L, Zurawski VR Jr, Knapp RC. 1983. A radioimmunoassay using a monoclonal antibody to monitor the course of epithelial ovarian cancer. *N Engl J Med* 309:883–887.

Berek JS, Hacker NF, Lagasse LD, Poth T, Resnick B, Nieberg RK. 1984. Second-look laparotomy in stage III epithelial ovarian cancer: Clinical variables associated with disease status. *Obstet Gynecol* 64:207–212.

Brenner DE, Shaff MI, Jones HW, Grosh WW, Greco FA, Burnett LS. 1985. Abdomino-pelvic computed tomography: Evaluation in patients undergoing second-look laparotomy for ovarian carcinoma. *Obstet Gynecol* 65:715–719.

Clarke-Pearson DL, Bandy LC, Dudzinski M, Heaston D, Creasman WT. 1986. Computed tomography in evaluation of patients with ovarian carcinoma in complete clinical remission: Correlation with surgical-pathologic findings. *JAMA* 255:627–630.

Coffin CM, Adcock LL, Dehner LP. 1985. The second-look operation for ovarian neoplasms: A study of 85 cases emphasizing cytologic and histologic problems. *Int J Gynecol Pathol* 4:97–109.

Cohen CJ, Bruckner HW, Goldberg JD, Holland JF. 1983. Improved therapy with cisplatin regimens for patients with ovarian carcinoma (FIGO III and IV) as measured by surgical end-staging (second-look surgery): The Mount Sinai experience. *Clin Obstet Gynaecol* 10:307–324.

Coleman M, Pasmantier MW, Silver RT. 1985. HAC-Cytoxan (cyclophosphamide) chemotherapy for ovarian carcinoma: Alternating chemotherapy with intensification. *Cancer* 55:2342–2347.

Copeland LJ. 1985. Second-look laparotomy in ovarian carcinoma. *Clin Obstet Gynecol* 28:816–823.

Copeland LJ, Gershenson DM, Wharton JT, Atkinson EN, Sneige N, Edwards CL, Rutledge FN. 1985. Microscopic disease at second-look laparotomy in advanced ovarian cancer. *Cancer* 55:472–478.
Curry SL, Zembo MM, Nahhas WA, Jahshan AE, Whitney CW, Mortel R. 1981. Second-look laparotomy for ovarian cancer. *Gynecol Oncol* 11:114–118.
Decker DG, Fleming TR, Malkasian GD Jr, Webb MJ, Jefferies JA, Edmonson JH. 1982. Cyclophosphamide plus *cis*-platinum in combination: Treatment program for stage III or IV ovarian carcinoma. *Obstet Gynecol* 60:481–487.
Dembo AJ, Chang P-L, Urbach GI. 1985. Clinical correlations of ovarian cancer antigen NB/70K: A preliminary report. *Obstet Gynecol* 65:710–714.
Donnell RM, Greco FA, Julian CG. 1980. Chemotherapy-induced histologic changes in ovarian epithelial tumors and adjacent tissue. *Lab Invest* 42:112.
Edwards CL, Herson J, Gershenson DM, Copeland LJ, Wharton JT. 1983. A prospective randomized clinical trial of melphalan and *cis*-platinum versus hexamethylmelamine, adriamycin, and cyclophosphamide in advanced ovarian cancer. *Gynecol Oncol* 15: 261–277.
Ehrlich CE, Einhorn L, Stehman FB, Blessing J. 1983. Treatment of advanced epithelial ovarian cancer using cisplatin, adriamycin and cytoxan: The Indiana University experience. *Clin Obstet Gynaecol* 10:325–335.
Gershenson DM, Copeland LJ, Wharton JT, Atkinson EN, Sneige N, Edwards CL, Rutledge FN. 1985. Prognosis of surgically determined complete responders in advanced ovarian cancer. *Cancer* 55:1129–1135.
Goldhirsch A, Triller JK, Greiner R, Dreher E, Davis BW. 1983. Computed tomography prior to second-look operation in advanced ovarian cancer. *Obstet Gynecol* 62:630–634.
Greco FA, Julian CG, Richardson RL, Burnett L, Hande KR, Oldham RK. 1981. Advanced ovarian cancer: Brief intensive combination chemotherapy and second-look operation. *Obstet Gynecol* 58:199–205.
Greer BE, Rutledge FN, Gallager HS. 1980. Staging or restaging laparotomy in early-stage epithelial cancer of the ovary. *Clin Obstet Gynecol* 23(1):293–303.
Hainsworth JD, Malcolm A, Johnson DH, Burnett LS, Jones HW III, Greco FA. 1983. Advanced minimal residual ovarian carcinoma: Abdominopelvic irradiation following combination chemotherapy. *Obstet Gynecol* 61:619–623.
Jacobs AJ, Kubitz RL, Scott JC Jr, Kessinger MA. 1983. Surgery following initial treatment of ovarian carcinoma: Restaging (second-look) and palliative operations. *J Surg Oncol* 24:59–63.
Jones ISC, Khoo SK, Whitaker SV. 1981. Evaluation of ovarian cancer by second-look laparotomy after treatment. *Aust NZ J Surg* 51:30–33.
Lewis JL, Cain JM, Pierce VK. 1983. The definition and role of "second-look" procedures. In *Carcinoma of the Ovary*, ed. E Grundmann, Cancer Campaign, vol. 7, pp. 147–150. Stuttgart: Gustav Fischer Verlag.
Luesley DM, Chan KK, Fielding JWL, Hurlow R, Blackledge GR, Jordon JA. 1984. Second-look laparotomy in the management of epithelial ovarian carcinoma: An evaluation of fifty cases. *Obstet Gynecol* 64:421–426.
Maggino T, Tredese F, Valente S, Marchesoni D, Brandes A, Menighetti M, Onnis GL. 1983. Role of second-look laparotomy in multidisciplinary treatment and follow-up of advanced ovarian cancer. *Eur J Gynaecol Oncol* 4:26–29.
Mangioni C, Mattioli G, Natale N. 1975. The "second-look" operation in long-term therapy of ovarian malignancies. In *Diagnosis and Treatment of Ovarian Neoplastic Alterations*, ed. H DeWatteville, PRJ Burch, pp. 153–155. New York: American Elsevier.
Mead GM, Williams CJ, MacBeth FR, Boyd IE, Whitehouse JMA. 1984. Second-look laparotomy in the management of epithelial cell carcinoma of the ovary. *Br J Cancer* 50:185–191.
Misset JL, Marnich R, Michel G, George M, Wolff JP, Mathe G. 1980. The management of

ovarian adenocarcinoma. "Second-look" surgical operation after chemotherapy. *Nouvelle Presse Medicale* 9: 1937–1939.

Pezner RD, Stevens KR Jr, Tong D, Allen CV. 1978. Limited epithelial carcinoma of the ovary treated with curative intent by the intraperitoneal installation of radiocolloids. *Cancer* 42:2563–2571.

Phibbs GD, Smith JP, Stanhope CR. 1983. Analysis of sites of persistent cancer at "second-look" laparotomy in patients with ovarian cancer. *Am J Obstet Gynecol* 147:611–617.

Phillips BP, Buchsbaum HJ, Lifshitz S. 1979. Reexploration after treatment for ovarian carcinoma. *Gynecol Oncol* 8:339–345.

Podratz KC, Malkasian GD Jr, Hilton JF, Harris EA, Gaffey TA. 1985. Second-look laparotomy in ovarian cancer: Evaluation of pathologic variables. *Am J Obstet Gynecol* 152:230–238.

Raju KS, McKinna JA, Barker GH, Wiltshaw E, Jones JM. 1982. Second-look operations in the planned management of advanced ovarian carcinoma. *Am J Obstet Gynecol* 144: 650–654.

Roberts WS, Hodel K, Rich WM, DiSaia PJ. 1982. Second-look laparotomy in the management of gynecologic malignancy. *Gynecol Oncol* 13:345–355.

Rocereto TF, Mangan CE, Giuntoli RL, Sedlacek TV, Ball HJ, Mikuta JJ. 1984. The second-look celiotomy in ovarian cancer. *Gynecol Oncol* 19:34–45.

Rorat E, Wallach RC. 1983. Clinical and pathologic findings at second-look surgery for ovarian carcinoma. *Eur J Gynaecol Oncol* 4:175–181.

Rutledge F, Burns BC. 1966. Chemotherapy for advanced ovarian cancer. *Am J Obstet Gynecol* 96:761–772.

Schwartz PE, Smith JP. 1980. Second-look operations in ovarian cancer. *Am J Obstet Gynecol* 138:1124–1130.

Smirz LR, Stehman FB, Ulbright TM, Sutton GP, Ehrlich CE. 1985. Second-look laparotomy after chemotherapy in the management of ovarian malignancy. *Am J Obstet Gynecol* 152:661–668.

Smith JP, Delgado G, Rutledge F. 1976. Second-look operation in ovarian carcinoma. Postchemotherapy. *Cancer* 38:1438–1442.

Stern J, Buscema J, Rosenshein N, Siegelman S. 1981. Can computed tomography substitute for second-look operation in ovarian carcinoma? *Gynecol Oncol* 11:82–88

Stuart GCE, Jeffries M, Stuart JL, Anderson RJ. 1982. The changing role of "second-look" laparotomy in the management of epithelial carcinoma of the ovary. *Am J Obstet Gynecol* 142:612–616.

Varia M, Fowler W, Walton L, Currie J, Halle J, White J. 1983. Intraperitoneal ^{32}P following second-look laparotomy for ovarian cancer (Abstract). *Int J Radiat Oncol Biol Phys* 9:98.

Wangensteen OH, Lewis FJ, Tongen LA. 1951. The "second-look" in cancer surgery: Patient with involved lymph nodes negative on "sixth look". *J Lancet* 71:303–307.

Wallach RC, Blinick G. 1970. The second-look operation for carcinoma of the ovary. *Surg Gynecol Obstet* 131:1085–1089.

Webb MJ, Snyder JA Jr, Williams TJ, Decker DG. 1982. Second-look laparotomy in ovarian cancer. *Gynecol Oncol* 14:285–293.

Webster KD, Ballard LA Jr. 1981. Ovarian carcinoma; second-look laparatomy postchemotherapy: Preliminary report. *Cleve Clin Q* 48:365–371.

Whitley N, Brenner D, Francis A, Kwon T, Villa Santa U, Aisner J, Wiernik P, Whitley J. 1981. Use of the computed tomographic whole body scanner to stage and follow patients with advanced ovarian carcinoma. *Invest Radiol* 16:479–486.

Wiltshaw E, Raju KS, Dawson I. 1985. The role of cytoreductive surgery in advanced carcinoma of the ovary: An analysis of primary and second surgery. *Br J Obstet Gynaecol* 92:522–527.

Annual Clinical Conference on Cancer, Vol. 29
Gynecologic Cancer: Diagnosis and Treatment Strategies
© 1987 by The University of Texas System Cancer Center

8. Hormonal Therapy for Epithelial Ovarian Cancer

Peter E. Schwartz, Arnold J. Eisenfeld, Neil J. MacLusky,
John S. Lazo, Richard B. Hochberg, and Fredrick N. Naftolin

Hormonal therapy has been employed to manage epithelial ovarian cancer for the past 30 years. Initial use of progestins, and to a much lesser extent estrogens, was based on the observations that hormonally sensitive cancers (e.g., cancers of the breast and endometrium) could respond to hormonal manipulation and that such therapy was associated with minimal toxicity. Hormonal therapy was generally administered after such standard therapy as surgery, radiation therapy, and cytotoxic chemotherapy failed to control the cancer. Recent interest in hormonal therapy for epithelial ovarian cancers is based on the detection of cytosol estrogen and progestin receptors in samples of epithelial ovarian cancer. This chapter will review steroid hormone receptor data, experiences with progestins and estrogens, combined estrogen and progestin therapy, antiestrogen therapy, and hormonal therapy in combination with cytotoxic chemotherapy, and indicate new approaches to be considered in the hormonal therapy of epithelial ovarian cancer.

Estrogen and Progestin Receptor Proteins

The past decade witnessed the identification of cytosol estrogen and progestin receptors in the common epithelial cancers of the ovary and gave further impetus to clinical investigation of hormonal therapy in the management of these cancers. Previous studies had demonstrated that hormonally sensitive breast cancers could be predicted by the presence of a macromolecular binding protein in the cytosol, the estrogen receptor protein, that had a high affinity and high specificity for estrogen (Jensen, Smith, and DeSombre 1976; Knight et al. 1977). Subsequent studies have suggested that the cytosol progestin receptor was a more sensitive indicator for response to hormonal manipulation, since the progestin receptor is a product of successful estrogen interaction with its receptor (Horwitz et al. 1975; Fisher et al. 1983). Progestin therapy for endometrial cancer was established before the biochemical identification of cytosol estrogen or progestin receptors (Kelley and Baker 1961). Recent studies have suggested that endometrial cancers most likely to respond to progestin administration have elevated levels of progestin receptors (Ehrlich, Young, and Cleary 1981; Martin et al. 1981; Benraad et al. 1980).

In 1978 Eisenfeld and I presented the first series of epithelial ovarian cancers to be specifically studied for the presence of estrogen-binding macromolecules consistent with classic cytosol estrogen receptors found in breast and endometrial cancers

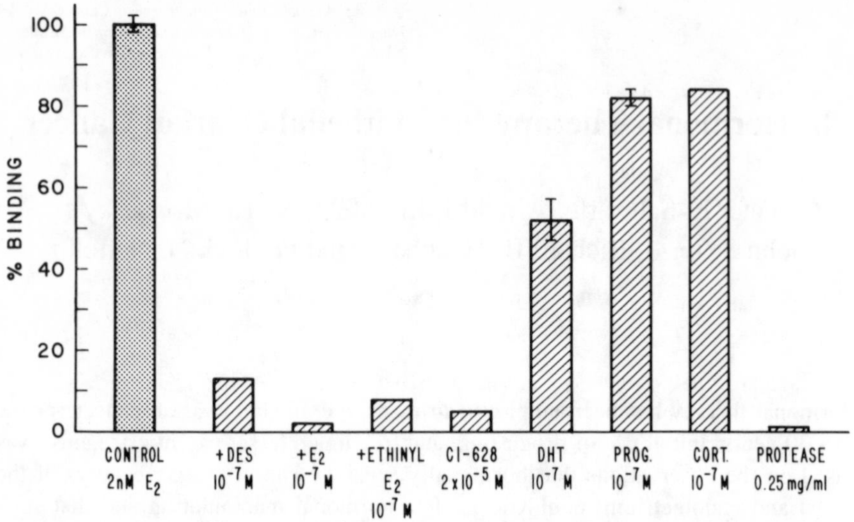

Fig. 8.1. Tritiated estradiol binding in cytosol of human ovarian cancer. Radioactive estradiol (2×10^{-9} M) was incubated with cytosol from a poorly differentiated serous ovarian carcinoma with and without a variety of nonradioactive compounds. Macromolecular-bound radioactivity in the control is 330 fmol/mg cytosol protein (DES, diethylstilbestrol; E_2, estradiol, CI-628, α-[p-[2-(1-pyrrolidino)ethoxyl]phenyl]-4-methoxy-α-nitrostilbene; DHT, dihydrotestosterone; PROG., progesterone; CORT., cortisol). Brackets indicate the standard error of the mean, unless it was too small to depict. Reprinted, by permission, from The American College of Obstetricians and Gynecologists from Schwartz PE, LiVolsi VA, Hildreth N, MacLusky NJ, Naftolin FN, Eisenfeld AJ, Estrogen receptors in ovarian epithelial carcinoma. *Obstet Gynecol* 1982; 59:229–238.

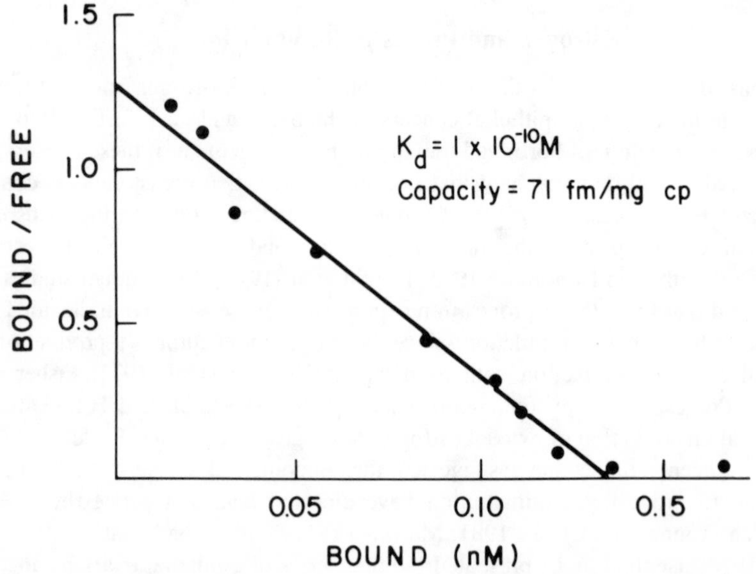

Fig. 8.2. Scatchard plot of estrogen binding in the cytosol of ovarian cancer. The cytosol was prepared from a serous, grade 3 ovarian cancer. The figure depicts the specific macromolecular binding after 24 hours incubation at 0°C.

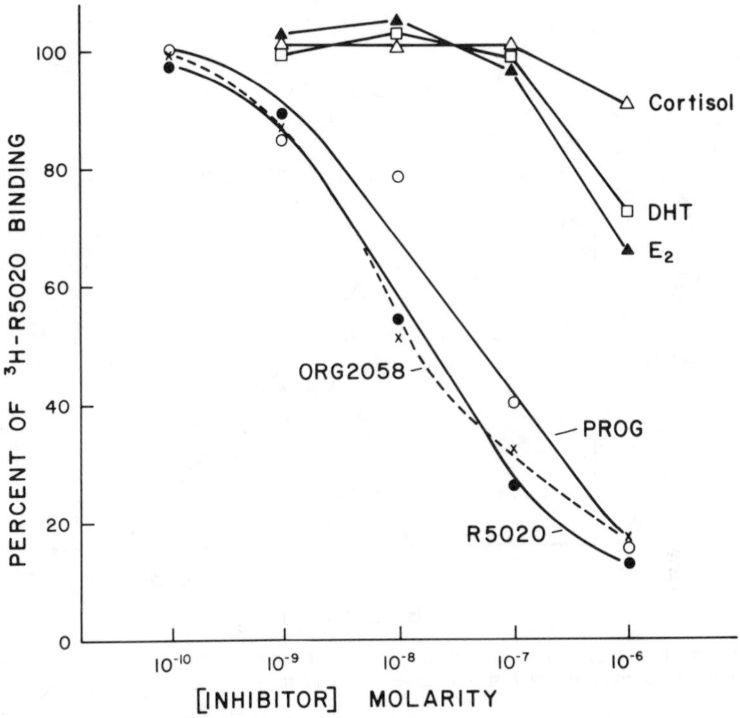

Fig. 8.3. Competition for tritiated R5020 macromolecular binding using a variety of nonradioactive steroids. Tritiated R5020(2 nM) was incubated with cytosol and a variety of competitors ranging in concentrations from 10^{-10} M to 10^{-6} M (PROG, progesterone; ORG2058, 16-α-ethyl-21-hydroxy-19-nor-4-pregnene-3,20-dione; E_2, estradiol; DHT, dihydrotestosterone). The specimen is a moderately differentiated mucinous ovarian carcinoma. The control progestin binding level is 786 fmol/mg cytosol protein, and the estrogen receptor value is 13 fmol/mg cytosol protein. Reprinted, by permission, from The American College of Obstetricians and Gynecologists from Schwartz PE, LiVolsi VA, Hildreth N, MacLusky NJ, Naftolin FN, Eisenfeld AJ, Estrogen receptors in ovarian epithelial carcinomas. *Obstet Gynecol* 1982; 59:229–238.

(Schwartz and Eisenfeld 1978). A subsequently published report of 30 previously untreated epithelial ovarian cancers confirmed the presence of an estrogen-binding macromolecule with the high specificity (fig. 8.1) and binding affinity (fig. 8.2) of classic estrogen receptor protein in 16 of 30 specimens studied (Schwartz et al. 1982b). A progestin-binding macromolecule with the binding specificity (fig. 8.3) and binding affinity (fig. 8.4) of a progestin receptor has also been identified (Schwartz et al. 1982b). Heterogeneity of the estrogen receptor content in primary ovarian cancer samples and metastases was also documented in the same report. Results of tumor analyses of multiple samples for the presence of estrogen receptors were consistent when the specimens were obtained from the primary site, but differences in cytosol receptor content were found when estrogen receptor content of metastases was compared with content levels in the primary cancer site (fig. 8.5). Pri-

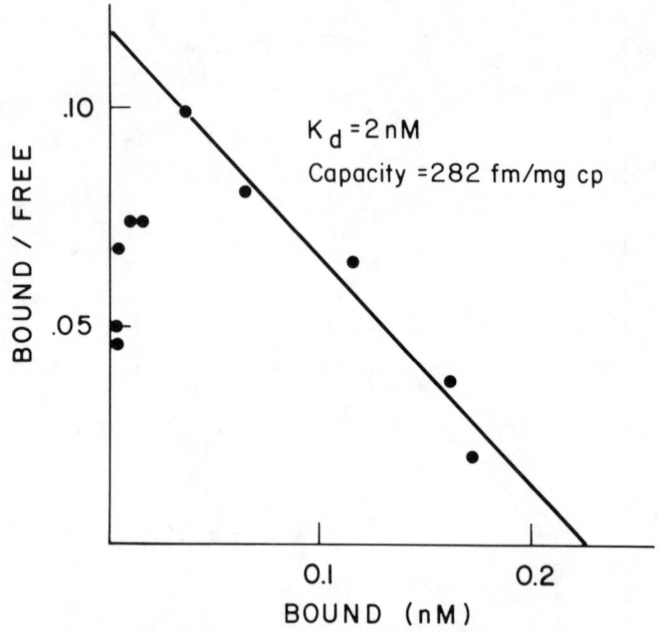

Fig. 8.4. Scatchard plot of progestin binding in the cytosol of ovarian cancer. The cytosol was prepared from a serous, grade 1 ovarian cancer specimen.

mary cancers rich in receptors may have receptor-poor metastases, and occasionally receptor-poor primary tumors may have receptor-rich metastases. Heterogeneity of estrogen receptor content has also been demonstrated by Holt et al. (1979).

A report of 113 primary epithelial ovarian cancers correlated multiple histological parameters (histological type and grade, necrosis, fibrosis, lymphocyte infiltration, mitoses, tumor giant cells, psammoma bodies, and stroma) with the estrogen and progestin receptor content (Schwartz et al. 1985). The only statistically significant findings were that grade 4 cancers had a statistically greater likelihood of containing estrogen receptors than did lower grade cancers (table 8.1), and grade 3 tumor samples containing abundant mitoses had a significantly greater number of estrogen receptor–negative cancers than did cancers containing no to moderate mitoses (table 8.1). Progestin receptor content was only statistically correlated with the presence of lymphocyte infiltration (table 8.2). Progestin receptors were significantly greater in samples containing no to minimal lymphocyte infiltration. Thus, with the exception of a small group of tumors (either grade 4 or grade 3 with mitoses), estrogen receptor content of epithelial ovarian cancers appears to be independent of all histological features studied, and similarly, with the exception of lymphocyte infiltration, progestin receptor content is independent of the histological parameters examined.

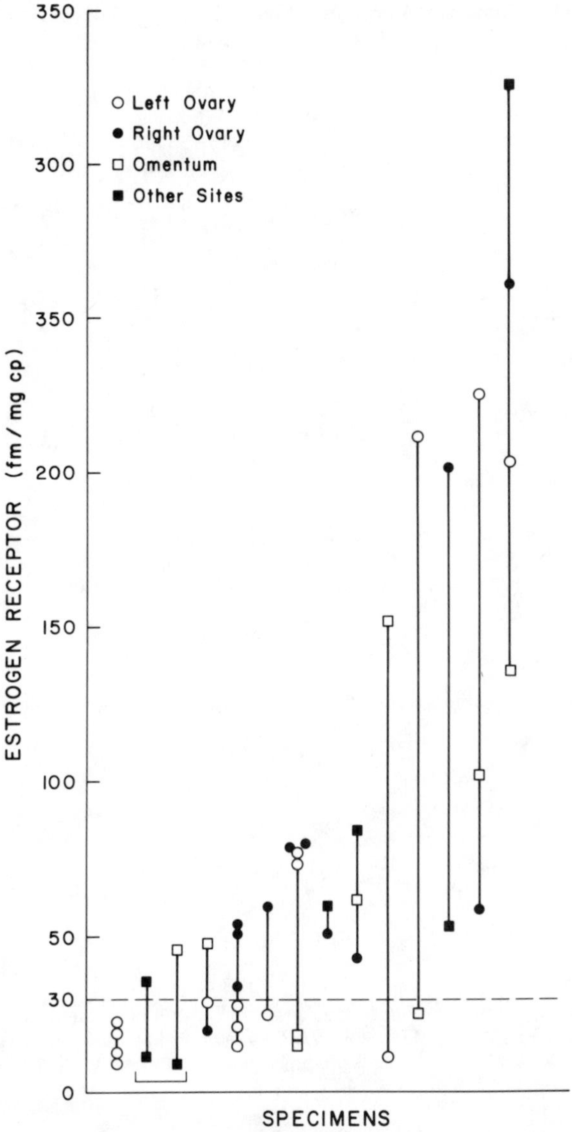

Fig. 8.5. Estrogen receptor values obtained from multiple sites of involvement in individual patients.

Table 8.1. *Significant Associations between Estrogen Receptor Content and Histological Parameters*

Histological Parameter		Estrogen Receptor Categories: Negative (<15 fmol) *N*	%	Borderline (15–30 fmol) *N*	%	Positive (>30 fmol) *N*	%	Total *N* (100%)
Grade	1	5	42	5	42	2	17	12
	2	12	50	3	12	9	38	24
	3	28	58	7	15	13	27	48
	4	4	22	3	17	11	61	18
Total[a]		49		18		35		102
Mitoses (Grade 3)	0,1+	0		1		1		2
	2+	3		3		5		11
	3+,4+	24	(88.9)	2	(33.3)	7	(53.9)	33
Total[b]		27		6		13		46

[a] $\chi^2_6 = 13.9; p = .03.$
[b] $\chi^2_4 = 11.2; p = .02.$
Source: Reprinted, by permission, from the American College of Obstetricians and Gynecologists from Schwartz PE, Merino MJ, LiVolsi VA, Lawrence R, MacLusky NJ, Eisenfeld A, Histopathologic correlations of estrogen and progestin receptor protein in epithelial ovarian carcinomas. *Obstet Gynecol* 1985; 66:428–433.

Table 8.2. *Lymphocyte Infiltration vs. Progestin Receptor Content*

Lymphocyte Infiltration	Progestin Receptor Content: <20 fmol *N*	%	>20 fmol *N*	%	Total *N* (100%)
0	22	37	38	63	60
1+	13	65	7	35	20
2+,3+	11	79	3	21	14
Total	46		48		94

$\chi^2_2 = 10.6; p = .005.$
Source: Reprinted, by permission, from the American College of Obstetricians and Gynecologists from Schwartz PE, Merino MJ, LiVolsi VA, Lawrence R, MacLusky NJ, Eisenfeld A, Histopathologic correlations of estrogen and progestin receptor protein in epithelial ovarian carcinomas. *Obstet Gynecol* 1985; 66:428–433.

Hormonal Therapy

Progestin Therapy

Progestin therapy has been used by various investigators for the past 30 years to treat epithelial ovarian cancers (table 8.3). Early reports tended to be vague in distinguishing objective tumor responses from subjective patient responses. Jolles presented the first series of ten patients to be treated with progestin therapy in 1962. One patient appeared to have had an objective response to intramuscular 17α-

hydroxyprogesterone caproate (Delalutin). That patient was noted to have had "a good reduction of tumor size" for at least three months. Another patient cleared pleural effusions for six months and ascites for three months. A third patient was noted to have "improvement" good for six months and a drying up of ascites. Subjectively, patients noted an increased sense of well-being associated with an increased appetite. Eight of ten patients in this series had recurrent disease following external beam radiation therapy. Two patients received primary progestin therapy, neither demonstrating an objective response.

Two subsequent series employing 17α-hydroxyprogesterone caproate revealed a similar experience. Varga and Hendrikson reported in 1964 one objective response among six patients receiving 17α-hydroxyprogesterone caproate. That patient experienced a clearing of ascites and edema along with a reduction in size of a pelvic mass such that the patient was considered possibly to be in remission. The patient died suddenly at home four months after therapy was initiated, and a postmortem examination was not performed. Ward in 1972 reported the largest series of patients to be treated with 17α-hydroxyprogesterone caproate. Three of 23 patients (13%) in this series experienced objective responses. Each of the three patients had reductions in the size of pelvic masses lasting three, two, and three months, the last two

Table 8.3. *Progestin Therapy in Advanced and Recurrent Ovarian Cancer*

Study	Year	Progestin[a]	Route of Administration[b]	*N*	Response *N*	Response %
Jolles	1962	Delalutin	IM	10	1	10
Varga and Henrikson	1964	Delalutin	IM	6	1	17
Ward	1972	Delalutin	IM	23	3	13
Kaufman	1966	Provera	PO	11	1	9
Malkasian et al.	1977	Provera	PO	19	1	5
Mangioni et al.	1981	Provera	PO	30	0	0
Aabo et al.	1982	Provera	PO	27	1	4
Slayton, Paygano, and Creech	1981	Provera	IM	19	0	0
Mangioni et al.	1981	Provera	IM	33	5	15
Trope et al.	1982	Provera	IM	25	1	4
Bergqvist et al.	1981	Provera	IM	4	3	75
Rendina, Donadio, and Giovannini[c]	1982	Provera	IM	31	17	55
Geisler	1985	Megace	PO	31	10	32
Ahlgren et al.	1985	Megace	PO	26	1	4
Malkasian et al.	1973	NSC 123018	PO	9	2	22
Timothy	1982	Depostat	IM	7	3	43

[a] Delalutin, 17α-hydroxyprogesterone caproate; Provera, medroxyprogesterone acetate; Megace, megestrol acetate; NSC 123018, 6-dehydro-6,17α-dimethylprogesterone; Depostat, gestonorone caproate.

[b] IM, intramuscular; PO, *per os* (by mouth).

[c] Each patient had an endometrioid ovarian carcinoma.

patients still responding at the time of submission for publication. No statistical relationship could be demonstrated between histological appearance and response to therapy. No toxicity was reported in any of these series employing 17α-hydroxyprogesterone caproate.

The progestational agent most commonly used for treating advanced, recurrent ovarian cancer is medroxyprogesterone acetate (Provera), an agent that has been administered orally and intramuscularly (table 8.3). Oral medroxyprogesterone acetate was initially reported to be associated with an occasional objective response (Kaufman 1966). One of 11 patients (9%) in Kaufman's series responded. That patient had previously failed radiation and cytotoxic chemotherapy but sustained a complete remission for 18 months on oral medroxyprogesterone acetate. Unfortunately, other investigators were unable to substantiate a high response rate to this preparation. Reports from a total of 76 patients treated with oral medroxyprogesterone acetate revealed only 2 patients who experienced an objective response (Malkasian et al. 1977; Mangioni et al. 1981; Aabo et al. 1982). No toxicity was reported with this mode of therapy.

Results with intramuscularly administered medroxyprogesterone acetate were no more encouraging than the oral preparation for the management of recurrent ovarian cancer (table 8.3). Three series employing intramuscular medroxyprogesterone acetate published in 1981 and 1982 and consisting of 77 patients demonstrated objective responses in only 6 (7.8%) patients (Mangioni et al. 1981; Slayton, Pagano, and Creech 1981; Trope et al. 1982). These series utilized more objective response criteria than the earlier series with 17α-hydroxyprogesterone caproate. Reported toxicity to intramuscular medroxyprogesterone acetate included two patients with deep vein thrombophlebitis, one with a gluteal abscess, and one who experienced hypertension in association with fluid retention.

Bergqvist, Kullander, and Thorell (1981) administered intramuscular medroxyprogesterone acetate to four patients with advanced, previously untreated ovarian cancer and observed objective responses in three patients. Each of three patients with mucinous carcinomas responded to progestin therapy, but a patient with a stage IV serous carcinoma had rapidly progressing cancer while receiving this therapy.

The well-documented observation that endometrial cancer may respond to progestin therapy led Rendina, Donadio, and Giovannini (1982) to study a series of 41 patients with endometrioid ovarian cancers employing high-dose intramuscular medroxyprogesterone acetate as the primary therapy. The dose of progestin was 1 g/day for five days each week for three months and then 2 g/wk for three to five months. Thirty patients had stage III disease and one had stage IV disease. Twenty-six of the 31 patients with advanced cancer had well-differentiated cancers. Cytosol estrogen receptor proteins were elevated in 81.3% of the primary tumors (entire series) and progestin receptors were elevated in 72.1% (entire series). Estrogen and progestin receptor content appeared to correlate with the histological grade. Only 5 of 38 well-differentiated cancers were estrogen and progestin receptor negative, whereas 3 of 5 poorly differentiated cancers were receptor negative. Among the patients, there were 3 patients with complete responses, 14 with partial responses, 8 with no change, and 6 with progression of disease. Ten of 15 patients with stage III cancer assessable at three years following diagnosis were alive. A relationship was established between the presence of steroid receptors and therapeutic efficacy. For the entire series, complete (8) and partial (15) responses to progestin therapy were observed only in that group of patients whose cancers contained estrogen receptors or estrogen and progestin receptors. Six of eight patients with steroid receptor–poor tumors demonstrated progressive disease, and the remaining two patients had stable disease. The results of this study clearly support the concept that endometrioid ovarian cancers, like endometrial cancers, are hormonally sensitive tumors, and responses to progestin therapy may be correlated to steroid receptor content of the primary cancer.

In 1983 Geisler reported on the use of very high dose oral megestrol acetate (Megace)—800 mg by mouth every day for a month and then 400 mg by mouth every day thereafter—in the management of advanced or recurrent ovarian cancer. The dose schedule was based on the anecdotal observation that a patient with endometrial cancer who failed to respond to standard doses of megestrol acetate responded to this high-dose regimen (Geisler 1983). The ovarian cancer series was subsequently updated (Geisler 1985). In total, 10 of 31 patients (32%) sustained an objective response. Six patients experienced a complete response lasting 5 to 36 months (mean, 16.5 months), and four patients sustained a partial response, the progression-free interval ranging from 4 to 10 months. Two patients received megestrol acetate as primary therapy, and each sustained a partial remission. Toxicity was not reported nor were progestin receptor values determined from tumor samples.

Ahlgren et al. (1985) reported on their experience employing the same dosage of megestrol acetate in 26 patients whose disease had failed to respond to prior cytotoxic chemotherapy. Only one objective partial response was observed lasting four months. One patient experienced neurotoxicity manifest by confusion and proximal muscle wasting, but her condition improved after discontinuation of therapy. Another patient died of a stroke that was of unknown relation to therapy.

I have treated 12 patients with high-dose megestrol acetate who had recurrent ovarian cancer and had not responded to previous combination chemotherapy (unpublished data). No objective responses were seen in this group of patients. One patient who initially responded to cisplatin and Adriamycin (doxorubicin HCl) but subsequently did not respond to the CHAP II regimen (cyclophosphamide, hexamethylmelamine, doxorubicin HCl, and cisplatin) was treated with a local radium implant for an isolated posterior vaginal wall recurrence. Immediately following the radiation treatment the patient was placed on high-dose megestrol acetate for control of presumed but not documented systemic disease. She has gained 31 pounds on megestrol acetate over 14 months and remains free of disease.

Another progestin that has been employed for treating advanced recurrent disease is the experimental agent NSC 123018 (6-dehydro-6, 17α-dimethylprogesterone) (Malkasian et al. 1973). Two of nine patients demonstrated an objective response lasting 30 and 45 months. No toxicity was reported. This agent is not currently available for clinical use.

Timothy (1982) reported on 15 patients receiving intramuscular gestonorone caproate (Depostat) as primary therapy. Seven patients with stages III or IV disease had progression-free intervals of 9, 9, 12, 12, 18, 24, and 48 months. Two patients appeared to have complete responses lasting 9 and 18 months, and one patient had a partial response allowing easy surgical excision and has survived 48 months. Additionally, eight patients with stage IB-IIB disease remain free of disease 6 to 72 months following diagnosis. Timothy was impressed with patients reporting an increased sense of well-being despite advanced disease.

This series' results are consistent with the results of other investigators and strongly suggest a role for progestins in first-line therapy for patients with epithelial ovarian cancer (Bergqvist, Kullander, and Thorell 1981; Rendina, Donadio, and Giovannini 1982). Unfortunately, data on cytosol steroid receptor content were not consistently available in the reports cited above (except for Rendina, Donadio, and Giovannini 1982), and a method for identifying those patients who might benefit from progestin therapy remains to be established.

Estrogen Therapy

There is a paucity of literature on the role of estrogen therapy in the management of advanced epithelial ovarian cancer. Long and Evans (1963) reported the only experience in the literature on the use of diethylstilbestrol as a chemotherapeutic agent for ovarian cancer. Fourteen patients with advanced metastatic ovarian cancer were given diethylstilbestrol by mouth at the high doses of 15–30 mg/day. Five of the patients were lost to follow-up once the medication was prescribed. Two of nine evaluable patients maintained an objective response for more than one year following initiation of therapy. One patient had a papillary adenocarcinoma with generalized metastases; the other had myxomatous peritonitis. Three patients noted an increased sense of well-being similar to that experienced with progestin therapy. At least one patient was thought to have had the disease aggravated by diethylstilbestrol therapy. Long and Evans suggest that suppression of gonadotropins by diethylstilbestrol administration may be the mechanism of action for the therapeutic effects observed with its administration.

Estrogen and Progestin Therapy

Recognition of the need for hormones to bind to their receptors in target tissue in order to evoke a hormone-induced response resulted in a study combining estrogen and progestins as second-line therapy in a series of patients who did not respond to cisplatin combination therapy (Jolles, Freedman, and Jones 1983). Eleven patients received 0.1 mg/day ethinylestradiol by mouth for 25 days of a 30-day cycle and 100 mg/day medroxyprogesterone acetate by mouth on days 8 to 25 of the cycle. No therapy was administered on days 26 to 30. Two patients demonstrated parital responses, each lasting two months, and two patients had stabilization of disease, each lasting three months. One patient sustained a cerebrovascular accident while receiving her first course of hormonal therapy. One patient who sustained a partial response was the only patient to discontinue therapy because of severe nausea. A patient with a vaginal apex recurrence was noted to have elevated levels of cytosol estrogen receptors but no detectable progestin receptors. High levels of progestin receptors were found after combined estrogen and progestin treatments, but when no objective regression of tumor was observed after three treatment cycles, therapy was discontinued.

Antiestrogen Therapy

Tamoxifen Therapy

The identification of cytosol estrogen receptors led to the establishment of a treatment program at Yale University School of Medicine designed to establish a possible role for the antiestrogen tamoxifen in managing epithelial ovarian cancers. Tamoxifen had already been successfully employed in treating patients with breast cancer, the patients most likely to respond having cancers rich in estrogen receptors (Legha, Davis, and Muggia 1978). Thirteen patients with advanced recurrent epithelial ovarian cancer were treated with oral tamoxifen (Schwartz et al. 1982a). All but one patient had previously undergone treatment in two separate chemotherapy regimens or radiation therapy followed by chemotherapy without improvement. The remaining patient had prolonged bone marrow suppression following a combination chemotherapy regimen. Each patient in this protocol had estrogen receptor determinations made from samples of her cancer prior to participating in the study. Patients initially received 10 mg tamoxifen twice a day, but those whose tumors failed to show an objective response had their doses doubled every four weeks to a maximum daily dose of 320 mg. A complete response was not observed in this study. One patient had a partial response that lasted two months, and four patients had stabilization of previously rapidly progressing cancer that lasted 11 to 30 weeks. Eight patients demonstrated no response to tamoxifen. Five of these patients had partial small bowel obstruction and may not have absorbed the tamoxifen, and each died within nine weeks of initiating tamoxifen therapy. Three patients whose disease failed to respond to the tamoxifen died 18 to 24 weeks after beginning tamoxifen therapy. The first death in a tamoxifen-treated patient whose disease stabilized was observed 25 weeks following initiation of therapy. The survival curves for these patients are presented in figure 8.6. Each patient who showed stabilization of disease on the tamoxifen regimen had a cancer rich in cytosol estrogen receptors (23–169 fmol/mg cytosol protein). However, estrogen receptor–rich tumors were also present in the group whose disease failed to respond to tamoxifen therapy. There was no difference in the two groups of patients regarding histological type, histological grade, or time from initial diagnosis to initiation of tamoxifen therapy.

A subsequent study of the direct cytotoxic and antiproliferative properties of tamoxifen was performed utilizing newly excised human ovarian carcinomas that were treated with tamoxifen and examined for colony formation in soft agar (Lazo et al. 1984). Nineteen of 46 tumor samples studied produced 15 or more colonies per 1×10^5 cells plated in soft agar. No significant decrement in colony formation of the tumor samples was seen when tumor samples were incubated with 0.2 μM tamoxifen for one hour. However, 8 of 18 (44%) of cancer samples tested demonstrated a decline in colony formation when exposed to continuous 2 μM tamoxifen. Only one of seven samples yielded a decrease in colony formation to 0.2 μM tam-

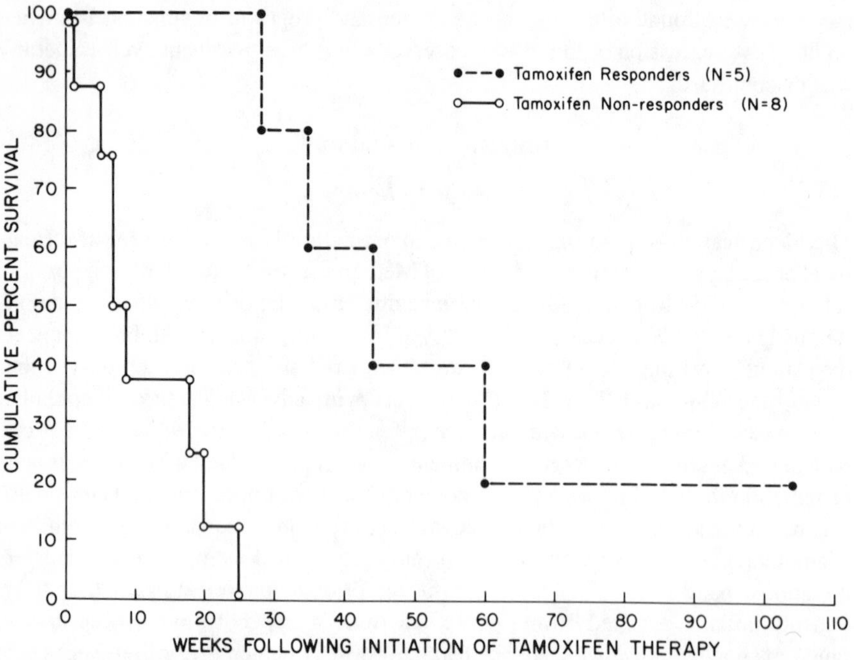

Fig. 8.6. Duration of patient survival following initiation of tamoxifen therapy. For this figure, "tamoxifen responders" includes one patient with a partial response and four with stabilization of disease. Solid circle, broken line = tamoxifen responders (N=5); open circle, solid line = tamoxifen nonresponders (N=8). Reprinted, by permission, from the American College of Obstetricians and Gynecologists from Schwartz PE, Keating G, MacLusky N, Naftolin FN, Eisenfeld A, Tamoxifen therapy for advanced ovarian cancer. *Obstet Gynecol* 1982; 59:583–588.

oxifen. Thus, brief exposure to tamoxifen had no effect, but continuous exposure, which more closely resembles the clinical pharmacokinetics of tamoxifen, produced antitumor effects. When colony formation was compared with receptor data, no tumor sample containing less than 30 fmol/mg cytosol protein estrogen receptor content showed a 50% decrease in colony formation when exposed to continuous 2 μM tamoxifen. (Reductions in colony formation of 50% or greater are associated with clinical responsiveness [Lazo et al. 1984].) These data suggested that the results reported by Schwartz et al. (1982a) with tamoxifen represented a direct effect of tamoxifen on ovarian cancer cells rather than an indirect effect on other organs or cell types.

A subsequent report by investigators at The University of Texas M. D. Anderson Hospital and Tumor Institute at Houston failed to demonstrate an objective response with tamoxifen therapy but confirmed the Yale University findings of stabilization of growth of advanced ovarian cancer in 19 of 23 patients whose disease had failed to respond to standard cytotoxic chemotherapy (Shirey et al. 1985). The disease remained stable for a mean duration of 17 weeks (range, 8–47 weeks). Stabilization of disease is not a dramatic response. Nevertheless, a previous study from U.T.

M. D. Anderson Hospital employing cytotoxic chemotherapy revealed only a 6% objective response rate and a 12.7% rate of stabilization of disease for second-line agents (Stanhope, Smith, and Rutledge 1977). Cisplatin (Pesando, Come, and Parker 1979) and hexamethylmelamine (Johnson et al. 1978) are each active as second-line therapy, but doxorubicin HCl does not appear to be active in such situations (Pesando, Come, and Parker 1979). These agents are now frequently incorporated into first-line therapy. Once cisplatin, hexamethylmelamine, doxorubicin HCl, and cyclophosphamide fail, there are no chemotherapeutic agents available that have significant activity.

Tamoxifen Combined with Cytotoxic Chemotherapy

The rationale for combining tamoxifen and cytotoxic chemotherapy for the management of epithelial ovarian cancer is as follows: (1) objective responses have been documented with cytotoxic chemotherapy, and tamoxifen has been shown to stabilize rapidly progressing ovarian cancer; (2) ovarian cancer is heterogeneous in regard to cell type and cell-to-cell estrogen receptor content; (3) cytotoxic chemotherapy and tamoxifen have different mechanisms of action and may thereby inhibit cancer cells with different biologic characteristics; (4) disease-free survival has been prolonged when cytotoxic and tamoxifen therapy have been combined as adjuvant therapy in patients with breast cancer; and (5) tamoxifen has minimal myelosuppression, making it unnecessary to reduce the dosage of cytotoxic chemotherapeutic agents used in combination with it (Schwartz et al. 1982a).

A prospective randomized trial employing tamoxifen in combination with cytotoxic chemotherapy has been initiated at the Yale University School of Medicine. Patients in this study were required to have stage III or IV ovarian cancers, as outlined by the staging system of the International Federation of Gynecology and Obstetrics (FIGO). Additionally, patients operated on at Yale–New Haven Hospital had tissue samples analyzed for cytosol estrogen and progestin receptor levels. Patients received 50 mg/m^2 of doxorubicin HCl and 50 mg/m^2 of cisplatin on day 1 of a 28-day cycle. Every 28 days the patient received each of these medications. The total number of treatments was 18. In addition, half of the patients were randomized to receive tamoxifen. Tamoxifen was taken orally (10 mg twice a day) throughout the entire 18 months of the treatment program.

Of the first 35 patients, 17 received cytotoxic chemotherapy alone and 18 received tamoxifen in combination with cytotoxic chemotherapy. The overall survival for the entire group is seen in figure 8.7. Patients receiving the combination of tamoxifen and cytotoxic chemotherapy had a slightly better disease-free survival rate than those receiving cytotoxic chemotherapy alone, but this difference in survival was not statistically significant. The only survival finding that was statistically significant was based on the volume of residual tumor at the initial operation. Patients having less than a 2-cm maximum residual tumor diameter at the end of the initial operation had an 82% two-year survival rate regardless of therapy employed, whereas those with more than a 2-cm residual diameter had a 25% two-year survival. The significance of residual tumor as an important prognostic factor is well established (Wharton, Edwards, and Rutledge 1984). Until more patients are in-

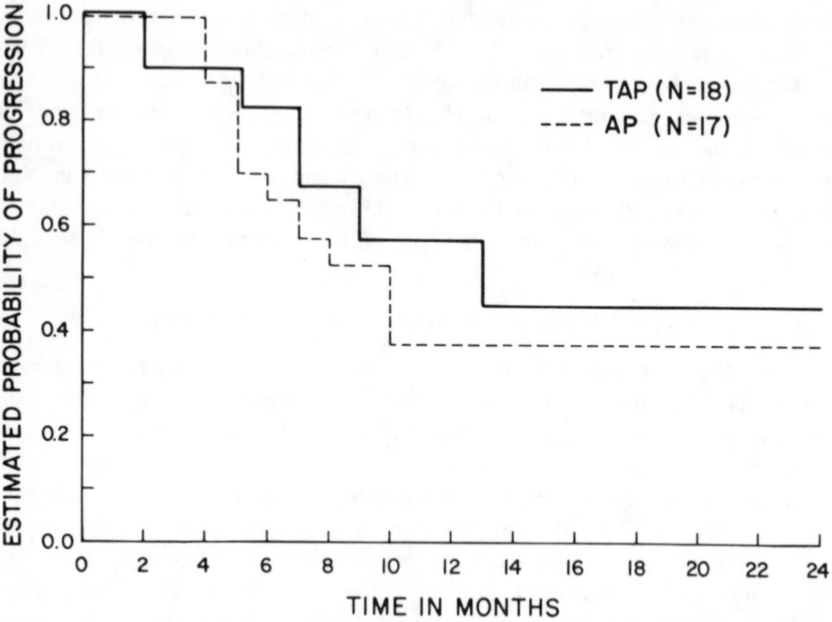

Fig. 8.7. Disease-free survival for patients with stage III or IV epithelial ovarian cancer randomized to receive either TAP (tamoxifen, Adriamycin [doxorubicin HCl], cisplatin) or AP (doxorubicin HCl and cisplatin).

cluded in this clinical trial, the significance of combined tamoxifen and cytotoxic chemotherapy cannot be determined.

Progestins Combined with Cytotoxic Chemotherapy

Intramuscular medroxyprogesterone acetate was used in combination with melphalan in treating 33 patients, 28 of whom had epithelial ovarian cancers (Bergqvist et al. 1981). Clinical details are incomplete for this group of patients, but overall 28 women were reported to have responded to treatment. The patient group treated included all stages of ovarian cancers. Details of the type of response and duration were not stated. Kahanpaa, Karkkainen, and Nieminen (1982) reported on ten patients (five with primary disease, five with recurrent) with advanced ovarian cancers who received medroxyprogesterone acetate (1 gm intramuscularly weekly) in combination with cisplatin, doxorubicin HCl, and cyclophosphamide. This group of patients was compared with ten patients who received the cytotoxic chemotherapy only. No objective responses were observed in patients receiving the combined progestin and cytotoxic chemotherapy, but two complete responses and one partial response were documented in the group receiving only the cytotoxic chemotherapy. The authors noted that the group of patients in this study had unfavorable therapeutic and prognostic factors, that no estrogen or progestin receptor levels were available, and that the study size was very small.

One report is available about utilizing oral medroxyprogestrone acetate (200 mg by mouth four times a day) in combination with cytotoxic chemotherapy (mitomycin and vinblastine) for managing recurrent epithelial ovarian cancer (Ozols et al. 1983). None of 13 patients in this trial demonstrated an objective response. Of interest were 5 of 13 patients (38%) who developed signs and symptoms consistent with drug-induced pulmonary toxicity, which was believed to be due to prior or current cytotoxic chemotherapy.

Potential Approaches for Hormonal Therapy

Aromatase Inhibitors

The presence of estrogen receptor proteins in epithelial ovarian cancers suggests that these cancers may be estrogen sensitive. A series of ovarian cancers were analyzed to determine whether they contained aromatase activity and were therefore capable of estrogen biosynthesis (Voit et al. 1982). Twenty-one primary ovarian cancers (ten serous, three undifferentiated, two clear cell, one endometrioid, one endodermal sinus tumor, and one steroid-producing) and two recurrent serous carcinomas were studied to determine if they could convert tritiated androstenedione to tritiated estrogen. Aromatase activity was detected in all but one of the tumors (a grade 3 serous primary). Eight tumor samples converted the androgen to estrogen at levels equal to or above the levels seen in normal postmenopausal ovarian tissue (fig. 8.8). Further work is necessary to determine whether local estrogen formation

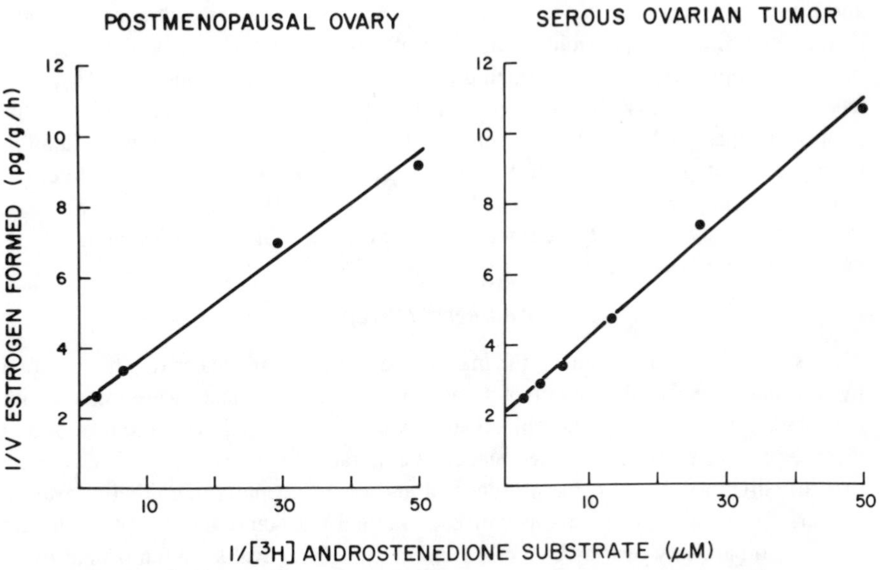

Fig. 8.8. Aromatase activity in the postmenopausal ovary and in a serous ovarian cancer as measured by the amount of tritiated estrogen formed when tissue specimens were exposed to tritiated androstenedione substrate.

may contribute to the growth of ovarian cancer and, if so, whether such aromatase inhibitors as aminoglutethimide may play a role in the treatment of ovarian cancer.

Luteinizing Hormone-Releasing Factor Analogues

The common epithelial ovarian cancers occur infrequently in young women but dramatically increase in incidence in women over age 45. This observation suggests the possibility that epithelial ovarian cancers may be gonadotropin-dependent. Rajaniemi et al. (1981) identified luteinizing hormone (LH), or human chorionic gonadotropin (HCG), receptors with HCG tagged with Iodine 125 in 38 benign and 26 malignant ovarian tumors. Eighteen percent of all benign and 27% of all malignant tumors were LH (HCG) receptor positive. Four of 12 (33%) benign serous tumors and 3 of 17 (18%) benign mucinous tumors showed definite binding of ^{125}I-labeled HCG. Two Brenner tumors were receptor negative. Three of ten serous cancers, one of three endometrioid, one of four adenocarcinomas, one of two cystadenocarcinomas, and neither of the two mucinous carcinomas bound ^{125}I-labeled HCG. Receptor levels were lower in the cancers than in follicular cells during the menstrual cycle in all but one cancer.

The lack of binding of ^{125}I-labeled HCG to the majority of tumor samples studied might be explained in part by the receptors being occupied or down-regulated by elevated levels of circulating gonadotropins. Heterogeneity of gonadotropin receptor–binding sites has yet to be evaluated, and there is no laboratory evidence establishing epithelial ovarian cancers as gonadotropin-dependent. Nevertheless, the overall poor survival results for patients with ovarian cancer of an advanced stage requires that these observations be further evaluated. The intriguing data of Long and Evans (1963) employing estrogen therapy in ovarian cancer treatment has yet to be duplicated, but the possible mechanism of estrogen action may be the reduction of gonadotropin secretion. Luteinizing hormone-releasing hormone (LHRH) agonists have been successfully employed in managing prostatic cancer (LaBrie, Dupont, and Belanger 1985). These agents decrease serum LH and follicle-stimulating hormone or antagonize gonadotropin action. Thus, LHRH agonists appear to effect a medical hypophysectomy selective for gonadotropins. It would be appropriate at this time to institute phase II clinical trials with LHRH agonists for managing advanced recurrent ovarian cancers.

Androgen Therapy

A possible role for androgens in the management of ovarian cancer was first studied by Kaufman (1966). Six patients with advanced recurrent cancer were treated with unspecified androgens, but no objective responses were noted. The author reported that the patients probably received inadequate therapy. Friberg et al. (1978) were the first investigators to report the presence of androgen receptors in epithelial ovarian cancers. Each of three mucinous cancers sampled had androgen receptors, as did one of two papillary ovarian cancers. Galli et al. (1981) evaluated ten primary epithelial ovarian cancer samples and identified androgen receptors in eight (80%). Eleven of 13 (85%) tissue samples from normal ovaries and each of five benign ovarian tumors contained androgen receptors (Galli et al. 1981). A role for androgen therapy in the management of epithelial ovarian cancer remains to be established. The presence of androgen receptors would support in vitro studies of human ovarian cancers as the first step in determining whether androgens have possible efficacy in treating epithelial ovarian cancers.

Corticosteroid Therapy

Scant literature exists regarding the use of corticosteroids in the treatment of patients with epithelial ovarian cancers. Kaufman (1966), in a broad review of the management of ovarian cancer, indicated that eight patients with very advanced disease had been unsuccessfully treated with corticosteroids at the Memorial Hospital–Sloan-Kettering Institute. A study of the occurrence of multiple steroid hormone receptors in disease-free and neoplastic human ovary (Galli et al. 1981) revealed corticosteroid receptors to be present in 12 of 13 (92%) normal (disease-free) ovaries, 2 of 4 (50%) benign ovarian tumors, and 8 of 9 (89%) primary ovarian cancers. In vitro studies of human ovarian cancers and of their response to corticosteroid therapy would be highly appropriate in helping to assess the possible role of corticosteroids in managing epithelial ovarian cancers.

Radiolabeled Estrogen Therapy

The identification of cytosol estrogen receptor proteins in approximately 50% of epithelial ovarian cancers (Schwartz et al. 1982b) and the synthesis of a gamma-emitting estrogen (16α-^{125}I-iodoestradiol) (Hochberg 1979) that bound with high affinity to the estrogen receptor led us to initiate a study at Yale University School of Medicine to determine whether such a compound might be useful in imaging estrogen receptor–rich cancers and subsequently might have a therapeutic role in managing these cancers. Eleven patients with epithelial ovarian cancers undergoing surgery for clinical indications had 0.3 mCi of 16α-^{125}I-iodoestradiol injected, and at specific times after administration of the tracer, portions of the cancer, control tissues (muscle, fat), and blood were removed and radioactivity counted. There was a strong correlation ($p < .005$) between estrogen receptor concentration in the cancer specimens and the amount of radioactivity. There was no correlation between the isotope in muscle and the cancer receptor and, as would be expected, none between the radioactivity in the tumor and that in fat or muscle. A substantial proportion (approximately 30%) of the radioactivity was present in the nuclear compartment of the cancers, consistent with a steroid receptor–mediated process. The nuclear radioactivity in the cancers correlated directly with their receptor content. Unfortunately, blood concentrations of radioactivity were high because circulating levels of the injected steroid metabolites produced low cancer-to-blood ratios. Rapid liver metabolism of this compound and an active enterohepatic circulation in humans precludes using this compound for routine imaging of estrogen receptor–rich cancers. The synthesis of 16α-iodoestradiol analogues that are sterically protected against inactivation by rapid metabolism may lead to compounds that will be of value for diagnostic imaging of estrogen receptor–rich ovarian cancers and subsequently for therapeutic purposes (Hochberg et al. 1985).

Conclusions

The efficacy of hormonal therapy in managing epithelial ovarian cancers has yet to be established; however, the inability to translate high objective response rates with cytotoxic chemotherapy regimens into high five-year disease-free survival rates justifies continued research in evaluating hormonal therapy for patients with epithelial ovarian cancers. Selected tumors (e.g., well-differentiated endometrioid carcinomas) might be as sensitive to hormonal therapy as to cytotoxic chemotherapy. Measurements of estrogen and progestin receptors might help to identify such patients, and these individuals might avoid the significant untoward side effects of cytotoxic chemotherapy. We are currently evaluating the combination of tamoxifen with standard cytotoxic chemotherapy for the treatment of advanced epithelial ovarian cancer. The role of LHRH agonists, androgens, and corticosteroids must be further evaluated in vitro before clinical trials. The clinical efficacy of hormonal therapy may not be defined until hormonal treatment is used as part of the initial treatment for patients with ovarian cancers. In the case of progestins, the scant data cited above suggest that they should be further evaluated as part of primary therapy for patients with epithelial ovarian cancers.

References

Aabo K, Pedersen AG, Hald I, Dombernowsky P. 1982. High dose medroxyprogesterone acetate (MPA) in advanced chemotherapy-resistant ovarian carcinoma: A phase II study. *Cancer Treat Rep* 66:407–408.

Ahlgren JD, Thomas D, Ellison N, Huberman N, Harvey J, Freeman A, Wilosky T, Gillings D, Zaloudek C, Browder H, Noble S. 1985. Phase II evaluation of high dose megestrol acetate in advanced refractory ovarian cancer (abstract). *Proceedings of the American Society of Clinical Oncology* 4:124.

Benraad TJ, Friberg LG, Koenders AJM, Kullander S. 1980. Do estrogen and progesterone receptors (E_2R and PR) in metastasizing endometrial cancers predict the response to gestagen therapy? *Acta Obstet Gynecol Scand* 59:155–159.

Bergqvist A, Kullander S, Thorell J. 1981. A study of estrogen and progesterone cytosol receptor concentration in benign and malignant ovarian tumors and a review of malignant ovarian tumors treated with medroxyprogesterone acetate. *Acta Obstet Gynecol Scand [Suppl]* 101:75–81.

Ehrlich CE, Young PEM, Cleary RE. 1981. Cytoplasmic progesterone and estradiol receptors in normal, hyperplastic and carcinomatous endometria: Therapeutic implications. *Am J Obstet Gynecol* 141:539–546.

Fisher B, Redmond C, Brown A, Wickerham DL, Wolmark N, Allegra J, Escher G, Lippman M, Savlov E, Wittliff J, Fisher ER. 1983. Influence of tumor estrogen and progesterone receptor levels on the response to tamoxifen and chemotherapy in primary breast cancer. *J Clin Oncol* 1:227–240.

Friberg LG, Kullander S, Persijn JP, Korsten CB. 1978. On receptors for estrogen (E_2) and androgens (DHT) in human endometrial carcinoma and ovarian tumors. *Acta Obstet Gynecol Scand* 57:261–264.

Galli MC, DeGiovanni C, Micoletti G, Grilli S, Nanni P, Prodi G, Gola G, Rocchetta R, Orlandi C. 1981. The occurrence of multiple steroid hormone receptors in disease-free and neoplastic human ovary. *Cancer* 47:1297–1302.

Geisler HE. 1983. Megestrol acetate for the palliation of advanced ovarian carcinoma. *Obstet Gynecol* 61:95–98.

Geisler HE. 1985. The use of high-dose megestrol acetate in the treatment of ovarian adenocarcinoma. *Semin Oncol* 12:20–22.

Hochberg RB. 1979. Iodine-125-labelled estradiol: A gamma-emitting analog of estradiol that binds to the estrogen receptor. *Science* 205:1138–1140.

Hochberg RB, MacLusky NJ, Chambers J, Eisenfeld AJ, Naftolin F, Schwartz PE. 1985. Concentration of (16α-^{125}I) iodoestradiol in human ovarian tumors *in vivo* and correlation with estrogen receptor content. *Steroids* 46:775–788.

Holt JA, Caputo TA, Kelly KM, Greenwald P, Chorost S. 1979. Estrogen and progestin binding in cytosols of ovarian adenocarcinomas. *Obstet Gynecol* 53:51–55.

Horwitz KB, McGuire WL, Pearson OH, Segaloff A. 1975. Predicting response to endocrine therapy in human breast cancer: A hypothesis. *Science* 189:726–727.

Jensen EV, Smith S, DeSombre ER. 1976. Hormone dependency in breast cancer. *J Steroid Biochem* 7:911–916.

Johnson BL, Fisher RI, Bender RA, DeVita VT Jr, Chabner BA, Young RC. 1978. Hexamethylmelamine in alkylating agent resistant ovarian cancer. *Cancer* 42:2157–2161.

Jolles B. 1962. Progesterone in the treatment of advanced malignant tumors of breast, ovary and uterus. *Br J Cancer* 16:209–221.

Jolles CJ, Freedman RS, Jones LA. 1983. Estrogen and progestogen therapy in advanced ovarian cancer: Preliminary report. *Gynecol Oncol* 16:352–359.

Kahanpaa KV, Karkkainen J, Nieminen U. 1982. Multi-agent chemotherapy with and without medroxyprogesterone acetate in the treatment of advanced ovarian cancer. *Excerpta Medica International Congress Series* 611:477–482.

Kaufman RJ. 1966. Management of advanced ovarian carcinoma. *Med Clin North Am* 50:845–856.

Kelley R, Baker WH. 1961. Progestational agents in the treatment of carcinoma of the endometrium. *N Engl J Med* 264:216.

Knight WA, Livingston RB, Gregory EJ, McGuire WL. 1977. Estrogen receptor as an independent prognostic factor for early recurrence in breast cancer. *Cancer Res* 37:4669–4671.

LaBrie F, Dupont A, Belanger A. 1985. Complete androgen blockade for the treatment of prostatic cancer. In *Important Advances in Oncology 1985*, ed. VT DeVita Jr, S Hellman, SA Rosenberg, pp. 193–217. Philadelphia: J. B. Lippincott.

Lazo JS, Schwartz PE, MacLusky NJ, Labaree DC, Eisenfeld AJ. 1984. Antiproliferative actions of tamoxifen to human carcinomas in vitro. *Cancer Res* 44:2266–2271.

Legha SS, Davis HL, Muggia FM. 1978. Hormonal therapy of breast cancer: New approaches and concepts. *Ann Intern Med* 88:69–77.

Long RTL, Evans AM. 1963. Diethylstilbestrol as a chemotherapeutic agent for ovarian carcinoma. *Mo Med* 60:1125–1127.

Malkasian GD, Decker DG, Jorgensen EO, Edmonson H. 1977. Medroxyprogesterone acetate for the treatment of metastatic and recurrent ovarian carcinoma. *Cancer Treat Rep* 61:913–914.

Malkasian GD, Decker DG, Jorgensen LO, Webb MJ. 1973. 6-Dehydro-6,17α-dimethylprogesterone (NSC123018) for the treatment of metastatic and recurrent ovarian carcinoma. *Cancer Chemother Rep* 57:241–242.

Mangioni C, Franceschi S, LaVecchia C, D'Incalci M. 1981. High-dose medroxyprogesterone acetate (MPA) in advanced epithelial ovarian cancer resistant to first- or second-line chemotherapy. *Gynecol Oncol* 12:314.

Martin PM, Rolland PH, Gammerre M, Serment H, Toga M. 1981. Estradiol and progesterone receptors in normal and neoplastic endometrium: Correlations between receptors, histopathological examination and clinical responses under progestin therapy. *Int J Cancer* 23:321–329.

Ozols RF, Hogan WM, Ostchega Y, Young RC. 1983. MVP (mitomycin, vinblastine, and progesterone): A second-line regimen in ovarian cancer with a high incidence of pulmonary toxicity. *Cancer Treat Rep* 67:721–722.

Pesando JM, Come SE, Parker LM. 1979. *Cis*-diamminedichloroplatinum (CDDP) therapy of advanced ovarian cancer (abstract). *Proceedings of the American Association for Cancer Research* 20:378.

Rajaniemi H, Kauppila A, Ronnberg L, Selander K, Pystynen P. 1981. LH (HCG) receptor in benign and malignant tumors of human ovary. *Acta Obstet Gynecol Scand [Suppl]* 101: 83–86.

Rendina GM, Donadio C, Giovannini M. 1982. Steroid receptors and progestinic therapy in ovarian endometrioid carcinoma. *Eur J Gynaecol Oncol* 3:241–246.

Schwartz PE, Eisenfeld A. 1978. Steroid receptor proteins in epithelial ovarian cancer. Paper presented at the Ninth Annual Meeting of the Felix Rutledge Society, 21–24 June, Washington, D.C.

Schwartz PE, Keating G, MacLusky NJ, Naftolin F, Eisenfeld A. 1982a. Tamoxifen therapy for advanced ovarian cancer. *Obstet Gynecol* 59:583–588.

Schwartz PE, LiVolsi VA, Hildreth N, MacLusky NJ, Naftolin FN, Eisenfeld AJ. 1982b. Estrogen receptors in human ovarian epithelial carcinoma. *Obstet Gynecol* 59:229–238.

Schwartz PE, Merino MJ, LiVolsi VA, Lawrence R, MacLusky N, Eisenfeld A. 1985. Histopathologic correlations of estrogen and progestin receptor protein in epithelial ovarian carcinomas. *Obstet Gynecol* 66:428–433.

Shirey DR, Kavanagh JJ Jr, Gershenson DM, Freedman R, Copeland LJ, Jones LA. 1985. Tamoxifen therapy of epithelial ovarian cancer. *Obstet Gynecol* 66:575–578.

Slayton RE, Pagano M, Creech RH. 1981. Progestin therapy for advanced ovarian cancer: A phase II Eastern Cooperative Oncology Group trial. *Cancer Treat Rep* 65:895–896.

Stanhope RC, Smith JP, Rutledge F. 1977. Second trial drugs in ovarian cancer. *Gynecol Oncol* 5:52–58.

Timothy I. 1982. Progestogen therapy for ovarian carcinoma. *Br J Obstet Gynaecol* 89: 561–563.

Trope C, Johnson JE, Sigurdsson K, Simonsen E. 1982. High-dose medroxyprogesterone acetate for the treatment of advanced ovarian carcinoma. *Cancer Treat Rep* 66:1441–1443.

Varga A, Henriksen E. 1964. Effect of 17-alpha-hydroxyprogesterone 17-n-caproate on various pelvic malignancies. *Obstet Gynecol* 23:51–62.

Voit R, MacLusky NJ, Schwartz PE, Eisenfeld AJ, Naftolin F. 1982. Aromatase activity in ovarian cancer (abstract). In *Society of Gynecologic Investigation Scientific Abstracts*, p. 138. New York: Society of Gynecologic Investigation.

Ward HW. 1972. Progestogen therapy for ovarian carcinoma. *Journal of Obstetrics and Gynaecology of the British Commonwealth*. 79:555–559.

Wharton JT, Edwards CL, Rutledge FN. 1984. Long-term survival after chemotherapy for advanced epithelial ovarian cancer. *Am J Obstet Gynecol* 148:997–1005.

Annual Clinical Conference on Cancer, Vol. 29
Gynecologic Cancer: Diagnosis and Treatment Strategies
© 1987 by The University of Texas System Cancer Center

9. Comparison of Immunologic and Steroid-Binding Assays for Estrogen Receptors in Human Ovarian Carcinomas

Lovell A. Jones, Michael F. Press, John A. Holt, H. Stephen Gallager, Ralph S. Freedman, and Creighton L. Edwards

The role of estrogen receptors (ER) and progesterone receptors (PR) in the management of gynecologic malignancies has begun to interest a number of investigators over the last few years (DeSombre et al. 1984; Freedman et al. 1986). Studies in our laboratory and others have demonstrated the presence of ER and PR in a large proportion of gynecologic malignancies, particularly in ovarian and endometrial carcinomas (Holt et al. 1979; Hoffman et al. 1980; Bergqvist, Kullander, and Thorell 1981; Ehrlich, Young, and Cleary 1981; Jones et al. 1983; Richardson and MacLaughlin 1983). Since gynecologic tissues, like breast tissue, are targets for steroid hormones, the presence of these receptors suggests that hormonal therapy may be useful in the clinical management of gynecologic malignancies.

Cancer of the ovary yields the highest death rate of all gynecologic cancers (Beral 1980). Although surgical techniques have improved and more effective chemotherapy is available, the mortality for the disease has not changed significantly over the past half century (Saul 1984). Ovarian cancer still claims more lives than endometrial and cervical cancers combined (Rosenshein and Rotmensch 1982). One in 70 women will develop this disease, making it the second most common gynecologic cancer (Bagshawe, Wass, and Searle 1980; Rosenshein and Rotmensch 1982).

The majority of patients with carcinoma of the ovary present with disease in an advanced state, when only palliative treatment is possible. The development in recent years of highly effective combination chemotherapy for advanced or recurrent ovarian carcinoma has markedly enhanced the frequency with which patients achieve complete clinical remission. Although a significant number of these patients experience remissions of several years and a few are even cured, the majority of patients either fail to respond to treatment or relapse after an initial regression of the disease. These patients will eventually die of recurrent disease. Therefore, it is important to identify a more effective form of therapy for such patients.

The fact that ovarian tumors contain ER and PR strongly suggests that hormonal therapy might offer a valid approach to treatment. However, only a few attempts have been made to correlate response with receptor status (Bergqvist, Kullander, and Thorell 1981; Creasman et al. 1981; Schwartz et al. 1982; Kauppila et al. 1983; Kauppila 1984; Freedman et al. 1986), and most of these looked at the frequency of ER and PR in tumors. A recent review by Thigpen et al. (1984) reported that, in 176 nonselected patients with advanced ovarian carcinoma who were treated with progestins in 10 different series, 22 objective responses were observed, yielding an overall response rate of approximately 12%. Most responses occurred in patients with serous or endometrioid histology. However, no conclusion regarding response duration, optimal choice of progestin, or dose-response relationship could be drawn from an analysis of available data.

A second set of compounds summarized in the same review (Thigpen et al. 1984) included triphenylethylene antiestrogens such as MER-25, clomiphene citrate, nafoxidine, and tamoxifen citrate. The demonstrated efficacy of tamoxifen citrate in breast carcinoma suggests that the antiestrogens might be an effective alternative to progestins in ovarian cancer. Although a few studies suggested that, analogous to breast cancer, ER–rich epithelial ovarian carcinomas might theoretically respond to antiestrogen therapy (Schwartz et al. 1982), recent studies in our laboratory indicate that tamoxifen produces only stability of the malignancy (Shirey et al. 1985), not complete or partial response as reported by others.

A common deficiency in most hormonal therapy studies is lack of adequate ER and PR information. In addition, the numbers of patients included in these trials have been too small to allow definitive conclusions regarding patient survival, disease-free intervals, or histological patterns. The suggested correlation between response and presence of ER and PR still raises the possibility of hormonal manipulation as a possible treatment. Several papers have appeared reporting the use of either estrogen or antiestrogen to increase synthesis of PR in both ovarian and endometrial carcinomas (Mortel et al. 1981; Jolles, Freedman, and Jones 1983; Carlson et al. 1984; Hamilton et al. 1984). The use of progestin therapy alone has produced varying results. One reason for this may rest with the effect of progestins on PR. Janne et al. (1980) have shown that four weeks of medroxyprogesterone acetate treatment alone significantly reduces the level of both ER and PR. Data that we will present, as well as findings of others, suggest that, to achieve full benefit from long-term progestin therapy, periodic treatment with estrogen or antiestrogen be used in conjunction with progestins (Jolles, Freedman, and Jones 1983; Hamilton et al. 1984; Freedman et al. 1986). Therefore, it appears that effective use of progestin therapy may rest on use of both estrogen and progestins. For this reason alone, further evaluation of combination hormonal therapy is warranted.

The recent production of a series of monoclonal antibodies against ER and PR from cytosolic extracts of MCF-7 human breast carcinoma cell lines (Greene et al. 1980; Geoffrey L. Greene and Michael F. Press, University of Chicago, personal communication, September 1985) may provide a new approach for characterizing ER and PR in neoplastic tissues. The monoclonal antibodies for ER recognize both estrogen-occupied and unoccupied receptors in different target tissues from a variety of mammals, including humans (Greene 1984; King and Greene 1984). This may allow the detection of the presence of ER and PR on tumor specimens too small to be analyzed by previous methods.

Materials and Methods

Estrogen receptor titers were obtained on a total of 87 ovarian tumor samples. Histologically, the 87 ovarian tumor samples reported here included 47 serous, 3 mixed, 9 mucinous, 11 endometrioid, 8 adeno-, 2 undifferentiated, and 3 stromal tumors, as well as 1 mixed teratoma, 1 teratoma, and 2 fibromas. The ER titers are summarized in table 9.1. Of those samples measured by biochemical analysis, 17 were measured by both an immunocytochemical and an immunobead analysis using a monoclonal antibody specific for ER (kindly provided by Dr. Geoffrey L. Greene, Ben May Laboratory for Cancer Research, University of Chicago, Chicago, Illinois).

Biochemical Receptor Assays

Biochemical receptor determinations were performed according to a previously published methodology (Jones et al. 1983). In brief, frozen tissue was powdered in a Thermovac stainless steel autopulverizer; the powder was weighed and added to ice-cold 0.01 M Tris-HCl/0.0015 M EDTA buffer (pH 7.4, room temperature) containing 0.5 mM dithiothreitol and 20 mM sodium molybdate with 10% glycerol (TEDG). The pulverized tissue was homogenized two times for ten seconds each with one-minute cooling periods, using a Polytron tissue homogenizer with a rheostat setting of 7. Fresh specimens were homogenized in 0.01 M TEDG buffer with an all-glass Kontes homogenizer with a motor-driven pestle.

Homogenates were centrifuged in a J6B Beckman low-speed centrifuge at 3,000 rpm for ten minutes at 2° C. The pellets were washed twice with 0.01 M TEDG buffer, and the supernatant from each spin was added to the 3,000-rpm supernatant. The pooled crude cytosol was centrifuged in an L5–65B ultracentrifuge at 50,000 rpm for one hour (2° C) using a Beckman type 65 rotor. The final concentration was made to equal 100 mg/ml by adding the appropriate amount of 0.01 M TEDG buffer.

Biochemical determination of cytosolic ER was performed by a G-25 Sephadex filtration assay (Jones et al. 1983). The assay was carried out by adding varying concentrations of ^{3}H-estradiol (E_2) dissolved in 200-proof ethanol along with 0.01 ml propylene glycol to 12 (75 mm) disposable test tubes that had been previously baked at 500° F for three to four hours. In addition, unlabeled 5α-dihydrotestosterone (DHT), 200 times the concentration of the $^3HE_2$, was added to each test tube. The ethanol was then evaporated under a stream of prepurified nitrogen. Cytosol (0.02 ml) was added and the tubes then incubated at 4° C for at least two hours. After incubation, an aliquot (0.02 ml) was removed to determine the concentration of ^{3}H-ligand present in each tube. The amount of bound ligand was determined by applying 100 μl to individual G-25 Sephadex columns (5″ Dispo pipettes). After a 40-μl TEDG buffer wash, 300 μl of TED (without glycerol) buffer was added and then the eluant was discarded. The bound ligand was eluted with 700 μl of TED buffer directly into 5-ml mini-vials.

Every assay was run with a control standard with a known ER titer. Our standards were made from human myoma. Our experience with this tissue has been quite satisfactory. Receptor results indicate that ER and PR titers remain stable for more than

Table 9.1. *Histology and Biochemical ER Content in Relation to Percentage of Tumor in Ovarian Cancers*

Tumor Histology	Cytosolic ER[a]	Percentage Tumor Content[b]
1. Serous	27.8	87
2. Endometrioid	38.2	90
3. Endometrioid	8.7	33
4. Serous	1.1	90
5. Mucinous	2.0	30
6. Serous	<1.0	0
7. Serous	<1.0	98
8. Mixed	25.6	39
9. Serous	8.4	75
10. Serous	8.8	77
11. Endometrioid	5.2	80
12. Mucinous	67.2	53
13. Mixed	7.9	61
14. Serous	2.4	25
15. Serous	2.3	80
16. Endometrioid	<1.0	8
17. Mucinous	<1.0	24
18. Serous	18.3	85
19. Mucinous	3.6	30
20. Serous	16.5	10
21. Serous	13.8	75
22. Serous	4.2	67
23. Serous	32.5	37
24. Serous	14.3	80
25. Mucinous	3.6	20
26. Serous	1.5	70
27. Serous	6.1	75
28. Serous	5.3	40
29. Mucinous	9.2	<1
30. Endometrioid	45.4	20
31. Mixed teratoma	<1.0	0
32. Endometrioid	1759.4[c]	90
33. Serous	135.4	80
34. Gran cell	70.5	60
35. Serous	48.8	60
36. OV fibroma	26.7	0
37. Adeno	19.2	75
38. Endometrioid	18.2	50
39. Serous	15.0	20
40. Serous	14.3	80
41. Serous	9.1	10
42. Serous	8.5	38
43. Adeno	8.1	38
44. Serous	6.1	40
45. Endometrioid	3.7	90
46. Serous	2.8	13
47. Adeno	2.5	50
48. Serous	1.4	13
49. Adeno	<1.0	30
50. Serous	3.2	40
51. Serous	<1.0	75

Table 9.1. (*continued*)

Tumor Histology	Cytosolic ER[a]	Percentage Tumor Content[b]
52. Endometrioid	846.5	50
53. Mixed	5.4	50
54. Serous	2.0	0
55. Serous	7.0	32
56. Serous	7.9	25
57. Serous	1.7	0
58. Mucinous	4.7	52
59. Serous	15.4	27
60. Serous	13.8	10
61. Serous	9.1	30
62. Endometrioid	6.3	75
63. Serous	9.1	<1
64. Serous	10.2	60
65. Serous	<1.0	80
66. Gran cell	13.1	—[d]
67. Serous	9.1	20
68. OV fibroma	<1.0	90
69. Serous	8.1	20
70. Teratoma	17.3	100
71. Stromal, gran cell	6.4	11
72. Serous	5.3	90
73. Serous	6.4	—
74. Serous	20.0	—
75. Adeno	16.0	—
76. Adeno	2.3	—
77. Serous	103.2	—
78. Undifferentiated	322.2	—
79. Adeno	9.7	—
80. Endometrioid	9.6	95
81. Serous	25.9	—
82. Serous	12.5	—
83. Adeno	<1.0	—
84. Serous	6.0	—
85. Mucinous	<1.0	—
86. Undifferentiated OV	<1.0	50
87. Mucinous	3.5	—

Note: ER, estrogen receptor; OV, ovarian; gran cell, granulosa cell.
[a] Values expressed as fmol/mg cytosol protein.
[b] Percentage tumor in specimen grossly determined by H. Stephen Gallager.
[c] Value expressed as fmol/mg wet tissue weight.
[d] Insufficient tissue for analysis by H. Stephen Gallager.

a year when stored at -190° C. Protein and DNA determinations were done using Bradford (1976) methodology and Burton (1956) methodology, respectively.

Binding data were analyzed according to the methods of Scatchard (1949) as modified by Rosenthal (1967). Correction for nonspecific binding was done as previously described by Seematter et al. (1979) and Hoffman et al. (1980). For single-point assays, specific binding was calculated as the difference in bound radioactivity between samples incubated with and without a 100-fold excess of unlabeled hormone.

Immunocytochemical Localization of Estrogen Receptors

The immunocytochemical technique for localizing ER, previously published elsewhere (Press and Greene 1984), was an indirect immunoperoxidase technique using the peroxidase-antiperoxidase technique of Sternberger (1979). Immunocytochemical localization of receptor involved the sequential application of three immune reagents to tissue sections and then incubation in diaminobenzidine-H_20_2 to identify the site of the immunoprecipitate. Each of these steps was followed by extensive washing in phosphate-buffered saline. The first immune reagent, the rat monoclonal antibody to ER (5–20 μg/ml), was applied in excess of the amount of receptor present in the tissue section (approximately 10^{-10} M) (Chamness, Mercer, and McGuire 1980). The second immune reagent was a goat antirat IgG, also called the bridging antibody because it binds both the first rat monoclonal antibody and the third immune reagent, which was a rat peroxidase-antiperoxidase (1:100) (Sternberger 1979). Horseradish peroxidase, present in the peroxidase-antiperoxidase complex, catalyzes the conversion of diaminobenzidine from soluble monomer to insoluble polymer in the presence of H_2O_2. This precipitate is recognized as a brown pigment by light microscopy.

Results and Discussion

All tumors with ER values of more than 1 fmol/mg cytosol protein were considered positive for ER. This definition of positive was arbitrary and based on the sensitivity of the biochemical assay. This approach was initiated because of the lack of sufficient clinical information needed to establish a minimum hormone-responsive ER titer similar to that set for breast cancer. Experiments were also done to compare varying amounts of tumor tissue from the same ovarian carcinoma. It was determined that the ER titer varied according to the percentage of tumor tissue present (Lovell A. Jones, unpublished data). Our initial studies were performed in histological sections and with specimens composed of more than 75% tumor tissue. More than 80% of all documented ovarian tumors assayed had more than 1 fmol ER/mg cytosol protein. Approximately 35% of the ovarian tumor samples assayed had 10 or more fmol ER/mg cytosol protein.

So far, the receptor results obtained by the different receptor assays correlate very well. Comparison of cytosolic ER content with immunocytochemical staining intensity (−, +, ++, +++) for ER can be correlated with increasing ER content by biochemical assay. Interestingly, no tumor with a titer greater than 20 fmol/mg cytosol protein was observed to be ER negative using the immunocytochemical localization of ER by monoclonal antibody. As shown in table 9.2, attempts are being made to establish range correlations. In addition, some of the cytosolic and nuclear extracts were also assayed, using an enzyme-linked immunosorbent assay (ELISA) incorporating monoclonal antibodies to ER. These results are summarized in table 9.3. Comparison of cytosolic ER content with staining intensity indicates

Table 9.2. *Comparison of Radioligand Assay and Immunologic Assay for Estrogen Receptors*

Titer Ranges (fmol/mg Cytosol Protein)	Staining Intensity[a] –	+	++	+++
<10	21 (66)	7 (22)	3 (9)	1 (3)
11–30	(0)	5 (38.5)	3 (23)	5 (38.5)
31–100	(0)	2 (40)	(0)	3 (60)
>100	— —	— —	— —	1 (100)

[a]Number of specimens (%).

Table 9.3. *Comparison of Biochemical, Immunocytochemical, ELISA, and Pathological Analysis of Ovarian Tumors*

Tumor Histology	Stage, Grade	CytER[a]	ImmunocytER Int	ImmunocytER fac (%)	ImmunocytER Tumor (%)[b]	EIA[c] ERc	EIA[c] ERn	Tumor (%)[d]
Ser	III, 3	8.4	–	0	20	821	33	75
Endo OV	—	5.2	+++	—	—	109	136	80
Endo OV	III, 3	<1	+++	77	8	21	0	5
Ser, adeno, OV	IV, 3	16.5	+	8	13	107	11	10
Adeno	III, 2	1,759.4[c]	+	29	67	1,737	167	90
Ser	III, 2	135.4	+++	72	84	4,368	48	80
Ser, adeno	III, 3	48.8	+++	74	54	1,832	242	60
OV fibroma	—	26.7	–	0	0	—	8	0
Adeno	III, 3	19.2	+	2	44	274	30	75
Endo	IV, 3	18.2	+++	54	11	295	23	50
Ser	III, 3	15.0	+++	75	64	2,046	52	20
Ser, adeno	III, 3	14.3	++	59	98	4,454	561	80
Ser, adeno	IIIB	9.1	–	0	11	27	11	10
Ser, cystad	III, 2	6.1	–	0	36	103	13	40
Endo	IA, 2	3.7	+	36	86	404	157	90
Adeno	III, 3	2.5	–	0	65	179	10	50
Adeno	III, 3	<1	+	55	14	397	146	30

Note: ELISA, enzyme-linked immunosorbent assay; ser, serous; endo, endometrioid; OV, ovarian; cystad, cystadenoma; cytER, biochemically determined ER; immunocytER, immunocytochemically determined ER; int, staining intensity; fac (%), percentage of tumor cells stained; EIA, estrogen immunobead assay; ERc, cytosolic estrogen receptors; ERn, nuclear extract estrogen receptors.
[a]Values expressed as fmol/mg cytosol protein.
[b]Percentage of tumor cells in specimen.
[c]Values expressed as fmol/g tissue.
[d]Percentage of tumor in specimen grossly determined by H. Stephen Gallager.

that, as staining intensity increases, cytosolic ER content by biochemical assay increases. In addition, comparison of cytosolic ER content also correlates with proportion of tumor cells immunocytochemically stained. Still unknown is how well both of these determinations correlated with hormonal therapy.

At the same time that we began our studies on ER in ovarian cancers, a clinical protocol based on the role that estrogen plays with regard to increased synthesis of

PR was initiated. Present results with the hormonal protocol indicate that sequential and combined administration of ethinyl estradiol and medroxyprogesterone acetate may offer an alternative to ovarian carcinoma patients who have failed optimum first-line chemotherapy. At present, 65 patients with advanced ovarian cancer have been registered in the study; of these, 17 were less than 50 years of age and therefore were considered premenopausal. In these patients, serous carcinoma was the most common histological type of tumor, with ten patients having endometrioid tumors. The initial group of patients with advanced ovarian cancer in our hormonal therapy study received ethinyl estradiol at a dose of 100 μg daily on days 1 through 25, and 50 μg of medroxyprogesterone acetate twice a day on days 8 through 25. No treatment was administered on days 26 through 30, and then the cycle was repeated. After the first 37 patients had been treated, a second protocol was started with the dose of ethinyl estradiol being reduced to 50 μg daily, whereas the dose of medroxyprogesterone acetate was increased to 50 mg four times a day. The treatment schedule remained the same.

To date, 28 patients have been treated utilizing this protocol. Statistical analysis found no differences between the two protocol treatment dosages in terms of response rate and survival; therefore, the data have been pooled. Unfortunately, ER titer determinations were made in only 17 of the initial cases. Based on 51 patients who have completed at least one full course of treatment, there was an 18% response rate, with 25% of the patients having stable disease and 57% showing progression (table 9.4). Older patients and those without ascites or intestinal dysfunction appear to be better candidates for this line of treatment. Of interest is the fact that only patients who had ER determinations of greater than 10 fmol/mg cytosol protein and PR determinations of greater than 25 fmol/mg cytosol protein responded to hormonal therapy (data not shown). Unfortunately, the number of patients who had ER determinations prior to hormonal therapy was small, but the results are supportive of further study. The mean survival is presently 5.2 months for

Table 9.4. *Response to Ethinyl Estradiol and Medroxyprogesterone Acetate*

		Numerators and Percentages			
		CR	PR	NC	PD
Denominators	*N*	*N* (%)	*N* (%)	*N* (%)	*N* (%)
Registered and treated	65				
Treatment no. 1	37	1 (3)	5 (13)	7 (19)	24 (65)
Treatment no. 2	28	0 (0)	3 (11)	6 (21)	19 (68)
Total		1 (2)	8 (12)	13 (20)	43 (66)
Registered and adequately treated	51[a]				
Treatment no. 1	30	(3)	(17)	(23)	17 (57)
Treatment no. 2	21	(0)	(14)	(29)	12 (57)
Total		(2)	(16)	(25)	(57)

Note: CR, complete response; PR, partial response; NC, no change; PD, progressive disease.
[a]14 patients unable to complete one course because of toxicity or disease progression.

the entire group, 13.6 months for the responding patients, 7.9 months for the patients with stable disease, and 3.7 months for the patients with progressive disease.

Summary

Thus, the presence of ER in ovarian cancers may serve as a marker of responsiveness to hormonal therapy. More than 35% of all ovarian tumors analyzed in our study had an ER titer above 10 fmol/mg cytosol protein. Immunocytochemical results indicate that the ER are localized in the nuclei of tumor cells from all types of ovarian cancers, and that nuclear localization correlates with biochemical ER determinations. As with breast cancer, histological determination of the percentage of tumor present in a specimen is required for accurate evaluation of ER determinations. Also as with breast cancer, there may be a need in the near future to analyze all ovarian tumor specimens for the presence of steroid receptors.

Acknowledgments

The authors gratefully acknowledge the technical assistance of Shahram Badrei, Joan Rooke, Wanza Scott, Mei Tan, Ronnie Van Dam, and Robert P. Verjan. This investigation was supported in part by Public Health Service grants CA 31382 and CA 27476, the National Cancer Institute, National Institutes of Health, U.S. Department of Health and Human Services.

References

Bagshawe KD, Wass M, Searle F. 1980. Markers in gynaecological cancer. *Arch Gynecol* 229:303–310.

Beral VJ. 1980. Menopausal oestrogen use and breast cancer (letter). *Br Med J [Clin Res]* 281:1638.

Bergqvist A, Kullander S, Thorell J. 1981. A study of estrogen and progesterone cytosol receptor concentration in benign and malignant ovarian tumors and a review of malignant ovarian tumors treated with medroxyprogesterone acetate. *Acta Obstet Gynecol Scand [Suppl]* 101:75–81.

Bradford MM. 1976. A rapid sensitive method for quantitation of protein using the principle of protein dye binding. *Anal Biochem* 72:248–254.

Burton K. 1956. A study of the conditions and mechanism of the diphenylamine reaction for the colorimetric estimation of deoxyribonucleic acid. *Biochem J* 62:315–326.

Carlson JA, Allegra JC, Day TG, Wittliff JL. 1984. Tamoxifen and endometrial carcinoma: Alterations in estrogen and progesterone receptors in untreated patients and combination hormonal therapy in advanced neoplasia. *Am J Obstet Gynecol* 149:149–153.

Chamness GC, Mercer WD, McGuire WL. 1980. Are histochemical methods for estrogen receptor valid? *J Histochem Cytochem* 28:792–797.

Creasman WT, Sasso RA, Weed JC Jr, McCarty KS Jr. 1981. Ovarian carcinoma: Histologic and clinical correlation of cytoplasmic estrogen and progesterone binding. *Gynecol Oncol* 12:319–327.

DeSombre ER, Greene GL, King WJ, Jensen EV. 1984. Estrogen receptors, antibodies, and hormone-dependent cancer. In *Progress in Clinical and Biological Research: Hormones and Cancer*, ed. E Gurpide, R Calandra, C Levy, R Soto, vol. 142, pp. 1–21. New York: Alan R. Liss.

Ehrlich CE, Young PC, Cleary RE. 1981. Cytoplasmic progesterone and estradiol receptors in normal, hyperplastic, and carcinomatous endometria: Therapeutic implications. *Am J Obstet Gynecol* 141:539–546.

Freedman RS, Saul PB, Edwards CL, Jolles CJ, Gershenson DM, Jones LA, Atkinson N, Dana WJ. 1986. Ethinyl estradiol and medroxyprogesterone acetate in patients with epithelial ovarian carcinoma: A phase II study. *Cancer Treat Rep* 70:369–373.

Greene GL. 1984. Application of immunocytochemical techniques to the analysis of estrogen receptor structure and function. In *Biochemical Actions of Hormones*, ed. G Litwack, vol. 2, pp. 207–239. New York: Academic Press.

Greene GL, Nolan C, Engler JP, Jensen EV. 1980. Monoclonal antibodies to human estrogen receptor. *Proc Natl Acad Sci USA* 77:5115–5119.

Hamilton TC, Young RC, Louie KG, Behrens BC, McKoy WM, Grotzinger KR, Ozols RF. 1984. Characteristics of a xenograft model of human ovarian carcinoma which produces ascites and intraabdominal carcinomatosis in mice. *Cancer Res* 44:5286–5290.

Hoffman PG, Jones LA, Kuhn RW, Siiteri PK. 1980. Progesterone receptors: Saturation analysis by a solid-phase hydroxylapatite adsorption technique. *Cancer* 46:2801–2804.

Hoffman PG, Siiteri PK. 1980. Sex steroid receptors in gynecologic cancer: A review. *Obstet Gynecol* 55:648–652.

Holt JA, Caputo TA, Kelly KM, Greenwald P, Chorost S. 1979. Estrogen and progestin binding in cytosols of ovarian endocarcinomas. *Obstet Gynecol* 53:50–58.

Janne O, Kauppila A, Syrjala P, Vihko R. 1980. Comparison of cytosol estrogen and progestin receptor status in malignant and benign tumors and tumor-like lesions of human ovary. *Int J Cancer* 25:175–179.

Jolles C, Freedman R, Jones LA. 1983. Estrogen and progesterone therapy in advanced ovarian cancer: Preliminary report. *Gynecol Oncol* 16:352–359.

Jones LA, Edwards CL, Freedman RS, Tan MT, Gallager HS. 1983. Estrogen and progesterone receptor titers in primary epithelial ovarian carcinomas. *Int J Cancer* 32:567–571.

Kauppila A. 1984. Progestin therapy of endometrial, breast and ovarian carcinoma. *Acta Obstet Gynecol Scand* 63:441–450.

Kauppila A, Vierikko P, Kivinen S, Stenback F, Vihko R. 1983. Clinical significance of estrogen and progestin receptors in ovarian cancer. *Obstet Gynecol* 61:320–326.

King WJ, Greene GL. 1984. Monoclonal antibodies localize estrogen receptors in the nuclei of target cells. *Nature* 307:745–747.

Mortel R, Levy C, Wolff JP, Nicolas JC, Robel P, Baulieu EE. 1981. Female sex steroid receptors in postmenopausal endometrial carcinoma and biochemical response to an antiestrogen. *Cancer Res* 41:1140–1147.

Press MF, Greene GL. 1984. An immunocytochemical method for demonstrating estrogen receptor in human uterus using monoclonal antibodies to human estrophilin. *Lab Invest* 50:480–486.

Richardson GS, MacLaughlin DT. 1983. Hormonal receptors in endometrial and ovarian neoplasia. In *Gynecologic Oncology*, ed. CT Griffiths, AF Fuller, pp. 81–101. Boston: Martinus Nijhoff.

Rosenshein NB, Rotmensch J. 1982. Combating postmenopausal gynecologic malignancy. *Geriatrics* 37:107–110, 115–116.

Rosenthal HE. 1967. A graphic method for the determination and presentation of binding parameters in a complex system. *Anal Biochem* 29:525–532.

Saul P. 1984. *Gynecologic Oncology Medical Student Training Manual*. Houston, Tex.: Department of Gynecology, M. D. Anderson Hospital Press.

Scatchard G. 1949. The attractions of proteins for small molecules and ions. *Ann NY Acad Sci* 51:660–672.

Schwartz PE, Keating G, MacLusky N, Naftolin F, Eisenfeld A. 1982. Tamoxifen therapy for advanced ovarian cancer. *Obstet Gynecol* 59:585–588.
Seematter RJ, Hoffman PG, Kuhn RW, Lockwood LC, Siiteri PK. 1979. Comparison of ^{3}H-progesterone and [6,7-^{3}H]17,21 dimethyl-19-norpregan-4, 9-diene-3, 20-dione for measurement of progesterone receptors in human malignant tissue. *Cancer Res* 38:2800–2805.
Shirey DR, Kavanagh J, Gershenson DM, Freedman RS, Copeland LJ, Jones LA. 1985. Tamoxifen therapy of epithelial ovarian cancer. *Obstet Gynecol* 66:575–578.
Sternberger LA. 1979. *Immunocytochemistry*. Englewood Cliffs, N.J.: Prentice-Hall.
Thigpen JT, Vance RB, Balducci L, Khansur T. 1984. New drugs and experimental approaches in ovarian cancer treatment. *Semin Oncol* 11:314–326.

Annual Clinical Conference on Cancer, Vol. 29
Gynecologic Cancer: Diagnosis and Treatment Strategies
© 1987 by The University of Texas System Cancer Center

10. Natural Killer Cell Antitumor Activity in Patients with Ovarian Carcinoma: Induction of Cytotoxicity by Viral Oncolysates and Interleukin-2

Eva Lotzová, Cherylyn A. Savary, Ralph S. Freedman, and James M. Bowen

One of the major therapeutic modalities for the treatment of patients with ovarian carcinoma is chemotherapy. However, a relatively low percentage of patients (approximately 20%–25%) with late stage ovarian cancer are responsive to this therapy (Silverberg and Lubera 1986). Consequently, it is imperative to investigate new avenues to the treatment of this disease. In recent years it has become quite obvious that the immune system plays an important role in defense against cancer. Moreover, it has been noted by our and other laboratories that patients with ovarian carcinoma experience impaired cell-mediated immunity (Lotzová et al. 1984; Allavena et al. 1981). The latter observation initiated our investigations on the anticancer immunity of patients with ovarian carcinoma and potentiation of such response by biologic response-modifying agents.

We elected to investigate the natural killer (NK) cell-mediated cytotoxicity profile of ovarian cancer patients because this arm of immunity appears to represent an important mechanism in defense against primary and metastatic tumors (Lotzová 1983, 1984; Herberman and Ortaldo 1981). The NK cell-mediated immune mechanism has several advantages over the defense mechanisms represented by T cells and macrophages: (1) NK cells do not require any intentional immunization and specific clone production for tumor-directed cytotoxic function, and thus kill tumor cells promptly; (2) NK cells recognize a broader repertoire of antigenic structures on tumor cells and consequently are independent of tumor-specific antigens, which are quite rarely expressed on most of the human tumors; and (3) NK cells can be grown and propagated in vitro and retain their tumor lytic activity after adoptive transfer in vivo to NK cell-compromised individuals (for review see Lotzová 1984).

Results and Discussion

NK Cell Activity of Ovarian Cancer Patients and Its Potentiation by Viral Oncolysates

Initially, we investigated the NK cell cytotoxic profile in peripheral blood and ascitic fluids of ovarian cancer patients against the highly NK cell–sensitive target cell line, K-562. The NK cytotoxic potential in ascitic fluids was of utmost interest

Table 10.1. *NK Lytic Activity of Normal Donors and Patients with Ovarian Carcinoma*

Source of Effector Cells	Mean $LU_{20}/10^7$ Cells ± S.E.[a]
Peripheral blood	
Normal donors	88.0 ± 15.6 (20)[b]
Cancer patients	29.4 ± 7.9 (17)
Ascitic fluid	
Cancer patients	< 1 (9)

Source: Lotzová et al. 1984.
Note: S.E., standard error.
[a]NK lytic activity against K-562 was measured in a 3-hour ^{51}Cr-release assay. Results are expressed in lytic units ($LU_{20}/10^7$ cells), and calculated by linear regression analysis using 1:50, 1:25, and 1:12 target-to-effector cell ratios.
[b]Number of individuals tested is shown in parentheses.

because this anatomical site coincides with tumor location, and thus more realistically reflects regional antitumor immunity. Results of our studies demonstrated that patients with ovarian cancer displayed low NK cell activity in peripheral blood and virtually no cytotoxicity in ascitic fluids (table 10.1). In the light of possible NK cell importance in cancer defense, we investigated whether NK cell activity could be induced in the peritoneal cavity after treatment with various immunomodulating agents.

In the first series of investigations, we studied the effect of regionally (intraperitoneally, i.p.) administered viral oncolysates on NK cell lytic potential in ascitic fluids of ovarian cancer patients. Viral oncolysates are extracts derived from allogeneic cultured ovarian tumor cells whose surface membranes were modified by the PR8-A-34 strain of influenza virus (for review see Freedman et al., in this volume). Peritoneal fluid of each patient was tested for NK cytotoxicity against K-562 target, before and after single or multiple injections with viral oncolysates. As observed previously, no NK cytotoxicity was manifested by mononuclear cells of the ascites in untreated ovarian cancer patients; however, high levels of cytotoxicity were induced in all patients after single or multiple i.p. injections with viral oncolysates (fig. 10.1). The impressive feature of such treatment was not only the high degree of potentiation of NK activity, but also its long-lasting duration, for 7 to 21 days after injection (fig. 10.2).

NK cells display characteristic morphology, such as quite large size, indented to renal-type nucleus, and azurophilic cytoplasmic granules. Based on these features, the cells were designated large granular lymphocytes (LGL) (Lotzová 1984; Herberman and Ortaldo 1981). The typical morphological characteristics of NK cells allowed us to analyze the change in the content of this lymphocyte subpopulation in the peritoneal cavity of ovarian cancer patients after treatment with viral oncolysates. Table 10.2 shows that low LGL content was seen in untreated patients; however, in parallel with augmentation of NK activity, an increase in LGL content was observed after viral oncolysate treatment. Figure 10.3 illustrates the LGL present in

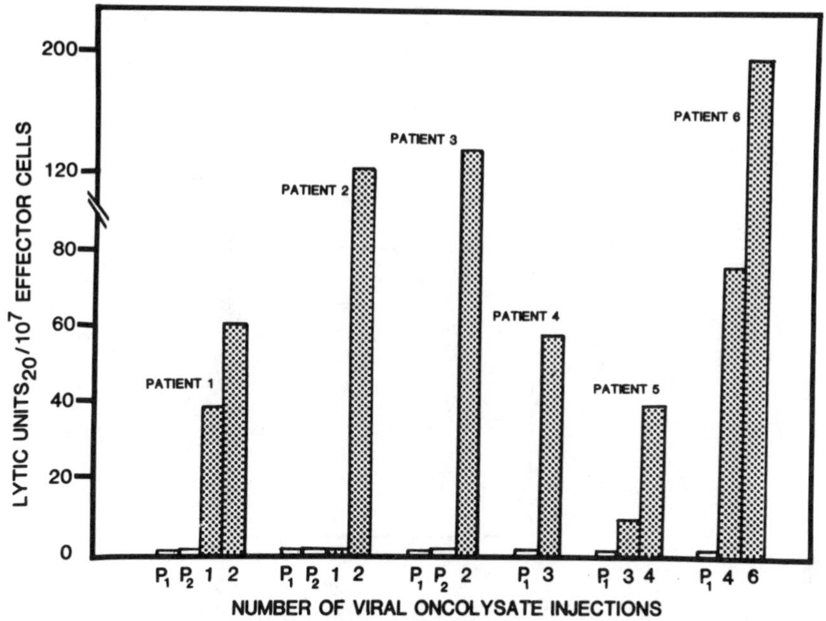

Fig. 10.1. Effect of regional injection of viral oncolysates on ascitic fluid NK cytotoxicity of ovarian cancer patients. Ficoll-Hypaque-separated effector cells in ascitic fluids were tested for cytotoxicity against K-562 as described in the legend of table 10.1. Cytotoxicity was evaluated before (P_1, P_2) and 24 hours (patients 1, 2, 5, and 6), 48 hours (patient 4), or 3 weeks (patient 3) after viral oncolysate treatment. Each injection consisted of 4.5 to 9 mg of viral oncolysates.

the peritoneal fluid of one of the ovarian cancer patients. It can be seen that the morphology of patients' LGL resembles that of normal donors.

One of the most clinically important questions that we raised during our studies was whether regional potentiation of NK lytic activity was reflected by regression of malignant ascites. Indeed, we noted close correlation between NK cell potentiation and regression of ascitic tumors in the peritoneal cavity (table 10.3). The reduction of malignant ascites after NK cell augmentation ranged from 58% to 100%. These data suggest that NK cells may be one of the components of the immune system playing a role in resistance to ovarian ascitic tumors. Subsequently, NK cell regional augmentation may represent an effective approach to the destruction of malignant ascites. The latter postulation is supported by the observation that peritoneal fluid–associated NK cells of oncolysate-treated patients displayed lysis of ascitic tumors (fig. 10.4).

Even though we considered the peritoneal cavity to be the most important representative site of immunity against ovarian cancer, we also studied systemic (peripheral blood) NK cytotoxicity after treatment with viral oncolysates. In the peripheral blood, the oncolysate treatment produced variable results. Increase in NK cytotoxicity was observed in some patients, whereas no potentiation was noted in others

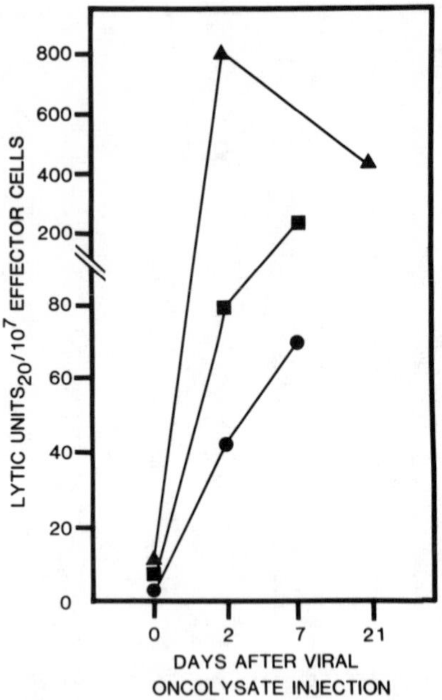

Fig. 10.2. Duration of NK cell augmentation after viral oncolysate treatment. NK cell lytic activity of effector cells from ascitic fluids of three ovarian cancer patients (indicated by symbols) was tested against K-562 before and 2 to 21 days after intraperitoneal injections of 6 mg (●), 9 mg (▲), or 12 mg (■) of viral oncolysates. The cytotoxicity test was the same as described in the legend of table 10.1.

Table 10.2. *Changes in NK Cell Cytotoxicity and LGL Content of Ovarian Cancer Patients After Treatment with Viral Oncolysates*

		Percentage [a]	
Patient No.	Treatment	Lysis	LGL
1	None	10.2	0.3
	Viral oncolysates	71.0	18.2
2	None	1.3	2.2
	Viral oncolysates	72.9	12.3

Source: Lotzová et al. 1985.
Note: LGL, large granular lymphocytes.
[a] Ficoll-Hypaque-separated effector cells from ascitic fluids of ovarian cancer patients were analyzed for NK cytotoxicity against K-562 in a 3-hour ^{51}Cr-release assay (1:50 target-to-effector ratio), before and 21 days (patient 1) or 24 hours (patient 2) after two intraperitoneal injections (9 mg) of viral oncolysates. The percentage of LGL was determined by analysis of May-Grünwald- and Giemsa-stained cytocentrifuge slides.

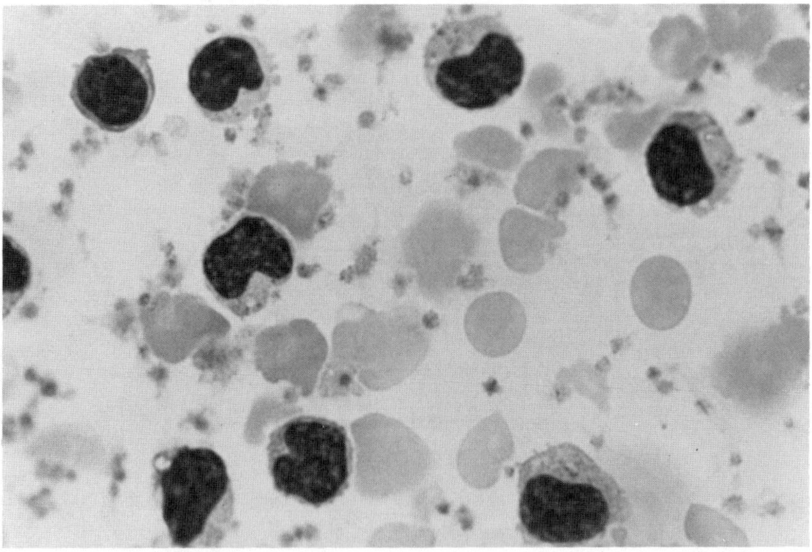

Fig. 10.3. Large granular lymphocytes in ascitic fluid of viral oncolysate-treated ovarian cancer patient. Ficoll-Hypaque-separated cells were analyzed 21 days after two intraperitoneal injections of 9 mg of viral oncolysates (at the time of highest NK augmentation).

Table 10.3. *Correlation Between Augmentation of NK Cell Cytotoxicity and Regression of Malignant Ascites*

Patient No.	Percentage of Cytotoxicity[a] Prior to Treatment	Percentage of Cytotoxicity[a] Post-treatment	Percentage of Reduction of Malignant Ascites[b]
1	3.5	65.1	100
2	1.6	69.5	87
3	3.8	55.2	67
4	6.2	43.3	75
5	−1.6	34.0	58

[a] Ficoll-Hypaque-separated effector cells from ascitic fluids of ovarian cancer patients were tested before and 24 hours to 21 days after intraperitoneal injection(s) of viral oncolysates for NK activity to K-562 in a 3-hour ^{51}Cr-release assay (1:50 target-to-effector ratio). Patients had received two to six injections of 6 to 9 mg of viral oncolysates.

[b] The percentage of malignant cells in the ascitic fluids was determined by cytological examination of ascitic fluid samples. Values represent the percentage of reduction in malignant ascitic cells after oncolysate treatment.

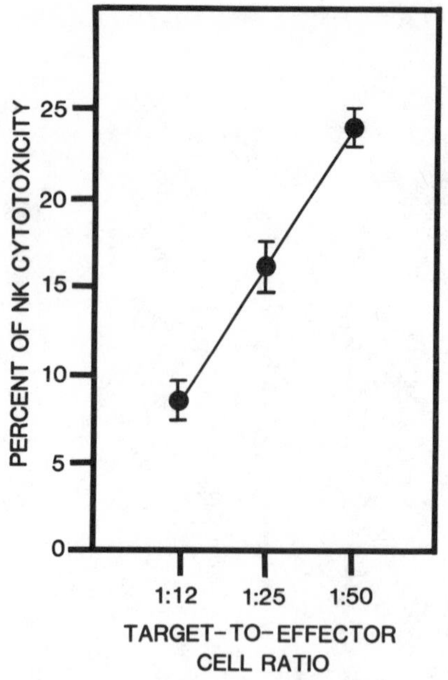

Fig. 10.4. Effect of viral oncolysates on NK cell activity against OV-2774. Ficoll-Hypaque-separated effector cells from ascitic fluid of ovarian cancer patients were tested for cytotoxicity in a 14-hour ^{51}Cr-release assay. The patient received 9 mg of viral oncolysates intraperitoneally, three weeks prior to the test.

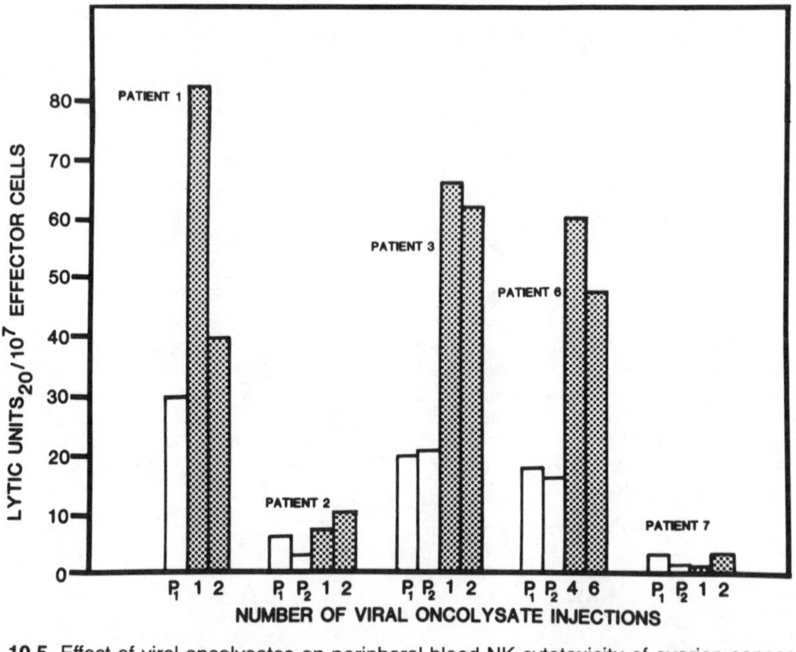

Fig. 10.5. Effect of viral oncolysates on peripheral blood NK cytotoxicity of ovarian cancer patients. Ficoll-Hypaque-separated cells from peripheral blood were tested against K-562. The cytotoxicity assay and treatment schedules for patients 1, 2, 3, and 6 were identical to those described in the legend of figure 10.1; patient 7 received 9 mg of viral oncolysates 24 hours prior to the test.

(fig. 10.5). This indicates that the peripheral blood does not always realistically reflect the regional antitumor immunity and its modulation.

Augmentation of NK Cell Cytotoxicity of Ovarian Cancer Patients by Interleukin-2

Because of the failure of viral oncolysates to augment peripheral blood NK cytotoxicity of patients with ovarian cancer reproducibly, we examined the effect of interleukin-2 (IL-2) on the lytic function of NK cells in the peripheral blood of these patients. Culture of functionally NK cell–inert peripheral blood with IL-2 for 1 to 14 days resulted in induction of high levels of cytotoxicity. The cytotoxicity was induced not only against the K-562 target, which is highly sensitive to NK lysis, but

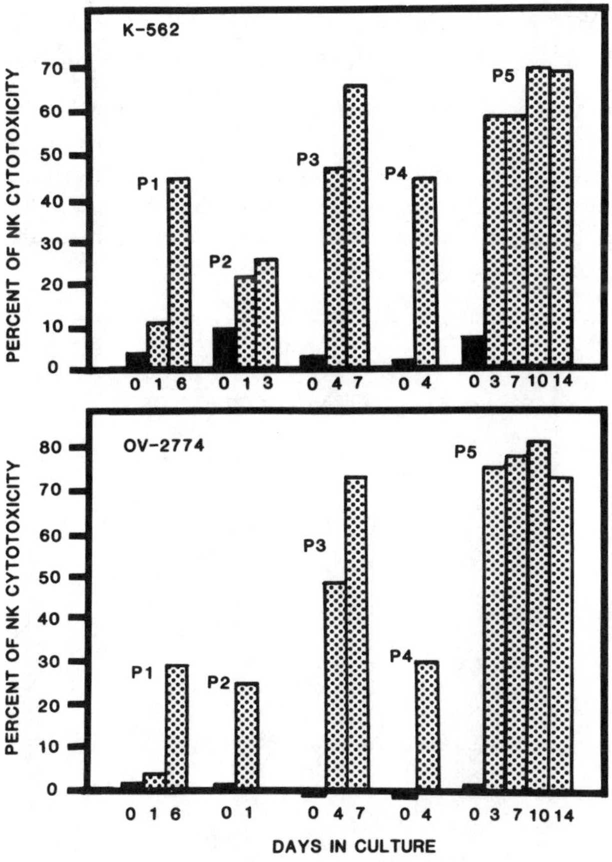

Fig. 10.6. Generation of cytotoxicity in peripheral blood of ovarian cancer patients by interleukin-2 (IL-2). Ficoll-Hypaque-separated cells from peripheral blood of five patients (P1–P5) were tested before (solid bar) and after (stippled bar) culture with IL-2 (Lotzová, Savary, and Herberman 1986). Cytotoxicity against K-562 was tested at 1:6 (patient 4), 1:12 (patients 2, 3, and 5), and 1:25 (patient 1), and against OV-2774 at 1:6 (patient 4), 1:12 (patient 3), 1:25 (patient 1), and 1:50 (patients 2 and 5) target-to-effector cell ratios (3-hour ^{51}Cr-release assay).

also against the NK cell-resistant line of ovarian carcinoma origin, OV-2774 (obtained and established from the patient's malignant ascites) (fig. 10.6).

Most important, cytotoxic activity was induced by IL-2 against fresh solid ovarian tumors of both autologous and allogeneic origins (fig. 10.7). The latter observation is quite important because it suggests that IL-2–activated NK cells have the ability to kill not only malignant ovarian ascites but also solid ovarian tumors. Another important observation made during our studies was the ability of IL-2 to activate the NK cells residing within the solid ovarian tumor. Specifically, Ficoll-Hypaque- or Percoll gradient-separated tumor-associated lymphocytes displayed lytic activity against ovarian tumors (fig. 10.8).

Morphological evaluation of IL-2-dependent cultures of cytotoxic cells showed that induction of cytotoxicity against ovarian tumors was associated with an increase in the LGL numbers. In contrast, no association was observed with monocytes (table 10.4).

Characterization of Cytotoxic Cells Against Ovarian Tumors

To determine whether NK cells were indeed the cell population involved in cytotoxicity against ovarian tumors, we used two experimental approaches. In the first set of studies, we separated peripheral blood lymphocytes on Percoll density gradient (Lotzová, Savary, and Herberman 1986) into LGL-enriched and LGL-depleted fractions and tested both fractions for NK cytotoxicity. In these studies, we used

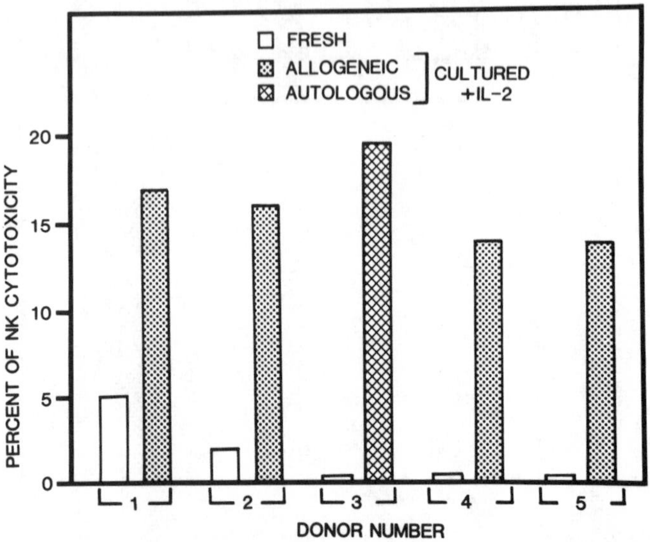

Fig. 10.7. Lysis of fresh ovarian tumors by interleukin-2 (IL-2)–activated peripheral blood cells. Cytotoxicity of Ficoll-Hypaque-separated effector cells of ovarian cancer patients (donors 1–3) and normal donors (donors 4 and 5) was tested before and 6 (patients 1 and 3) or 15 days (patient 2 and normal donors) after culture with IL-2 against solid ovarian tumor cells (3-hour ^{51}Cr-release assay at target-to-effector cell ratios of 1:12, patient 1; 1:50, patient 3; and 1:100, patient 2 and normal donors).

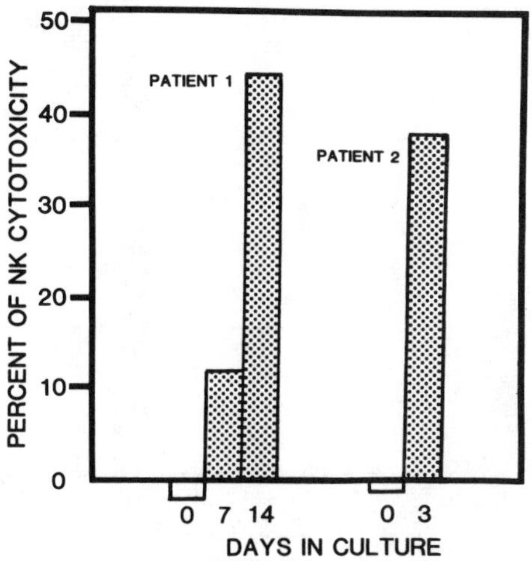

Fig. 10.8. Interleukin-2 (IL-2)–induced cytotoxicity of tumor-derived lymphocytes. Tumor cells were separated from mononuclear cells of solid ovarian tumors by Percoll or Ficoll-Hypaque density gradient (patients 1 and 2, respectively) and tested before (solid bar) and after (stippled bar) culture with IL-2 against OV-2774 (3-hour ^{51}Cr-release assay, 1:12 and 1:50 target-to-effector cell ratio for patients 1 and 2, respectively).

Table 10.4. *Correlation between LGL Content and NK Activity in Peripheral Blood Cultures of Ovarian Cancer Patients*

		Percentage[a]		
Patient No.	Culture (Weeks)	Lysis	LGL	Monocytes
1	0	3	8	1
	1.5	71	21	9
2	0	9	17	11
	1	26	28	3
3	0	3	67	19
	1	66	80	3
4	0	2	28	7
	0.5	45	38	1
5	0	7	9	42
	2	70	42	0

Note: LGL, large granular lymphocytes.
[a] Ficoll-Hypaque-separated effector cells were tested before and after culture with IL-2 against K-562 in a 3-hour ^{51}Cr-release assay (target-to-effector [T:E] ratio was 1:12 in all patients, with the exception of patient 4, who was tested at a 1:6 T:E ratio). Content of LGL and monocytes was determined by analysis of May-Grünwald- and Giemsa-stained cytocentrifuge slides.

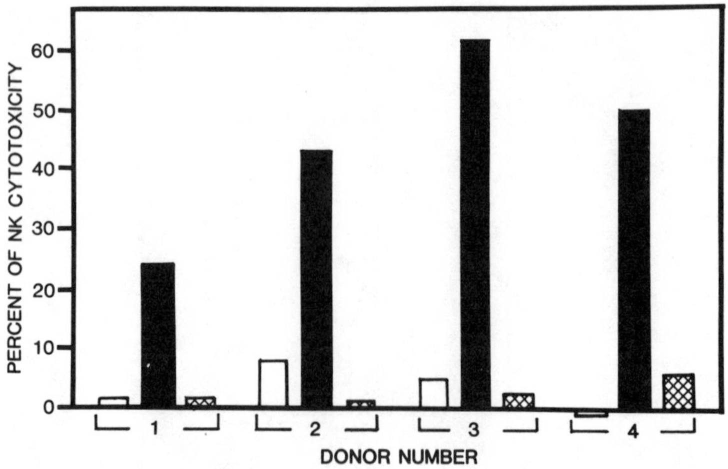

Fig. 10.9. Cytotoxic activity against malignant ascites is mediated by large granular lymphocytes (LGL). Peripheral blood cells of normal donors were nylon wool–filtered (open bar) or separated on Percoll density gradients and tested for cytotoxicity to OV-2774 in a 3-hour (donors 1 and 2) or 14-hour (donors 3 and 4) ^{51}Cr-release assay. (LGL-enriched, solid bar; LGL-depleted, hatched bar).

peripheral blood of normal donors rather than that of cancer patients to be certain that the tested NK cells were fully active. It can be clearly seen in figure 10.9 that only the LGL-enriched fraction displayed cytotoxicity against ovarian ascites, whereas the LGL-depleted fraction did not exhibit any activity. In another set of experiments, we tested the effect of NK cell-associated antibody, Leu-11b, on the tumor-directed activity of cytotoxic cells. These studies demonstrated that peripheral blood cytotoxic activity was abolished by Leu-11b antibody and complement treatment (fig. 10.10). Similarly, the lytic potential of cytotoxic cells residing in ascitic fluid of oncolysate-treated patients was significantly decreased after treatment with Leu-11b antibody (fig. 10.10). These two observations indicate clearly that NK cells can kill ovarian tumors.

Next, we investigated the effect of Leu-11b antibody on IL-2–activated peripheral blood cytotoxicity against K-562 and ovarian tumor cell line OV-2774. The depletion of cytotoxic activity with the latter antibody indicates that IL-2–stimulated effector cells are activated NK cells (fig. 10.11). To determine whether the precursors of IL-2–activated NK cells were LGL, we cultured LGL-depleted or -enriched populations for six days with IL-2 and tested for cytotoxicity against a K-562 and NK-resistant ovarian cell line. Active cytotoxic cells could be generated only from LGL-enriched but not from LGL-depleted fractions (fig. 10.12).

Studies on the Mechanism of Cytotoxicity Against Ovarian Tumors

Using the conjugate assay on the cytocentrifuge slides (Lotzová, Savary, and Herberman 1986), we determined that the majority of cells binding to ovarian and

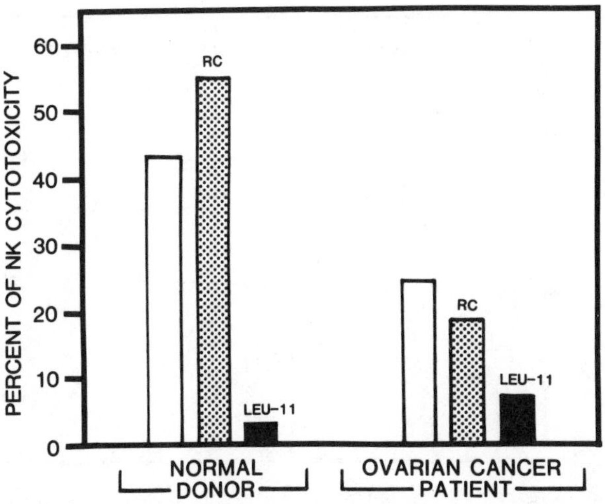

Fig. 10.10. Effect of Leu-11 monoclonal antibody treatment on cytotoxic activity against ovarian tumors. Peripheral blood large granular lymphocytes of a normal donor and effector cells separated by Ficoll-Hypaque density gradient from ascitic fluid of ovarian cancer patient (three weeks after intraperitoneal injection of 9 mg of viral oncolysates) were either untreated (open bar), treated with rabbit complement (RC; stippled bar), or treated with Leu-11 antibody and RC (solid bar) (Lotzová, Savary, and Herberman 1986). Cytotoxicity was tested against OV-2774 in a 3-hour (normal donor) or 14-hour (patient) ^{51}Cr-release assay.

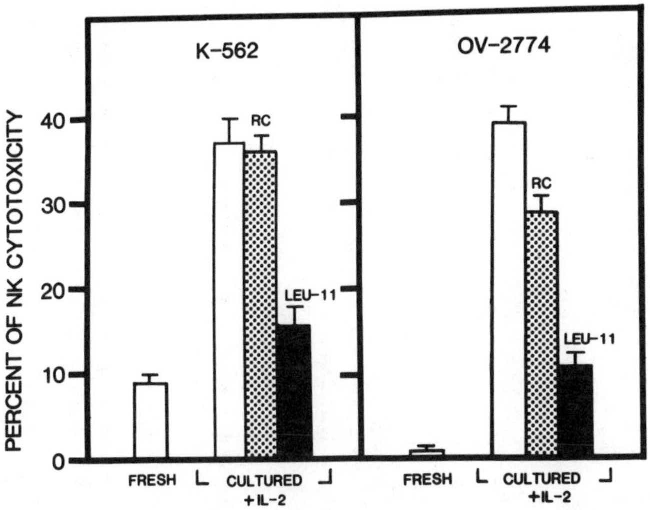

Fig. 10.11. Effect of Leu-11 monoclonal antibody treatment on cytotoxic activity of IL-2–activated peripheral blood effector cells. Nylon wool–filtered effector cells of normal donors were tested before and three to five days after culture with IL-2 against K-562 (1:12 target-to-effector cell ratio) and OV-2774 (1:25 target-to-effector cell ratio) in a 3-hour ^{51}Cr-release assay. Cells were untreated (open bar), treated with rabbit complement (RC; stippled bar), or treated with Leu-11 and RC (solid bar) (Lotzová, Savary, and Herberman 1986). Bars represent mean percentage of cytotoxicity ± the standard error of two experiments.

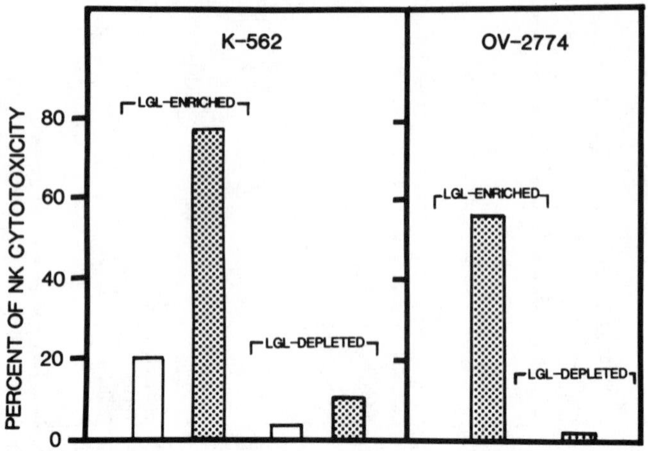

Fig. 10.12. Generation of tumor-directed cytotoxicity in culture with IL-2. Large granular lymphocyte (LGL)-enriched and LGL-depleted peripheral blood effector cells of normal donors were tested prior to (open bar) and six days after culture (stippled bar) with IL-2 against K-562 and OV-2774 in a 3-hour ^{51}Cr-release assay (1:6 target-to-effector cell ratio).

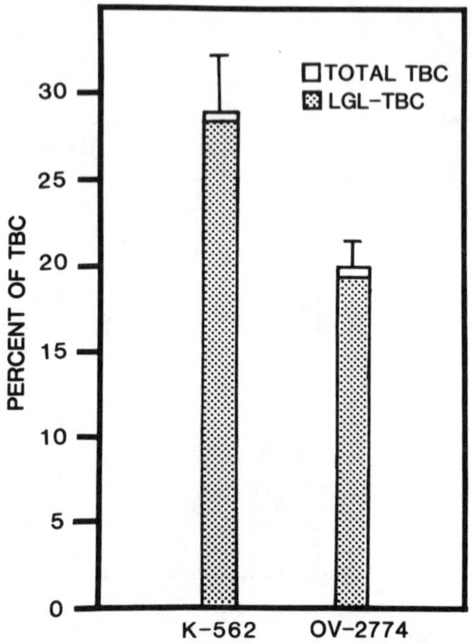

Fig. 10.13. Tumor-binding capacity of peripheral blood large granular lymphocytes (LGL). The morphology of nylon wool–filtered cells binding to K-562 and OV-2774 was analyzed in a slide conjugate assay (Lotzová, Savary, and Herberman 1986). Bars represent mean percentage of tumor-binding cells (TBC) ± the standard error of three normal donors.

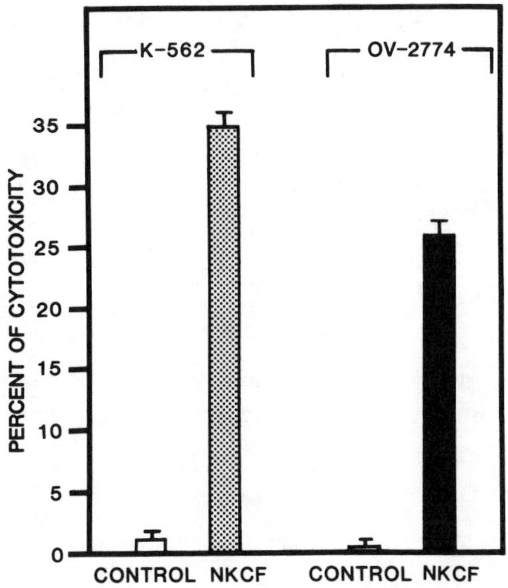

Fig. 10.14. Effect of NK cell cytotoxic factor (NKCF) on K-562 and malignant ascites. Supernatants obtained by co-culture of nylon wool–filtered peripheral blood effector cells of normal donors with K-562 or OV-2774 for 24 hours (1:50 target-to-effector cell ratio) were tested for NKCF activity in a 40-hour microsupernatant test (Lotzová, Savary, and Herberman 1986). Controls consisted of supernatants derived from cultures of effector cells alone. Bars represent mean percentage of cytotoxicity ± the standard error of triplicate determinations.

K-562 tumors were of LGL morphology (fig. 10.13), supporting the contention that the NK-LGL are the cells with reactivity against ovarian tumors.

Analysis of the mechanism of cytotoxicity showed that similar to K-562 tumors, activity against ovarian tumors could be mediated by the factor generated after incubation of peripheral blood effector cells of normal donors with the ovarian malignant ascitic cell line (fig. 10.14).

Summary

We have shown that NK cells (LGL) of normal donors can lyse cultured and fresh ovarian cancer cells. In contrast, patients with ovarian carcinoma displayed low or no NK cell cytotoxicity against both the NK highly sensitive line, K-562, and ovarian tumors. However, NK cell activity of these patients could be corrected by two approaches. The first was the in vivo regional treatment of patients with viral oncolysates, which induced high levels of NK cell activity in ascitic fluids; such treatment had a potentiating effect on systemic (peripheral blood) NK cell activity of some, but not all, patients. Second, NK cell activity in peripheral blood could be generated in in vitro culture with IL-2.

Both endogenous and IL-2–activated cytotoxic cells, as well as the precursors of the latter population, displayed LGL morphology. Furthermore, cytotoxic activity of the effector cells was depleted with NK-associated antibody, Leu-11. All of these observations indicate that NK cells are the cytotoxic cells and that these cells may play an important role in resistance against ovarian cancer. Consequently, regional potentiation of NK activity by viral oncolysates, the adoptive transfer of IL-2 in vitro-activated, autologous peripheral blood NK cells, or a combination of these approaches, may represent new modalities in the treatment of patients with ovarian carcinoma.

Acknowledgments

This work was supported by grant CA 39632 from the National Cancer Institute.
The expert secretarial assistance of Ann Childers is greatly appreciated.

References

Allavena P, Introna M, Mangiori C, Mantovani A. 1981. Inhibition of natural killer activity by tumor-associated lymphoid cells from ascites of ovarian carcinomas. *J Natl Cancer Inst* 67:319–325.

Herberman RB, Ortaldo JR. 1981. Natural killer cells: Their role in defenses against disease. *Science* 214:24–30.

Lotzová E. 1983. Function of natural killer cells in various biological phenomena. *Surv Synth Path Res* 2:41–46.

Lotzová E. 1984. The role of natural killer cells in immune surveillance against malignancies. *Cancer Bull* 36:215–226.

Lotzová E, Savary CA, Freedman RS, Bowen JM. 1984. Natural killer cell cytotoxic potential of patients with ovarian carcinoma and its modulation with virus-modified tumor cell extract. *Cancer Immunol Immunother* 17:124–129.

Lotzová E, Savary CA, Herberman RB. In press. Antileukemia reactivity of endogenous and IL-2 activated NK cells. In *NK Cells, Cancer and Other Diseases*, ed. E Lotzová, RB Herberman. Basel:S. Karger.

Lotzová E, Savary CA, Keating MJ, Hester JP. 1985. Defective NK cell mechanism in patients with leukemia. In *Mechanisms of Cytotoxicity by NK Cells*, ed. RB Herberman, pp. 507–519. New York: Academic Press.

Silverberg E, Lubera J. 1986. Cancer statistics. *CA* 36:9–25.

Annual Clinical Conference on Cancer, Vol. 29
Gynecologic Cancer: Diagnosis and Treatment Strategies
© 1987 by The University of Texas System Cancer Center

11. Virus Augmentation as a Biologic-Modifier Approach: Experience with Intracavitary Virus-Augmentation Therapy

Ralph S. Freedman, James M. Bowen, Eva Lotzová, Creighton L. Edwards, Errol Lewis, and Ruth L. Katz

Viruses can be used in different ways to destroy tumors (Austin and Boone 1979; Kobayashi 1982). The evolution of virus-augmented therapy in experimental tumor systems is illustrated in figure 11.1. "Viral oncolysis" (Koprowski, Love, and Koprowski 1957; Lindenmann and Klein 1967) refers to the virus-induced destruction of tumors that may follow the complete infection of a tumor with a particular virus type, usually one expressing neurotropism. A similar effect was observed after therapeutic attempts to infect human tumors with several virus types (Austin and Boone 1979). This approach may have limited application therapeutically since it is necessary to achieve complete infection of the tumor and its metastases before antiviral immunity has had an opportunity to develop. It was observed, however, that animals rendered tumor free through successfully induced viral oncolysis were immune to challenge with the identical tumors (Lindenmann and Klein 1967; Boone 1974). This phenomenon has been called "postoncolytic immunity"; the observation was logically followed by experiments that used homogenates derived from either the collapsed in vivo infected tumor or in vitro infected cultured tumor cells to induce a similar state of immunity against transplantable tumors (Lindenmann and Klein 1967; Gillette and Boone 1976). This approach has been referred to as "virus-augmented therapy" and has served as the model for several previous clinical studies (Freedman et al. 1983; Freedman, Rutledge, and Wharton 1983; Cassel, Murray, and Phillips 1983; Green, Pratt, and Webster 1976; Murray et al. 1977; Sauter, Cavalli, and Lindenmann 1978; Sinkovics et al. 1974, 1978; Sinkovics, Plager, and McMurtrey 1980; Sinkovics 1977; Wallack et al. 1983; Livingston et al. 1985), as well as for our current studies in ovarian cancer.

The most frequently used viruses in preclinical studies have included vesicular stomatitis virus (VSV), influenza, vaccinia, and Newcastle disease virus (Austin and Boone 1979). The preclinical studies used syngeneic, immunogenic tumors in most instances. Autologous human tumors are more difficult to work with since virus adaptation to the tumor cells appears to be needed in most cases, whereas allogeneic tumor cell lines are more readily infected. All of the above viruses were shown to promote tumor prophylaxis experimentally; nevertheless, each has characteristics (table 11.1) that could determine differences in efficacy or safety when any route of administration is used.

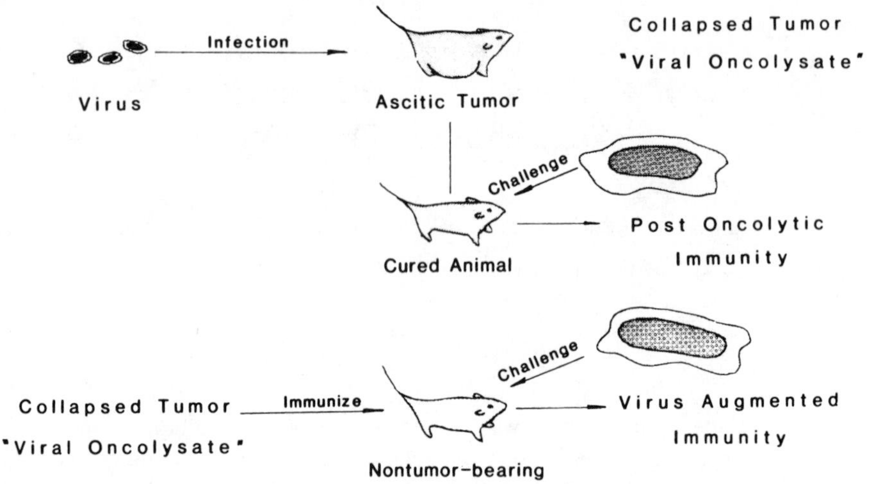

Fig. 11.1. Evolution of virus-augmentation therapy.

The virus-modified extracts are commonly referred to as "viral oncolysates." Influenza may be of particular interest because this virus has the largest number of optimum characteristics, including surface-budding and antigenicity, and has also been shown to confer greater immunogenicity than VSV (Gillette and Boone 1976). In another study, viral oncolysates (VOs) prepared with influenza were able to prolong the survival of animals with established, incompletely resected tumors (Boone 1974). Another reason for using influenza is that there have been no significant toxic effects when attenuated type A strains were used in clinical studies (Sinkovics 1977; Sinkovics, Plager, and McMurtrey 1980; Freedman et al. 1983; Freedman, Rutledge, and Wharton 1983).

The immunologic basis for virus augmentation is suggested by experiments that show (1) transferability of tumor prophylaxis through lymphocytes of immunized animals, and sometimes passively with serum (Lindenmann and Klein 1967); (2) abrogation of the tumor prophylaxis effect by admixing VO preparations with antibody to the modifying virus or through induction of tolerance to the virus; and

Table 11.1. *Characteristics of Some Augmenting Viruses*

	Complete Replication	Surface-Budding	Neuraminidase	Immunogenicity
Influenza	+	+	+	+[a]
VSV	+	+	−	+
NCDV	−	+	+	+
Vaccinia	+	−	+	+

Note: VSV, vesicular stomatitis virus; NCDV, Newcastle disease virus.
[a]100X VSV.

(3) enhancement of tumor prophylaxis by preimmunizing animals with the virus incorporated in the VO preparation (Lindenmann and Klein 1967; Lindenmann 1974), although the opposite result has also been observed (Austin and Boone 1979).

Viral oncolysates prepared for experimental animal and clinical studies are currently crudely prepared materials. Nevertheless, progress is being made toward a determination of their biologic activity and characteristics. This situation is not too dissimilar from earlier studies with human leukocyte interferon, which is only 1% pure, although the clinical activity and toxicity associated with its use are similar to the experience with the newer recombinant materials.

Viral oncolysates showing tumor protection in preclinical studies were also observed to mediate enhanced delayed-type hypersensitivity reactions (DTH) when injected intradermally into footpads of mice (Boone 1974). These studies preceded patient testing with VOs (Boone et al. 1978; Austin et al. 1982; Freedman et al. 1984). Augmented skin-test reactivity was demonstrated in patients with malignant melanoma who were injected with VSV-modified allogeneic extracts, as compared with responses observed with unmodified extracts (Boone et al. 1978). Similar results were observed in patients with carcinoma of the breast (Austin et al. 1982), and in ovarian cancer (Freedman et al. 1984) using extracts derived from two characterized and cultured ovarian carcinoma cell lines after they had been infected with influenza A/PR8/34. We selected PR8 influenza virus for the ovarian studies because of our previous safety experience with PR8-modified extracts and because preclinical studies indicated that influenza might have better attributes than other systems. Our earlier studies had also demonstrated the antigenicity of the virus (Freedman et al. 1983), which was a prerequisite to tumor prophylaxis in the preclinical studies.

Intracavitary Viral Oncolysates in the Treatment of Ovarian Cancer

In examining the need for new strategies in the treatment of ovarian cancer, it is necessary to consider that less than 40% of patients with this disease can anticipate a survival of five years or more (Silverberg and Lubera 1986). Furthermore, the five-year survival is only 20% to 25% for the more common stages III and IV. Combination chemotherapy is the most frequently used adjuvant therapy, but a variety of experimental approaches, including radiation, hormones, and agents called "biologic-response modifiers" (BRMs), are being evaluated. A review of earlier studies with BRMs, which include substances formerly referred to as "immunotherapeutic" agents, is somewhat disappointing for ovarian cancer (Freedman 1985). There has, however, been renewed enthusiasm in particular for the intracavitary administration of BRMs in ovarian cancer (Webb, Oaten, and Pike 1978; Mantovani et al. 1982; Bast et al. 1983; Rambaldi et al. 1985).

The intraperitoneal (i.p.) approach is especially attractive for ovarian cancer, which is typically an intraperitoneal disease that sometimes spreads across the diaphragm to involve the pleural cavity and infrequently spreads outside of the abdominal and pleural cavities. Moreover, our own studies and those of others have demonstrated impaired natural immunity in the peritoneal cavity of patients with ovarian cancer (Lotzová et al. 1984; Mantovani et al. 1980). This impairment can be reversed by i.p. injection with certain immune modulators, including interferon-beta (Rambaldi et al. 1985) and i.p. VOs (Lotzová et al. 1984). The kinetics of this enhanced natural killer cell (NK cell) cytotoxicity response to i.p. VOs has been outlined (for details, see Lotzová et al. in this volume).

Since initial studies of escalating dose response were performed (Lotzová et al. 1984), we have conducted a study of i.p. VOs at fixed doses, but with different frequencies during the first month of treatment, in patients with advanced ovarian cancer (Freedman RS, Edwards CL, Bowen JM, Lotzová E, Katz R, Lewis E, Atkinson N, Adams S. Intracavitary viral oncolysates in ovarian cancer. Unpublished data.) The agents' clinical activity, toxicity, and biologic effect were evaluated in these patients.

Methods

Preparation of Viral Oncolysates for Clinical Studies

Viral oncolysates were prepared from characterized ovarian carcinoma cell lines MDAH 2774 (Freedman et al. 1978) and $CaOV_3$. The former was kindly supplied by J. Sinkovics, St. Joseph's Community Cancer Center, Tampa, Florida; the latter by J. Fogh, Memorial Sloan-Kettering Cancer Center, New York. The kinetics of virus infection of these cell lines has been determined using influenza A/PR8/34 as the infecting virus.

The cells were grown in L-15 medium supplemented with *L*-glutamine and 10% fetal bovine serum. Contamination by *Mycoplasma* was excluded by regular examination in a Mycotrim® (Hanna Media Incorporated, Berkeley, California) culture system and by electron microscopy.

Type A influenza virus PR8/34 (Francis and Magill 1934) was used to infect the ovarian carcinoma cells. The virus was attenuated and was originally obtained from Flow Laboratories, Rockville, Maryland. The virus had been maintained by several passages in leukosis-free embryonated hens' eggs. Limiting dilutions of the virus in phosphate-buffered saline (PBS) were injected into the allantoic cavities of ten-day-old embryos and incubated at 35° C and 500 *g*, after which they were titrated for viral hemagglutinin, dispensed into small ampules, flash-frozen, and stored at −70° C. Virus of all preparations was routinely monitored by titrating hemagglutinin, using a standard tube dilution technique read by the Salk pattern method after the virus dilutions had been incubated with 0.4% washed, pooled chicken erythrocytes (Salk 1944).

The kinetics of PR8/A virus infection of the cell lines was studied in the ovarian cell lines as follows: Viral replication was detected by titrating culture fluid for hemagglutination of chicken red blood cells. Peak antigen-modification of the cell membrane was measured by cell-membrane immunofluorescence developed by polyvalent rabbit anti-PR8 serum and was maximum at 20 hours.

For preparation of the lysates, cells were seeded into T-150 plastic tissue culture flasks in L-15 medium supplemented with 10% fetal bovine serum. When the monolayers were barely subcontiguous, they were washed free of growth medium and incubated for a further 72 hours in L-15 without serum. No antibiotics were used in these cultures at any time. After incubation in serum-free medium, the monolayers were washed again in sterile pH 7.3 PBS and infected with 5 ml/flask of a dilution of frozen-stock virus in PBS sufficient to give approximately $10^5 EID_{50}$ (50% egg infective dose) per flask. The infected cultures were incubated at 35° C. After the 20-hour incubation, cells were scraped from the flasks with a sterile rubber policeman. The resulting suspensions were aseptically pooled and centrifuged at 300 *g*, and the supernatants were discarded. The cell pellets were resuspended in PBS and washed by a further centrifugation step.

Next, the washed cell pellets were resuspended in an equal volume of 0.001 M $MgCl_2$. A volume of DNase (Worthington, Freehold, New Jersey) 1 mg/ml equal to the volume of the cell pellet was added, followed by the addition of a volume of 1.8 N NaCl equal to that of the cells plus DNase. The resulting suspension was sonicated for three minutes in a Raytheon cup sonicator with an output of 310 kHz. Sonications were carried out in small plastic tubes packed in ice in the sonicator cup. Ultraviolet irradiation of the sonicates was carried out as follows: A homogenate layer of less than 4 mm in a sterile 50-mm petri dish was irradiated in a hood with a shortwave ultraviolet lamp, set to deliver 40 erg/sec/m^2. The irradiated lysates were pooled, adjusted to uniform protein concentrations, and dispersed into sterile precapped serum vials at concentrations of 1.5 and 4.5 mg/10 ml NaCl. Material derived from the MDAH 2774 cell line was designated "OV1," and that from $CaOV_3$, "OV2." The material was stored at −70° C. All vials were appropriately labeled.

Quality-Control Studies

Bacterial Sterility

Aliquots of each preparation were thawed and assayed for sterility by Dr. Roy L. Hopfer of the Department of Laboratory Medicine of our institution according to the procedure described in the *Federal Register*, vol. 38:P, 32056, paragraph 610,12. Preparations were not used until they had been shown to be free of bacteria on repeated subculture.

Assay for Residual Viable Virus

Undiluted lysate plus serial dilutions was injected into embryonated eggs and treated as for virus stocks, except that three sequential blind passages of undiluted fluid and serial dilutions were made, with each passage being titrated for influenza virus hemagglutination. In the preparation of VOs, tumor cells are disrupted when there is only one tenth of the virion output. Ultraviolet irradiation further reduces any live virus by a factor of 10 logs.

Antigen Complement

A standardized enzyme-linked immunosorbent assay (ELISA), described by Chan (1985), was used to check oncolysate preparations for viral antigens specific to

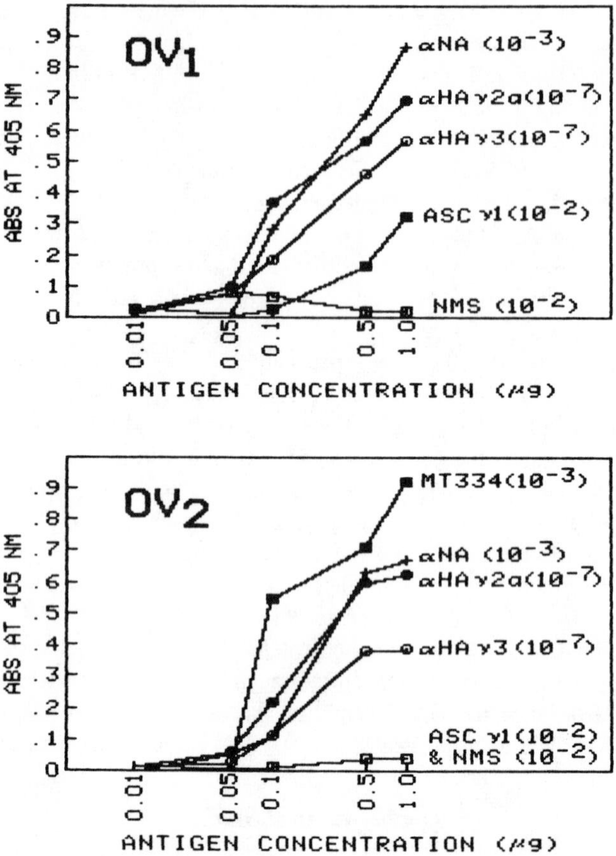

Fig. 11.2. Reactivity of monoclonal antibodies with viral oncolysates by enzyme-linked immunosorbent assay (ELISA). NA, neuraminidase; HA, hemagglutinin antibody; ASC, monoclonal antibody derived from MDAH 2774; NMS, normal mouse serum; MT334, monoclonal antibody reactive with ovarian carcinoma cells.

PR8/A/34, using murine monoclonal antibodies reactive with specific hemagglutinin and neuraminidase antigens of the virus (Staudt and Gerhard 1983). Other murine monoclonal antibodies that are reactive with ovarian carcinoma cells were used to detect the presence of ovarian tumor-associated antigen (TAA) in the VO preparation (Mattes et al. 1984). Monoclonal antibodies were kindly provided by M. Herlyn and W. Gerhard, of the Wistar Institute, Philadelphia, and J. Mattes, of Memorial Sloan-Kettering Cancer Center, New York. A typical ELISA results analysis of the two ovarian VO preparations is shown in figure 11.2; antigens derived from both the viral and nonviral TAA components of VOs were detected in both VO preparations in this example, although there appear to be qualitative differences between the two preparations.

Cytokine Content

The oncolysates were assayed for cytokines by Jim Klostergaard of our institution, using his previously published procedures (1985), and for interferon-alpha and interferon-gamma by Herbert A. Fritsche, Jr., of our institution, using commercially available radiometric procedures. Neither cytokines nor interferons were found.

Administration of Viral Oncolysates

Viral oncolysates were administered i.p. to all patients. The peritoneal cavity was easily entered in patients with ascites, and in those without ascites an ultrasound-guided procedure was used. In the latter cases, the peritoneal cavity was identified by instilling 100 to 200 ml of normal saline into the abdominal cavity and monitoring the location of fluid by ultrasound (figs. 11.3 and 11.4). Most of the patients were injected i.p. with a 1:1 combination of OV1 and OV2 extracts with a protein equivalent of 9.0 mg. For intrapleural injection, a dose of 3 mg of the combined extract was used. During the first month, patients received either a single injection, biweekly injections, or weekly injections; thereafter, treatment was given monthly.

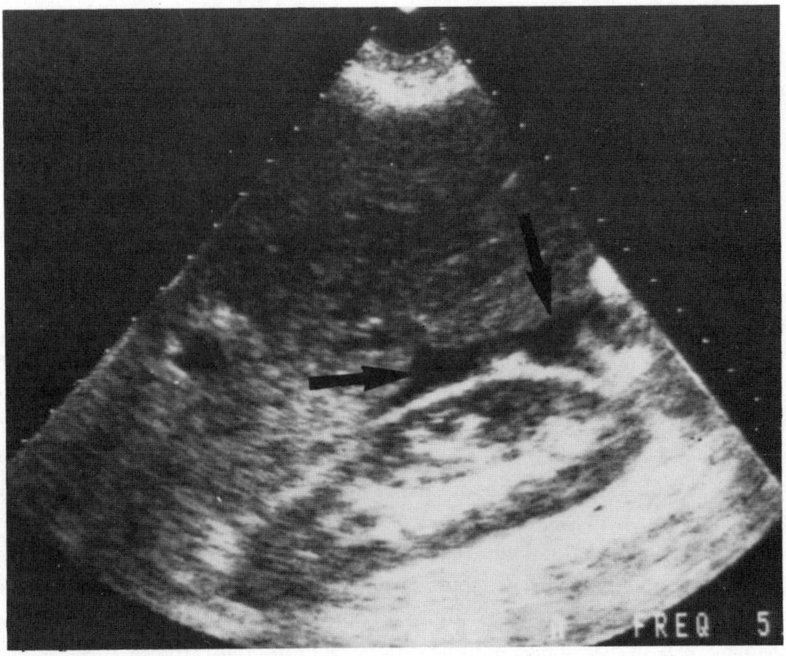

Fig. 11.3. Ultrasound examination showing intraperitoneal localization of fluid.

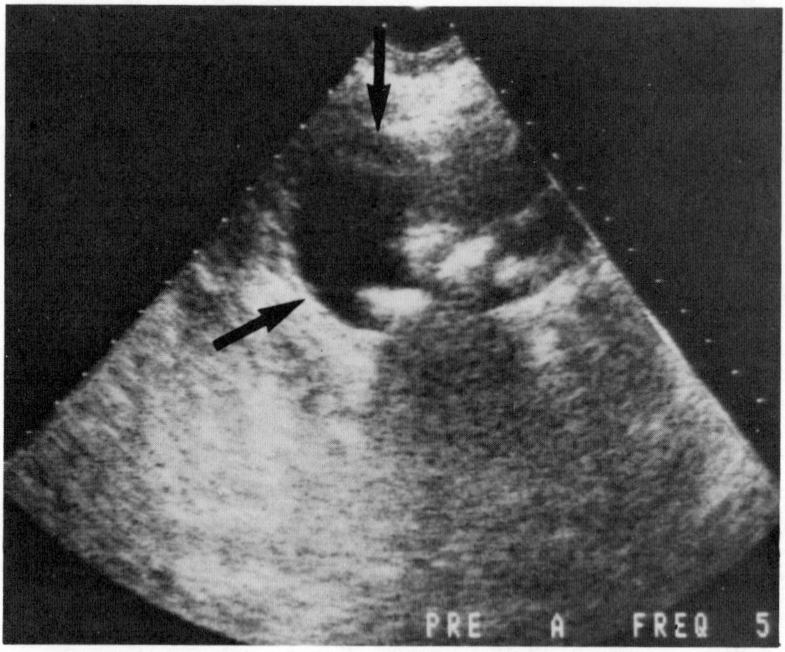

Fig. 11.4. Ultrasound examination showing intraperitoneal localization of fluid.

Results

A detailed analysis of this study has been submitted for publication. Clinical activity was evidenced in 9 of 40 patients with advanced-stage progressive disease; this activity included regression of malignant ascites and of pleural effusions and partial regression of the solid tumor component in some patients.

Case Studies

The four case histories reported here illustrate the clinical responses observed in several patients with advanced ovarian cancer and the changes in their immune profiles over the period of treatment.

Case 1

This 39-year-old woman had removal of a mucinous cystadenoma in 1978. By December 1981, malignant ascites had accumulated, and she underwent surgery again. Diffuse carcinomatosis was found and chemotherapy with cisplatin, doxorubicin HCl, cyclophosphamide, and tamoxifen was administered until August 1982, when malignant ascites began to reaccumulate. Hexamethylmelamine was added to her therapy until October 1982, but without a response. Repeated monthly abdominal paracentesis was performed without additional therapy until March 1983.

Between March 1983 and April 1984, the patient received monthly i.p. injections of VO derived from the two ovarian carcinoma cell lines, the dose being escalated from 6.0 to 9.0 mg. During the first month, fluid accumulation decreased dramatically, which was associated with a marked improvement in the patient's symptoms. Malignant cells disappeared from the ascites as its level decreased, and a 50% decrease in carcinoembryonic antigen levels in the ascitic fluid was observed. By the second month, there was no detectable ascites. Pelvic masses decreased slightly, according to two observers. The response remained stable for 19 months. Side effects following treatments included fever to 40° C, abdominal pain, nausea, and occasional vomiting. Symptoms occurred after six hours but seldom persisted beyond 48 hours. The patient was able to resume her usual activities and occupation between treatments. The frequency of i.p. injections was reduced to alternate months at the end of the first year, but after 19 months of treatment the patient developed a left-sided pleural effusion. The effusion was successfully pleurodesed with tetracycline instilled through a chest tube. Two courses of i.p. chemotherapy with cisplatin were administered for recurrent ascites and progressive abdominal pelvic disease, but without effect. The patient died at 41 months from progressive disease.

Immune response studies were performed before and after i.p. injections with VO (fig. 11.5). In previous published data on this patient (Lotzová et al. 1984), we showed that after i.p. administration of VO there was a significant enhancement of cytotoxicity to NK cells in the ascitic fluid. Furthermore, DTH reactions were markedly increased after i.p. injections. Notably, the response to unmodified extracts of the ovarian carcinoma cells was converted from negative to strongly positive. A standardized T mitogen–induced lymphocyte blastogenesis assay (relative proliferation index [RPI] method) was used to determine T-cell responsiveness of the patients' lymphocytes in comparison with the mean of three normal standards.

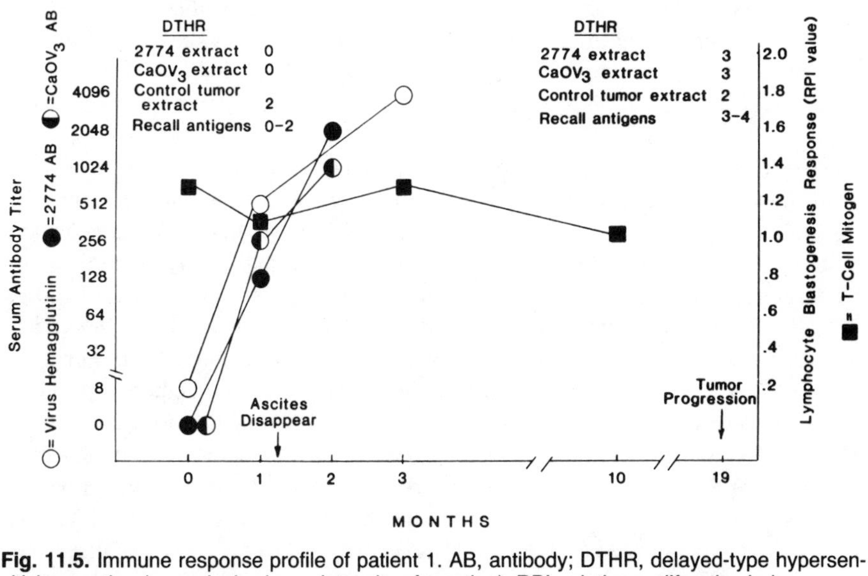

Fig. 11.5. Immune response profile of patient 1. AB, antibody; DTHR, delayed-type hypersensitivity reaction (numerical value = intensity of reaction); RPI, relative proliferation index.

The T-cell response index remained within the 90th percentile range (> 0.58) following treatment (fig. 11.5). Humoral responses to viral and TAA-associated components on the extracts were also apparent, with marked increases in antibody titer to the PR8 virus and to surface-antigen determinants on two ovarian carcinoma cell lines used in the preparation of VO (fig. 11.5). These assays were described in a previous publication (Freedman et al. 1983).

Case 2

This 32-year-old woman underwent surgical exploration in October 1979. A stage III serous carcinoma was found. The patient received alkylating agents for 12 months and, at reexploratory surgery in 1981, diffuse small macroscopic disease was found. Six courses of cisplatin and cyclophosphamide were administered until June 1981, and there was no clinical evidence of disease until June 1983, when symptoms recurred and increasing disease was confirmed at exploratory surgery. The patient declined further treatment at that time.

The patient presented at U.T. M. D. Anderson Hospital in March 1984 complaining of fatigue, abdominal swelling, and anorexia. In addition to ascites, the patient had large abdominopelvic cystic masses. In May 1984, the first i.p. injection of VO, consisting of both OV1 and OV2, was administered. Before the second treatment course, the patient underwent emergency abdominal surgery following a stabbing incident. The surgeon repaired a gastric laceration and confirmed ascites and extensive unresectable carcinomatosis, which was shown on pathology to be derived from a grade II papillary serous carcinoma. No tumor debulking was performed. Within a month of the surgery, the ascites returned and the patient continued on i.p. VO injections. The second i.p. injection was associated with abdominal pain and some intraperitoneal bleeding, suggestive in retrospect of tumor necrosis. This was followed by disappearance of the ascites apart from two small fluid collections. Intraperitoneal injections continued at monthly intervals into the cystic areas. Repeated cytological examination of the cyst fluid showed only degenerate tumor cells and a background inflammatory response that included lymphocytes and macrophages (figs. 11.6 and 11.7).

After four months, less than 150 ml of cyst fluid could be removed, from only one of the cystic areas, at each monthly visit. Injections were continued into this site. Generalized ascites did not recur and the abdominal pelvic masses remained stable for ten months. At ten months, a large left-sided malignant pleural effusion that was bloodstained occurred. This was partially drained by thoracentesis, and a single 3-mg dose of VO (including both ovarian extracts) was injected into the pleural cavity without the use of a chest tube. The procedure was associated with minimal discomfort. The effusion regressed completely following the procedure (fig. 11.8). The patient was fully functional and without recurrence of her ascites or pleural effusions for 20 months. Abdominal and pelvic masses appeared to be stable during this time. At 20 months, progression of the pleura-based lesion was noted without recurrence of the effusion, and tamoxifen therapy was begun. The patient declined further chemotherapy and is alive at 31 months with slowly progressing disease.

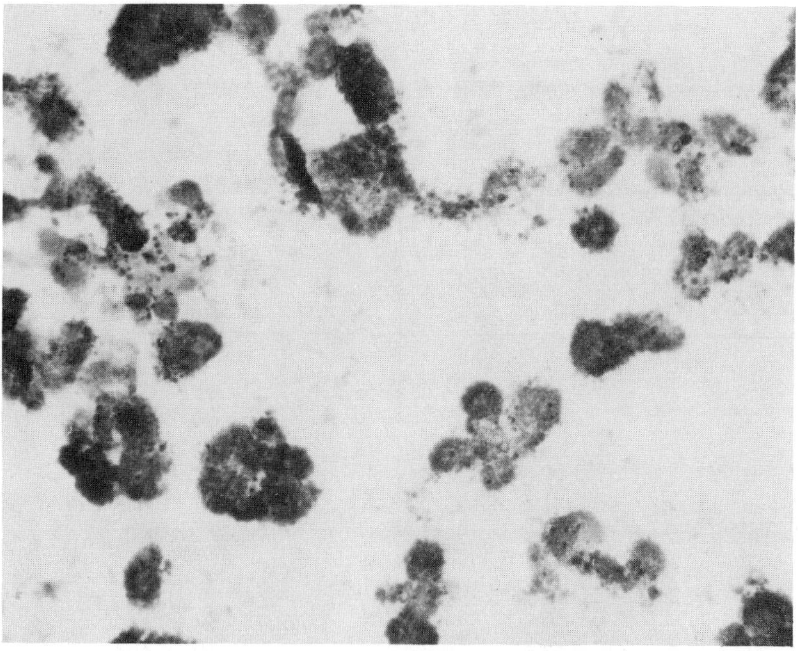

Fig. 11.6. Ascitic fluid cytology before administration of viral oncolysate.

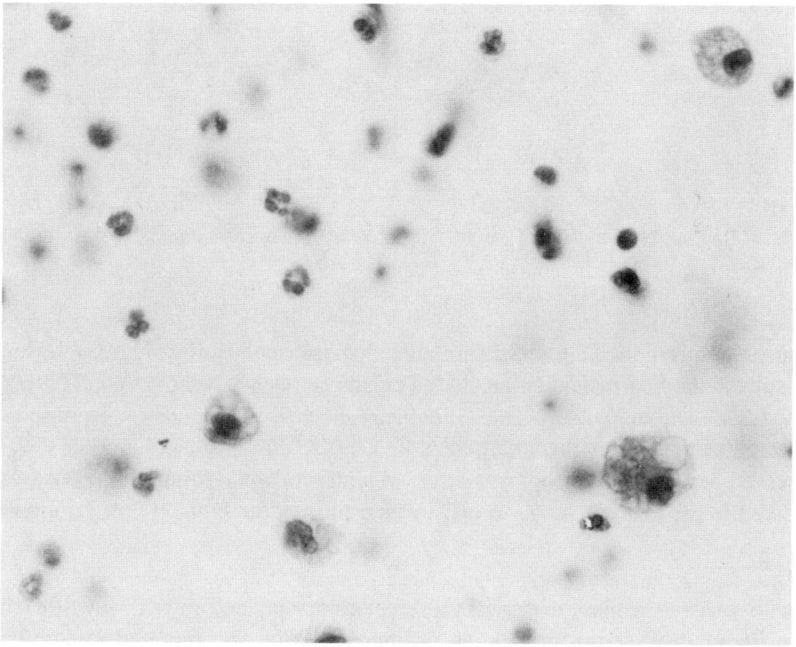

Fig. 11.7. Ascitic fluid cytology after viral oncolysate.

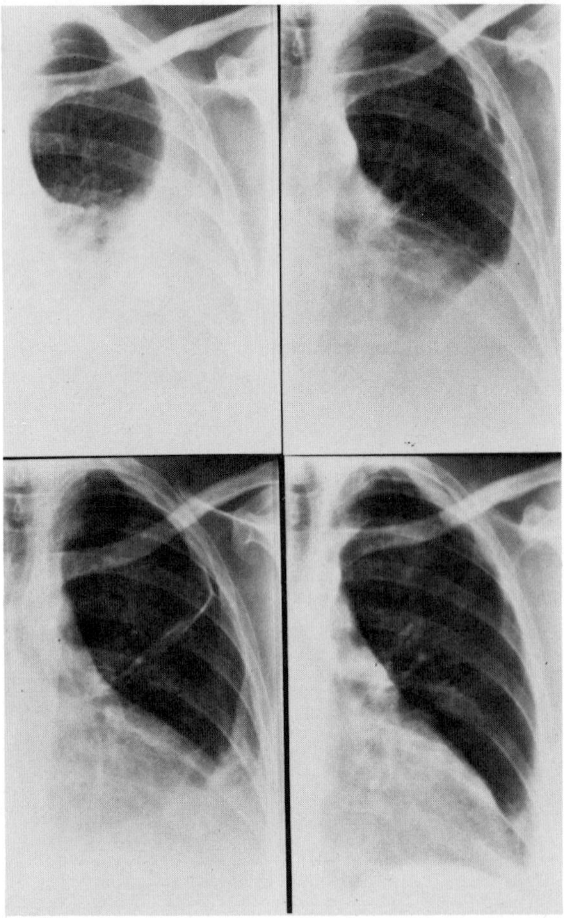

Fig. 11.8. Regression of malignant pleural effusion after viral oncolysate (chest radiograph from patient 2).

Observations in the longitudinal immune response studies (fig. 11.9) were similar to results in the first patient and included enhanced responsiveness to one of the two unmodified ovarian extracts. The T mitogen–induced blastogenesis response index studies remained within the 90th percentile (> 0.58) for this assay, but those values decreased before the development of the pleural effusion. Humoral responses were observed to the PR8 virus and to cell surface antigens on both VO preparations.

Case 3

This 26-year-old woman underwent an exploratory laparotomy in May 1981 for a stage III, grade I, serous carcinoma. Tumor reduction that required a large bowel resection was performed. Surgery was followed by 12 courses of cisplatin and cyclophosphamide until June 1982, and then megestrol acetate for 10 courses. In

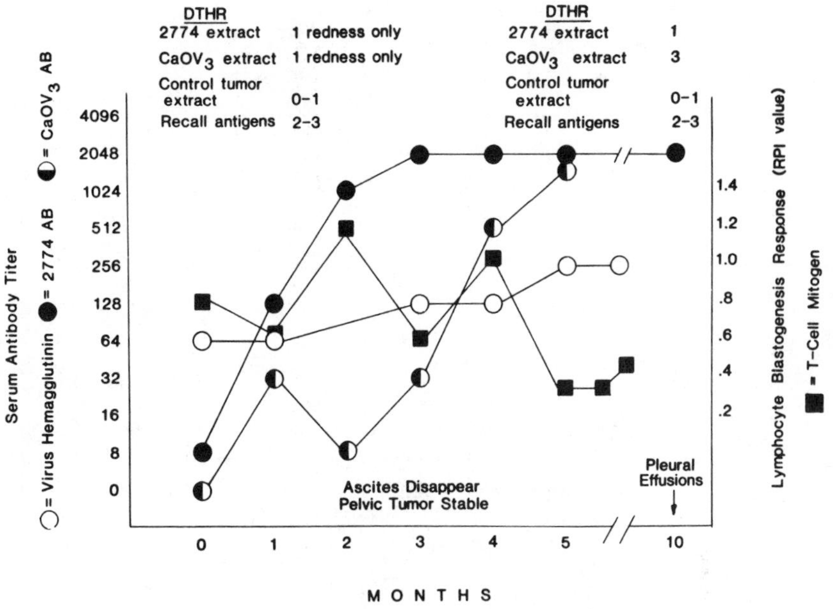

Fig. 11.9. Immune response profile of patient 2. Abbreviations as in figure 11.5.

August 1983, the patient presented with small bowel obstruction and left ureter blockage associated with a significant regrowth of the original tumor. A side-to-side bypass was performed, with placement of a ureteral stent in the obstructed ureter, and the patient was referred to U.T. M. D. Anderson Hospital in October 1983. Palpation showed large abdominopelvic masses without ascites; these findings were confirmed by palpation while the patient was under general anesthesia. A Tenckhoff catheter was implanted into the peritoneal cavity, and the patient received 12 i.p. treatments of the combined VO preparation. During the succeeding months, the abdominal tumor could no longer be palpated, and diameters of the pelvic tumor decreased by greater than 50%. These observations were confirmed by three independent examiners. The patient was fully functional and virtually without symptoms for 12 months, at which time increasing constipation was the first evidence of progression of the pelvic component. Pelvic irradiation was administered for palliative control. Perforation of the bowel occurred 3 months later, and the patient died 15 months after the first i.p. treatment. The autopsy confirmed the diagnosis and extent of disease. It was attended by the surgeon who had performed her previous operations, who determined that the abdominal disease was less than had been observed at the last surgery for small bowel obstruction. There was also no evidence of fibrosis induced by the i.p. VO administration.

Apart from flulike symptoms, there had been no other toxic effects from the i.p. treatments. The longitudinal immune studies (fig. 11.10) showed a stable response pattern in the T-mitogen assay and in the standard recall antigen response. Unlike the results in the first two patients, augmentation of skin-test reactivity to the un-

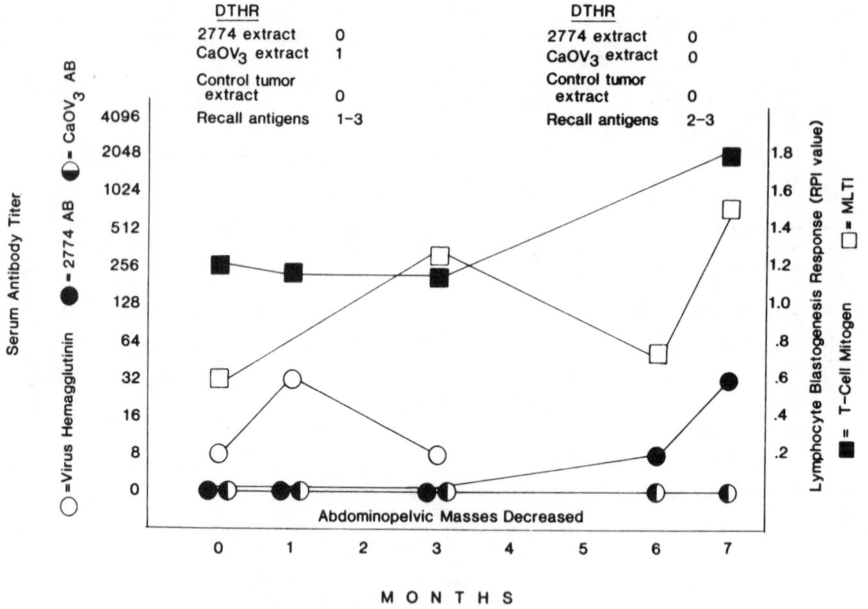

Fig. 11.10. Immune response profile of patient 3. MLTI, mixed leukocyte–tumor cell interaction. Other abbreviations as in figure 11.5.

modified tumor cell extracts was not observed and humoral responses to VO preparations were delayed or absent. The lymphocyte blastogenesis response (RPI method) to mitomycin C–inactivated $CaOV_3$ cells was increased in postimmunization lymphocytes using previously published methods (Davis et al. 1983–84). This demonstrated a responsiveness to cells used in the preparation of the oncolysates.

Case 4

This 72-year-old woman presented in 1979 with a stage III, grade III, ovarian carcinoma. She underwent initial exploration and biopsy only. The patient received combination chemotherapy with cyclophosphamide, doxorubicin HCl, and 5-fluorouracil for six months. Chemotherapy was discontinued, and the patient remained in remission for just over one year.

In January 1982, she underwent reexploration and persistent disease was found. The patient underwent a total abdominal hysterectomy and a bilateral salpingo-oophorectomy. She then received seven courses of cisplatin combined at times with hexamethylmelamine and methotrexate. In October 1982, a computerized tomography (CT) scan revealed a possible lesion in the right lobe of the liver. In December 1982, reexploration was done, and the patient was found to have small tumors in the left paracolic sulcus, the pelvic peritoneum, the diaphragm, and the liver. A biopsy of the liver was positive for metastatic carcinoma. The parenchymal liver lesion was also documented on repeat CT scan.

The patient was referred to U.T. M. D. Anderson Hospital in January 1983 for further therapy and was enrolled in an experimental protocol of ethinyl estradiol and medroxyprogesterone. She underwent 20 months of treatment, until September 1984. During this time, the liver lesion became calcified and smaller, and there was no other clinical evidence of disease. In December, the patient developed epigastric discomfort and ascites, new lesions appeared on the liver CT scan, and a small tumor nodule was palpated in the pelvis. The patient received two courses of combination chemotherapy and returned to U.T. M. D. Anderson Hospital complaining of weakness, weight loss, and clinical ascites. Two liters of clear fluid was removed and a CT scan showed a peripancreatic mass. From March 1985 onwards, the patient received monthly i.p. injections of VO, derived from both OV1 and OV2. The

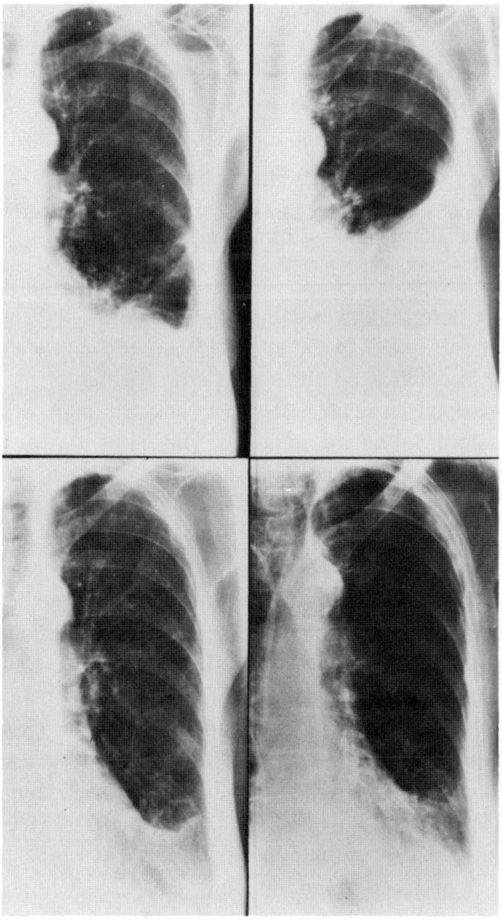

Fig. 11.11. Regression of malignant pleural effusion after viral oncolysate treatment (chest radiograph from patient 4).

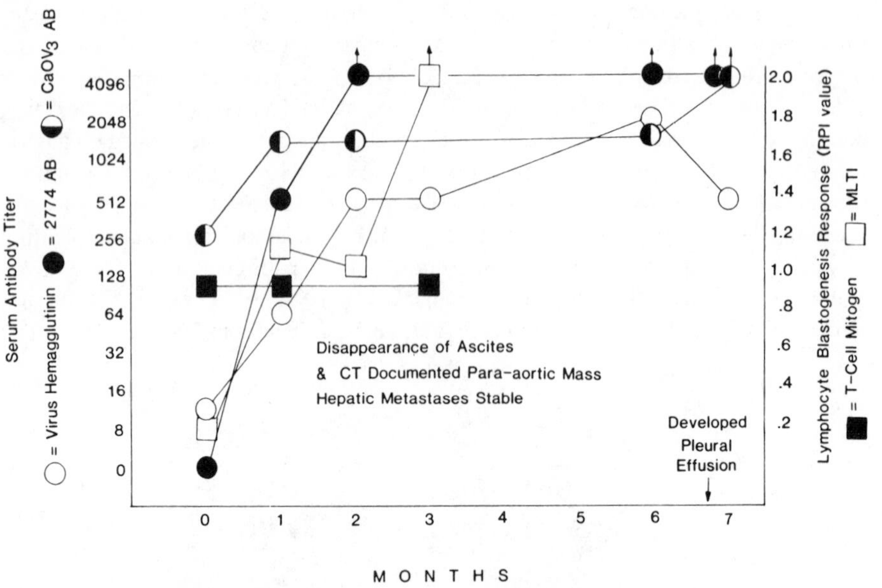

Fig. 11.12. Immune response profile of patient 4. CT, computed tomography; MLTI, mixed leukocyte–tumor cell interaction. Other abbreviations as in figure 11.5.

patient experienced considerable tiredness and malaise, but, within one month, there was a dramatic decrease in the amount of ascites and also in the number of malignant cells. At two and one-half months after the initial i.p. treatment, the patient suddenly developed an acute left-sided backache and abdominal distention. Two liters of bloodstained fluid was removed. This incident was similar to that experienced by the second patient described here.

Because of the patient's poor appetite, feeding by Dobhoff tube was commenced and replaced one month later by feeding with a percutaneous gastrostomy tube. On this regimen, the patient gained 10 kg without recurrence of her ascites, and the i.p. VO program was continued using ultrasound to localize the abdominal cavity. No abdominal masses were palpated and the liver metastases remained unchanged on CT. The previously recognized peripancreatic mass was no longer visible and no new lesions were seen. After seven months of treatment, the patient suddenly developed a left-sided pleural effusion and required continuous oxygen support. A thoracentesis was performed and was positive for malignant cells. A single intrapleural treatment with VO was administered. The pleural fluid disappeared and there was no further need for paracentesis or oxygen assistance (fig. 11.11).

The patient is presently 11 months out from the first i.p. injection without any effusions or evidence of disease other than the stable CT-documented liver metastases and a persistent small nodule on the left side of the pelvis that was detected 15 months earlier. The tube-feeding program has maintained her weight at prechemotherapy levels, but she still has malaise and restricted activity, considered to be a toxic effect of the VO, aggravated by a preexisting, chronic obstructive airways disease.

The longitudinal immune studies (fig. 11.12) in this patient are interesting in that they demonstrate the apparent existence of an antibody to the $CaOV_3$ ovarian carcinoma cells prior to the initiation of therapy. Following therapy, there was no change in the titer of this antibody, whereas a marked increase in titer to the MDAH 2774 cell line occurred. There was also a marked increase in antibody titer to the PR8 virus. An increased lymphocyte blastogenesis response to the T-cell mitogen and to the $CaOV_3$ cells was also observed.

Conclusions

Patients with ovarian cancer who present with disease that is refractory to standard chemotherapy or who develop late-onset recurrent ascites infrequently respond to other conventional therapies. Survival is usually shorter than four months in patients with late-onset ascites (Currie et al. 1983), but such cases may still offer an opportunity to evaluate new types of therapy. These new approaches include biologic agents (BRMs) such as bacterial products and the interferons (Webb, Oaten, and Pike 1978; Currie et al. 1983; Bast et al. 1983; Rambaldi et al. 1985; Mantovani et al. 1982; Uchida and Micksche 1983).

Viral oncolysates could prove useful because they are immunogenic preparations that can produce local and regional immune responses in both animals and man, which in turn may have a beneficial effect on host-tumor responses (Austin and Boone 1979; Boone 1974; Austin et al. 1982; Freedman et al. 1984; Lotzová et al. 1984). Viral oncolysates were prepared for our clinical studies using attenuated influenza virus A/PR8/34 to infect cultured ovarian carcinoma cell lines. We were able to demonstrate influenza virus–induced hemagglutinins and neuraminidase on the extracts as well as antigens that may be found on both tumor-derived ovarian carcinoma cells and allogeneic cultured ovarian carcinoma cells. The in vivo and in vitro cell-mediated and in vitro humoral immune responses that were observed following i.p. VO suggest that the ovarian patients had developed an augmented response to both the ovarian and the artificially introduced virus-related antigens. These findings confirm the antigenicity of the virus and give support to the virus "helper" or virus augmentation concept proposed in the preclinical studies (Austin and Boone 1979) and also observed in the virus-augmented skin-test studies (Freedman et al. 1984). Future studies on the characterization and purification of VO would be greatly assisted if the virus-augmented antigen response to TAA on the cultured ovarian carcinoma cell lines could also be demonstrated against antigens present on in vivo carcinoma cells.

Clinical studies with VOs using influenza PR8/A/34 have been conducted in patients with other malignancies, including malignant melanoma (Sinkovics, Plager, and McMurtrey 1980), soft tissue sarcoma (Sinkovics et al. 1974, 1978; Sinkovics, Plager, and McMurtrey 1980; Sinkovics 1977), bone sarcoma, and squamous carcinoma of the genital tract (Freedman et al. 1983; Freedman, Rutledge, and Wharton 1983). Data from these studies have shown enhanced in vivo and in vitro cell-mediated and humoral immune responses in immunized patients (Sinkovics, Plager, and McMurtrey 1980; Freedman et al. 1983); VO preparations appeared to be safe and improved survivals were suggested when VOs were used as adjuvants in treatment for high-risk primary disease. The ovarian study is the first to examine the effects of regional therapy with VOs. For ethical and other practical reasons, patients with advanced disease were selected for our initial studies.

Antitumor activity was evidenced in patients with advanced ovarian carcinoma when ovarian oncolysates as described previously were injected into the peritoneal cavity. Clinical activity was seen in 9 of 40 patients following i.p. VO. Several examples of responders in this patient group were discussed in this chapter. Responses included the disappearance of malignant ascites, resolution of pleural effusions, and reduction of some tumor masses. Life-threatening toxicity was not observed after i.p. VO, and no significant complications were attributed to repeated injections through instantly removable catheters. The results are comparable to those observed with i.p. *Corynebacterium parvum* in similar patients with advanced ovarian cancer (Webb, Oaten, and Pike 1978; Mantovani et al. 1982). The use of *C. parvum* has also been associated with significant abdominal symptoms, but increased stimulation of NK cells was not observed in a patient population similar to ours. The same investigators did, however, observe increases in the activity of NK cells after i.p. interferon. In this respect, we have observed significant levels of interferon-gamma in several patients who have received repeated injections of i.p. VO (unpublished observations). There could also be a relationship between the high and prolonged NK-cell activity reported by Lotzová et al. (1984) and regional production of lymphokines; this aspect is being investigated further.

Selective augmentation of DTH responses to unmodified ovarian carcinoma cell extracts and increased lymphocyte blastogenesis responses to phytohemagglutinin and the inactivated ovarian carcinoma cells used to prepare VO also suggest a role for the T-cell response. Humoral responses to the viral and tumor-associated determinants on the immunizing cell extracts indicate the antigenicity of the modifying virus and the modifying cell extracts and have been confirmed by other investigators (Savage et al. 1986). Since allogeneic cells are used mainly in the preparation of VOs, it has been difficult to prove that the serological activity to the surface antigens includes a specific response to determinants also present on the patient's own tumor (Livingston et al. 1985; Savage et al. 1986). Hybridoma methods could be used to address this problem. Peripheral blood lymphocytes of patients after immunization can be fused with suitable human lymphoblastoid cell lines (Glassy et al. 1983) to produce stable human antibody–secreting hybridomas. Indeed, tumor cell–reactive human monoclonal antibodies have been produced using the peripheral blood lymphocytes of actively immunized patients with colorectal carcinoma (Haspel et al. 1985). Preliminary results suggest that a similar approach is feasible in patients who are receiving VOs in therapeutic protocols. These antibodies might be used in the characterization and isolation of TAA on VO preparations, as mentioned previously. Observations from ELISA studies on ovarian VO preparations have indicated the presence of antigens common to the in vivo ovarian tumors. Moreover, since ovarian tumor cell–reactive antibodies can be produced by human hybridomas derived from immunized patients, we may also have an opportunity to develop antibodies for clinical application with reduced risks of an allergic response as compared with murine monoclonal antibodies.

Virus augmentation is an approach that appears to have potential value for clinical and biologic research. Our studies indicate clinical activity with minimal toxicity when VOs are injected into the peritoneal cavity of patients with advanced ovarian carcinomatosis. Although further studies on clinical activity and mechanisms of action are indicated, there is already evidence that VOs might be responsible for important biologic responses involving both cell-mediated and humoral immunity. Further experience with VOs can be expected to contribute to a better understanding of human tumor immunity and to determine a therapeutic role in various malignancies.

Acknowledgment

The authors wish to thank the Blum Kovler Foundation for their financial support.

References

Austin FC, Boone CW. 1979. Virus augmentation of the antigenicity of tumor cell extracts. *Adv Cancer Res* 30:301–345.

Austin FC, Boone CW, Levin DL, Cavins JA, Djerassi I, Rosner D, Case R, Klein E. 1982. Breast cancer skin test antigens of increased sensitivity prepared from vesicular stomatitis virus–infected tumor cells. *Cancer* 49:2034–2042.

Bast RC Jr, Berek JS, Obrist R, Griffiths CT, Berkowitz RS, Hacker NF, Parker L, Lagasse LD, Knapp RC. 1983. Intraperitoneal immunotherapy of human ovarian carcinoma with *Corynebacterium parvum*. *Cancer Res* 43:1395–1401.

Boone CW. 1974. Augmented immunogenicity of tumor cell homogenates infected with influenza virus. In *Recent Results in Cancer Research*, ed. G Mathe, R Weiner, pp. 394–400. New York: Springer-Verlag.

Boone CW, Austin FC, Gail M, Case R, Klein E. 1978. Melanoma skin test antigens of improved sensitivity prepared from vesicular stomatitis virus–infected tumor cells. *Cancer* 41:1781–1787.

Cassel WA, Murray DR, Phillips HS. 1983. A phase II study on the postsurgical management of stage II malignant melanoma with a Newcastle disease virus oncolysate. *Cancer* 52: 856–860.

Chan JC. 1985. A monoclonal antibody generated against MSV-induced transformation related proteins (MC). *Monoclonal Antibody News* 2:7.

Currie JL, Gall S, Weed JC, Creasman WT. 1983. Intracavitary *Corynebacterium parvum* for treatment of malignant effusions. *Gynecol Oncol* 16:6–14.

Davis JW, Freedman RS, Atkinson N, Bowen JM. 1983–84. Augmentation of in vitro lymphocyte blastogenesis and cytotoxicity responses by tumor cells modified with dodecanoyl cytochrome C. *Nat Immun Cell Growth Regul* 3:203–209.

Francis T, Magill TP. 1934. Transmission of influenza by a filterable virus. *Science* 80: 457–459.

Freedman RS. 1985. Recent immunologic advances affecting the management of ovarian cancer. In: *Clinical Obstetrics and Gynecology*, ed. JT Wharton, vol. 28, pp. 853–871. Philadelphia: Harper & Row.

Freedman RS, Bowen JM, Atkinson EN, Scott W, Wagner S. 1984. Virus-augmented delayed hypersensitivity skin tests in gynecological malignancies. *Cancer Immunol Immunother* 17:142–146.

Freedman RS, Bowen JM, Herson JH, Wharton JT, Edwards CL, Rutledge FN. 1983. Immunotherapy for vulvar carcinoma with virus-modified homologous extracts. *Obstet Gynecol* 62:707–714.

Freedman RS, Pihl E, Kusyk C, Gallager HS, Rutledge F. 1978. Characterization of an ovarian carcinoma cell line. *Cancer* 42:2352–2359.

Freedman RS, Rutledge FN, Wharton JT. 1983. Adjunctive immunotherapy with VMTCE in patients with high-risk squamous carcinoma of the uterine cervix (abstract). *Am J Clin Oncol* 6:155–156.

Gillette RW, Boone CW. 1976. Augmented immunogenicity of tumor cell membranes produced by surface budding viruses: Parameters of optimal immunization. *Int J Cancer* 18:216–222.

Glassy MC, Handley HH, Hagiwara H, Royston I. 1983. UC 729-6, a human lymphoblastoid B-cell line useful for generating antibody-secreting human-human hybridomas. *Proc Natl Acad Sci USA* 80:6327–6331.

Green AA, Pratt C, Webster RB. 1976. Immunotherapy of osteosarcoma patients with virus-modified tumor cells. *Ann NY Acad Sci* 277:396–411.

Haspel MV, McCabe RP, Pomato N, Janesch NJ, Knowlton JV, Peters LC, Hoover HC Jr, Hanna MG Jr. 1985. Generation of tumor cell–reactive human monoclonal antibodies using peripheral blood lymphocytes from actively immunized colorectal carcinoma patients. *Cancer Res* 45:3951–3961.

Klostergaard J. 1985. A rapid, extremely sensitive, quantitative microassay for cytotoxic cytokines. *Lymphokine Res* 4:309–317.

Kobayashi H. 1982. Modification of tumor antigenicity in therapeutics: Increase in immunologic foreignness of tumor cells in experimental model systems. In *Immunological Approaches to Cancer Therapeutics*, ed. E Mihich, pp. 405–440. New York: John Wiley & Sons.

Koprowski H, Love R, Koprowski I. 1957. Enhancement of susceptibility to viruses in neoplastic tissues. *Texas Reports on Biology and Medicine* 15:559–576.

Lindenmann J. 1974. Viruses as immunological adjuvants in cancer. *Biochim Biophys Acta* 355:49–75.

Lindenmann J, Klein PA. 1967. Viral oncolysis: Increased immunogenicity of host cell antigen associated with influenza virus. *J Exp Med* 126:93–108.

Livingston PO, Albino AP, Chung TJC, Real FX, Houghton AN, Oettgen HF, Old LJ. 1985. Serological response of melanoma patients to vaccines prepared from VSV lysates of autologous and allogeneic cultured melanoma cells. *Cancer* 55:713–720.

Lotzová E, Savary CA, Freedman RS, Bowen JM. 1984. Natural killer cell cytotoxic potential of patients with ovarian carcinoma and its modulation with virus-modified tumor cell extract. *Cancer Immunol Immunother* 17:124–129.

Mantovani A, Allavena P, Biondi A, Sessa C, Introna M. 1982. NK activity in human ovarian carcinoma. In *Natural Killer Cells*, ed. B Serrou, C Rosenfeld, RB Herberman, p. 123. Amsterdam: Elsevier/Biomedical Press.

Mantovani A, Allavena P, Sessa C, Bolis G, Mangioni C. 1980. Natural killer activity of lymphoid cells isolated from human ascitic ovarian tumors. *Int J Cancer* 25:573–582.

Mattes MJ, Cordon-Cardo C, Lewis JL Jr, Old LJ, Lloyd KO. 1984. Cell surface antigens of human ovarian and endometrial carcinoma defined by mouse monoclonal antibodies. *Proc Natl Acad Sci USA* 81:568–572.

Murray DR, Cassel WA, Torbin AH, Olkowski Z, Moore ME. 1977. Viral oncolysate in the management of malignant melanoma. *Cancer* 40:680–686.

Rambaldi A, Introna M, Colotta F, Landolfo S, Colombo N, Mangioni C, Mantovani A.

1985. Intraperitoneal administration of interferon beta in ovarian cancer patients. *Cancer* 56:294–301.
Salk JE. 1944. A simplified procedure for titrating hemagglutinating capacity of influenza virus and corresponding antibody. *J Immunol* 49:87–98.
Sauter C, Cavalli F, Lindenmann J. 1978. Viral oncolysis: Its application in maintenance treatment of acute myelogenous leukemia: Study analysis at 2.5 years. Current Chemotherapy Proceedings at the 10th International Congress in Chemotherapy in Zurich. *International Society of Chemotherapy*, vol. 2.
Savage HE, Rossen RD, Hersh EM, Freedman RS, Bowen JM, Plager C. 1986. Antibody development to viral and allogeneic tumor cell–associated antigens in patients with malignant melanoma and ovarian carcinoma treated with lysates of virus-infected tumor cells. *Cancer Res* 46:2127–2133.
Silverberg E, Lubera J. 1986. Cancer statistics. *CA* 36:9–25.
Sinkovics JG. 1977. Immunotherapy with viral oncolysates for sarcoma (letter). *JAMA* 237:869.
Sinkovics JG, Plager C, McMurtrey M. 1980. Adjuvant chemoimmunotherapy for malignant melanoma. In *Neoplasm Immunity: Experimental and Clinical*, ed. RG Crispen, pp. 481–519. New York: Elsevier/Biomedical Press.
Sinkovics JG, Plager C, Papadopoulos N, McMurtrey MJ, Romero JJ, Waldinger R, Romsdahl MM. 1978. Immunology and immunotherapy of human sarcomas. In *Immunotherapy of Human Cancer*, pp. 267–288. The University of Texas System Cancer Center M. D. Anderson Hospital and Tumor Institute 22nd Annual Clinical Conference on Cancer. New York: Raven Press.
Sinkovics JG, Thota H, Loh KK, Gonzalez F, Campos LT, Romero JJ, Kay HD, King DK. 1975. Prospectives for immunotherapy for human sarcomas. In *Cancer Chemotherapy — Fundamental Concepts and Recent Advances*, pp. 417–443. The University of Texas System Cancer Center M. D. Anderson Hospital and Tumor Institute 19th Annual Clinical Conference on Cancer. Chicago: Year Book Medical Publishers.
Staudt LM, Gerhard W. 1983. Generation of antibody diversity in the immune response of BALB/c mice to influenza virus hemagglutinin. I. Significant variation in repertoire expression between individual mice. *J Exp Med* 157:687–704.
Uchida A, Micksche M. 1983. Intrapleural administration of OK432 in cancer patients: Activation of NK cells and reduction of suppressor cells. *Int J Cancer* 31:1–5.
Wallack MK, Meyer M, Bourgoin A, Dore JF, Leftheriotis E, Carcagne J, Koprowski H. 1983. A preliminary trial of vaccinia oncolysates in the treatment of recurrent melanoma with serologic responses to the treatment. *J Biol Response Mod* 2:586–596.
Webb HE, Oaten SW, Pike CP. 1978. Treatment of malignant ascitic and pleural effusions with *Corynebacterium parvum*. *Br Med J [Clin Res]* 1:338–340.

Annual Clinical Conference on Cancer, Vol. 29
Gynecologic Cancer: Diagnosis and Treatment Strategies
© 1987 by The University of Texas System Cancer Center

12. Cancer Therapy by Biologic-Response Modifiers

Ronald B. Herberman

Biologic-response modifiers (BRMs) have been defined as those agents or approaches that modify the relationship between the tumor and host by modifying the host's biologic response to tumor cells, with resultant therapeutic effects (Vanky and Argov 1980). Biologic-response modifiers may modify the host responses in several ways: (1) by increasing the host's antitumor response by augmentation or restoration of effector mechanisms or mediators of the host's defenses, or decreasing a component of the host's reactions that may interfere with antitumor responses; (2) by administering natural or recombinant, genetically engineered effectors or mediators of antitumor responses; (3) by augmenting the sensitivity of the host's tumor cells to endogenous mechanisms for control of tumor growth; (4) by decreasing the transformation or increasing the differentiation of tumor cells; and (5) by increasing the ability of the host to tolerate damage by conventional cancer treatments, particularly chemotherapy or radiotherapy.

A major category of BRMs includes the agents called immunomodulators; therapeutic approaches with such agents could be defined as immunotherapy. Immunomodulators include both chemical and biologic agents, which can modify immunologic resistance mechanisms of the host that might be important in control of tumor growth or metastasis. There are a variety of different agents in this category. These include chemical or synthetic, as well as natural, agents that affect the immune response; antigens on cells or isolated from them; immunologic effector cells or antibodies with tumor effects; and soluble factors produced by various cells that may affect the immune system (referred to as cytokines). A type of nonimmunologic BRM that could favorably affect host resistance to tumors would be a protective agent that, in some way, could overcome or lessen the damage produced by chemotherapy or radiotherapy and thereby facilitate the actions of the host's effector mechanisms.

Another category of BRMs includes cellular products, particularly products made by components of the immune system, that could have direct antitumor effects. For example, cytotoxic antibodies and some cytokines (e.g., lymphotoxin and tumor necrosis factor) can have direct cytotoxic activity against tumor cells. Similarly, some immunologic effector cells (e.g., cytotoxic T cells, natural killer [NK] cells, and macrophages) have substantial cytotoxic reactivity against a variety of tumor cells. There is also the potential for various cellular products to influence tumor growth, not by being directly cytotoxic, but by decreasing the state of transformation or increasing the differentiation of the tumor cells (optimally, to a terminal, nonproliferative mature form) or, in some way, changing the sensitivity of the tumor cells to control by intrinsic effector mechanisms in the host.

A major problem is that most BRMs are pleiotropic in their actions. It was hoped for some time that in the transition from relatively crude microbial agents (e.g., bacille Calmette Guérin [BCG] or *Corynebacterium parvum*) to chemically defined, purified, even homogeneous substances, particularly those with low molecular weight, only one function or action in the host would be observed. However, it has usually been found that low-molecular-weight homogeneous chemicals tend to be pleiotropic in their effects on the immune system or on other host functions.

What are the biologic effects of a BRM on which we should focus? In considering the use of agents for therapeutic efficacy, it seems reasonable to place a strong emphasis on effector cells, which can have cytotoxic effects on tumor cells. In classic immunologic terms, cytotoxic T lymphocytes (CTL) would be considered the main candidate for mediation of specific and potent resistance against tumor growth and progression. However, CTL would only be relevant for tumors with immunogenic, tumor-associated transplantation antigens. The proportion of human tumors that fall in this category remains unclear. Although CTL with apparent specificity, with restriction to autologous and not allogeneic tumors, have been generated from lymphocytes from some cancer patients (Vanky and Argov 1980; Vose and Bonnard 1982), it has been technically difficult to extend such approaches to large numbers of patients with a wide variety of tumor types. In addition, studies with spontaneous tumors in rodents have often failed to detect tumor-associated transplantation antigens. This is in contrast with earlier positive results with tumors induced by oncogenic viruses or chemical carcinogens. Because almost all human tumors, in the absence of a clearly defined etiology, are considered to be spontaneous, the negative results obtained with spontaneous rodent tumors have often been considered to be more clinically relevant (Hewitt 1982). There has also been considerable evidence against a central role for immune T cells in protection against a variety of tumors. For example, the incidence of spontaneous or chemical carcinogen–induced tumors has generally been the same in nude or neonatally thymectomized mice as in euthymic mice (Stutman 1979).

There is a large amount of data to indicate that NK cells may be quite important for resistance against metastases from tumors (for reviews see Herberman in press; Herberman 1980; Hanna in press). If the NK cell activity of mice or rats is depressed by various treatments, including nonspecifically with drugs, such as cyclophosphamide, or more selectively with antibodies such as antiasialo GM_1, or by use of beige mice, which have a selective immunologic deficit on NK activity, one sees considerably more metastases than in control animals with normal levels of NK activity. More direct evidence that NK cells are required for resistance against metastases from some tumors has come from experiments with a rat mammary adenocarcinoma (Barlozzari et al. 1985). Rats pretreated with antiasialo GM_1 developed a large increase in the number of lung metastases as compared with controls treated with normal serum. However, when NK activity was selectively restored by adoptive transfer of a purified population of large granular lymphocytes (LGL)—the small subpopulation of lymphocytes that account for virtually all NK activity—

there was a concomitant restoration of resistance to the development of metastases.

Another issue that was raised by studies in experimental animals is whether monitoring of NK cell and other immunologic parameters only in the central and convenient sources of lymphocytes, i.e., blood or spleen, is sufficient. Most metastases occur in the major organs such as the lungs or liver. The important questions then are: What is the effector activity in these organs, and is that affected in the same way by a BRM as effector cells in the blood or spleen? Procedures have been developed to isolate LGL from the lungs and liver of mice. After administration of a variety of BRMs, including MVE-2, a pyran copolymer, or *C. parvum*, or interferon, there was a large increase in the number of LGL accumulating in these organs, accompanied by a marked increase in NK activity (Wiltrout et al. 1984). This is encouraging because it shows that specific types of effector cells can be increased in the organs where metastases might be present. It also seems important to consider effector cell activity in such sites. This is because repeated doses of a BRM such as MVE-2 may cease to stimulate augmented NK activity in the spleen but still continue to stimulate high levels of NK activity in the liver or lungs (Talmadge et al. 1985). This has potentially quite important implications for clinical studies, where it is generally preferred that the agent be given repeatedly over a prolonged period of time. Monitoring of NK activity in the peripheral blood of patients receiving repeated high doses of alpha interferon has indicated a hyporesponsiveness to augmentation of NK activity. It would be quite helpful to develop the ability to also sample effector cells from tissue sites, to determine the degree of correlation with blood levels.

For each BRM, it would be very desirable to determine which effector mechanism is actually responsible for the agent's antitumor effects. This would allow a focus of monitoring effects on that parameter. This question is difficult to answer, even in experimental tumor systems; however, it has been approached with MVE-2, which, as noted above, can augment NK activity and can also strongly augment macrophage-mediated cytotoxic activity. Experiments have been performed with mice treated with antiasialo GM_1 in addition to the BRM. When sufficient antiserum was given to ablate NK activity in the liver or lungs, MVE-2 lost its ability to protect against the development of metastases (Wiltrout et al. 1985). This supports the conclusion that the NK activity was, in fact, quite important in the protection afforded by MVE-2 against this tumor. It will be important to extend such an approach to other BRMs and other tumor systems, to determine to what extent augmented NK activity is responsible for therapeutic efficacy.

Ideally, one would like to have all promising BRMs evaluated in depth for their in vivo immunologic and antitumor effects in rodents and to determine the effector cells required for their therapeutic efficacy. However, a variety of potentially useful BRMs do not cross the species barrier. They might have potent effects, either directly on human tumor cells or indirectly on patients' effector mechanisms, but be entirely ineffective in rodents. For such BRMs (e.g., most human interferons and monoclonal antibodies against human tumors), it has been necessary to rely on in vitro preclinical assessments and on studies of human tumor xenografts in nude mice.

Interferons

As an example of some of the issues to be faced in studies with BRMs, it is worthwhile to consider some of the lessons learned from studies with the interferons. A family of proteins that induce antiviral resistance in cells, interferons represent the BRMs that have been most extensively evaluated over the last few years. With the advent of recombinant DNA technology, it has been possible to produce large, essentially unlimited quantities of homogeneous materials for clinical use. However, it has become very clear that each of the interferons that have been examined has quite pleiotropic effects. On one hand, interferons can directly inhibit the growth of certain tumor cells, and this could be an important mechanism by which they might be useful therapeutically. On the other hand, the interferons are very potent immunomodulators. They can augment NK cell activity and activate macrophages for antitumor cytotoxic activity. They can modulate specific T cell immunity and change various cell surface structures (e.g., tumor-associated antigens and antigens of the major histocompatibility complex), which can be quite important in immune responses against tumors. Any one of these possible effects might account for therapeutic efficacy in some circumstances.

For the last several years, the interferons have been in phase I and II clinical trials, and, by now, hundreds of patients have been treated. It has become reasonably clear that certain types of tumors, particularly lymphomas and hairy cell leukemia, are highly responsive to interferon (Foon et al. in press; Quesada et al. 1984). It is quite possible that the high degree of responsiveness that has been seen in these tumors may be related to a direct antitumor effect of interferon. There are at least some hints that higher doses are more effective than lower doses, but some excellent clinical responses have been observed with low doses. In other tumor types in which clinical responses have been seen only infrequently, it seems possible that interferons have little direct antitumor effect but might be effective if they induced potent immunomodulation. The current clinical protocols that are being used with interferon have not been shown to have optimal—or even good—immunomodulatory effects on parameters that would be expected to be strongly affected as shown in past in vitro studies with human peripheral blood mononuclear cells and studies in animal model systems (Maluish et al. 1983). A major concern is that one might draw a premature negative conclusion about the lack of efficacy of a BRM such as interferon when it has not been adequately tested under the appropriate circumstances. For evaluation of the potential therapeutic benefit of interferon through some of its immunomodulatory effects, it seems essential to develop protocols and schedules of administration that produce the desired alterations in the patients' immune functions. Until that has been achieved, the hypothesis that interferons can have therapeutic efficacy by their ability to augment immunologic effector mechanisms will not be adequately tested.

Interleukin-2

Another example of some current problems in the evaluation of BRMs has come from studies with another cytokine, interleukin-2 (IL-2). This cytokine is a product of T cells and LGL that can stimulate the growth and function of T cells and NK cells; by either one of these effects, it might be quite useful therapeutically. The Biological Response Modifiers Program (BRMP) of the National Cancer Institute decided last year to become actively involved in clinical trials with IL-2, and as a first step it organized an in-depth preclinical evaluation of the effects of IL-2. In addition, most IL-2 preparations, including the recombinant materials, have recently been found to have macrophage or monocyte-activating properties. This indicates an additional functional effect of IL-2 that might have therapeutic implications and will need to be monitored during clinical trials with IL-2. Preclinical evaluation of IL-2 has been easier than that of interferons because human IL-2 is active in mice and rats as well as in humans. Thus, it can be extensively tested, both in vitro and in vivo, in rodents as well as in humans. Recombinant IL-2 alone was found to have substantial efficacy against pulmonary metastases from B16 melanoma in mice. Significant effects were observed with modest doses of IL-2, as well as with very high doses. This indicates that phase I clinical trials should cover a wide dose range and not be restricted to very high and toxic dose levels.

In addition to the assessment of a variety of parameters in animal model systems, one needs to consider which IL-2 preparation to utilize. One question was whether to perform studies with natural IL-2, produced by lymphoid cells, or to proceed immediately to studies with the recombinant protein. On one hand, recombinant IL-2 was preferred because of the potential availability of unlimited quantities of homogeneous factor. Natural IL-2 preparations, on the other hand, are difficult to make in large amounts and to purify to homogeneity. However, one might expect that the lack of glycosylation of the recombinant protein and possible differences in its physical form might make it appreciably different from natural IL-2 in terms of biodistribution or functional activities. Upon surveying possible supplies of IL-2, we soon became aware of 12 different products—six natural and six recombinant. Since clearly it would not be practical to perform clinical trials with more than one or two of these preparations, a series of preclinical studies was performed to directly compare the potency of the different products in various functional assays and to examine them for possible contaminants or unexpected effects (Thurman et al. 1986).

To adequately evaluate the relative potency of the various IL-2 preparations, we first had to standardize them in terms of their activity in assays of growth promotion of T cell lines. When the preparations were all compared to a BRMP standard preparation of IL-2, it was obvious that a unit of IL-2 from one company was considerably different from a unit of IL-2 from another company. Overall, there was greater than a 100-fold variation in the preparations in regard to the relationship between the companies' stated units of activity and the BRMP reference units that were actually measured. To adequately compare the results of the various trials with different IL-2 preparations, it will obviously be important to achieve standardization of the units of activity. Beyond the standardization of the potency, another issue was to determine the possible presence of contaminants in the preparations. Although it is desirable to work only with homogeneous materials, there were no completely homogeneous natural IL-2 preparations available. It was therefore necessary to screen for a number of other cytokine activities and other materials that might have been contaminating the IL-2. Endotoxin was detected in some of the natural and recombinant preparations, which would clearly have been undesirable for clinical use. Some of the natural products were found to have interferon activity, and if these were used in clinical trials it would be difficult to determine whether any therapeutic effects were due to the IL-2 or to the interferon. In addition, after the IL-2 preparations were standardized to have the same potency in terms of their ability to grow T cells, they were still found to vary in regard to other biologic activities. For example, there was much heterogeneity—greater than 50-fold—in the ability of the preparations to augment NK cell activity, another important property of IL-2. Even among the recombinant IL-2 preparations, there was a 50-fold difference among the preparations in NK cell–augmenting activity.

Lymphokine-Activated Killer Cells

The combination of IL-2 administration with the adoptive transfer of large numbers of lymphokine-activated killer (LAK) cells has recently been reported to have therapeutic efficacy in some patients with advanced metastatic disease (Rosenberg et al. 1985). These encouraging preliminary results raise many important questions; for example, what is the nature of the LAK cells responsible for the in vivo antitumor effects? What is the optimal way to generate high levels of activity and maximal proliferation in vitro and in vivo of the effector cells? What doses and schedules for administration of IL-2 and LAK cells are optimal for therapy, and can one develop a protocol that will be effective and yet avoid the serious toxicity associated with the initial trial? Will systemically administered LAK cells circulate sufficiently well and reach all of the sites of tumor involvement, or could direct administration of effector cells into the tumor area be required instead of, or in addition to, systemic administration in order to achieve long-lasting therapeutic benefits?

In regard to the nature of LAK cells, it was initially thought that these effector cells must be distinct from NK cells because fresh solid tumor cells are rather resistant to NK cell activity of unfractionated lymphoid cells (Grimm et al. 1983). However, studies in several laboratories have indicated that isolated human or mouse LGL have substantial NK cell activity against autologous or syngeneic, as well as allogeneic, fresh tumor cells (Serrate et al. 1982; Uchida and Yanagawa 1984). In addition, recent studies have indicated that the cytotoxic activity of NK cells is strongly augmented by IL-2 (Ortaldo 1984)—at least a large proportion of LAK activity is derived from lymphocytes with NK cell–associated markers (e.g., Itoh et al. 1985).

To gain insight into some of the other issues raised above, experiments have been performed on a mouse tumor model, involving the inoculation of a transplantable renal cell carcinoma under the kidney capsule (Salup, Herberman, and Wiltrout 1985). This tumor followed a course of growth that was very similar to that seen clinically. After initial growth in the kidney, there was local invasion through the capsule into the perinephric area, then regional lymph node and venous metastastic involvement, followed by distant metastatic growth. When therapy was initiated at one week after tumor inoculation, nephrectomy was not curative, indicating the early presence of occult metastases. Treatment with IL-2 plus IL-2–stimulated spleen cells also failed to result in long-term survival. Chemotherapy also was not particularly effective because only a small percentage of the animals showed long-term survival (Salup and Wiltrout in press). In contrast, when combined therapy was performed with Adriamycin for cytoreduction along with IL-2 plus IL-2–stimulated spleen cells, the majority of the mice showed long-term survival and, in fact, could be shown to be cured of their disease. When treatment was delayed until visible metastases were present (Salup and Wiltrout 1986), more extensive combination therapy was required. A high percentage of long-term survivors could only be obtained in mice treated by surgical removal of the primary tumor and by intraperitoneal as well as intravenous administration of chemotherapy plus adoptive immunotherapy with IL-2 and IL-2–stimulated cells. These results emphasize several points:

1. Immunotherapy is likely to be very effective only when there is a low tumor burden and may have no detectable benefits when given alone to individuals with extensive, advanced disease. Thus, immunotherapeutic efforts should be directed toward the treatment of residual disease after reduction of tumor burden by surgery, chemotherapy, or radiotherapy.
2. Treatment directed at tumor involvement in each of several compartments may be needed for curative effects, presumably due to problems of access of the administered cells (or other agents) to all of the tumor cells when only systemic administration is utilized.
3. Dramatic therapeutic results with this approach can be achieved with relatively modest and nontoxic doses of IL-2 and cells.
4. Recent evidence indicates that most (or all) of the effector cells in this experimental model have markers of NK cells and not of CTL as has been noted by R. Salup, M.D. (personal communication, March 1986).

Phase I Clinical Trials

Another major issue to be considered is the design of phase I clinical trials with BRMs. Currently, clinical trials with BRMs are being performed along lines very similar to those utilized for trials with chemotherapeutic agents. Phase I trials with both BRMs and chemotherapeutic agents are performed in patients with advanced cancer in whom other therapies have failed. The major emphasis in the phase I trials has been to evaluate toxicity and to determine the maximum tolerated dose (MTD). To get some information about the immunologic or other biologic effects of the BRMs, assays have been performed to determine possible biologic responses in the context of the dose-escalation studies. A major goal in the phase I trials with BRMs is to not only determine the MTD but also to determine the optimal biologic response modifying dose (OBRMD, namely, the dose that would have the optimal or maximum effects on the immunologic or other biologic parameters that would be expected to be most important for therapeutic efficacy). Unfortunately, with current trial design, one regularly gets the information about toxicity and MTD, but often inadequate information is gathered to determine the OBRMD. For example, in the studies with interferon, although hundreds of patients now have been put into phase I and II trials, the OBRMD has yet to be determined. This has resulted in the design of phase II trials with doses close to the MTD. Since the interferons might have therapeutic effects as a result of their ability to modify biologic responses, it would be highly desirable to also perform phase II therapeutic trials with the OBRMD, which might be considerably different from the MTD. Unfortunately, it is becoming increasingly clear that a phase I trial that is designed primarily to obtain MTD and toxicity information may not be adequate to get sufficient information about the OBRMD.

Another major problem to consider in this regard is that the effects of BRMs on the immune system or on other biologic responses in previously treated patients with advanced disease and large tumor burdens might not be comparable to the effects of the same materials, even at the same doses, on patients with lower tumor burdens. As discussed above, there is also considerable evidence from animal model systems that many, if not most, BRMs would have therapeutic efficacy only in individuals with low tumor burdens and would be ineffective in individuals with extensive, widespread disease. Therefore, with the current design of phase I and II clinical trials with BRMs, immunomodulatory and positive clinical effects of potentially valuable BRMs might be completely missed.

Yet another problem is that of adequate systemic delivery of the agents to the tumor sites. A number of BRMs are labile, have a short half-life in the circulation, and do not distribute evenly throughout the body. As discussed above, IL-2 is an example of this problem. After intravenous inoculation, the half-life of IL-2 in the serum is only a few minutes, and it may not accumulate in sufficient levels in the lymphoid organs or at sites of tumor growth where its effect would hopefully be mediated.

What are the possible solutions to the problems that I have raised? One would be to have a greater emphasis in the phase I trials on determining the OBRMD. The OBRMD may be defined as the safe route, dose, and schedule that induce sustained or repeated alterations in a maximum number of the desired parameters, particularly immunologic functions that would be expected to have direct effector activity against the tumor. One could also examine the biologic response modifying aspects in phase I trials in patients with lower tumor burden and even in patients with minimal or no detectable disease who have not received chemotherapy or radiotherapy. Alternatively, or in addition, one could perform phase I trials with BRMs in combination with cytoreductive therapy, since these combinations may be most useful for therapy, and it would be important to first determine the biologic response modification that could be induced in this context.

The sequence of clinical studies with BRMs that I have proposed, which has been supported quite enthusiastically by the NCI BRMP's Decision Network Committee, would be to divide phase I into two stages: phase I-A and I-B. Phase I-A trials would first be performed in patients with advanced cancer, primarily to get the necessary information on toxicity and possibly to determine the MTD. Immunologic and other biologic studies would be performed in those patients, but as in current studies, this would be a secondary objective. At the conclusion of the phase I-A trial, a phase I-B trial would be performed in which the main focus would be on determining the OBRMD. Such studies would be performed in patients with minimal, or perhaps even undetectable, tumor burden. Then the established OBRMD would be used to examine therapeutic efficacy in phase II trials in patients at the same stage of disease as the patients utilized in the phase I-B trial.

This is clearly a more complicated study design than that currently used. Only certain types of patients would be suitable for the phase I-B or phase II trials that I am proposing. Unfortunately, however, there are several major tumor types in which after surgical resection of tumor, there is a relatively low tumor burden but a high probability of rapid recurrence of tumor growth and metastases and refractoriness to currently available forms of therapy. For example, patients with non–small cell carcinoma of the lung or Dukes' C colorectal carcinoma would seem to be good candidates for phase I-B and II studies with BRMs. Alternatively, as discussed above, for the mouse model of renal cell carcinoma, these dose-finding efforts could be performed in trials combining the BRM with a cytoreductive and well-tolerated schedule of chemotherapy.

Conclusions

BRMs appear to have considerable promise for therapy of malignant disease. This conclusion is based mainly on many positive therapeutic results with a wide variety of BRMs in experimental animal tumor systems. The major challenge appears to be how to translate such therapeutic efficacy into a clinically applicable setting. As discussed above, it seems that empirically designed clinical studies, even with highly promising BRMs, will be unlikely to produce even close to optimal therapeutic efficacy. Rather, it will probably be essential to systemically evaluate the range of biologic effects of each agent, particularly on antitumor effector cells, determine the OBRMD in well-designed phase I-A and I-B studies, and only then perform the appropriate phase II and III therapeutic trials.

References

Barlozzari T, Leonhardt J, Wiltrout R, Herberman RB, Reynolds CW. 1985. Direct evidence for the role of LGL in the inhibition of experimental tumor metastases. *J Immunol* 134:2783–2789.

Foon KA, Sherwin SA, Abrams PG, Longo DL, Fer MF, Stevenson HC, Ochs JJ, Bottino GC, Schoenberger CS, Zeffren J, Jaffe ES, Oldham RK. 1984. Treatment of advanced non-Hodgkin's lymphoma with recombinant leukocyte A interferon. *N Engl J Med* 311: 1148–1152.

Grimm EA, Ramsey KM, Mazumder A, Wilson DJ, Djeu JY, Rosenberg SA. 1983. Lymphokine-activated killer cell phenomenon. II. Precursor phenotype is serologically distinct from peripheral T lymphocytes, memory cytotoxic thymus-derived lymphocytes, and natural killer cells. *J Exp Med* 157:884–897.

Hanna N. In press. Review of evidence for the role of NK cells in immunoprophylaxis of metastasis. In *Immune Responses to Metastases*. ed. RB Herberman, RH Wiltrout, E Gorelik. Boca Raton:CRC Press.

Herberman RB. In press. Antimetastasis and immunoregulatory functions of NK cells. Federation Proceedings.

Herberman RB (ed.). 1980. *Natural Cell-Mediated Immunity Against Tumors*. New York: Academic Press.

Hewitt HB. 1982. Animal tumor models and their relevance to human tumor immunology. *J Biol Response Mod* 1:107–119.

Itoh K, Tilden AB, Kumagai K, Balch CM. 1985. Leu 11^+ lymphocytes with natural killer (NK) activity are precursors of recombinant interleukin 2 (or IL-2)–induced activated killer (AK) cells. *J Immunol* 134:802–807.

Maluish AE, Leavitt R, Sherwin SA, Oldham RK, Herberman RB. 1983. Effects of recombinant interferon-alpha on immune function in cancer patients. *J Biol Response Mod* 2:470–481.

Ortaldo JR, Mason L, Gerard JP, Henderson LE, Farrar W, Hopkins RF III, Herberman RB, Rabin H. 1984. Effects of natural and recombinant IL-2 on regulation of IFN production and natural killer activity: Lack of involvement of the TAC antigen for these immunoregulatory effects. *J Immunol* 133:779–783.

Quesada JR, Reuben J, Manning JR, Hersh EM, Gutterman JU. 1984. Alpha interferon for induction of remission in hairy cell leukemia. *N Engl J Med* 310:15–18.

Rosenberg SA, Lotze MT, Muul LM, Leitman S, Chang A, Ettinghausen SE, Matory YL, Skibber JM, Shiloni E, Vetta JT, Seipp CA, Simpson C, Reichart CM. 1985. Observations on the systemic administration of autologous lymphokine activated killer cells and recombinant IL-2 to patients with metastatic cancer. *N Engl J Med* 313:1485–1492.

Salup R, Herberman RB, Wiltrout R. 1985. Role of NK activity in development of spontaneous metastases in murine renal cell cancer. *J Urol* 134:1236–1241.

Salup R, Wiltrout R. 1986. Adjuvant immunotherapy of established murine cancer by interleukin 2–stimulated cytotoxic lymphocytes. *Cancer Res* 46:3358–3363.

Salup R, Wiltrout R. 1986. Chemoimmunotherapy of advanced murine renal carcinoma. In *Leukocytes and Host Defense*, ed. JJ Oppenheim, B Jacobs, pp. 457–464. New York: Alan R. Liss.

Serrate SA, Vose BM, Timonen T, Ortaldo JR, Herberman RB. 1982. Association of human natural killer cell activity against human primary tumors with large granular lymphocytes. In *NK Cells and Other Natural Effector Cells*, ed. RB Herberman, pp. 1055–1060. New York: Academic Press.

Stutman O. 1979. Chemical carcinogenesis in nude mice. Comparison between nude mice from homozygous matings and heterozygous matings and effects of age and carcinogen dose. *JNCI* 62:353–358.

Talmadge JE, Herberman RB, Chirigos MA, Schneider MA, Adams JS, Phillips H, Thurman GB, Varesio L, Long CW, Oldham RK, Wiltrout RH. 1985. Augmentation of induction of hypo-responsiveness of murine natural killer cell activity in different anatomical compartments by various immunomodulators including recombinant interferons and interleukin 2. *J Immunol* 135:2483–2491.

Thurman GB, Maluish AE, Rossio J, Schlick E, Onozaki K, Talmadge J, Procopio A, Ortaldo J, Ruscetti F, Stevenson H, Cannon G, Iyer S, Herberman RB. 1986. Comparative evaluation of multiple lymphoid and recombinant human IL-2 preparations. *J Biol Resp Mod* 5:85–107.

Uchida A, Yanagawa E. 1984. Natural killer cell activity and autologous tumor killing activity in cancer patients: Overlapping involvement of effector cells as determined in a two-target conjugate cytotoxicity assay. *JNCI* 73:1093–1100.

Vanky F, Argov S. 1980. Human tumor-lymphocyte interaction *in vitro* VII. Blastogenesis and generation of cytotoxicity against autologous tumor biopsy cells are inhibited by interferon. *Int J Cancer* 26:405–411.

Vose BM, Bonnard GD. 1982. Antigens of human tumours defined by cytotoxicity and proliferative responses of cultured lymphoid cells. *Nature* 296:359–361.

Wiltrout RH, Herberman RB, Zhang SR, Chirigos MA, Ortaldo JR, Green MA Jr, Talmadge JE. 1985. Role of organ-associated NK cells in decreased formation of experimental metastases in lung and liver. *J Immunol* 134:4267–4275.

Wiltrout RH, Mathieson BJ, Talmadge JE, Reynolds CW, Zhang SR, Herberman RB, Ortaldo JR. 1984. Augmentation of organ-associated natural killer activity by biological response modifiers: Isolation and characterization of large granular lymphocytes from the liver. *J Exp Med* 160:1431–1449.

Annual Clinical Conference on Cancer, Vol. 29
Gynecologic Cancer: Diagnosis and Treatment Strategies
© 1987 by The University of Texas System Cancer Center

13. Pathology of Ovarian Tumors of Low Malignant Potential

Henry J. Norris and Philip M. Mount

Ovarian epithelial neoplasms account for a significant proportion of the clinically significant tumors in women. Gynecologists and pathologists have long recognized that the clinical and pathological features of these lesions exhibit a broad spectrum ranging from benign to overtly malignant. Between these two extremes there are gradations in the biologic potential of epithelial tumors. Malignant potential is not sharply defined, but is possessed by tumors in varying amounts. This makes it difficult to achieve a precise, accurate, and replicable pathological classification and to reliably predict the prognosis and select a rational therapy. Any classification should allow recognition of the fact that tumors have variable biologic potential. Diagnostic criteria must be well known and uniformly applied. Historically, these criteria have been poorly understood and unevenly applied by both pathologists and clinicians. This is particularly true with regard to intermediate epithelial tumors that are variously termed *proliferative tumors*, *borderline tumors*, *borderline carcinoma*, *tumors of low malignant potential (LMP)*, and *well-differentiated* or *grade 1 carcinomas*.

Taylor (1929) first called attention to this group when he reported a series of papillary ovarian tumors with histological features of malignancy, some of which had peritoneal implants, but which nonetheless tended to behave in a benign manner. These tumors were termed *semimalignant*. Although this intermediate category did not gain immediate acceptance, it became apparent that the category was needed if the natural history and therapeutic responses of ovarian carcinoma were to be understood. In 1971 the International Federation of Gynecology and Obstetrics (FIGO) adopted a classification that divided epithelial tumors into three groups: benign cystadenomas, cystadenocarcinomas of LMP, and cystadenocarcinomas. The World Health Organization classification, which appeared two years later, also recognized a carcinoma of LMP (Serov, Scully, and Sobin 1973). The intermediate nature of these neoplasms is supported by other than clinical and microscopic grounds. Carcinoembryonic antigen levels and DNA content are intermediate between benign and malignant (Dietel 1982).

Terminology

As indicated above, the terminology applied to the intermediate group of neoplasms is varied. The term *carcinoma* should be avoided because it implies a more rapid growth potential and promotes a more aggressive approach to therapy. This is of particular importance to the younger patient who may desire to retain fertility. The terms *borderline* and *proliferative* are more neutral, but they fail to convey the fact that a proportion of intermediate tumors behave aggressively and may prove fatal. Accordingly, the term *tumor of low malignant potential* is favored because it is the one most descriptive of behavior.

Criteria for Diagnosis

To arrive at a reliable pathological diagnosis, thorough sampling of each neoplasm is required because wide variation in histology is frequent in epithelial tumors. The determination of benign, LMP, or malignant is based on the least differentiated area. To obtain reasonable sampling, a block of tissue for microscopic examination should be taken for each 1 to 2 cm of maximal tumor diameter. Solid areas, the base of papillary processes, and regions adjacent to the surface should be given special attention.

Tumors are classified with respect to cell type (serous, mucinous, endometrioid, clear cell, Brenner or transitional cell, and mixed), the amount of fibrous stroma (adenofibroma family), and the center of growth (surface or cystic). Neoplasms with malignant growth potential are identified by the presence of cellular stratification, increased mitotic activity, and cytological atypia with detachment of atypical cell clusters. By definition, tumors of LMP lack the stromal infiltration that characterizes carcinoma. Stromal invasion is often subtle in mucinous and endometrioid tumors. A ragged epithelial border, associated with inflammatory cells in the stroma or a desmoplastic alteration of the stroma may by the only clue of invasion.

Mestastasis may occur in tumors of LMP as well as with carcinoma. In fact, about 15% have spread beyond the ovary at the time of initial surgery. Thus, metastasis is not a criterion that separates the tumor of LMP from carcinoma. The separation is based entirely on the presence or absence of stromal invasion within the primary tumor. This point is often misunderstood by clinicians and pathologists and requires frequent reemphasis.

Staging

Once it has been determined that a particular neoplasm has malignant potential, a crucial determinant of prognosis is the stage of disease. Survival figures and the efficacy of various therapeutic modalities are frequently compared on this basis. Accurate staging includes cytological examination of ascitic fluid or peritoneal washings; inspection and biopsy of peritoneal surfaces, including the diaphragm; generous omental resection, biopsy, or dissection of lymph nodes; and palpation of the liver, with biopsy as indicated. In the past, these procedures have not been vigorously applied. A current report indicates that gynecologists incompletely stage almost half of their patients and that this figure rises to two thirds when the patients undergo operations by general surgeons (McGowan et al. 1985). Because of variations in the extent of staging, it is difficult to evaluate and compare reports on ovarian epithelial tumors. Obviously, improved staging will lead to increased survival rates for patients with stage I lesions because understaged tumors will be excluded. Similarly, the survival time of higher-stage tumors will increase because some will be detected earlier in their course and should be more amenable to therapy. Accurate staging also will allow more reliable multivariate analysis of independent prognostic features such as histological type and tumor grade (Swenerton et al. 1985).

Miscellaneous Aspects

Tumors of LMP are recognized in all of the major epithelial cell types. The proportion of benign to malignant, and of tumors of LMP to malignant, varies with the cell type. Especially common in stage I, tumors of LMP comprise 14% to 16% of ovarian epithelial tumors. They tend to occur in a younger age group (mean age in the late 40s) than do cystadenocarcinomas (mean age in the mid-50s). Because the serous and mucinous variants are most commonly encountered, these types are better understood. Information concerning endometrioid, clear cell, and the Brenner or transitional cell variants is increasingly available. Adenofibromatous neoplasms with epithelial atypia must also be considered because they often appear clinically distinct from tumors of LMP despite sharing some histological features. When strict criteria are followed, most tumors of LMP are distinct entities and are easily identified. Mixtures of cell types occur less frequently than with the carcinoma category.

Serous Tumors of Low Malignant Potential

Serous tumors are composed of epithelium which resembles that of the fallopian tube. They may arise directly from the ovarian surface epithelium (a modified peritoneal mesothelium) or from epithelial inclusions trapped within the substance of the ovary. Serous tumors may arise from cells of any type that retain the ability to develop into epithelium. Characteristically, serous tumors of LMP are papillary and cystic.

Frequency

In most series (Russell 1979a, 1979b; Purola 1963), serous tumors of LMP account for approximately 15% of all serous neoplasms. Carcinomas account for about 35% of all serous tumors, whereas 50% are benign. Aure and colleagues (1971) found that 21% of ovarian serous malignancies were of LMP, and Santesson and Kottmeier (1968) placed one third of their cases into the LMP category. The median age of patients with serous LMP (45–48 years) is about 7 years less than the age of patients with carcinoma (Aure, Hoeg, and Kolstad 1971; Russell 1979b). Bilaterality occurs in approximately one third of serous LMP tumors (Russell 1979a). Extraovarian spread was recognized in only about 15% of Russell's cases (1979a), but was seen in 45% of patients reported by Katzenstein et al. (1978).

Diagnostic Criteria

The studies of Katzenstein et al. (1978) and of Russell (1979a, 1979b) contain the most detailed clinical and pathological analyses of serous tumors of LMP. The tumors are typically cystic (fig. 13.1) and are composed of complex, branching papillary fronds lined by several layers of cells. Lining cells are heaped into tufts and

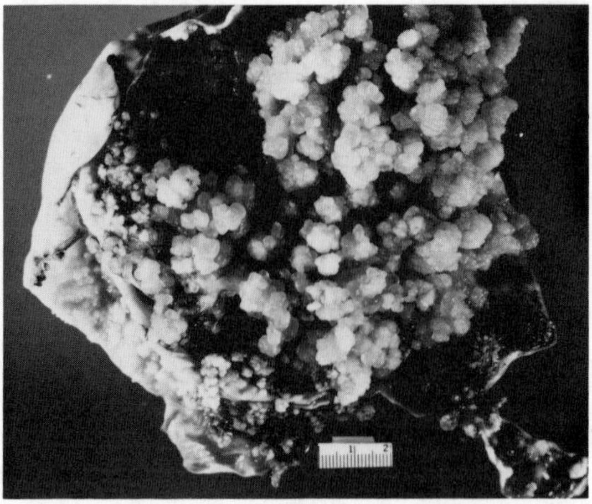

Fig. 13.1. Serous tumor of LMP. Papillary processes extending from the inner surface are shown.

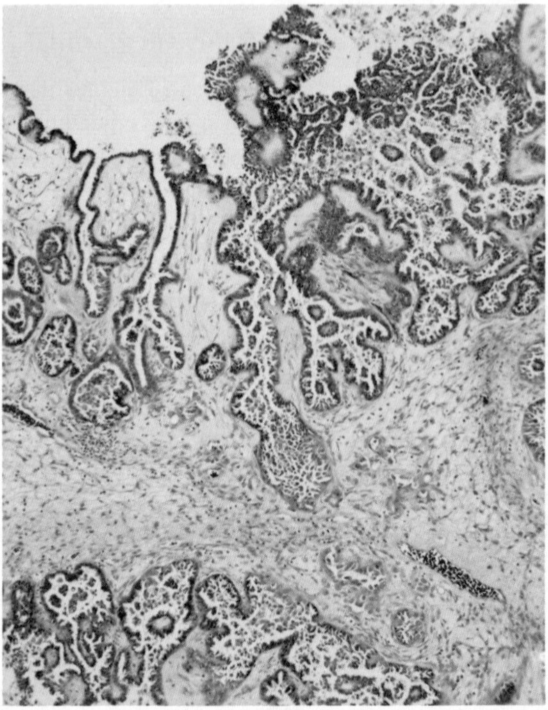

Fig. 13.2. Serous tumor of LMP. The tumor is characterized by stratified cells with detachment of atypical cell clusters.

form buds of four or more cells that lack a supporting fibrovascular stalk (fig. 13.2). The buds are often detached and free-floating within the cyst. Epithelial disorganization with loss of cellular polarity of cells is seen. Cytological atypia, characterized by nuclear pleomorphism, hyperchromatism, and enlarged, prominent nucleoli, is present in all cases. These features have been graded by Russell (1979b). Atypia is usually only mild to moderate, but may be severe in up to 25% of cases. Mitotic activity is present; however, only 6% of cases have had more than five mitotic figures per ten high-power fields (Katzenstein et al. 1978). Cribriform glandular patterns, tumor necrosis, stromal inflammation, and psammoma bodies may be seen.

All of the histological features described above are seen in serous carcinomas as well but are more prominent in carcinomas than in serous tumors of LMP. The only histological finding that separates the two neoplasms is stromal invasion. By definition, destructive invasion is lacking in serous tumors of LMP. Invasion is identified by irregular, destructive epithelial projections into the stroma. Invasion is not only associated with irregular glandular margins, but also with signs of destruction—inflammation, edema, and stromal fibrosis. Early invasion or microinvasion by individual cells (fig. 13.3) may or may not alter the prognosis. Glands, isolated within the stroma, with or without a cribriform growth pattern, do not represent invasion and usually are a result of tangential cutting.

Serous tumors of LMP should also be distinguished from serous cystadenoma with atypia. The latter contains focal areas with cellular proliferation and atypia,

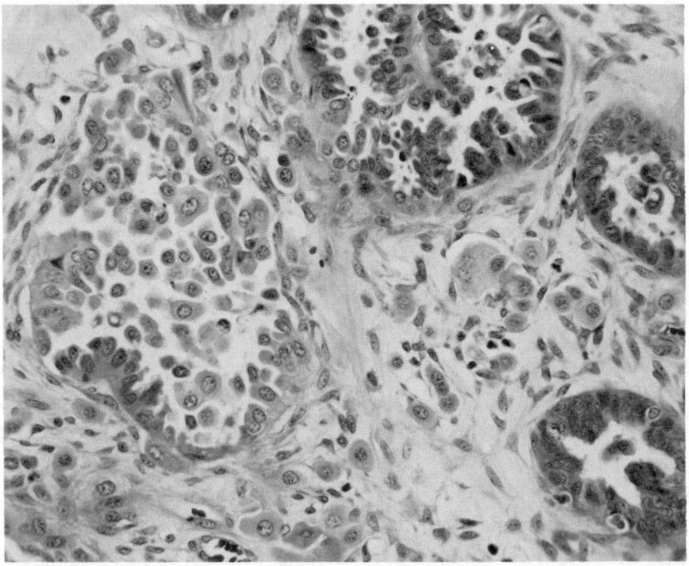

Fig. 13.3. Serous tumor of LMP with microinvasion of the stroma. It is unclear whether this type of neoplasm should be designated as *overt carcinoma*. A paraaortic lymph node contained similar cells.

but it lacks the complex epithelial tufting and intracystic budding with detachment of atypical cell clusters that characterize the serous tumor of LMP.

Mucinous Tumors of Low Malignant Potential

Benign mucinous cystadenomas are formed by epithelium resembling that of the endocervix. The cells are columnar with basally oriented nuclei. Intracytoplasmic mucin is present. As the mucinous tumor progresses in the spectrum toward malignancy, the cells tend to lose the capacity for mucin production and resemble benign or adenomatous intestinal epithelium (Fenoglio, Ferenczy, and Richart 1976). Goblet cells and vacuoles of intracytoplasmic mucin are formed. In mucinous tumors of LMP, mixtures of both cell types (endocervical and intestinal) occur.

Frequency

Hart and Norris (1973) studied 688 stage I mucinous tumors. Of these, 80% were benign, 14% were of LMP, and 6% were carcinomas. Russell's series (1979a, 1979b) included 362 mucinous tumors, of which 15% were of LMP and 5% were carcinomas. In both of these reports, the median age of patients with mucinous tumors of LMP was 48 years—4 years younger than patients with carcinoma. The frequency of bilateral involvement was 6% and 8% in the two series. This contrasts with mucinous carcinoma, in which nearly half are bilateral. Fifteen percent of mucinous tumors of LMP have extended beyond the ovary at the time of discovery (Russell 1979a).

Diagnostic Criteria

The criteria for the identification of mucinous tumors of LMP are similar to those of serous tumors of LMP (Hart and Norris 1973). Mucinous tumors of LMP are characteristically cystic. The median size is 17 cm and most have a smooth external surface. Numerous secondary cysts and short papillary infoldings are usually present. The epithelial lining is stratified and exfoliation of small groups of cells is common (fig. 13.4). True cribriform intraglandular bridging is uncommon, but this pattern may be simulated by tangential sectioning, which obscures fine fibrovascular stalks. Cytological atypia is expressed by pleomorphism, nuclear hyperchromasia, and prominent nucleoli. The atypia is usually mild to moderate but may be severe. Two or more mitotic figures are often seen per ten high-power fields.

The microscopic features of mucinous tumors are notoriously variable. Histologically benign areas, zones of LMP, and regions of carcinoma may coexist within the same neoplasm. Accordingly, all mucinous tumors must be well sampled to ensure reliable histological evaluation. As in serous carcinoma, invasion is a diagnostic hallmark of malignancy. Many carcinomas are readily separated from tumors of LMP by the presence of single cells or nests and cords of cells infiltrating the stroma. The presence of solid sheets of atypical epithelium that spans more than half the diameter of a 4.2-mm low-power field without intervening stroma is regarded by some workers as indicative of invasion (Colgan and Norris 1983). In some tumors, tangential sectioning and complex subgland formations can obscure

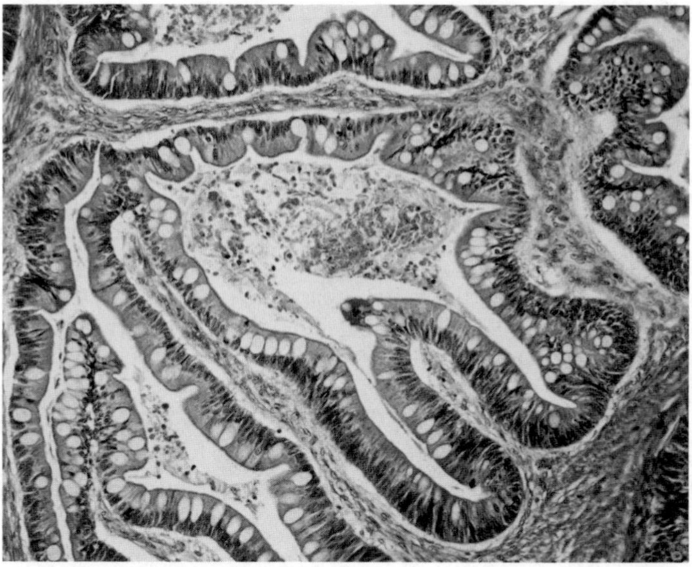

Fig. 13.4. Mucinous tumor of LMP. Moderate atypia, a minor degree of stratification, and goblet cells produce an "intestinal" appearance.

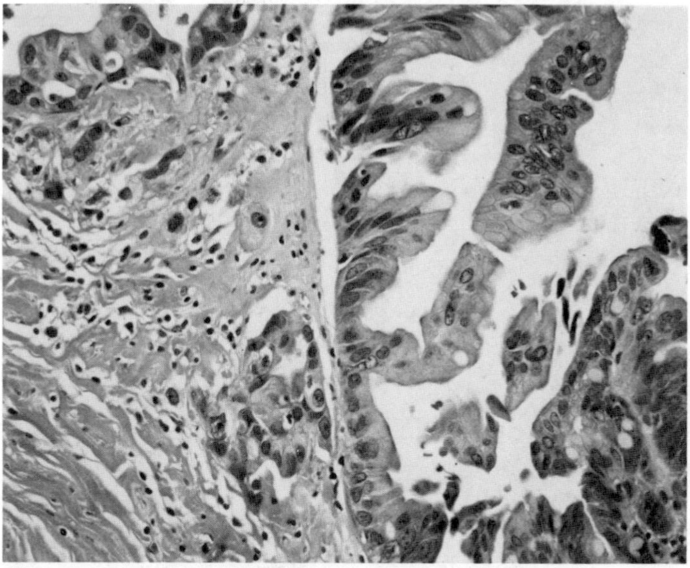

Fig. 13.5. Mucinous tumor of LMP (*right*) and invasion of stroma (*left*). This illustrates that mucinous tumors of LMP have invasive capability. When invasion is present, the tumor should be classified as a carcinoma.

the presence or absence of invasion. Additional sections of such tumors are sometimes needed to establish a diagnosis. An irregular, gland-stroma interface and lymphoplasmacytic infiltrates are features of early invasion. Dissection of mucin into the ovarian stroma (pseudomyxoma ovarii) occurs in almost 25% of cases but does not indicate stromal invasion (Russell 1979b). Destructive invasion is shown in figure 13.5.

An additional criterion for the identification of mucinous carcinoma was proposed by Hart and Norris (1973). These investigators found that mucinous tumors that lacked unequivocal stromal invasion but had moderate-to-marked cytological atypia and cellular stratification of four or more cell layers showed sufficiently aggressive clinical behavior to justify a diagnosis of carcinoma (fig. 13.6). This approach was not accepted by Russell (1979b), who believed that this criterion unnecessarily complicated pathological evaluation and could not be justified by an increased precision or by a difference in prognosis. Support for the Hart and Norris (1973) criteria recently has been provided by the study of Chaitin, Gershenson, and Evans (1985). This group determined that patients with mucinous carcinoma lack-

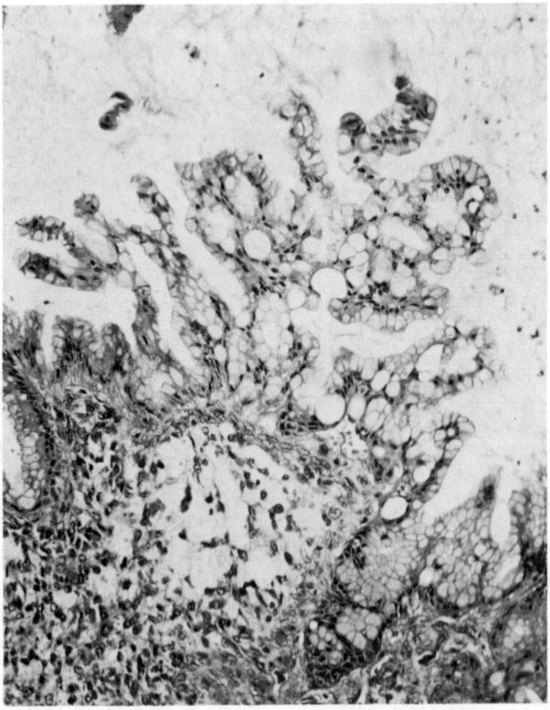

Fig. 13.6. A mucinous tumor with filigree papillae and detached clusters of cells. This type of mucinous tumor usually contains stratification of four or more cells and has an invasive and metastatic nature. Therefore, mucinous neoplasms with a filigree pattern should be designated as carcinomas.

ing stromal invasion (as defined above) had an overall survival intermediate between that of patients with a mucinous tumor of LMP and patients with a carcinoma with stromal invasion. Most of the carcinomas without stromal invasion were stage I at the time of surgery and could be expected to have a better prognosis. When stage was taken into account, there was little difference in survival, with or without stromal invasion.

Endometrioid Tumors of Low Malignant Potential

Endometrioid tumors are characterized by the presence of nonciliated stratified or pseudostratified epithelium that resembles endometrial epithelium. They may be divided into four categories: benign endometrioid tumors (usually endometrioid adenofibromas), atypical endometrioid adenofibromas, endometrioid tumors of LMP (proliferative endometrioid tumor, borderline endometrioid tumor), and endometrioid carcinoma. More cases of atypical and LMP endometrioid tumors must be studied to clarify the behavior and nomenclature of neoplasms encountered in this category.

Frequency

The majority of endometrioid tumors are malignant. Endometrioid tumors of LMP and benign endometrioid tumors are uncommon and reported cases are few. Russell's series (1979a) included only 14 cases, and Bell and Scully (1985) reported an additional 20 patients. Reports of proliferating endometrioid adenofibromas (Roth, Czernobilsky, and Langley 1981) and endometrioid adenofibromas with atypia (Kao and Norris 1978) include only four and three cases. Also, some of these cases would be regarded as "proliferative" or of LMP, depending on whether the epithelium was cytologically malignant and formed cribriform or closely packed glands. The epithelium in the "proliferative" variety is not cytologically malignant or as crowded as it is in the endometrioid LMP. This distinction may be too subjective to obtain wide acceptance, however.

Studies indicate that between 4% and 19% of endometrioid tumors are in the LMP category (Aure et al. 1971; Russell 1979a). Endometrioid tumors account for only 2% to 10% of all LMP neoplasms (Creasman et al. 1982; Russell and Merkur 1979). The mean age of patients with an endometrioid LMP is 48 years, whereas the mean age is 55 for patients with carcinoma and 40 for those with a benign endometrioid tumor (Russell 1979a). In Russell's series, only 1 of 14 patients had bilateral tumors. In two patients, the neoplasm had extended beyond the ovary at the time of operation. All of the 20 tumors described by Bell and Scully (1985) were confined to one ovary, and none had surface involvement.

Diagnostic Criteria

Two basic growth patterns are characteristic of endometrioid tumors of LMP. By definition, the epithelium in both types resembles that of the endometrium. In one type, there is a major fibrous stromal component. This solid type appears to be an

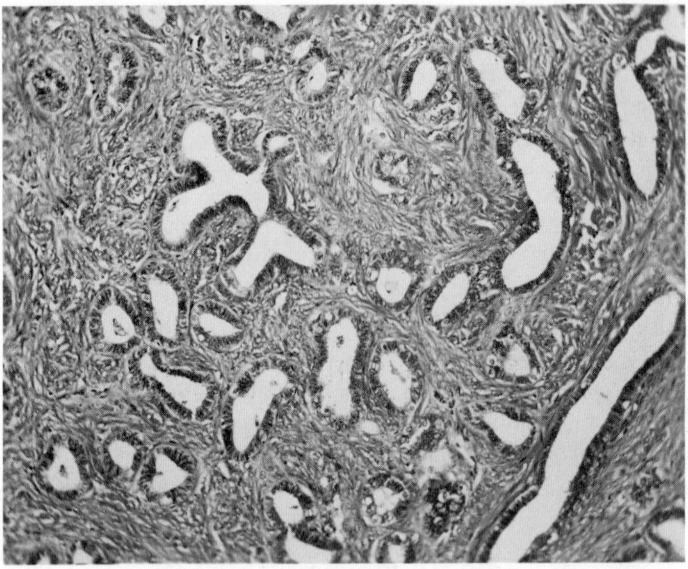

Fig. 13.7. Endometrioid adenofibroma. The fibrous stromal background composes most of the neoplasm. The epithelium is not complex and resembles inactive endometrial glands.

overgrowth of endometrioid epithelium in an adenofibroma. It is distinguished from an adenofibroma (fig. 13.7) by the presence of epithelial atypia (fig. 13.8). Kao and Norris (1978) acknowledged that endometrioid tumors with fibrous stroma and epithelial atypia correspond to tumors of LMP but classified them as endometrioid adenofibromas with atypia. Subsequently, Bell and Scully (1985) proposed a modification of the diagnostic criteria for endometrioid adenofibromas. These authors regarded tumors with epithelial atypia as atypical adenofibromas. Lesions that contain foci of closely opposed glands or epithelial islands with a cribriform growth pattern and cells with a low nuclear grade (grade 1, scale of 3) are classified as "borderline" (LMP) endometrioid adenofibromas (fig. 13.9). However, the neoplasms are regarded as malignant if they have a high nuclear grade (2 to 3, scale of 3) and epithelial crowding in the absence of stromal invasion.

The second type of endometrioid tumor of LMP is mainly epithelial in character. This type is reminiscent of an adenomatous endometrial hyperplasia. The stromal contribution is relatively minor and consists only of columns and papillary supportive processes lined by epithelium.

In both types of endometrioid tumor of LMP, the epithelial proliferations are characterized by irregular glandular structures lined by pseudostratified or stratified columnar cells. Nuclear atypia is usually mild but may be more advanced. The glands may contain papillary processes or cribriform formations. The extent of glandular crowding is variable, but there is no evidence of invasion. Squamous metaplasia is seen in one third to one half of cases (Bell and Scully 1985; Russell 1979b).

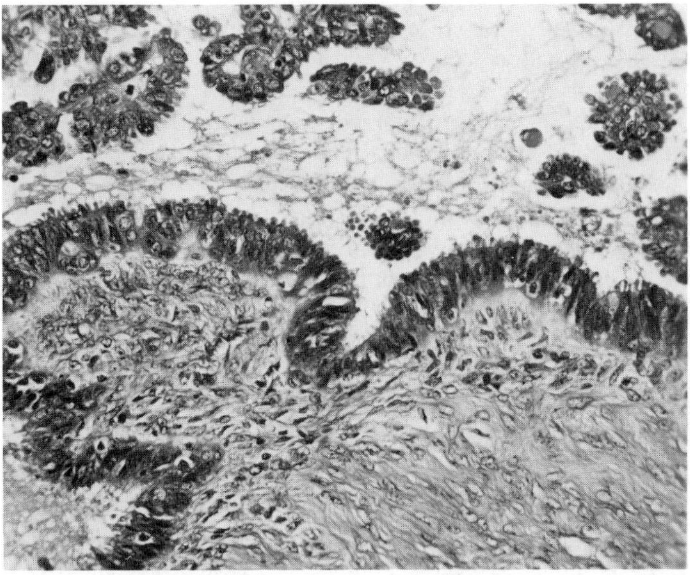

Fig. 13.8. Endometrioid adenofibroma with atypia. The epithelium, although atypical, is not clearly cytologically malignant. If it were cytologically malignant and lacked invasion, it would be classified as an adenofibroma of LMP.

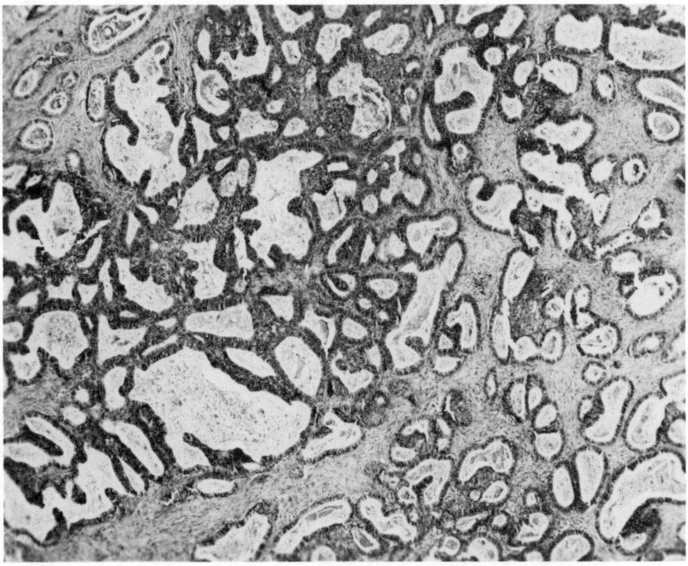

Fig. 13.9. Endometrioid tumor of LMP with extensive squamous metaplasia. Elsewhere this neoplasm was mostly solid and consistent with the characteristics of an adenofibroma.

Miscellaneous Features

Endometriosis is present in 15% to 30% of the patients. Associated endometrial abnormalities are present in a surprisingly high proportion of cases. In the Bell and Scully (1985) group, the endometrium was examined in 12 cases. Four of the patients had endometrial hyperplasia, and three had an adenocarcinoma. Of the 14 patients described by Russell (1979b), 3 had endometrial adenocarcinoma. However, the ovarian and endometrial tumors were discovered simultaneously in only one patient. Cases with associated endometrial pathology are more likely to have stromal luteinization within the ovarian tumor (Bell and Scully 1985).

Clear Cell Tumors of Low Malignant Potential

Clear cell neoplasms are characterized by cuboidal, columnar, or hobnail cells with clear or pale eosinophilic granular cytoplasm. The cells typically contain glycogen, and mucicarmine-positive material may be seen in secretions and at the luminal border of the cells. Like endometrioid tumors, clear cell neoplasms can be divided into four categories: clear cell adenofibroma, adenofibroma with atypia, clear cell tumor of LMP (proliferative clear cell tumor), and clear cell carcinoma.

Frequency

Clear cell tumors of LMP are very rare, and only a small number have been reported. Russell's series (1979a, 1979b) contained 33 cases of clear cell tumors: three (8%) were classified as tumors of LMP, whereas the remainder were malignant. Roth and associates (1984) collected 17 cases of clear cell adenofibromatous neoplasms but did not report the incidence. In their group, 2 were benign, 3 were of LMP, and 12 were carcinomas with an adenofibromatous growth pattern. Three benign clear cell adenofibromas were described by Kao and Norris (1979). The mean age of the patients reported by Russell (1979a) was 44 years, but those of Roth et al. (1984) had a mean age of 67 years. The median age was 53 years for ordinary clear cell carcinoma.

Diagnostic Criteria

All of the well-documented cases of clear cell tumor of LMP have had sufficient stroma to qualify as being adenofibromatous in nature. Cases without a prominent stroma are said to exist but are exceedingly rare (Roth et al. 1984). The adenofibromatous clear cell variant consists of irregular tubules or microcysts lined by one or more layers of clear and hobnail cells set in a cellular fibrous stroma (figs. 13.10 and 13.11). Nuclear atypia is moderate to marked. Occasional mitotic figures (< 1 per 10 high-power fields) are seen. Cysts with internal budding, scattered solid nests, or cords of cells may be present. It can be difficult to distinguish a well-differentiated clear cell carcinoma from a clear cell tumor of LMP unless both are well sampled. The presence of papillary processes, glomerulus-like tufts, or sheets of cells are indicative of malignancy. Benign clear cell cystadenofibromas have little or no nuclear atypia, and their tubules and cysts are lined by single- or double-cell layers (Kao and

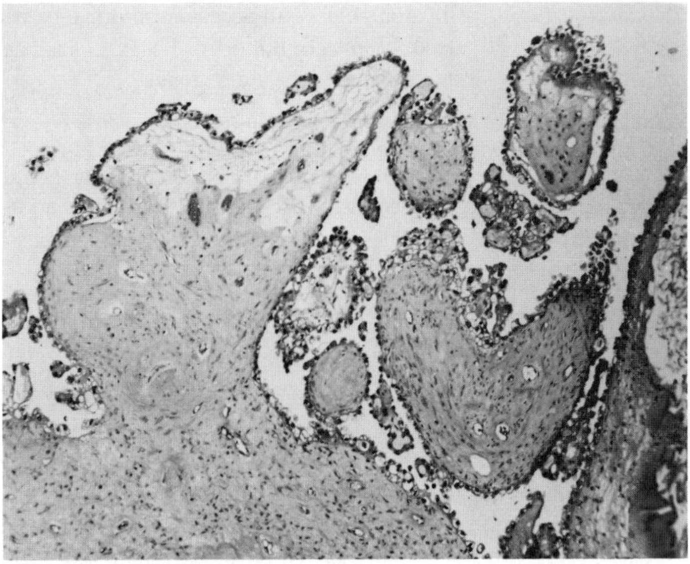

Fig. 13.10. Clear cell adenofibroma of LMP.

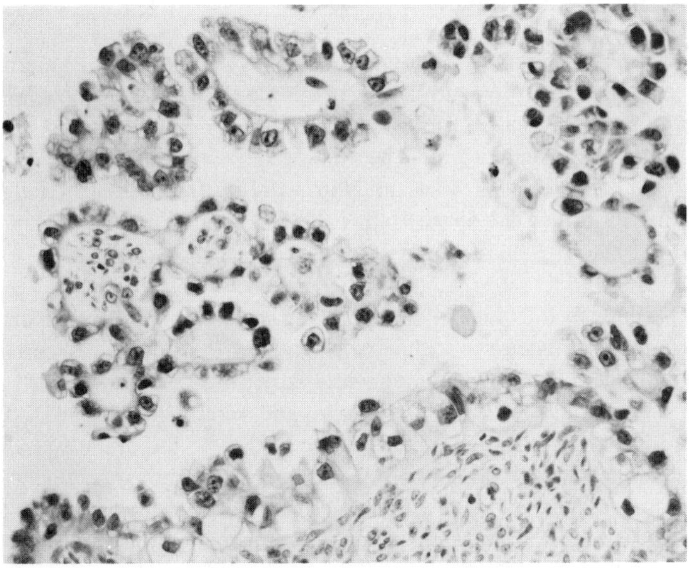

Fig. 13.11. Higher view of the clear cell adenofibroma of LMP shown in figure 13.10. The cells have atypical nuclei and are stratified and frequently detached.

Norris 1979). Because clear cell carcinomas with an adenofibromatous pattern are more common than clear cell adenofibromas or tumors of LMP, all such neoplasms must be well sampled to avoid overlooking high-grade areas.

Miscellaneous Features

Clear cell carcinomas are frequently associated with endometriosis, and this association was seen in three of the six cases reported by Russell (1979a) and Roth et al. (1984). Postmenopausal bleeding was a common presenting complaint.

Brenner Tumors of Low Malignant Potential

Brenner tumors are formed by epithelium resembling transitional epithelium of the urinary tract. Mucinous and squamous differentiation is common in proliferative Brenner tumors, however. In the past, the proliferative Brenner tumor has been regarded as a borderline Brenner or Brenner tumor of LMP, although aggressive behavior has not been described. More recently, Roth, Dallenbach-Hellweg, and Czernobilsky (1985) recommended subdivision of Brenner tumors into benign, proliferative, metaplastic, LMP, and malignant. The intermediate varieties will be discussed under the heading of "proliferative Brenner tumor" for convenience because the older literature does not distinguish between subtypes. When a distinction is possible, it will be made in the discussion.

Frequency

Proliferating Brenner tumors (including the Brenner tumor of LMP) are rare. The largest series consist of 10 (Woodruff et al. 1981) and 14 (Roth, Dallenbach-Hellweg, and Czernobilsky 1985) cases. Russell and Merkur (1979) found only 1 among 144 tumors of LMP. All were unilateral. The average age of patients has varied in different series from the early 50s (Miles and Norris 1972) to the late 60s (Hallgrimsson and Scully 1972; Roth, Dallenbach-Hellweg, and Czernobilsky 1985).

Diagnostic Criteria

As originally described (Roth and Sternberg 1971), the proliferative Brenner tumor bears a striking resemblance to a low-grade papillary transitional cell carcinoma of the urinary bladder. The tumor is frequently large (average diameter, 20 cm) and partially cystic (Roth, Dallenbach-Hellweg, and Czernobilsky 1985). Papillary fronds lined by transitional cell epithelium protrude into the cystic spaces. If tangentially cut, they appear as circumscribed sheets or nests of cells within the stroma. Characteristically, a benign Brenner component with typical histological features is present in adjacent areas, but this is not essential for the diagnosis (Roth, Dallenbach-Hellweg, and Czernobilsky 1985). This is in contrast to the malignant Brenner tumor where most authors require the presence of a benign or proliferative Brenner component to make the diagnosis (Roth and Czernobilsky 1985). Proliferative activity in the intermediate form of Brenner tumor is identified by the presence of moderate mitotic activity and cellular stratification of 20 or more layers. Cysts are lined by stratified transitional cell epithelium. Mild-to-moderate cytological atypia is present in most lesions. Mucinous and squamous metaplasia is common in proliferating Brenner tumor. A mucinous cystadenoma may also be present.

In an attempt to better define the natural history of the intermediate form of Brenner tumors, and in recognition of the histological variability of these types of lesions, Roth, Dallenbach-Hellweg, and Czernobilsky (1985) proposed that the tumors be divided into three groups: metaplastic, proliferating, and LMP. The metaplastic variant is usually cystic. Formerly included in the proliferative category, the metaplastic Brenner tumor has few or absent papillary fronds and no nuclear atypia. Mucinous metaplasia is prominent, and complex glandular patterns may be seen within the epithelium. The proliferating variant is typical of the original descriptions of the proliferating Brenner tumor as described above. The cytological features of the proliferating Brenner tumor are low grade. The tumor of LMP resembles the proliferating type but differs in that it contains areas with high-grade cytological atypia corresponding to a grade 3 or 4 in situ transitional cell carcinoma or to in situ squamous carcinoma.

This approach toward defining a Brenner tumor of LMP is deserving of acceptance. Prior to this, investigators have found difficulty in identifying stromal invasion in Brenner tumors and have preferred to classify neoplasms with high-grade cytological features as being malignant (Colgan and Norris 1983). Roth, Dallenbach-Hellweg, and Czernobilsky (1985), however, believe that invasion often can be identified. Their criteria for determining invasion include irregularity of epithelial nests, large or confluent epithelial masses, and, occasionally, a desmoplastic stromal reaction (Roth, Dallenbach-Hellweg, and Czernobilsky 1985). Certainly, these features reflect an aggressive neoplasm.

Survival of Patients with Neoplasms of Low Malignant Potential

Implicit in the concept of the tumor of LMP is that there are improved survival rates—stage for stage—compared with carcinoma of the ovary. Russell (1979a, 1979b) and Russell and Merkur (1979) found some correlation between tumor recurrence and behavior and the degree of cytological and architectural atypia. Other investigators, however, have found no consistent relationship between histological features and patient outcome within the category of LMP (Katzenstein et al. 1978; Bostwick et al. 1985).

In all major series, the five-year survival rate for patients with stage I serous tumor of LMP is 95% or better (Julian and Woodruff 1972; Katzenstein et al. 1978; Russell 1979a; Creasman et al. 1982; Bostwick et al. 1985). Reports of rapidly progressive stage I tumors should raise the suspicion of incomplete sampling of the primary tumor or of understaging. Just how many patients with stage I neoplasms treated by unilateral oophorectomy will develop a recurrence or second primary tumor in the contralateral ovary is unknown, but it probably exceeds 10%.

The ten-year survival rate for patients with stage I neoplasms also appears to exceed 90% (Aure, Hoeg, and Kolstad 1971; Russell and Merkur 1979). Collected series of cases of higher-stage lesions contain only a small number of patients. In Katzenstein and associates' series (1978), the seven patients who died of disease and the three patients who were alive with tumor had stage IIb or stage III disease at initial presentation. Thirty-eight percent of patients in stage III died of disease; the average survival was nine years. Similarly, the four patients reported by Russell and Merkur (1979) who died of serous tumor of LMP had stage II or stage III disease. Half of the patients with stage II disease died. These findings are consistent with the general experience with ovarian malignancy in which higher-stage lesions have poorer prognosis. Serous tumors of LMP may recur after decades (Aure, Hoeg, and Kolstad 1971). Recurrences may be in the opposite ovary or within the peritoneum in conservatively treated stage Ia disease (Bostwick et al. 1985). Although stated here as a "recurrence," it is uncertain what proportion of these "recurrences" represent metastatic disease as opposed to multifocal primary neoplasia of the peritoneum (Russell 1985; Woodruff, Solomon, and Sullivant 1985).

A majority of the larger series of mucinous tumors of LMP have included only patients with stage I disease (Hart and Norris 1973; Chaitin, Gershenson, and Evans 1985; Bostwick et al. 1985). Evidence of extraovarian spread at the initial staging of mucinous tumor of LMP is found in 12% to 15% of patients (Aure, Hoeg, and Kolstad 1971; Russell 1979a; Russell and Merkur 1979). Survival rates ranging from 90% to 100% have been reported in the stage I series, with a median follow-up of 8.6 years. The best survival rate was reported by Bostwick et al. (1985), who found no recurrences in 30 stage I mucinous neoplasms over a mean follow-up period of seven years. Because of the histological variations typical of mucinous tumors, some of the stage I tumor deaths may well represent understaged or underdiagnosed carcinomas (Hart and Norris 1973). The stage I tumors that caused deaths in the series reported by Russell (1979a) and Russell and Merkur (1979) were high-grade lesions that might have qualified as carcinoma by the criteria of Hart and Norris (1973). Higher-stage lesions were seen in 8 of 52 patients with mucinous tumors reported by Russell (1979b) and Russell and Merkur (1979). All were stage III lesions with histologically typical pseudomyxoma peritonei judged to be owed to leakage from the ovarian primary. Two of those patients died of disease within one year. Hart and Norris (1973) indicated that, in most cases, pseudomyxoma peritonei is the result of a coexisting appendiceal mucocele or a low-grade mucinous carcinoma originating outside the ovary. These authors also described 11 patients with ruptured mucinous tumors of LMP. None of the 11 developed pseudomyxoma peritonei in a follow-up period ranging from 3 to 19 years.

The low incidence of endometrioid tumors of LMP and the lack of well-accepted and generally recognized diagnostic criteria have hindered understanding of their behavior. The cases reported by Roth, Czernobilsky, and Langley (1981) as "proliferative," by Kao and Norris (1978) as "atypical," and by Bell and Scully (1985) as "tumors of LMP" have all proved to be stage Ia clinically benign lesions. All of these lesions have fallen into the adenofibromatous category, and some investigators believe they may have less malignant potential than tumors without a prominent stromal component (Kao and Norris 1978). It is logical to assume that neoplasms with a greater epithelial surface are likely to have greater malignant potential. The higher-grade endometrioid tumors of LMP described by Russell (1979b) were of the papillary variety. One of eight patients with grade 4 tumor died of disease; this patient had a stage I neoplasm at initial diagnosis. Two patients with stage II and stage III lesions survived.

The clear cell tumors of LMP described by Russell (1979b) and Roth et al. (1984) also had adenofibromatous patterns. All were stage Ia and clinically benign. The diagnosis of tumor of LMP was based on cytological features that were similar to those of overt malignancies. Eleven of the clear cell adenofibromatous tumors reported by Roth et al. (1984) contained invasive areas and were classified as carcinoma. It is of interest to speculate that the LMP variants represent in situ lesions that might have progressed to overt invasion had they not been removed (Russell 1984). Additional cases need to be accumulated to better understand the natural history of these rare neoplasms.

All of the proliferative Brenner tumors have proved to be clinically benign. Similarly, the four Brenner tumors of LMP described by Roth et al. (1985) did not behave aggressively; however, additional cases of this type must be studied to be certain of their biologic potential. Roth et al. (1985) noted a general progression in the degree of epithelial abnormality from benign through metaplastic, proliferating, and LMP. They suggested that the risk of malignant transformation increases as the degree of epithelial abnormality increases. Six of the nine malignant Brenner tumors reported by Roth and Czernobilsky (1985) had an associated proliferating or LMP component.

Benign and Malignant Proliferations of the Peritoneum

The histological evaluation of peritoneal biopsies and lymph nodes taken during staging procedures and second-look laparotomies is complicated by the existence of benign epithelial inclusions, with or without reactive changes, that may be interpreted as metastatic disease. This may result in overstaging and unnecessarily aggressive therapy.

Epithelial inclusions are found in the omentum of fewer than 15% of patients and occur in the pelvic lymph nodes in 4% to 14% of women not having an underlying tumor (Farhi and Silverberg 1982; Zinsser and Wheeler 1982; Hsu et al. 1980; Karp and Czernobilsky 1969; Ehrmann, Federschneider, and Knapp 1980). These inclusions have been ascribed to a variety of origins, including congenital rests, endometriosis, endosalpingiosis, mesothelial metaplasia, and "müllerianosis." Müllerianosis (Bassis 1960) refers to the origin of müllerian epithelium directly from the peritoneum, as a form of metaplasia.

A number of features are useful to distinguish benign inclusions from tumors (Coffin, Adcock, and Dehner 1985; Farhi and Silverberg 1982; Ehrmann, Federschneider, and Knapp 1980). Benign inclusions are usually in the form of solitary, round-to-oval nonsecreting glands with an intact lumen. The epithelium is usually one layer thick but may exceed one cell layer in the absence of an irregular piling up of cells. A peripheral basement membrane is usually present and cilia are prominent. The nuclei are basally situated, mitotic activity is absent, and the cytological

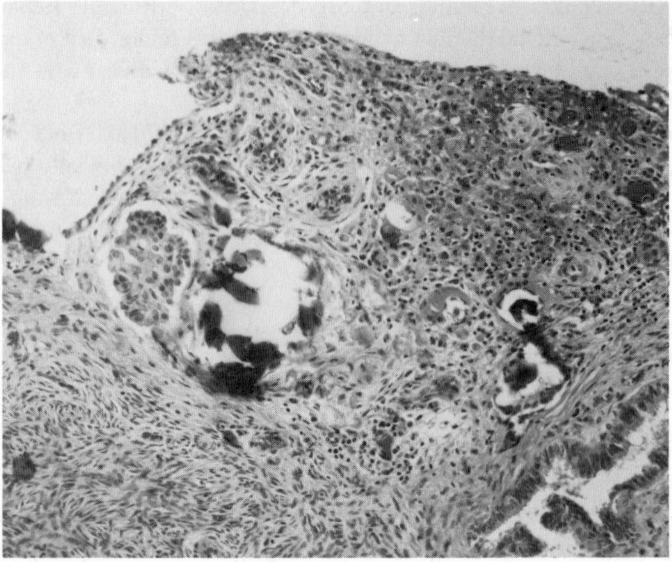

Fig. 13.12. Epithelial inclusions of peritoneum. Note papillary formation, psammoma bodies, and inflammation.

features are bland. The presence of psammoma bodies, papillary infoldings, and small clusters of cells can make it difficult to distinguish inclusions from a serous LMP. Serous mesothelial inclusions are usually found beneath the peritoneal surface rather than as surface implants typical of metastasis (fig. 13.12). A reactive desmoplastic stroma may be present in benign inclusions and metaplasia, as well as with metastatic implants from a neoplasm of LMP. Inflammation probably serves to embed peritoneal metaplastic inclusions, giving the appearance of invasion. Implantation metastases from endometrioid tumors are distinguished from endometriosis by the absence of endometrial stroma and lack of hemorrhage suggestive of cyclic hormone dependence.

Reactive mesothelial proliferations may also simulate malignancy, particularly inasmuch as reactive mesothelium commonly differentiates by metaplasia to serous epithelium (fig. 13.13). In some situations, endometrioid, squamous, and mucinous metaplasia occurs. Peritoneal washings may show a variety of features (fig. 13.14). Neoplastic proliferations are characterized by cytological atypia, mitotic activity, and irregular cellular stratification and should be histologically similar to a known primary tumor. Metastatic lesions may or may not be associated with a desmoplastic stromal response. Psammoma bodies are formed in response to inflammatory and other benign conditions and have no significance.

Peritoneal carcinomatosis of a microscopic type typical of ovarian carcinoma may occur in the absence of a dominant ovarian primary neoplasm (Russell 1985). Traditionally, these lesions have been regarded as metastatic from a small superficial carcinoma of the ovary. Because of minimal or absent ovarian involvement in some

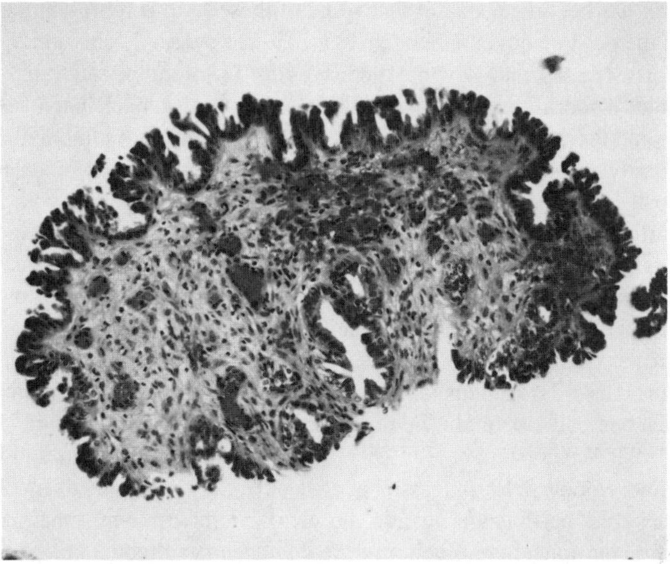

Fig. 13.13. Papillary peritoneal metaplasia. The stratification of the cells, detachment, and mild atypia are consistent with the characteristics of a serous tumor of LMP developing on the peritoneal surface.

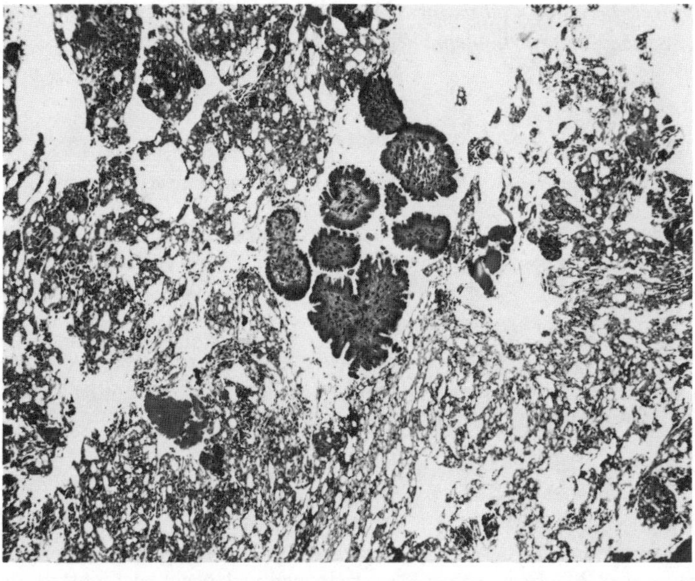

Fig. 13.14. Cell block of peritoneal washings from a patient with serous papillary metaplasia of the peritoneum. Without evidence of cytological malignancy, these structures are benign.

instances, it has become apparent that some of these lesions represent primary carcinoma of the peritoneum (Kannerstein et al. 1977; Foyle, Al-Jabi, and McCaughey 1981; August, Murad, and Newton 1985; Woodruff, Solomon, and Sullivant 1985). Parmley and Woodruff (1974) have held this view for years. Bilateral ovarian involvement and disseminated peritoneal disease in patients with tumors of LMP does not necessarily imply metastatic disease, but in some instances represents multifocal tumorigenesis. It seems probable that a proportion of patients with late recurrences, particularly those with stage I disease initially, can be explained on this basis. Certainly, there has been evidence to suggest that carcinoma may arise from the peritoneum. In two studies, patients with a strong family history of ovarian cancer developed an ovarian type of carcinoma in the pelvis years after prophylactic removal of the ovaries (Tobacman et al. 1982; Chen, Schooley, and Flam 1985). Other reports describe patients who developed an ovarian type of carcinoma in the pelvic area but had no tumor involvement in the ovaries (Ulbright, Roth, and Stehman 1983; Kannerstein et al. 1977). Multiple superficial in situ foci also occur (Parmley and Woodruff 1974; Russell et al. 1985). Serous tumors of LMP probably arise from pelvic peritoneum outside the ovary more commonly than carcinomas do. When the peritoneal mesothelium differentiates to carcinoma or an LMP tumor, the neoplasm formed usually is serous in character. The resemblance is probably due to the contribution of coelomic mesothelium to the embryonic development of the ovary and müllerian ducts.

The opinions and assertions contained herein are the private views of the authors and are not to be construed as official or as representing the views of the Department of the Army or the Department of Defense.

References

August CE, Murad TM, Newton M. 1985. Multiple focal extraovarian serous carcinoma. *Int J Gynecol Pathol* 4:11–23.

Aure JC, Hoeg K, Kolstad P. 1971. Clinical and histologic studies of ovarian carcinoma. *Obstet Gynecol* 37:1–9.

Bassis ML. 1960. An embryologically derived classification of ovarian tumors. *JAMA* 174:1316–1320.

Bell DA, Scully RE. 1985. Atypical and borderline endometrioid adenofibromas of the ovary. *Am J Surg Pathol* 9:205–214.

Bostwick DG, Tazelaar HD, Ballon SC, Hendrickson MR, Kempson RL. 1986. Ovarian tumors of low malignant potential: Clinicopathologic study of 109 cases. *Cancer* 58: 2052–2065.

Chaitin BA, Gershenson DA, Evans HL. 1985. Mucinous tumors of the ovary. A clinicopathologic study of 70 cases. *Cancer* 55:1958–1962.

Chen KTK, Schooley JL, Flam MS. 1985. Peritoneal carcinomatosis after prophylactic oophorectomy in familial ovarian cancer syndrome. *Obstet Gynecol* 66(Suppl 3):93s–94s.

Coffin CM, Adcock LL, Dehner LP. 1985. The second-look operation for ovarian neoplasms: A study of 85 cases emphasizing cytologic and histologic problems. *Int J Gynecol Pathol* 4:97–109.

Colgan TJ, Norris HJ. 1983. Ovarian epithelial tumors of low malignant potential: A review. *Int J Gynecol Pathol* 1:367–382.
Creasman WT, Park R, Norris HJ, DiSaia PH, Morrow P, Hreshchyshyn MM. 1982. Stage I borderline ovarian tumors. *Obstet Gynecol* 59:93–96.
Dietel M. 1982. Facultative malignant ovarian tumors (tumors of borderline malignancy). In *Ovarialtumoren*, ed. G Dallenbach-Hellweg, pp. 181–193. New York: Springer-Verlag.
Ehrmann RL, Federschneider JM, Knapp RC. 1980. Distinguishing lymph node metastases from benign glandular inclusions in low-grade ovarian carcinoma. *Am J Obstet Gynecol* 136:737–746.
Farhi DC, Silverberg SG. 1982. Pseudometastases in female genital cancer. *Pathol Ann* 17:47–76.
Fenoglio CM, Ferenczy A, Richart RM. 1976. Mucinous tumors of the ovary. II. Ultrastructural studies of mucinous cystadenocarcinomas. *Am J Obstet Gynecol* 125:990–999.
Foyle A, Al-Jabi M, McCaughey WTE. 1981. Papillary peritoneal tumors in women. *Am J Surg Pathol* 5:241–250.
Hallgrimsson J, Scully RE. 1972. Borderline and malignant Brenner tumors of the ovary. *Acta Pathol Microbiol Immuno Scand [A]* 80(Suppl 233):56–66.
Hart WR, Norris HJ. 1973. Borderline and malignant mucinous tumors of the ovary. *Cancer* 31:1031–1045.
Hsu YK, Parmley TH, Rosenshein NB, Bhagavan BS, Woodruff JD. 1980. Neoplastic and non-neoplastic mesothelial proliferations in pelvic lymph nodes. *Obstet Gynecol* 55: 83–88.
Julian CG, Woodruff JD. 1972. The biologic behavior of low-grade papillary serous carcinoma of the ovary. *Obstet Gynecol* 40:860–867.
Kannerstein M, Churg J, McCaughey WTE, Hill DP. 1977. Papillary tumors of the peritoneum in women. Mesothelioma or papillary carcinoma. *Am J Obstet Gynecol* 127:306–314.
Kao GF, Norris HJ. 1978. Cystadenofibromas of the ovary with epithelial atypia. *Am J Surg Pathol* 2:357–363.
Kao GF, Norris HJ. 1979. Unusual cystadenofibromas: Endometrioid, mucinous, and clear cell types. *Obstet Gynecol* 54:729–736.
Karp LA, Czernobilsky B. 1969. Glandular inclusions in pelvic and abdominal para-aortic lymph nodes. *Am J Clin Pathol* 52:212–218.
Katzenstein AA, Mazur MT, Morgan TE, Kao M. 1978. Proliferative serous tumors of the ovary. *Am J Surg Pathol* 8:339–355.
McGowan L, Lesher LP, Norris HJ, Barnett M. 1985. Misstaging of ovarian cancer. *Obstet Gynecol* 65:568–572.
Miles PA, Norris HJ. 1972. Proliferative and malignant Brenner tumors of the ovary. *Cancer* 30:174–186.
Parmley TH, Woodruff JD. 1974. The ovarian mesothelioma. *Am J Obstet Gynecol* 120: 234–241.
Purola E. 1963. Serous papillary ovarian tumors. *Acta Obstet Gynecol Scand* 42(Suppl 3): 1–77.
Roth LM, Czernobilsky B. 1985. Ovarian Brenner tumors. II. Malignant. *Cancer* 56:592–601.
Roth LM, Czernobilsky B, Langley FA. 1981. Ovarian endometrioid adenofibromatous and cystadenofibromatous tumors: Benign, proliferating, and malignant. *Cancer* 48:1838–1845.
Roth LM, Dallenbach-Hellweg G, Czernobilsky B. 1985. Ovarian Brenner tumors. I. Metaplastic, proliferating and of low malignant potential. *Cancer* 56:582–591.
Roth LM, Langley FA, Fox H, Wheeler JE, Czernobilsky B. 1984. Ovarian clear cell adenofibromatous tumors. *Cancer* 53:1156–1163.

Roth LM, Sternberg WH. 1971. Proliferating Brenner tumors. *Cancer* 27:687–693.
Russell P. 1979a. The pathological assessment of ovarian neoplasms. I: Introduction to the common "epithelial" tumours and analysis of benign "epithelial" tumours. *Pathology* 11:5–26.
Russell P. 1979b. The pathological assessment of ovarian neoplasms. II: The proliferating tumours. *Pathology* 11:251–282.
Russell P. 1984. Borderline epithelial tumours of the ovary: A conceptual dilemma. *Clin Obstet Gynaecol* 11:259–277.
Russell P. 1985. Multifocal tumorigenesis in the upper female genital tract—Implications for staging and management. *Int J Gynecol Pathol* 4:192–210.
Russell P, Merkur H. 1979. Proliferating ovarian "epithelial" tumours: A clinicopathological analysis of 144 cases. *Aust NZ J Obstet Gynaecol* 19:45–51.
Santesson L, Kottmeier HL. 1968. General classification of ovarian tumors. In *Ovarian Cancer*, Vol 11 of *UICC Monograph Series*, ed. F. Gentil, AC Junquerira, pp. 1–8. New York: Springer-Verlag.
Serov SF, Scully RE, Sobin LH. 1973. Histological typing of ovarian tumours. No. 9 of *International Histological Classification of Tumours*. Geneva: World Health Organization.
Swenerton KD, Hislop TG, Spinelli J, LeRiche JC, Yang N, Boyes DA. 1985. Ovarian carcinoma: A multivariate analysis of prognostic factors. *Obstet Gynecol* 65:264–270.
Taylor HC. Malignant and semimalignant tumors of the ovary. 1929. *Surg Gynecol Obstet* 48:702–712.
Tobacman JK, Tucker MA, Kase R, Greene MH, Costa J, Fraumeni JF Jr. 1982. Intra-abdominal carcinomatosis after prophylactic oophorectomy in ovarian-cancer prone families. *Lancet* 2:795–797.
Ulbright TM, Roth LM, Stehman FB. 1984. Secondary ovarian neoplasia. *Cancer* 53:1164–1174.
Woodruff JD, Dietrich D, Genadry R, Parmley TH. 1981. Proliferative and malignant Brenner tumors: Review of 47 cases. *Am J Obstet Gynecol* 141:118–125.
Woodruff JD, Solomon D, Sullivant H. 1985. Multifocal disease in the upper genital canal. *Obstet Gynecol* 65:695–698.
Zinsser KR, Wheeler JE. 1982. Endosalpingiosis in the omentum: A study of autopsy and surgical material. *Am J Surg Pathol* 6:109–117.

CERVICAL AND VULVAR CANCER

Annual Clinical Conference on Cancer, Vol. 29
Gynecologic Cancer: Diagnosis and Treatment Strategies
© 1987 by The University of Texas System Cancer Center

14. Herpes Simplex and Human Papilloma Viruses in Lower Genital Tract Neoplasia

Raymond H. Kaufman and Ervin Adam

An association between herpes simplex virus type 2 (HSV-2) and human papilloma virus (HPV) in carcinoma of the lower genital tract has been repeatedly demonstrated during the last two decades; however, the etiologic relationship of HSV-2 and HPV infections with lower genital tract cancer has not been definitely established. The frequency of antibodies to HSV-2 in cases of cervical carcinoma has yielded equivocal results in various geographic areas in that the prevalence of antibodies to HSV-2 has varied from 31% to 100% (Plummer and Masterson 1971; Pridan and Lilienfeld 1971; Rawls, Adam, and Melnick 1972). In some studies, no significant differences in antibody distribution were noted between cancer cases and comparison groups (Pridan and Lilienfeld 1971; Rawls, Adam, and Melnick 1972; Vonka et al. 1984). These findings have led us to question the role of HSV-2 in the pathogenesis of cervical neoplasia. It has also been suggested that cervical cancer is caused by multiple etiologic factors. There has been increasing evidence of an association between HPV infection and the development of squamous cell neoplasia of the lower genital tract (Meisels, Morin, and Casas-Cordero 1982; zur Hausen 1977, 1982; Orth et al. 1977; Laverty et al. 1977; Hills and Laverty 1979; Reid et al. 1980; Reid 1983; Shah et al. 1980; Woodruff et al. 1981; Kurman, Jenson, and Lancaster 1983; Schlehofer and zur Hausen 1982; Durst et al. 1983; Ostrow et al. 1983; Syrjänen et al. 1984; Fu et al. 1983; Kreider et al. 1985). The findings of Prakash et al. (1985) suggested that multiple etiologies rather than synergism between these factors as postulated by zur Hausen (1982) may be related to the development of cervical carcinoma. We will present data regarding the presence of HSV-induced nonstructural antigens in cells of lower genital tract carcinoma as well as information from a prospective study of 959 women in whom the development of antibodies to HSV-1 and HSV-2 was studied. In the same group, the development of HPV changes over a period of time was also investigated.

Herpesvirus-Induced Antigens

Infected cell–specific protein 11/12 (ICSP 11/12) and ICSP 34/35 have been characterized as early nonstructural HSV-2–specified proteins. An HSV-2 viral protein 143 (VP 143) has also been characterized. Antibodies to all three viral proteins were generated in rabbits. In addition, we prepared an antiserum to highly purified HSV-2 virions that were grown in baby rabbit kidney cells and medium containing only rabbit serum.

Cervical and vulvar tissues were obtained from women with various degrees of genital neoplasia; normal cervical and vulvar tissues were also obtained. The immunologic and histological staining procedures were carried out, using parallel tissue sections. An immunoperoxidase staining procedure was carried out on selected sections of tissue. Adsorption of the antiserum with HSV-2–infected cells blocked the reaction. The aspects of the staining pattern that showed positive results were similar to the cytoplasmic reaction of HSV-2–transformed hamster cells stained with anti-VP 143, and a cytoplasmic reaction was also observed in a human cervical cancer cell line stained with all three antisera. Tissues that demonstrated positive results from staining showed negative results when stained with antibody prepared against HSV-2 virions. Infectious virus was not recovered from tissues examined by cocultivation.

Biopsy specimens were taken from 51 women who had varying degrees of vulvar disease, and cervical biopsy specimens were obtained from 169 women. Serum specimens were collected from selected patients in both groups. The specimens were collected according to previously described procedures (Dreesman et al. 1980; Kaufman et al. 1981). The primary sera used in the staining procedures included anti-HSV-2, a rabbit antiserum prepared by immunization with purified HSV-2 that had been grown in rabbit kidney cells with media supplemented with normal rabbit serum; anti-ICSP 34/35 and anti-ICSP 11/12, rabbit antisera to HSV-2–infected cell-specific proteins 34/35 and 11/12, respectively; and a normal rabbit serum obtained from a nonimmunized animal. The preparation of specific antisera to the HSV-2 DNA–binding proteins ICSP 11/12 and ICSP 34/35 has been described in detail (Purifoy and Powell 1976; Powell and Purifoy 1976). The conjugation of goat anti-rabbit IgG antibody with horseradish peroxidase was performed as described previously (Cabral et al. 1978). The specificity of the reactivity for HSV DNA–binding protein antigen was demonstrated as follows: (*a*) preinoculation rabbit serum gave no reaction; (*b*) absorption of anti-ICSP 34/35 serum with HSV-2–infected cell lysate blocked the reaction; (*c*) adsorption with uninfected HEp-2 cell lysates did not alter the reactivity; (*d*) tissues with no pathological changes were negative; and (*e*) the results were identical when the reactivity tests were performed using peroxidase-conjugated and fluorescein-labeled agents.

Results of staining with ICSP 34/35 were positive in 18 of 35 specimens (51%) that demonstrated carcinoma in situ or severe dysplasia of the vulva (table 14.1). Seven of those specimens also demonstrated staining to the ICSP 11/12 antisera. Antibodies to HSV-2 were detected in five of nine women in the group. In two women in whom tissue specimens showed positive results from staining, there was no detection of antibodies to HSV-1 or HSV-2. Prakash et al. (1985) also made a similar observation in noting an absence of HSV-2 antibodies in a case of advanced cervical cancer in which there were positive results for HSV-2 sequences in the tumor specimen. In two of four women with vulvar intraepithelial neoplasia, grades 1 and 2, there were positive results from staining to ICSP 34/35, and in two of three women with epithelial hyperplasia without atypia, the results were similar. Specimens from two of eight women with condyloma acuminata of the vulva demonstrated positive staining, although none of the 29 specimens of normal tissue dem-

Table 14.1. *HSV Antigens in Vulvar Neoplasms by Immunoperoxidase Staining*

		Antigens to HSV-2 (Antibodies/Sera Tested)	
Diagnosis	No. Tested	ICSP 11,12	ICSP 34,35
Carcinoma in situ or severe dysplasia	35	7 (2/4)	18 (5/9)[a]
Moderate dysplasia	1	—	1 (1/1)
Mild dysplasia	3	—	1 (1/1)
Epithelial hyperplasia	3	—	2 (0/1)[b]
Hyperkeratosis	1	—	—
Condyloma	8	1	2 (1/1)
Normal	29	—	—

Source: Kaufman and Adam 1986.
Note: ICSP, infected cell–specific protein.
[a]Two women did not have antibodies to HSV-1 or HSV-2.
[b]No antibodies to HSV-1 or HSV-2.

onstrated staining with either antigen. All of the normal tissue biopsy specimens were taken from areas adjacent to carcinoma in situ of the vulva. Negative results were obtained in all of these cases—even in the 18 instances in which positive staining was found in the vulvar lesions.

In table 14.2, the findings from cervical biopsy specimens taken from 169 women are shown. In 7 of 24 patients (29%) with invasive carcinoma of the cervix or cervical intraepithelial neoplasia (CIN-III), there were positive results from staining with anti-ICSP 34/35. Positive results were also noted in 12% of women with moderate dysplasia and in 10% of women with mild dysplasia. In 4 of 48 women with squamous metaplasia and in 1 of 9 with chronic inflammation, ICSP 34/35 was present within the cells. There was no evidence of these antigens in any of the 23 samples with normal biopsy results.

These studies indicate that selected cells of malignant tissue can preferentially express the production of early nonstructural proteins in the absence of viral structural antigens or infectious virus. This is in close agreement with the observations of other research groups that have demonstrated the presence of HSV-2–specific RNA sequences in similar types of malignant tissue (Eglin et al. 1981; Maitland et al. 1981; McDougall, Galloway, and Fenoglio 1980). In one patient, there was a temporal association between genital herpesvirus infection and the development of carcinoma in situ of the vulva and cervix. In this patient, carcinoma in situ of the vulva and cervix developed six weeks after an initial HSV-2 infection of the vulva.

Staining reactions were entirely cytoplasmic, yet the two antisera utilized reacted exclusively with the nuclei of infected HEp-2 cells, as has been shown in previous

Table 14.2. *HSV Antigens in Cervical Neoplasms by Immunoperoxidase Staining*

Diagnosis	No. Tested	Antigens to HSV-2 (Antibodies/Sera Tested)	
		ICSP 11,12	ICSP 34,35
Invasive carcinoma	4	—	1 (50/1)
Carcinoma in situ or severe dysplasia	20	3 (1/3)	6 (4/6)[a]
Moderate dysplasia	25	—	3 (1/2)
Mild dysplasia	40	1 (0/1)	4 (2/4)[a]
Metaplasia	48	—	4 (2/4)
Inflammation	9	—	1 (1/1)
Normal	23	—	—

Source: Kaufman and Adam 1986.
Note: ICSP, infected cell–specific protein.
[a]One woman did not have antibodies to HSV-1 or HSV-2.

studies (Dreesman et al. 1980; Flannery, Courtney, and Schaffer 1977; Cabral et al. 1980). Cabral and coworkers have also detected cytoplasmic staining of cervical neoplastic tissue using anti-VP 143 serum. In addition, G. R. Dreesman and coworkers have recently demonstrated that a cell derived from a carcinoma in a human being yielded a cytoplasmic reaction when stained with anti-ICSP 11/12 (G.R. Dreesman, R.H. Kaufman, and E. Adam unpublished data).

HSV and HPV in Cervical Neoplasia

Most studies of the association of HSV and HPV with lower genital tract neoplasia have been retrospective. It has been evident, however, that prospective studies are needed for more definitive information. Such a study was initiated in Prague, Czechoslovakia, in 1975 (Vonka et al. 1984). An opportunity to institute a prospective study also developed in the United States in 1975 when the National Cancer Institute initiated a multicenter cooperative study of associated diethylstilbestrol (DES) exposure in utero and cancer risk in 5,000 women (Adam et al. 1977; Labarthe et al. 1978; Melnick and Adam 1978). The center in Houston was able to arrange for the collection of serum specimens as well as cytology and biopsy specimens. The current data present results of this prospective study, looking at the relationship of both HSV and HPV infections to the development of intraepithelial neoplasia of the cervix. The 959 women enrolled in the study were predominantly white, of middle or upper socioeconomic level, and had been exposed to DES in utero. Enrollment in the study began in April 1975 and continued through June

1983. Two hundred ninety-six women in the study were identified by review of the prenatal records in which exposure to DES was documented. These women were classified as "record reviews." Six hundred sixty-three other women were either referred by their physicians to the DES center or initiated enrollment themselves and were classified as "referrals" and "walk-ins," respectively. The study also included 175 women who had not been exposed to DES. These women were either siblings of the exposed "record-review" women or were pair-matched by age and by their mothers' ages with DES-exposed women from the same data source. Only women with no history of genital neoplasia and with no such findings at the time of baseline examination were enrolled in the study.

Documentation on the study patients included basic demographic data, prenatal and postnatal history, sexual and reproductive history variables, and information on oral and genital herpes. Each woman had a gynecologic examination consisting of breast examination, vaginal inspection, and colposcopic examination of the vagina and cervix, and iodine staining of the vagina and cervix. Cytological preparations were taken from the vagina and cervix, and colposcopically directed biopsies were taken in women with vaginal adenosis or other vaginal or cervical epithelial changes. All findings were carefully documented. The participants were periodically examined, usually at yearly intervals, during a follow-up period of five to seven years. All of the examinations were uniform, and information on interval changes and the pertinent history as well as objective findings were again documented on special forms.

Biopsy specimens showing evidence of neoplasia were reviewed by all diethylstilbestroladenosis (DESAD) project pathologists, and the diagnosis reached by consensus was computed. Histological evidence of viral infection was not emphasized in these evaluations. If a diagnosis of neoplasia was made by the patient's private physician, then the biopsy slides were obtained for review by the DESAD project pathologists. A blood sample was drawn at the time of entry, and other samples were drawn periodically thereafter for future serological studies. The serum samples were stored at −35° C. During the period of study, squamous cell cervical intraepithelial neoplasia (CIN) was diagnosed by biopsy in 24 women. Six of those women had been classified as "record reviews" (four had CIN grade I; one, CIN II; and one, CIN III), and 17 were from the "walk-in" and "referral" groups (eight had CIN I; four, CIN II; and five, CIN III) (Adam et al. 1985). One unexposed control patient was found to have moderate dysplasia. That patient refused to give consent for blood drawing. The 23 women who had been exposed to DES and had CIN were pair-matched with other DES-exposed women by method of enrollment, age at the time of entry, and time of enrollment as close as feasible to the date when the women who later developed CIN had entered the study.

A series of cervical biopsy specimens were available for reevaluation of histological evidence of papilloma virus infection. These included (1) specimens with evidence of CIN from 23 women, 11 of whom had biopsy specimens available prior to the development of CIN; (2) specimens obtained from the matched DES-exposed group, which consisted of 11 women who underwent cervical biopsy close to the time of diagnosis of CIN in the previous group. Eight of these latter 11 women had an earlier biopsy specimen available for study.

New paraffin block sections were prepared from 18 samples from the CIN cases. In ten of those cases, biopsy specimens taken prior to the development of CIN were available for study. Similar specimens were prepared from ten DES-exposed matched controls. Earlier biopsy specimens from five of those women were also available. The new sections were evaluated for the presence of structural antigens of papilloma virus. A parallel section of each tissue was stained by hematoxylin and eosin for verification of the histological diagnosis. The slide reviews were performed under code.

The micro-solid-phase radioimmunoassay (micro-SPRIA) was used for the detection of HSV type-specific antibodies of the IgG class (Matson et al. 1983; Adler-Storthz et al. 1983) using two major glycoprotein populations, VP 123 for HSV-1 and VP 119 for HSV-2. In addition, optimal dilutions for HSV-1 and HSV-2 virus stocks were used as coating antigens. The glycoproteins present in the VP 119 and VP 123 preparations were identified by Dr. R. Courtney (Department of Microbiology, University of Tennessee, Knoxville, Tennessee) as mainly gC-1 and gC-2 and also gB-1 and gB-2. Sera obtained from individuals with documented infections by HSV-1 and HSV-2 only reacted primarily with the type-specific antigens. The sera were also tested by the microneutralization test (Rawls, Adam, and Melnick 1970) for antibodies to HSV-1 and HSV-2. An index of greater than or equal to 85 was considered significant for evidence of HSV-2 infection. The peroxidase-antiperoxidase technique (Jenson et al. 1980; Kurman et al. 1981; Morin et al. 1981) was used to detect papilloma virus antigens.

Six (2.0%) CIN cases were observed in the 296 "record reviews." Seventeen of 663 (2.6%) "walk-ins" and "referrals" developed CIN. Only one of 175 (0.57%) nonexposed women developed neoplasia. Taking into consideration the maximal observation interval during which any CIN developed, the approximate estimate of incidence per 1,000 women per year in the DES-exposed women was 3.12 for CIN I, 1.3 for CIN II, and 1.56 for CIN III. The incidence of CIN II in women not exposed to DES was 1.14.

The characteristics of the women who had CIN and women in the comparison group are presented in table 14.3. The mean age of 21.6 years in both groups is a reflection of the matching. No substantial differences were observed in relation to marital status or estimated number of sexual partners. There was a slightly higher number of virgins and a lower number of divorcees in the comparison group. Although not statistically significant, this observed difference reflects a trend compatible with the findings of several preceding epidemiological studies. Thirteen of 46 women (28%; mean age, 21.6) in the study were virginal. Among the sexually active women, the mean number of sexual partners exceeded four. Increases in sexual activity during the study period were similar for both groups.

Two serum samples from each woman were selected for antibody studies. In the women who developed CIN, the first sample was obtained at the time of enrollment in the study, and the second sample was obtained at the time of diagnosis of neoplasia. The serum samples selected from the comparison group were obtained at the time of enrollment and at the time closest to diagnosis of CIN in the matched women. The mean time interval between the two samples was 27.3 months (range,

Table 14.3. *Characteristics of the Study Population*

Characteristic	CIN (*N* = 23) Enrollment	CIN (*N* = 23) Follow-up	Controls (*N* = 23) Enrollment	Controls (*N* = 23) Follow-up
Mean age (years)	21.6		21.6	
SD	3.09		3.02	
Range	16–28		16–28	
Marital status				
Single	17	13	17	15
Married	4	7	6	8
Divorced	2	3	—	—
Virginal	5	0	8	2
Sex partners/participant[a]	4.2	5.3	4.3	5.7
SD	5.5	5.7	4.8	7.2
Range	1–25	1–27	1–16	1–30
N	18	21[b]	15	19[c]

Source: Adam et al. 1985.
Note: CIN, cervical intraepithelial neoplasia; SD, standard deviation.
[a]Number of sex partners estimated by questionnaire.
[b]Of two women who refused information, one earlier reported having one sex partner and the other, five.
[c]Two women refused to give information; earlier, one reported being virginal and the other reported one sex partner.

12–77 months) in women with CIN and 22.6 months (range, 5–61 months) in the comparison group (not statistically significant). Both serum samples from each woman were simultaneously tested by micro-SPRIA. The second serum sample was also tested for antibody by the microneutralization technique.

Antibodies to individual HSV-1 and HSV-2 as assayed by the micro-SPRIA test are demonstrated in table 14.4. There were no significant differences between the study groups in the frequency of antibodies to HSV-2 (9% compared with 9%, first sample; 30% compared with 35%, second sample). However, the rate of antibodies to HSV-1 was higher in both samples in women with CIN than in the comparison group. The frequency of development of antibodies to HSV-2 was higher than to HSV-1 over the time period studied.

Histological findings associated with papilloma virus infection were found in 14 of 17 CIN I and CIN II cases and in 3 of 6 CIN III cases (table 14.5). Thus, 74% of women with CIN had histological changes compatible with papilloma virus infection. Antibodies to HSV-2 were noted in the 3 CIN III cases with HPV changes, although there were no HSV-2 antibodies detected in the enrollment serum samples. Only 2 of 14 CIN I and CIN II cases had simultaneous antibodies to HSV-2 (no antibodies were detected in the first serum samples).

Biopsy specimens from earlier procedures were available for review from 11 women with CIN. There was no evidence of papilloma virus infection in these early specimens. In 7 of the 11 women (64%), there was evidence of HPV infection with CIN changes in the second biopsy specimens. Eleven women of the comparison group had biopsy specimens taken at the approximate time that CIN was diagnosed

Table 14.4. *Antibodies Detected by Micro-SPRIA to HSV in 23 CIN Cases and Matched Controls*

Antibodies to HSV	CIN I–II	Controls	CIN III	Controls	All CIN	All Controls
First sample						
Negative	9	12	2	4	11 (48)	16 (70)
HSV-1 only	7	3	3	2	10 (44)	5 (22)
HSV-2 only	—	2	—	—	—	2 (9)
HSV-1 and HSV-2	1	—	1	—	2 (9)	—
All HSV-1	8 (47)	3 (18)	4	2	12 (52)[b]	5 (22)
All HSV-2	1 (6)	2 (12)	1	—	2 (9)	2 (9)
Second sample						
Negative	8	7	1	4	9 (39)	11 (48)
HSV-1 only	6	3	1	1	7 (30)	4 (17)
HSV-2 only	1	6			1 (4)	6 (26)
HSV-1 and HSV-2	2	1	4	1	6 (26)	2 (9)
All HSV-1	8 (47)	4 (23)	5 (83)	2 (33)	13 (57)[b]	6 (26)
All HSV-2	3 (18)	7 (41)	4 (67)[a]	1 (17)	7 (30)	8 (35)
N	17	17	6	6	23	23

Source: Adam et al. 1985.
Note: CIN, cervical intraepithelial neoplasia. Numbers in parentheses are percentages.
[a] Difference between CIN III and CIN I–II: $p<0.05$ (Fisher).
[b] CIN control difference: $p<0.05$ one-sided (Pike and Morrow chi-square for matched pairs).

Table 14.5. *Antibodies to HSV in Relation to Histological Findings Associated with HPV Infection*

HPV Changes	CIN I–II		CIN III	
	HSV-1 Only	HSV-2 (±HSV-1)	HSV-1 Only	HSV-2 (±HSV-1)
Present	4/14 (29)	2/14 (14)	0/3	3/3
Absent	2/3	1/3	1/3	1/3
N	17		6	

Source: Adam et al. 1985.
Note: Antibodies were measured by micro-SPRIA. Numbers represent number having antibodies per number tested. Numbers in parentheses are percentages.
[a] Difference from the corresponding CIN I–II: $p<.05$ (Fisher).

in the other group. Histological findings compatible with papilloma virus infection were noted in only one (9%) of the control group. Eight women in the control group had had previous biopsy specimens taken. There was also no evidence of papilloma virus infection in these early specimens.

We present in table 14.6 the results of histological diagnosis compared with the immunocytological detection of papilloma virus structural antigen in the same tissues from CIN cases and controls (12 of the 13 CIN cases had histological evidence of HPV infection). Papilloma virus structural antigen was detected in three of ten CIN I and CIN II cases and in none of the CIN III cases. Papilloma virus structural antigen was identified in one of three specimens with a histological diagnosis of HPV infection, whereas cases diagnosed as squamous metaplasia were all negative. Two of the three CIN cases with detectable HPV structural antigen present had serological evidence of HSV-1 infection.

Biopsy specimens obtained at the time of enrollment were available for 10 of 18 women of the CIN group and for 5 of 10 women in the comparison group. No epithelial cells were present in one specimen of the CIN group. Squamous metaplasia was diagnosed without evidence of HPV infection by either of the techniques used in the other 14 tissue samples.

The incidence of CIN II and CIN III was 2.64 per 1,000 women per year of observation. The only comparable cohort was recorded in a prospective HSV study carried out in Prague, Czechoslovakia (Vonka et al. 1984), in which biopsy-proven CIN II and CIN III cases were listed from women who did not demonstrate atypia at the time of enrollment or during the observation period. Vonka and coworkers found an incidence of 0.82 per 1,000 women per year. This is close to that found in our group of women who had not been exposed to DES (1.14 per 1,000 women per year). The differences observed could be a reflection of the substantially different sizes of the cohorts in each study or, more important, they could suggest that women exposed to DES in utero indeed have a higher rate of CIN than a comparable group from the general population (Robboy et al. 1984).

We were unable to demonstrate differences between the study groups in the rate or levels of antibodies to HSV-2 by either of the detection techniques utilized. Differences were found, however, in the prevalence of antibodies to HSV-1 between women with CIN and the matched control group as measured by the micro-SPRIA method. A similar trend was observed by the microneutralization test: 43.5% of women with CIN and 26% of women in the comparison group had antibodies to HSV-1.

The simplest explanation for these findings is that they occurred on the basis of chance because of the small numbers in each group. It can be speculated that there is a higher frequency of genital herpes associated with HSV-1 than is generally expected. In a comparable population in Houston (without exposure to DES), the fre-

Table 14.6. *Papilloma Virus Structural Antigen in Biopsy Specimens of Women with CIN and Women in the Comparison Group*

		HPV Infection		
Histological Diagnosis	No. of Cases	Histological Evidence	Structural Evidence	Controls
CIN I	9	8	2	—
CIN II	2	2	1	—
CIN III	2	2	0	—
HPV	3	3	1	—
Squamous metaplasia	2	0	0	10[a]
Women studied (*N*)	18	15	4	10

Source: Adam et al. 1985.
[a]HPV infection was not observed by either method of investigation.

quency of genital HSV-1 infection was found to be 12% (Kaufman et al. 1978). In Japan, one third to over one half of genital isolates were identified as HSV-1 (Kawana and Yoshino 1974; Ozaki et al. 1980; Ishiguro et al. 1982) and reports from England suggest an increasing frequency of genital herpes infection by HSV-1 (Peutherer, Smith, and Robertson 1982).

This hypothesis is not supported by our finding a minimal interval increase in the incidence of antibodies to HSV-1, while the frequency of antibodies to HSV-2 increased substantially. On the other hand, discrepancies between detection of antibodies to HSV by the two tests occurred in the CIN cases. Five women did not have antibodies to HSV by the micro-SPRIA test. However, three of five had neutralizing antibodies compatible with HSV-1 infection, and one had neutralizing antibodies compatible with HSV-2 infection. In one case, antibodies to HSV were detected by the micro-SPRIA using intact virus-coated wells. If we included these results in the case-control evaluation, the differences between the study groups in frequency of antibodies to HSV-1 would further increase.

The most striking feature in our study is the high rate of morphological evidence of HPV infection found in association with cervical intraepithelial neoplasia—82% in CIN I and CIN II and 50% in CIN III cases—as well as a lack of similar findings in biopsy specimens preceding the development of neoplasia. Serologically diagnosed HSV infections were observed at a lower rate, independent of the presence or absence of HPV-associated morphological changes. However, anti-HSV activity usually preceded evidence of HPV infection. No association was observed between morphological changes associated with HPV infection and the presence of vaginal or cervical changes assumed to be related to DES exposure. Therefore, a possible changed disposition to HPV infection related to exposure to DES remains speculative. If the cells containing virus particles are representative of an ongoing infection, the question arises about whether the neoplastic tissue is more sensitive to an HPV infection. The findings of Kreider et al. (1985) have demonstrated morphological transformation of human tissues with human papilloma virus under controlled experimental conditions, suggesting that indeed the papilloma virus can induce morphological changes compatible with CIN in previously normal tissue.

The large-scale prospective study conducted by Vonka et al. (1984) in Prague did not confirm the results of their previous retrospective study that indicated a higher prevalence of antibodies to HSV-2 in cervical neoplasia cases than in matched control groups. Our study of a smaller population yielded results that are similar to the above findings in relationship of antibodies to HSV-2 and cervical neoplasia. A substantial difference between these studies is that, in our study, compared with women in the matched control group, women with CIN had an increased rate of antibodies to HSV-1. Interpretation of this observation remains speculative. Morphological evidence of HPV infection in CIN cases furthers the importance of continuous studies of the association between both HSV and HPV and squamous neoplasia of the female genital tract.

The seroepidemiological studies of women with cervical neoplasia and women from control groups have demonstrated an association between sexual activity and the development of lower genital tract neoplasia. Although HSV infection has been studied most often, it is obvious from epidemiological studies that whether or not HSV plays any role in human oncogenesis, it does not appear to be the sole agent responsible for the development of cervical neoplasia in women. In most recent reports, specific HPV strains have been designated as causative agents in cervical neoplasia (Ostrow et al. 1983; Crum et al. 1984; zur Hausen 1977, 1982; zur Hausen, Gissman, and Schlehofer 1984; Durst et al. 1983; Syrjänen et al. 1984; Boshart et al. 1984). It is of interest that the frequency of identification of papilloma virus structural protein has been in inverse relation to the degree of cervical neoplasia (Kurman, Jenson, and Lancaster 1983). A working hypothesis on cervical oncogenesis was proposed by zur Hausen (1982) who suggested that the HPV represents the promoter factor in neoplasia after an initiating HSV infection with mutogenic potential. The findings of Prakash et al. (1985) suggest multiple etiologies rather than synergism between the factors. From these findings, all we can determine with certainty is that an association does exist between HPV and HSV infections and lower genital tract neoplasia.

References

Adam E, Decker DJ, Herbst AL, Noller KL, Tilley BC, Townsend DE. 1977. Vaginal and cervical cancers and other abnormalities associated with exposure in utero to diethylstilbestrol and related synthetic hormones. *Cancer Res* 37:1249–1251.

Adam E, Kaufman RH, Adler-Storthz K, Melnick JL, Dreesman GR. 1985. A prospective study of association of herpes simplex virus and human papillomavirus infection with cervical neoplasia in women esposed to diethylstilbestrol in utero. *Int J Cancer* 35:19–26.

Adler-Storthz K, Matson D, Adam E, Dreesman GR. 1983. A micro solid-phase radioimmunoassay for detection of herpesvirus type specific antibody: Specificity and sensitivity. *J Virol Methods* 6:85–97.

Boshart M, Gissman L, Ikenberg H, Kleinheinz A, Scheurlen W, zur Hausen H. 1984. A new type of papillomavirus DNA, its presence in genital cancer biopsies and in cell lines derived from cervical cancer. *EMBO J* 3:1151–1157.

Cabral GA, Gyorkey F, Gyorkey P, Melnick JL, Dreesman GR. 1978. Immunohistochemical and electron microscopic detection of hepatitis B surface and core antigens. *Exp Mol Path* 29:156–169.

Cabral GA, Marcino-Cabral F, Fry D, Lumpkin CK, Mercer L, Goplerud D. 1982. Expression of herpes simplex virus type 2 antigens in premalignant and malignant human vulvar cells. *Am J Obstet Gynecol* 143:611–619.

Crum CP, Ikenberg H, Richart RM, Gissman L. 1984. Human papilloma virus type 16 and early cervical neoplasia. *N Engl J Med* 310:880–883.

Dreesman GR, Burek J, Adam E, Kaufman RH, Matson DO, Powell KL, Purifoy DJM, Melnick JL. 1980. Expression of herpesvirus-induced antigens in human cervical cancer. *Nature* 28:591–593.

Durst M, Gissmann L, Ikenberg H, zur Hausen H. 1983. A papillomavirus DNA from a cervical carcinoma and its prevalence in cancer biopsy samples from different geographic regions. *Proc Natl Acad Sci USA* 80:3812–3815.

Eglin RP, Sharp F, MacLean AB, Macnab JCM, Clements JB, Wilkie NM. 1981. Detection of RNA complementary to herpes simplex virus DNA in human cervical squamous cell neoplasms. *Cancer Res* 41:3597–3603.

Flannery VL, Courtney RJ, Schaffer PA. 1977. Expression of an early, non-structural antigen of herpes simplex virus in cells transformed *in vitro* by herpes simplex virus. *J Virol* 21:284–291.

Fu YS, Lancaster WD, Richart RM, Reagan JW, Crum CP, Levine RU. 1983. Cervical papillomavirus infection in diethylstilbestrol-exposed progeny. *Obstet Gynecol* 61:59–62.

Hills E, Laverty CR. 1979. Electron microscopic detection of papilloma virus particles in selected koilocytotic cells in a routine cervical smear. *Acta Cytol* 23:53–56.

Ishiguro T, Ozaki Y, Matsunami M, Funakoshi S. 1982. Clinical and virological features of herpes genitalis in Japanese women. *Acta Obstet Gynecol Scand* 61:173–176.

Jenson AB, Rosenthal JD, Olson C, Pass F, Lancaster WD, Shah K. 1980. Immunologic relatedness of papillomaviruses from different species. *JNCI* 64:495–500.

Kaufman RH, Adam E. 1986. Herpes simplex virus and human papilloma virus in the development of cervical carcinoma. *Clin Obstet Gynecol* 29:678–692.

Kaufman RH, Adam E, Mirkovic RR, Melnick JL, Young RL. 1978. Treatment of genital herpes simplex infection with photodynamic inactivation. *Am J Obstet Gynecol* 132:861–869.

Kaufman RH, Dreesman GR, Burek J, Korhonen MO, Matson DO, Melnick JL, Powell KL, Purifoy DJM, Courtney RJ, Adam E. 1981. Herpesvirus-induced antigens in squamous-cell carcinoma *in situ* of the vulva. *N Engl J Med* 305:483–488.

Kawana T, Yoshino K. 1974. Typing of herpes simplex virus strains of genital and urogenital origins. *Japanese Journal of Microbiology* 18:235–241.

Kreider JW, Howett MK, Wolfe SA, Bartlett GL, Zaino RJ, Sedlacek TJ, Mortel R. 1985. Morphological transformation *in vivo* of human uterine cervix with papillomavirus from condyloma acuminata. *Nature* 317:639–641.

Kurman RJ, Jenson AB, Lancaster WD. 1983. Papilloma virus infection of the cervix. II. *Am J Pathol* 7:39–52.

Kurman RJ, Shah KH, Lancaster WD, Jenson AB. 1981. Immunoperoxidase localization of papillomavirus antigens in cervical dysplasia and vulvar condylomas. *Am J Obstet Gynecol* 140:931–935.

LaBarthe D, Adam E, Noller KL, O'Brien PC, Robboy SJ, Tilley BC, Townsend DE, Barnes AB, Kaufman RH, Decker DG, Fish CR, Herbst AL, Gundersen J, Kurland LT. 1978. Design and preliminary observations on National Cooperative Diethylstilbestrol Adenosis (DESAD) Project. *Obstet Gynecol* 51:453–458.

Laverty CR, Russell P, Hills E, Booth N. 1977. The significance of non-condylomatous wart virus infection of the cervical transformation zone: A review with discussion of two cases. *Acta Cytol* 22:195–201.

Maitland NJ, Kinross JH, Busuttil A, Ludgate SM, Smart GE, Jones KW. 1981. The detection of DNA tumor virus-specific RNA sequences in abnormal human cervical biopsies by *in-situ* hybridization. *J Gen Virol* 55:123–137.

Matson D, Adler-Storthz K, Adam E, Dreesman G. 1983. A micro solid-phase radioimmunoassay for detection of herpesvirus type-specific antibody: Parameters involved in standardization. *J Virol Methods* 6:71–83.

McDougall JK, Galloway DA, Fenoglio CM. 1980. Cervical carcinoma: Detection of herpes simplex virus RNA cells undergoing neoplastic change. *Int J Cancer* 25:1–8.

Meisels A, Morin C, Casas-Cordero M. 1982. Human papillomavirus infection of the uterine cervix. *Int J Gynecol Pathol* 1:75–94.

Melnick JL, Adam E. 1978. Epidemiological approaches to determining whether herpesvirus is etiological agent of cervical cancer. *Progress in Tumor Research* 21:49–69.

Morin C, Braun L, Casas-Cordero M, Shah KV, Roy M, Fortier M, Meisels A. 1981. Confirmation of the papillomavirus. Etiology of condylomatous cervix lesions by the peroxidase-antiperoxidase technique. *JNCI* 66:831–835.

Orth G, Breitburd F, Favre M, Croissant O. 1977. Papillomaviruses: Possible role in human cancer. In *Origins of Human Cancer*, ed. J Watson, pp. 1043–1068. Cold Spring Harbor, New York: Cold Spring Harbor.

Ostrow RS, Watts S, Bender M, Niimura M, Seki T, Kawashima M, Pass F, Faras AJ. 1983. Identification of three distinct papillomavirus genomes in a single patient with epidermodysplasia verruciformis. *J Am Acad Dermatol* 8:398–404.

Ozaki Y, Ishiguro T, Ohashi M, Kimura EM. 1980. Relationship between antigenic type of virus and antibody response in female patients with herpes genitalis. *J Med Virol* 5:249–256.

Peutherer JF, Smith IW, Robertson DHH. 1982. Genital infection with herpes simplex virus type 1. *J Infect* 4:33–35.

Plummer G, Masterson JG. 1971. Herpes simplex virus and cancer of the cervix. *Am J Obstet Gynecol* 111:81–84.

Powell KL, Purifoy DJM. 1976. DNA-binding proteins in cells infected by herpes simplex virus type 1 and type 2. *Intervirology* 7:225–239.

Prakash SS, Reeves WC, Sisson GR, Brenes M, Godoy J, Bacchetti S, de Britton RC, Rawls WE. 1985. Herpes simplex virus type 2 in human papillomavirus type 16 in cervicitis, dysplasia, and invasive cervical carcinoma. *Int J Cancer* 35:51–57.

Pridan H, Lilienfeld AM. 1971. Carcinoma of the cervix in Jewish women in Israel, 1960–1967. An epidemiological survey. *Isr J Med Sci* 7:1465–1470.

Purifoy DJM, Powell KL. 1976. DNA-binding proteins induced by herpes simplex virus in HEp-2 cells. *J Virol* 19:717–731.

Rawls WE, Adam E, Melnick JL. 1972. Geographic variation in the association of antibodies to herpesvirus type 2 and carcinoma of the cervix. In *Oncogenesis and Herpesviruses*, ed. PM Biggs, G de-The, LN Payne, pp. 424–427. No. 2 of Scientific Publications. Lyons, France: International Agency for Research on Cancer.

Reid R. 1983. Genital warts and cervical cancer. II. Is human papillomavirus infection the trigger to cervical carcinogenesis? *Gynecol Oncol* 15:239–252.

Reid R, Laverty CR, Coppleson M, Isarangkul W, Hills E. 1980. Noncondylomatous cervical wart virus infection. *Obstet Gynecol* 55:476–483.

Robboy SJ, Noller KL, O'Brien P, Kaufman RH, Townsend D, Barns AB, Gundersen J, Lawrence WD, Bergstrahl E, McGorray S, Tilley BC, Anton J, Chazen G. 1984. Increased incidence of cervical and vaginal dysplasia in 3,980 diethylstilbestrol-exposed young women. *JAMA* 252:2979–2983.

Schlehofer JR, zur Hausen H. 1982. Induction of mutations within the host cell genome by partially inactiviated herpes simplex virus type 1. *Virology* 122:471–475.

Shah KH, Lewis MG, Jenson AB, Kurman RJ, Lancaster WD. 1980. Papillomavirus and cervical dysplasia. *Lancet* 2:1190.

Syrjänen K, Mäntyjarvi R, Väyrynen M, Cashréen O, Yliskoski M, Saarikoski S, Pyrhönen S. 1984. Herpes simplex virus infection of females with human papilloma-virus lesions in the uterine cervix. *The Cervix and Lower Female Genital Tract* 2:25–32.

Vonka V, Kaňka J, Hirsch I, Závadová H, Krčmář M, Suchánková A, Rezáčová D, Brouček J, Press M, Domorázková E, Svoboda B, Havránková A, Jelínek J. 1984. Prospective study on the relationship between cervical neoplasia and herpes simplex type-2 virus. II. Herpes simplex type-2 antibody presence in sera taken at enrollment. *Int J Cancer* 33:61–66.

Woodruff JD, Braun L, Cavalieri R, Gupta P, Pass F, Shah KV. 1981. Immunological identification of papillomavirus antigen in paraffin-processed condyloma tissues from the female genital tract. *Obstet Gynecol* 198:727–732.

zur Hausen H. 1977. Human papilloma viruses and their possible role in squamous cell carcinomas. *Curr Top Microbiol Immunol* 78:1–30.

zur Hausen H. 1982. Human genital cancer: Synergism between two virus infections or synergism between a virus infection and initiating events? *Lancet* 2:1370–1372.

zur Hausen, Gissmann L, and Schlehofer JR. 1984. Viruses in the etiology of human genital cancer. *Prog Med Virol* 30:170–186.

Annual Clinical Conference on Cancer, Vol. 29
Gynecologic Cancer: Diagnosis and Treatment Strategies
© 1987 by The University of Texas System Cancer Center

15. The Outpatient Management of Cervical Intraepithelial Neoplasia

R. Michael Shier and A. Dennis De Petrillo

In the first half of this century, carcinoma of the cervix was a chief cause of cancer deaths in women throughout the world. Because of effective screening programs that can detect and eliminate the disease in its intraepithelial stage and because of improved therapies, this fact, fortunately, is no longer true. However, carcinoma of the cervix does remain the leading cause of cancer deaths among women in the Caribbean and in some Latin American countries that do not utilize modern medical technologies (Hart 1985).

Detection of this disorder in its preinvasive stage only became common in North America after George Papanicolaou published his treatise on cytology in 1943 (Papanicolaou and Traut 1943). For a while thereafter, the literature stressed the utilization of unsophisticated methods of diagnosis, including blind multiple cervical biopsies, Schiller's iodine-directed biopsies, and in-hospital methods such as cervical amputation and cold knife cervical conization (Scott, Welch, and Blake 1960; Crisp, Shalauta, and Bennett 1968). Cone biopsy was also relied upon for diagnosis during pregnancy, with significant attendant morbidity (Hannigan et al. 1982). The in-hospital setting was also required for therapy, which usually consisted of wide cone biopsy or hysterectomy (Topek 1967).

In 1925 Hans Hinselman invented the colposcope, but it has only been in the last 15 years in North America that colposcopy has become the cornerstone in the management of patients with abnormal cervical cytology. The modern colposcopic method has been popularized by a number of North American authors (among them, Townsend et al. 1970; Stafl 1975; and De Petrillo et al. 1975) and has allowed for the evolution of effective but conservative outpatient therapies (Lickrish and Fortier 1977).

The ambulatory management of patients with abnormal cytology reaps tremendous benefits. Not only are there major savings in costs and efficiency in time utilization, but the patient may be treated in a comfortable outpatient setting, without general anesthesia, and with better preservation of the cervix for future reproductive performance. This latter finding is particularly important in light of the increased number of women presenting with the preinvasive form of this disease at an earlier age, often prior to having children (Draper and Cook 1983). A number of epidemiological factors that are considered likely to be responsible for this trend have been identified. These include an earlier age of beginning intercourse (Boyes 1983; Rotkin 1973); an increased number of sexual partners over time (Harris et al. 1980);

increased incidence of DNA virus infections, including herpes type 2 cytomegalovirus; and, more important, a virtual epidemic of human papilloma virus (HPV) infections (Becker 1984). Other factors are an increased use of immunosuppressive therapy, maternal diethylstilbestrol (DES) exposure, smoking (Lyon et al. 1983), and male factors (Campion et al. 1985).

This chapter stresses that the outpatient management of these patients relies heavily on the clinician's ability to distinguish between invasive cancer and its precursors and requires a skilled and experienced colposcopist for complete and proper diagnosis. Once this critical determination has been made, therapy may be individualized based on the nature, size, and distribution of the patient's lesion.

Terminology

The traditional histopathologic terminology that describes preinvasive lesions of the cervix utilizes the categories of dysplasia and carcinoma in situ. This terminology has been particularly favored by pathologists. However, there is little to recommend this system as there is no meaningful difference between severe dysplasia and carcinoma in situ in either prognosis or methods of management. In 1968, Richart and Sciarra recommended the term *cervical intraepithelial neoplasia* (CIN), and the classification system that uses this term is employed by most clinical services reporting in the literature today. Grade I CIN comprises neoplastic proliferations involving up to one-half of the thickness of the epithelial surface. Grade II CIN lesions may involve from one half to three fourths of the thickness of the epithelium, and grade III CIN lesions involve from three fourths to the full thickness of the epithelium. Thus, grade I CIN is equivalent to mild dysplasia, grade II CIN is equivalent to moderate dysplasia, and grade III CIN is equivalent to severe dysplasia and carcinoma in situ grouped together.

Detection

Papanicolaou initially presented a paper on the cytological detection of cervical cancer in 1928, but he was largely ignored. However, he continued to work on this project, and 15 years later he and Traut published their now-classic monograph, *The Diagnosis of Uterine Cancer by the Vaginal Smear* (1943). He could not have imagined how extensively this test would be employed or that it would become the prototype of the methods of preventive medicine. Although Hinselman had intended that colposcopy be used as a screening technique, as indeed it is in Europe, and more recently Adolf Stafl has suggested cervicography (Stafl 1983), neither method has gained wide acceptance in North America.

Although the false-positive Papanicolaou smear is a rare event, a major drawback to the test has been its variable rate of false-negative findings. Approximately half of the time, results of the latter kind arise from cytolaboratory error. For the technique to be reliable, it is important that the cytologists not only be well trained but see samples of sufficient number to maintain their expertise. It is also important that the laboratory have an adequate quality-control system. We strongly recommend that cytopathologists abandon the old Papanicolaou cytology classification and use a descriptive reporting system that incorporates into its framework the CIN classification. Richart (1967) outlines an approach whereby, if cytological findings are neither within normal parameters nor inadequate for diagnosis, atypical cells are specified, with grading done according to the criteria for grades I, II, or III CIN and classification given as HPV infection, invasive squamous cell carcinoma, adenocarcinoma, endometrial carcinoma, or another specific cancer.

The other 50% of false-negative Papanicolaou smears are related to clinical errors, particularly to an inability to adequately sample the endocervical canal. This inability becomes of increasing importance with age and gravity, as the squamocolumnar junction migrates cephalad (Ostergard 1977). Also, the clinician cannot accurately pinpoint with the naked eye the location of the squamocolumnar junction (Garite and Feldman 1978).

Different cervical cell collection techniques were explored by Richart and Vaillant in 1965. For carcinoma in situ, they found a 6% detection failure rate by sampling with the Ayre spatula and 4% using endocervical aspiration alone. Failure rates for dysplasia were 28% for the spatula and 17% with endocervical aspiration. When both techniques were used, only a 1% false-negative rate was noted for all neoplasias in the study. The vaginal pool sample had a very high false-negative rate of 55%.

Some authors have advised the use of cotton-tipped applicators combined with exocervical scraping, but false-negative rates remain in the range of 13% to 18% with this strategy (Shen et al. 1984). Rubio (1977) and Townsend (1977), among others, have advised an aspiration technique that uses a pipette with an attached rubber bulb (such as the Accu-pap, Unimar) to reduce the trapping of malignant cells within cotton fibers. It is our preference to sample the exocervix with either a wooden or plastic spatula, followed by sampling of the endocervical canal with a cervical brush such as the Cytobrush by Medscand. We find that the cervical brush provides excellent endocervical cell samples, even in cases of the relative cervical stenosis that can occur after cryotherapy or conization (Ros et al. 1983; Trimbos JB, Ahrentz N. 1984. The efficiency of collecting endocervical cells in cervical smears: The cotton swab versus the brush. Unpublished paper. Departments of Gynecology and Pathology, University of Leiden Medical Center, Leiden, The Netherlands). Cytological samples are only taken from the vagina in DES-exposed offspring (smears are taken from all quadrants) and to detect vaginal HPV infection. In both instances, the vaginal samples are spread on a slide separate from that of the cervical samples.

Now that organized screening programs have increased vigilance for cervical cancer, it is unfortunate that so many different recommendations as to the timing of Papanicolaou tests have been put forward by such diverse groups as the National Institutes of Health of the U.S. Department of Health and Human Services, the American College of Obstetricians and Gynecologists, the American Cancer Society, and the Canadian Task Force on Cervical Cancer Screening Programs (Walton 1976; Walton 1982). The 1982 Canadian Task Force recommendation was that women who have had sexual intercourse should be advised to have screening annually between the ages of 18 and 35 years and thereafter every five years until age 60, if all tests have been negative. Beyond this age, women who have had repeatedly normal smears may leave the screening program. Others have related the peak incidence of CIN to the age of onset of intercourse and have suggested that the most comprehensive screening be carried out during the first 20 to 25 years after the beginning of sexual intercourse, then every 5 years until age 60, at which point screening could be discontinued (Wright and Riopelle 1982). In the midst of this confusion, our own recommendations regarding screening are based on the following observations.

First, all evidence points to the conclusion that squamous carcinoma of the cervix is a sexually transmitted disease. A number of studies have implicated the "high-risk male" (Beral 1974). Women whose husbands have at some time been married to a woman with cervical neoplasia are four times more likely to develop cervical cancer than are matched controls (Kessler 1976). Women whose sexual partners have penile condylomata acuminata are at high risk for developing cervical neoplasias (Campion et al. 1985). There is also a higher-than-expected incidence of cervical cancer in wives whose husbands have had penile cancer (Martinez 1969). It would appear that the carcinogenic factor is carried on the skin of the penis or in the anterior urethra rather than in semen (Richardson and Lyon 1981). Thus, cancer of the cervix is likely initiated in susceptible women by a sexually transmitted factor. This susceptibility may be based in genetic predisposition, as studies of lymphocyte chromosomes suggest that the incidence of chromosome 1C band heteromorphism is significantly higher among patients with grade III CIN or invasive carcinoma than in controls (Atkin and Brito-Babapulle 1983; Haneen, Habib, and Rohme 1980).

Further, the incidence of cervical neoplasia is increasing, particularly in young women (Draper and Cook 1983), and thus it seems foolish not to advise annual screening in this age group. However, sexual mores are changing in older women as well and it has been noted that women at age 35 and above are having many more sexual contacts than this age group had previously. It has been reported that as many as 60% of U.S. married women and 80% of U.S. married men have had at least one extramarital sexual experience and that this contact often takes place later in life. Others have found that carcinoma of the cervix is now developing in women who were not previously considered to be at high risk, including those over the age of 60 (Bain and Crocker 1983).

Thus, we believe that women who have never had sexual intercourse do not require screening, whereas those who are or who have been sexually active do. Until the prevalence of the disease is more stable, we simply advise annual screening for all sexually active women.

It is mandatory that all women with abnormal cytology be carefully evaluated. For those with mildly abnormal cytology (compatible with grade I CIN), it is acceptable to simply perform follow-up in two to three months with repeat cytological assessment. In the interim, any infection with organisms such as *Chlamydia* species, HPV, or *Trichomonas vaginalis* should be treated. If indicated by atrophic effects and secondary inflammation, estrogen therapy may be locally or systemically administered in the postmenopausal patient. If possible, repeat cytological samples should be taken during the "cleaner" proliferative phase of the hormonal cycle. Repeat sampling should not follow the previous smear by any less than four to six weeks; an earlier second smear could be unreliable because exfoliative material may have been swept away by the first sampling (Koss 1978). If there is a visible lesion, biopsy or colposcopy should supersede cytological assessment. Patients with any persistent atypia, even of mild degree and certainly if a more significant abnormality is present on even one occasion, should be referred to a unit specializing in this problem.

Diagnosis

Expert colposcopy is essential for the outpatient management of patients with abnormal cytology. The colposcope is simply an operating microscope that has been adapted to a special purpose. Although we have several different models in our unit, we most often employ one that has an attached beam-splitter and video camera so that we can both make a record of the patient's lesion and use a television monitor to help the patient better understand her disorder (a complete system is pictured in figure 15.1). The method of colposcopy has been well described elsewhere (Stafl 1975; Cartier 1984). Our standard method of triage is depicted diagrammatically in figure 15.2. The colposcopic diagnosis is based on the evaluation of a number of cervical characteristics, including the surface contour, whether there is a regular or irregular vascular pattern present, the caliber of the vessels, the whiteness of the epithelium, the intercapillary distance, the sharpness of borderline against adjacent tissue, whether satellite lesions are present, and whether there are any atypical vessels present. Alterations in the capillary vascular network of the cervix reflect local biochemical and metabolic changes related to rapid cellular proliferation.

The colposcopic terminology used in our unit is shown in table 15.1. The colposcopic grading system that we employ is modified after Coppleson, Pixley, and Reid (1971). In our system, grade I is assigned when the epithelium is flat, the vascular pattern regular, and the vessels of fine caliber. In grade II, the epithelium is still flat but whiter, the vascular pattern irregular, and the vessels more dilated. In grade III, the epithelium is white and irregular, the vascular pattern irregular, and the vessels coarse or varied in caliber (atypical vessels and papillary exophytia suggest possible invasion).

Unsatisfactory colposcopy associated with an inability to visualize the entire transformation zone is reported in 12.8% (Stafl and Mattingly 1973) to 15% of cases (Townsend et al. 1970); this compares with cone biopsy failure rates that vary from 5.6% (Stafl and Mattingly 1973) to 15% (Donohue and Meriwether 1972). The high degree of accuracy of colposcopically directed biopsy has been demonstrated by several authors. Stafl and Mattingly found a false-negative rate of only 0.3%, whereas the directed biopsy was more than one degree out of phase with the correct diagnosis in the same series (Stafl and Mattingly 1973). Veridiano, Delke, and Tancer (1981) examined 3,680 patients; directed biopsies yielded findings less severe than the actual diagnosis in 6.5% of cases, and no occult invasive carcinomas were underdiagnosed.

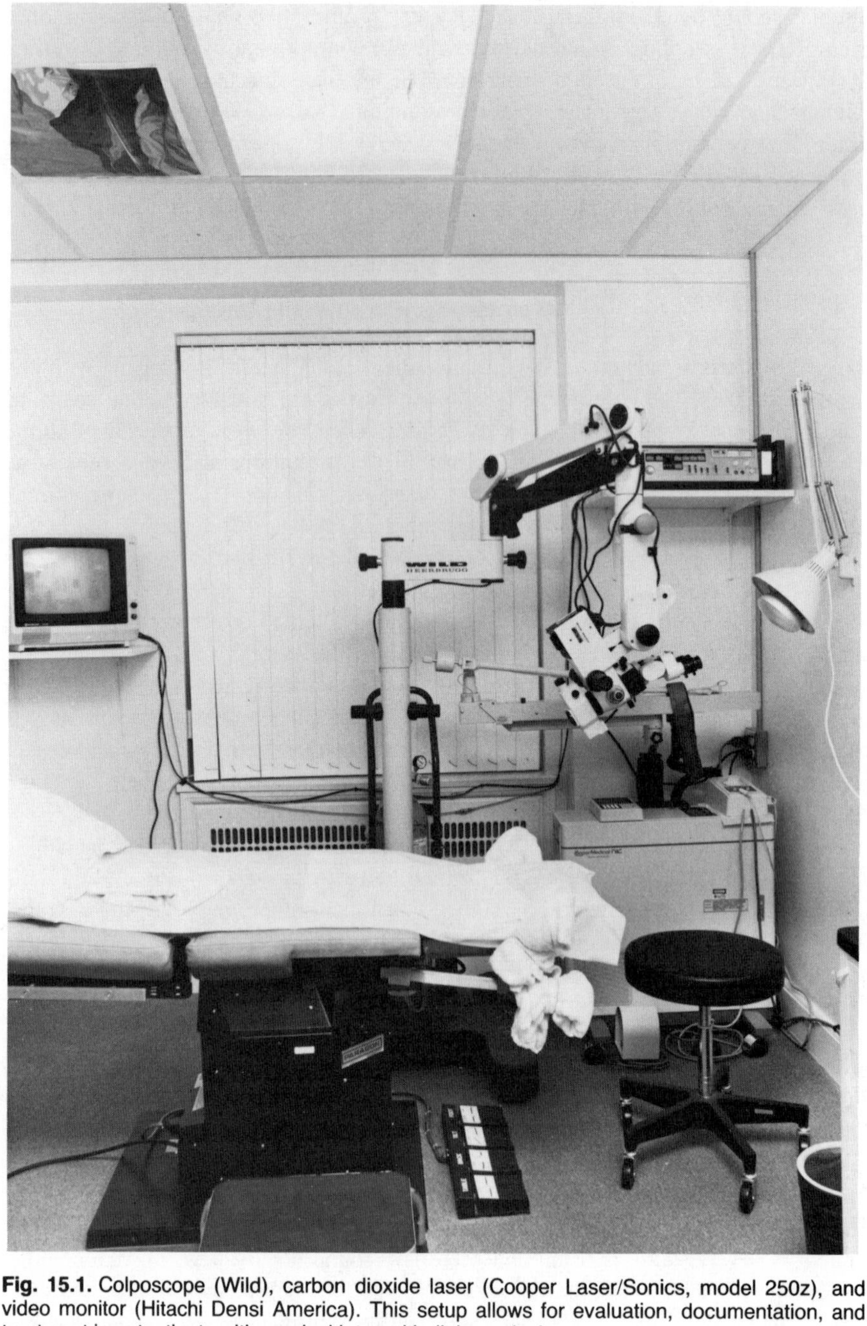

Fig. 15.1. Colposcope (Wild), carbon dioxide laser (Cooper Laser/Sonics, model 250z), and video monitor (Hitachi Densi America). This setup allows for evaluation, documentation, and treatment in outpatients with cervical intraepithelial neoplasia.

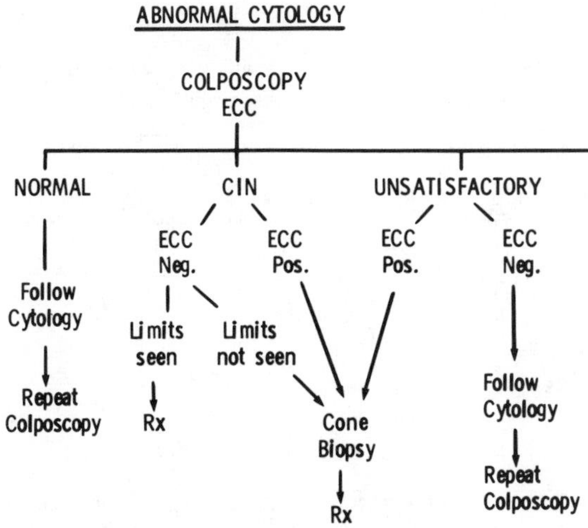

Fig. 15.2. Wellesley Hospital Colposcopy Unit diagrammatic representation of method of evaluation and treatment following finding of abnormal cervical cytology (ECC, endocervical curettage; CIN, cervical intraepithelial neoplasia; CA, carcinoma).

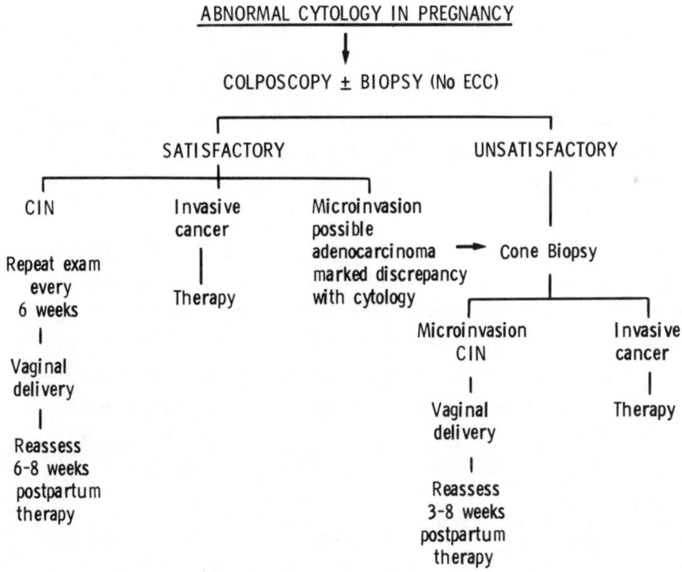

Fig. 15.3. Wellesley Hospital Colposcopy Unit diagrammatic representation of method of evaluation and treatment following finding of abnormal cervical cytology in pregnancy (ECC, endocervical curettage; CIN, cervical intraepithelial neoplasia).

Table 15.1. *Colposcopy Terminology*

- I. Normal colposcopic findings
  - A. Original squamous epithelium
  - B. Columnar epithelium
  - C. Transformation zone
- II. Abnormal colposcopic findings
  - A. Atypical transformation zone
    1. Mosaic
    2. Punctuation
    3. White epithelium
    4. Keratosis
    5. Atypical vessels
  - B. Suspected frank invasive carcinoma
- III. Unsatisfactory colposcopic findings
- IV. Miscellaneous
  - A. Inflammation
  - B. Atrophy
  - C. True erosion
  - D. Human papilloma virus effects

We rely heavily on the use of endocervical curettage with the Kevorkian curette. This technique is of particular importance in cases in which examination results were unsatisfactory or in which no lesion was observed (Hatch et al. 1985). Failure to carry out endocervical curettage and the subsequent failure in diagnosis often lead to patients developing invasive cancer following outpatient evaluation and therapy for cervical disease (Townsend and Richart 1981).

Colposcopy is invaluable in following patients who are pregnant and who have abnormal cervical cytology: our approach in these cases is diagramed in figure 15.3. The eversion of the cervix in pregnancy usually affords excellent colposcopic visualization of the entire transformation zone. Hacker (1982) reviewed 1,064 examinations and found a false-negative rate of 0.5%, with only a 0.6% complication rate. This accuracy virtually eliminates the need for cone biopsy during pregnancy. One study of cone biopsy in pregnancy revealed a mean blood loss of 216 ml, with 12.4% of patients losing more than 500 ml; cervical lacerations in 18% of cases; perinatal fetus mortality in 4.4%; and residual disease in 52% (Hannigan et al. 1982).

Colposcopy of DES-exposed daughters requires special expertise, as atypical squamous metaplasia may be overdiagnosed by the inexperienced clinician, giving rise to a high false-positive colposcopic rate (Welch et al. 1978).

Also, the gynecologist must be thoroughly familiar with the nuances of the various colposcopic appearances of HPV infections. Through the techniques of endonuclease analysis and molecular hybridization, our unit will soon be able to identify specific HPV DNA types. This will allow us to distinguish those lesions associated with HPV 6 and 11 from those related to types 16 and 18, which likely have greater potential for invasion.

Women who are at high risk for harboring invasive carcinoma include those over the age of 35; those with a wide, abnormal transformation zone in the cervix, particularly if that zone's area is greater than 40 mm^2 (Rome, Urcuyo, and Nelson 1977); those with either a highly irregular surface contour or atypical vessels in the cervix; and those who are symptomatic.

Patients with CIN may be treated on an outpatient basis by a destructive technique if there are visualization of the entire lesion and transformation zone; a high degree of correlation between cytological, colposcopic, and colposcopically directed biopsy findings; endocervical curettage results negative for disease; and patient reliability for follow-up. Patients whose cases do not fulfill these criteria must be further evaluated by knife or laser conization, which in addition is often therapeutic.

Outpatient Therapy

Management of diagnosed CIN can be categorized into four basic methods: observation, destruction, excision, or a combination of destruction and excision. A number of different modalities or combinations of modalities can be used to accomplish the operator's therapeutic goals.

Observation

Although minor degrees of dyplasia, especially those associated with HPV, may undergo spontaneous regression, it is at present impossible for the colposcopist to distinguish these from more aggressive lesions. Furthermore, allowing HPV lesions to persist may risk spreading the virus to other locations within the lower genital tract or to sexual partners. Thus, we advise active therapy whenever possible.

Local Excision

Several authors have noted that colposcopically directed biopsies may be curative (Ahlgren, Lindberg, and Nordqvist 1977; Einerth 1978; Atkinson 1984). Others have been more restrictive and recommended local excision only for early CIN that occupies less than one quadrant of the cervix (Townsend 1977). However, other authors have noted a high failure rate if the entire transformation zone is not treated along with the local visible lesion. Bellina (1981) noted a 16% failure rate of therapy for CIN when only the apparent lesion was treated with carbon dioxide laser, compared with a 5% failure rate when the entire transformation zone was removed.

It is our usual practice to ablate the entire transformation zone unless the patient is a DES-exposed daughter. This subgroup of patients may have a higher rate of cervical stenosis after traditional therapy (such as cryotherapy), and thus we either follow them closely without therapy or treat the lesion focally (Schmidt and Fowler 1980).

Destruction

Destruction of the lesion may be accomplished through the use of chemotherapeutic agents, electrocautery, cryotherapy, or laser therapy.

Chemotherapy

Topical 5-fluorouracil has been the most widely used chemotherapeutic agent for lower genital neoplastic lesions. It has been particularly useful in the treatment of patients with lower genital neoplastic syndrome with multiple sites of involvement

(Sillman, Sedlis, and Boyce 1985). This agent has been used infrequently and with less enthusiasm in cases of pure CIN, because of a high residual disease rate in endocervical crypts (Pride and Chuprevich 1982). We have used it mostly as ancillary therapy in cases of CIN associated with either widespread vaginal intraepithelial neoplasia or diffuse vaginal HPV lesions (Reid 1984).

Electrocautery

The term "electrocauterization" has come through common usage to refer to several diverse procedures. It includes hot cauterization or diathermy of the cervix, which may be accomplished by using an element that supplies intense heat (e.g., National electrocautery unit); by unipolar spark-gap electrocautery (e.g., Bovie electrosurgical unit); by diathermy-loop excision, which has the advantage of providing a pathology specimen (Atkinson 1984); or by caloric, or so-called cold, coagulation (e.g., Semm coagulator).

Hunner first described cervical electrocauterization in 1906, and the approach has been used extensively for the treatment of benign cervical disease since that time. Hot cautery is associated with a sensation of heat being transmitted to the vaginal wall, significant crampy uterine pain, unpleasant odor, and smoke formation. It has been shown that the cervix heals much more slowly after hot cauterization than after cryosurgery (Ostergard, Townsend, and Hirose 1969). Despite these drawbacks, some units still use hot cautery as their primary outpatient treatment of CIN, reporting an initial cure rate of 86% and no significant cervical scarring or stenosis, as well as excellent cost effectiveness (Schuurmans and Carmichael 1984).

Richart and Sciarra (1968) utilized electrocautery and reported an 89% eradication rate after initial therapy. However, 7.6% of the patients had significant complications, including cervical stenosis, cervicovaginal cicatrices, and postoperative bleeding. Chanen and Hollyock (1971) reported a 90% cure rate with electrocautery, but their patients all required general anesthesia. Other authors have confirmed that significant pain is produced by the procedure (Creasman and Parker 1975).

Whereas electrocautery and hot electrodiathermy destroy the affected tissue through high-temperature roasting, the cold (Semm) coagulator achieves its effect by boiling water molecules at approximately 100° C (Semm 1966). "Cold" coagulation is a misnomer; "caloric" coagulation more accurately describes the method, which has an effect on tissue similar to that of the carbon dioxide laser. Duncan (1983) reported on 592 CIN patients who were treated with caloric coagulation and found a primary success rate of 95% after one treatment and of 99.5% after two treatments (when required). The procedure is rapid, with the usual treatment time ranging between 40 and 100 seconds, and it entails a 1% rate of cervical stenosis requiring subsequent dilatation. There seems to be little discomfort during the procedure and healing is rapid.

Cryotherapy

For centuries it was known that cold had therapeutic properties, but it was the physician James Arnott in 1845 who first made the distinction between cooling and freezing human tissue when he described the use of an ice brine solution to palliate cancer. He referred to his technique of freezing tissue as "congelation." Crisp was the first to use cryosurgery for the treatment of CIN (Crisp, Asadourian, and Romberger 1967). There soon followed numerous reports of successful treatment of CIN by cryosurgery, without anesthesia and with few complications (Creasman et al. 1973).

The refrigerants used in cryotherapy have included liquid nitrogen (Ostergard, Townsend, and Hirose 1968), but more usually they are gaseous substances. These gases must have a boiling point in the cryogenic range. The freezing temperature varies with the gas used: with freon 22, it is −81° C; carbon dioxide, −78° C; and, more recently, nitrous oxide, −89° C. The gas under a high pressure ranging from 750 to 900 pounds per square inch is expanded through a small orifice in the probe tip into a low-pressure area, causing the surrounding temperature to substantially drop by the Joule-Thompson effect.

Contact freezing of the cervical surface causes cells to equilibrate by dehydration as water is removed from solution, resulting in concentration of intracellular and extracellular electrolytes. This effect is followed by crystallization, with rupture of cell membranes and denaturation of liquid protein molecules within the cell membranes, followed by surrounding vascular stasis (Charles and Savage 1980).

The reported cure rates for CIN range from 27.3% (Nielsen and Stakeman 1973) to 96% (Popkin, Scali, and Ahmed 1978). Anesthesia is usually not required, as typically only mild cramping is encountered. The major associated postoperative morbidity is a heavy, watery discharge, which usually lasts from three to five weeks. Bleeding and infection are rare complications, although pyometra has been reported, especially if therapy was carried out while an intrauterine device was in situ (Curry, Weed, and Creasman 1972). Cryotherapy has no significant effect on fertility or on the outcome of labor and delivery (Benrubi, Young, and Nuss 1984). Cytological findings in the cervix often are bizarre for about 12 weeks, requiring caution in interpretation (Crisp 1972). Reepithelialization of the cervix is usually complete by ten weeks; unfortunately, this occurs through a mechanism of squamous metaplastic activity, which usually moves the squamocolumnar junction inside the cervical os, making follow-up evaluation more difficult.

To reduce the freeze failure rate, our unit has developed several principles for the application of cryosurgery:

1. Endocervical extension of the lesion and endocervical curettage positive for disease are each an absolute contraindication to cryosurgery (Kaufman and Irwin 1978).
2. An adequate freeze temperature must be maintained throughout therapy; this is best accomplished by using a large tank (a "K" tank) of nitrous oxide.
3. The extent of freezing must be adequate, with the iceball effect observed to extend 5 mm beyond the periphery of the lesion. Simply freezing for an empiric time interval is to be condemned.
4. A flat probe without an endocervical extension should be used to avoid cervical stenosis. We most commonly use tips of 2 cm or 2.5 cm in diameter.
5. A double-freeze technique with an interposed rapid thaw with a heating lamp is used. Bryson, Lenehan, and Lickrish (1985) noted a 3.8% primary failure rate

after double freezing with a −75° C probe temperature, compared with a 13.2% rate with single freezing at that temperature. Numerous other authors have reported similar findings (Creasman and Parker 1975; Schantz and Thormann 1984).

6. The cure rate in large lesions that occupy more than two quadrants of the cervix is approximately 60% (Arof, Gerbie, and Smeltzer 1984), so that these lesions are probably better treated by carbon dioxide laser.

Laser Vaporization

The first use in gynecology of the carbon dioxide laser was in 1973 for the treatment of benign cervical ectropion (Kaplan, Goldman, and Ger 1973). Other early papers on this subject included those by Bellina in 1974 and Stafl, Wilkinson, and Mattingly in 1977.

LASER is the acronym for the term *light amplification by stimulated emission of radiation*. The carbon dioxide laser is a gas molecular laser. The laser chamber is a tube equipped with mirrors at each end, one of which is totally reflective, the other only partially reflective and allowing photons to exit from the tube. The carbon dioxide laser medium consists of the atoms of nitrogen, helium, and carbon dioxide. The electrons orbiting around the nucleus of the atom are stimulated to a high-energy state by either high-voltage electricity or radiofrequency waves. Hydrogen atoms through collision with other atoms are raised to metastable states and energy is transferred to carbon dioxide molecules, causing them to vibrate from ground state to high-energy levels. When the carbon dioxide electrons drop to transitional levels, they emit photons in the infrared portion of the electromagnetic spectrum. The helium atoms return the molecules to ground state, so the process may repeat itself. The protons then bounce back and forth between the mirrors, in waves, colliding with other molecules, producing more photons traveling in the same direction and frequency. The light stimulated by the small initial amount of spontaneous emission stimulates additional light, and thus the intensity of the light increases with each passage through the active medium.

Laser light differs from ordinary light in that it is of a single color, coherent in space and time, luminous (very bright), collimated (all rays are virtually parallel), and capable of being focused on a fine spot size by the lens system of an operating microscope. For the treatment of CIN, the focal length is generally between 250 and 400 mm, with spot sizes between 0.2 and 2 mm. Because the carbon dioxide laser beam is invisible to the naked eye, a harmless, visible helium-neon laser is used as a tracer beam. Laser light is absorbed by superficial tissues, causing their water molecules to vaporize and thus destroying the tissue. The depth of the wound created is related to the power of the absorbed beam in watts and the spot diameter of the beam in centimeters and is expressed as power density in terms of watts per square centimeter. Necrosis of surrounding tissue is caused by transfer of heat; it is purely a function of time—that is, it is independent of the power of the beam. Thus, when created by the skilled surgeon, the laser wound is very akin to a scalpel wound in terms of injury to surrounding tissue. It tends also to be a bloodless wound, as the laser beam is capable of sealing most vessels up to 1 mm in diameter.

Cervical crypt involvement by intraepithelial neoplasia has been studied by several authors. Anderson and Hartley (1980) found the mean depth of involved crypts to be 1.24 mm, with destruction to a tissue depth of 3.8 mm eradicating all of the involved crypts in 99.7% of patients. The mean depth of uninvolved crypts in their series was 3.38 mm, and to eradicate all uninvolved crypts in 99.7% of patients would have required a depth of destruction of 6.3 mm. Other authors have confirmed these findings (Abdul-Karim et al. 1982) and provided further scientific impetus for the use of the laser, in particular further emphasizing the importance of precise depth of tissue destruction, which is uncertain with modalities such as electrocoagulation and cryotherapy.

Cure rates of CIN with single therapy have ranged from a low of 76% (Anderson 1982) to a high of 99% (Berget and Lenstrup 1985). Using repeated treatments, a number of authors have reported very high cure rates, from 96% (Baggish 1983) to 100% (Wright, Davies, and Riopelle 1983). Townsend and Richart (1983) conducted a controlled comparison of cryotherapy and carbon dioxide laser for the management of CIN and found no significant difference in cure rates, but they did find that the cervices healed more rapidly after laser treatment. Wright and Davies (1981) compared the two modalities for treatment of CIN and found the overall rate of disease persistence after cryosurgery to be 14.5%, compared with 3.1% for laser. The results in patients with grade III CIN were even more divergent, with a 25% persistence rate after cryosurgery, but only a 7.7% rate following laser treatment. The major drawbacks reported by most authors include an increased incidence, vis-à-vis cryotherapy, of postoperative hemorrhage, the high capital cost of the equipment, and the extensive training required for all personnel.

In our unit, we have adopted laser guidelines to provide for both reduced treatment failures and for high operational safety. These guidelines are:

1. The surgeon must be well trained, both in the principles of laser physics and in practical aspects of using the laser.
2. The equipment must be carefully selected and in excellent working order, and regular maintenance must be carried out. A variable spot diameter is very helpful for coagulating bleeders. A computer-based unit that tests for system faults quickly and accurately is desirable. Safety precautions must be exactingly maintained. To reduce fire hazard, there should either be no drapes or flame-retardant drapes. To reduce inadvertent beam deflection, only nonreflective instruments and specula should be used. All personnel in the room except for the operator (whose eyes are shielded by the microscope lens) must wear protective glasses. The aperture should be closed except when the laser is in actual use. An excellent plume-evacuation system should be utilized.
3. The patient must receive adequate anesthesia and analgesia to reduce inadvertent movement and provide comfort. To block cervical prostaglandin release, our patients receive 550 mg of naproxen sodium a half hour prior to the procedure. Local anesthesia is provided by paracervical block through the use of a high-velocity, carbon dioxide–driven injecting gun (fig. 15.4). With the use of this device, only 2 to 3 ml of 1% lidocaine HCl is necessary to rapidly produce cervical anesthesia.

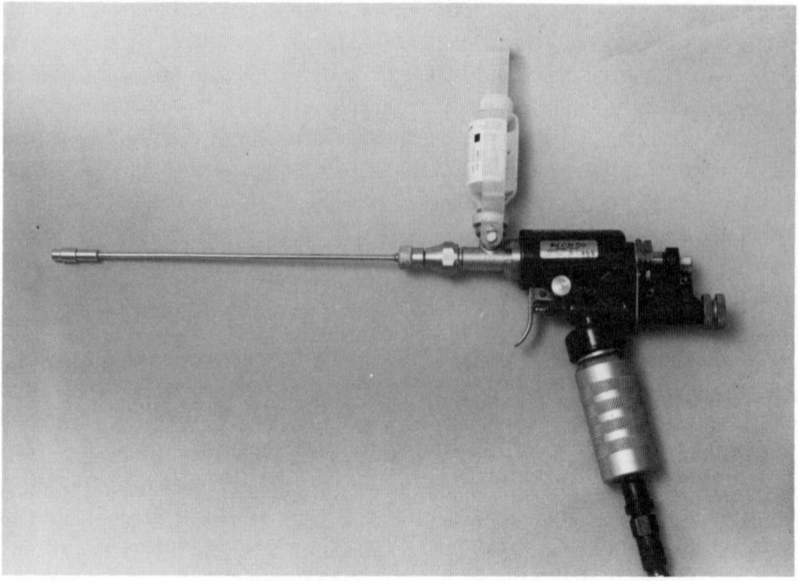

Fig. 15.4. Local-anesthetic gun for paracervical block (Med-E-Jet Corporation).

4. It is important to remove the entire transformation zone to a depth of 5 to 7 mm (Anderson and Hartley 1980). Jordan (1980) vaporized to depths varying from 1 to 7 mm and demonstrated that persistent disease varied inversely with depth of destruction. We often ablate to a depth of 1 cm or more near the central canal and usually 7 to 8 mm peripherally.
5. Treatment must also extend to 5 mm beyond the periphery of the lesion, since the site of recurrent disease is most frequently noted at the original treatment margin (Benedet, Nickerson, and White 1981).
6. The utilization of power densities approximating 1,000 W/mm^2 produces less carbon formation and thermal injury, with increased patient comfort.
7. We believe that at the conclusion of the procedure an endocervical button should be created by grooving the stroma surrounding the canal to a depth of about 2 mm. This facilitates follow-up colposcopic and cytological examination, as the new squamocolumnar junction will form on the exocervix. This approach is controversial, and some investigators prefer the new squamocolumnar junction be located inside the canal, where they believe it will be better protected from possible carcinogenic agents (Reid et al. 1984).

Excision

The excision of the entire transformation zone can be accomplished in several ways.

Laser and Knife Conization

Among 78 patients who underwent diagnostic conization at the colposcopy unit at Wellesley Hospital in Toronto, the indication for the procedure was endocervical curettage findings positive for disease in 30 (38.5%); incomplete visualization of the lesion upon colposcopic examination in 28 (35.9%); the finding of a complex lesion (indicating possible invasion) in 9 (11.5%); recurrence of a confusing lesion after therapeutic conization, laser therapy, or cryotherapy in 8 (10.2%); poor correlation between cytological findings, colposcopic findings, and biopsy pathology in 2 (2.6%); and the finding of microinvasion upon biopsy in 1 (1.3%) (Shier 1983).

All knife conizations at this unit are carried out in the operating theater, with the patient under general anesthesia, by a technique that leaves the cone bed open, as previously described (De Petrillo 1983). Sturmdorf sutures are not employed, as cytological follow-up of the transformation zone is then less likely to be adequate (Trimbos, Heintz, and van Hall 1983). Knife conization is particularly suitable for patients in whom a major part of the lesion is within the endocervical canal; in these cases, it may be advantageous to microcolpohysteroscopically control the depth of the incision to avoid leaving residual disease at the apex (Fenton et al. 1984).

A number of laser conizations or combination laser conization-vaporizations (fig. 15.5) performed in our hospital have been done in the colposcopy unit with the patient under local anesthesia. The high-velocity local-anesthetic gun greatly facilitates these procedures. In addition to the technique described for vaporization, we use relatively small spot diameters (0.8–1 mm), black-mat cervical tenacula to prevent light deflection, and lidocaine HCl with 1/100,000 epinephrine for hemostasis at the cone apex. Our instructions for the patient after laser therapy are listed in table 15.2. Other investigators have used narrower spot diameters and very high power densities with success, but their procedures require general anesthesia (Larsson, Gullberg, and Grundsell 1983). Laser vaporization-conization seems to have no adverse effects on fertility or subsequent pregnancy and delivery (Anderson, Horwell, and Broby 1984). The squamocolumnar junction is fully visible post-

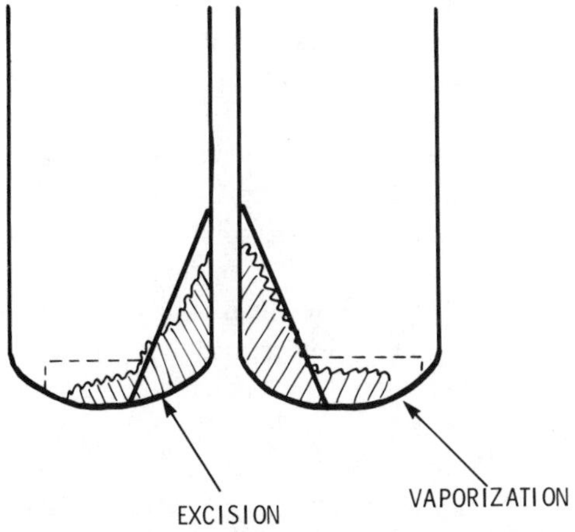

Fig. 15.5. Schematic of combination conization-vaporization of cervix (sagittal view). This combined method allows the operator to rapidly and easily ablate the abnormal tissue that has been adequately assessed by the colposcopic method, and also provides a pathology specimen of the endocervical portion of the tissue that has not been completely assessed.

Table 15.2. *Written Instructions Given to Patients at the Colposcopy Unit of Wellesley Hospital, Toronto, after Outpatient Cervical Laser Therapy*

1. Do not use tampons for two months following laser therapy.
2. Do not have intercourse for three to five weeks following laser therapy, depending on your doctor's specific instructions.
3. Do not douche for three months after laser therapy.
4. Use Sultrin Triple Sulfa Cream (Ortho Pharmaceutical Corporation) daily in the vagina for two weeks.
5. You may have a vaginal discharge or bleeding for several weeks after laser therapy.
6. Please return for a repeat Pap test three months after the therapy. It is important that you do not have a Pap test elsewhere before that visit.
7. If you have any problems, call the Wellesley Hospital Colposcopy Unit (416-926-4827), and the doctor or nurse will be pleased to talk to you.

operatively in 66% of cases, as compared with full visibility after only 39% of cold knife conizations performed without the use of sutures (Bostofte et al. in press).

Continuing Care

Patients are seen in follow-up at four- to six-month intervals for the first two years after therapy, as 75% of recurrent and residual disease will become apparent during that time (Richart et al. 1980; Berget and Lenstrup 1985). At each visit, colposcopic and cytological sampling are undertaken. If the squamocolumnar junction is inside the cervical canal (as is often the case after cryotherapy), endocervical brushings with or without endocervical curettage are done.

Patients should be encouraged to learn about their disease and to join interested consumer groups and research registries if applicable (e.g., DES Action or the Ontario DES Research Registry). Many excellent information pamphlets that help to allay patients' fears are available—among them, "The Pap Smear and Your Cervix," available from the Wellesley Hospital Colposcopy Unit, and the Ontario DES Research Registry's DES-awareness pamphlet ("Were You Born between 1941–1971?").

Preventive factors are stressed. If the original disease was associated with HPV, it is advised that condoms be used for at least six months. The use of condom therapy for other CIN lesions is controversial but advised by some authors (Richardson and Lyon 1981). Smoking has been identified as an epidemiological risk factor for cervical neoplasia (Clarke, Morgan, and Newman 1982). Lyon et al. (1983) found that smoking increased the risk of developing cervical carcinoma in situ by a factor of 3 over controls. Richardson and Lyon (1981) commented on the exceedingly similar histological sequence of events between bronchogenic carcinoma of the lung and carcinoma of the cervix. Women who have been treated for cervical cancer are four times more likely to develop lung cancer as a second primary than are controls (Clarke, Kreiger, and Spengler 1984). This evidence has led us to believe that a program to stop smoking should be part of therapy for CIN (Shier 1984). We provide our patients with a program called "Time to Quit," developed by the Canadian

Cancer Society and the Health Promotion Directorate of Health and Welfare of Canada (Health and Welfare Canada, 1983). In the past, celibacy and monogamy have not been popular methods of cervical cancer prevention, but the current widespread concern about the sexual spread of the causative virus of acquired immune deficiency syndrome may change this perspective.

Conclusion

There are many effective outpatient treatments for the patient with CIN. There are advantages and disadvantages to each. More definitive statements about their relative merits await the results of further, properly randomized, prospective trials. It should also be stressed that adequate therapy, together with avoidance of the disaster of missing or undertreating an invasive cancer, is completely dependent on accurate diagnosis and places a high degree of responsibility on the clinician-colposcopist.

References

Abdul-Karim FW, Fu YS, Reagan JW, Wentz WB. 1982. Morphometric study of intraepithelial neoplasia of the uterine cervix. *Obstet Gynecol* 60:210–214.

Ahlgren M, Lindberg LG, Nordqvist SRB. 1977. Management of carcinoma in situ of the cervix by selective local excision. *Acta Obstet Gynecol Scand* 56:531–536.

Anderson MC. 1982. Treatment of cervical intraepithelial neoplasia with the carbon dioxide laser: Report of 543 patients. *Obstet Gynecol* 59:720–725.

Anderson MC, Hartley RB. 1980. Cervical crypt involvement by intraepithelial neoplasia. *Obstet Gynecol* 55:546–552.

Anderson MC, Horwell DH, Broby Z. 1984. Outcome of pregnancy after laser vaporization-conization. *Journal of Colposcopy and Gynecological Laser Surgery* 1:35–40.

Arof HM, Gerbie MV, Smeltzer J. 1984. Cryosurgical treatment of cervical intraepithelial neoplasia: A four-year experience. *Am J Obstet Gynecol* 150:865–869.

Atkin NB, Brito-Babapulle V. 1983. Chromosome 1 C-band heteromorphisms in patients with carcinoma in situ and invasive carcinoma of the cervix uteri. *Aust NZ J Obstet Gynaecol* 23:73–76.

Atkinson K. 1984. Symposium on cervical neoplasia: Diathermy loop excision. *Journal of Colposcopy and Gynecological Laser Surgery* 1:285–289.

Baggish MS. 1983. Laser management of cervical intraepithelial neoplasia. *Clin Obstet Gynecol* 26:980–995.

Bain RW, Crocker DW. 1983. Rapid onset of cervical cancer in an upper socioeconomic group. *Am J Obstet Gynecol* 146:366–371.

Becker TM. 1984. Genital warts—A sexually transmitted disease epidemic? *Journal of Colposcopy and Gynecological Laser Surgery* 1:193–197.

Bellina JH. 1974. Gynecology and the laser. *Contemporary Ob/Gyn* 4:24–32.

Bellina JH. 1981. The carbon dioxide laser in gynecology. Part 1. *Current Problems in Obstetrics and Gynecology* 4:1–34.

Benedet JL, Nickerson KG, White GW. 1981. Laser therapy for cervical intraepithelial neoplasia. *Obstet Gynecol* 58:188–192.

Benrubi GI, Young M, Nuss RC. 1984. Intrapartum outcome of term pregnancy after cervical cryotherapy. *J Reprod Med* 29:251–254.

Beral V. 1974. Cancer of the cervix—A sexually transmitted disease (letter). *Lancet* 2:1037.

Berget A, Lenstrup C. 1985. Cervical intraepithelial neoplasia. Examination, treatment, and follow-up. *Obstet Gynecol Surv* 40:545–552.

Bostofte E, Berget A, Falck Larsen J, Hjorkjaer Pedersen P. In press. Conization by carbon dioxide laser or cold knife in the treatment of cervical intraepithelial neoplasia. *Acta Obstet Gynecol Scand.*

Boyes DA. 1983. Cervical neoplasia. Paper read at Current Concepts Symposium, 4 May, at the University of Toronto.

Bryson PC, Lenehan P, Lickrish GM. 1985. The treatment of grade 3 cervical intraepithelial neoplasia with cryotherapy: An 11-year experience. *Am J Obstet Gynecol* 151:201–206.

Campion MJ, Singer A, Clarkson PK, McCance DJ. 1985. Increased risk of cervical neoplasia in consorts of men with penile condylomata acuminata. *Lancet* 1:943–946.

Cartier R. 1984. *Practical Colposcopy*. Paris: Laboratoire Cartier.

Chanen W, Hollyock VE. 1971. Colposcopy and electrocoagulation-diathermy for cervical dysplasia and carcinoma in situ. *Obstet Gynecol* 37:623–628.

Charles EH, Savage EW. 1980. Cryosurgical treatment of cervical intraepithelial neoplasia. *Obstet Gynecol Surv* 35:539–548.

Clarke EA, Kreiger N, Spengler RF. 1984. Second primary cancer following treatment for cervical cancer. *Can Med Assoc J* 131:553–556.

Clarke EA, Morgan RW, Newman AM. 1982. Smoking as a risk factor in cancer of the cervix: Additional evidence from a case-control study. *Am J Epidemiol* 115:59–66.

Coppleson M, Pixley E, Reid R. 1971. *Colposcopy*. Springfield, Ill.: Charles C Thomas.

Creasman WT, Parker RT. 1975. Management of early cervical neoplasia. *Clin Obstet Gynecol* 18:233–242.

Creasman WT, Weed JC, Curry SL, Johnston WM, Parker RT. 1973. Efficacy of cryosurgical treatment of severe intraepithelial neoplasia. *Obstet Gynecol* 41:501–506.

Crisp WE. 1972. Cryosurgical treatment of neoplasia of the uterine cervix. *Obstet Gynecol* 39:495–499.

Crisp WE, Asadourian L, Romberger W. 1967. Application of cryosurgery to gynecologic malignancy. *Obstet Gynecol* 30:668–672.

Crisp WE, Shalauta H, Bennett WA. 1968. Shallow conization of the cervix. *Obstet Gynecol* 6:755–758.

Curry SL, Weed JC, Creasman WT. 1972. Pyometra, a complication of cervical cryosurgery. *Obstet Gynecol* 40:499–501.

De Petrillo AD. 1983. Examining patients who have had conization or hysterectomy. *Contemporary Ob/Gyn* 22:99–111.

De Petrillo AD, Townsend DE, Morrow CP, Lickrish GM, DiSaia PJ. 1975. Colposcopic evaluation of the abnormal Papanicolaou test in pregnancy. *Am J Obstet Gynecol* 121: 441–444.

Donohue L, Meriwether D. 1972. Colposcopy as a diagnostic tool in the investigation of cervical neoplasias. *Am J Obstet Gynecol* 113:107–112.

Draper GJ, Cook GA. 1983. Changing patterns of cervical cancer rates (editorial). *Br Med J [Clin Res]* 287:510–512.

Duncan ID. 1983. The Semm cold coagulator in the management of cervical intraepithelial neoplasia. *Clin Obstet Gynecol* 26:996–1006.

Einerth Y. 1978. Cryosurgical treatment of dysplasia and carcinoma in situ of the cervix uteri (abstract). *Acta Obstet Gynecol Scand* 57:361.

Fenton DW, Soutter WP, Sharp F, Mann M. 1984. Preliminary experience with microcolpohysteroscopically controlled cone biopsies. *Journal of Colposcopy and Gynecological Laser Surgery* 1:167–172.

Garite TJ, Feldman MJ. 1978. An evaluation of cytologic sampling techniques. A comparative study. *Acta Cytol (Baltimore)* 22:83–87.

Hacker NF, Berek JS, Lagasse LD, Charles EH, Savage EW, Moore JG. 1982. Carcinoma of the cervix associated with pregnancy. *Obstet Gynecol* 59:735–746.

Haneen WK, Habib ZA, Rohme D. 1980. Heteromorphism of constitutive heterochromatin in carcinoma and dysplasia of the uterine cervix. *Experimental Journal of Obstetrical and Gynecological Reproductive Biology* 10:173–182.

Hannigan EV, Whitehouse HH, Atkinson WD, Becker SN. 1982. Cone biopsy during pregnancy. *Obstet Gynecol* 60:450–455.

Harris RW, Brinton LA, Cowdell RH, Skegg DC, Smith PG, Vessey MP, Doll R. 1980. Characteristics of women with dysplasia or carcinoma in situ of the cervix uteri. *Br J Cancer* 42:358–369.

Hart GD. 1985. The World Health Organization and cancer. *Can Med Assoc J* 133:269–271.

Hatch KD, Shingleton HM, Orr JW, Gore H, Soong S. 1985. Role of endocervical curettage in colposcopy. *Obstet Gynecol* 65:403–408.

Health and Welfare Canada. 1983. *Time to Quit*. Ottawa: Supply and Services Canada.

Hunner GL. 1906. The treatment of leukorrhea with the actual cautery. *JAMA* 46:191–195.

Jordan JA. 1980. Laser treatment of cervical intraepithelial neoplasia. *Cancer Cytology* 20:12–16.

Kaplan I, Goldman J, Ger R. 1973. The treatment of erosions of the uterine cervix by means of the CO_2 laser. *Obstet Gynecol* 41:795–800.

Kaufman RH, Irwin JF. 1978. The cryosurgical therapy of cervical intraepithelial neoplasia. III. Continuing follow-up. *Am J Obstet Gynecol* 131:381–386.

Kessler II. 1976. Human cervical cancer as a venereal disease. *Cancer Res* 36:783–791.

Koss LG. 1978. Dysplasia: A real concept or a misnomer? *Obstet Gynecol* 51:374–380.

Larsson G, Gullberg B, Grundsell H. 1983. A comparison of complications of laser and cold knife conization. *Obstet Gynecol* 62:213–217.

Lickrish GM, Fortier M. 1977. Conservative management of intraepithelial cervical neoplasia. *Can Med Assoc J* 116:641–643.

Lyon JL, Gardner JW, West DW, Stanish WM, Hebertson RM. 1983. Smoking and carcinoma in situ of the uterine cervix. *Am J Public Health* 73:558–562.

Martinez I. 1969. Relationship of squamous cell carcinoma of the cervix to squamous cell carcinoma of the penis. *Cancer* 24:777–780.

Nielsen NC, Stakeman G. 1973. Cryosurgery for carcinoma in situ of cervix. *Lancet* 2: 627–628.

Ostergard DR. 1977. The effect of age, gravity, and parity on the cervical squamocolumnar junction. *Am J Obstet Gynecol* 129:59–61.

Ostergard DR, Townsend DE, Hirose FM. 1968. Treatment of chronic cervicitis by cryotherapy. *Am J Obstet Gynecol* 102:426–432.

Ostergard DR, Townsend DE, Hirose FM. 1969. Comparison of electrocauterization and cryosurgery for the treatment of benign disease of the uterine cervix. *Obstet Gynecol* 33:58–63.

Papanicolaou GN, Traut HF. 1943. *Diagnosis of Uterine Cancer by the Vaginal Smear*. New York: New York Commonwealth Fund.

Popkin DR, Scali V, Ahmed MN. 1978. Cryosurgery for cervical intraepithelial neoplasia. *Am J Obstet Gynecol* 130:551–554.

Pride GL, Chuprevich TW. 1982. Topical 5-fluorouracil treatment of transformation zone intraepithelial neoplasia of cervix and vagina. *Obstet Gynecol* 60:467–472.

Reid R. 1984. Laser safety. I. Avoidance of surgical misadventure with the CO_2 laser. *Journal of Colposcopy and Gynecological Laser Surgery* 1:117–139.

Reid R, Atkinson K, Chanen W, Coppleson M, Creasman W, Jordan J. 1984. Symposium on cervical neoplasia. Differing views. *Journal of Colposcopy and Gynecological Laser Surgery* 1:299–306.

Richardson AC, Lyon JB. 1981. The effect of condom use on squamous cell cervical intraepithelial neoplasia. *Am J Obstet Gynecol* 140:909–913.

Richart RM. 1967. Natural history of cervical intraepithelial neoplasia. *Clin Obstet Gynecol* 10:748–760.

Richart RM, Sciarra JJ. 1968. Treatment of cervical dysplasia by out-patient electrocauterization. *Am J Obstet Gynecol* 101:200–204.

Richart RM, Townsend DE, Crisp W, De Petrillo AD, Ferenczy A, Johnson G, Lickrish G, Roy M, Villa Santa U. 1980. An analysis of 'long-term' follow-up results in patients with intraepithelial neoplasia treated by cryotherapy. *Am J Obstet Gynecol* 137:823–826.

Richart RM, Vaillant HW. 1965. Influence of cell collection techniques upon cytological diagnosis. *Cancer* 18:1474–1476.

Rome RM, Urcuyo R, Nelson JH. 1977. Observations on the surface area of the abnormal transformation zone associated with intraepithelial and early invasive squamous cell lesions of the cervix. *Am J Obstet Gynecol* 129:565–570.

Ros E, Jimenez AM, Vilaplana E, Saiz-Pardo F, Lorite L, Navarro E, Rodriguez C. 1983. [New technique for endocervical cytological sampling with Stormby's brush. Preliminary results.] *Citologia* 3:9–20.

Rotkin ID. 1973. A comparison review of key epidemiological studies in cervical cancer related to current searches for transmissible agents. *Cancer Res* 13:1353–1358.

Rubio CA. 1977. A trap for atypical cells. *Am J Obstet Gynecol* 128:687–690.

Schantz A, Thormann L. 1984. Cryosurgery for dysplasia of the uterine ectocervix. A randomized study of the single and double freeze techniques (abstract). *Acta Obstet Gynecol Scand* 63:417.

Schmidt G, Fowler WC. 1980. Cervical stenosis following minor gynecologic procedures on DES-exposed women. *Obstet Gynecol* 56:333–335.

Schuurmans SN, Carmichael JA. 1984. Treatment of cervical intraepithelial neoplasia with electrocautery: Report of 426 cases. *Am J Obstet Gynecol* 148:544–546.

Scott JW, Welch WB, Blake TF. 1960. Bloodless technique of cold knife conization (ring biopsy). *Am J Obstet Gynecol* 79:62–66.

Semm K. 1966. New apparatus for the cold coagulation of benign cervical lesions. *Am J Obstet Gynecol* 95:963–968.

Shen JT, Nalick RH, Schlaerth JB, Morrow CP. 1984. Efficacy of cotton-tipped applicators for obtaining cells from the uterine cervix for Papanicolaou smears. *Acta Gynaecologica* 28:541–545.

Shier RM. 1983. Current concepts in the diagnosis of cervical intraepithelial neoplasia—Indications for cone biopsy. Paper read at Current Concepts Symposium, 4 May, at the University of Toronto.

Shier RM. 1984. Carbon dioxide laser therapy in the management of patients with abnormal cervical cytology. *Wellesley Hospital 15th Annual Clinical Day*. Program abstracts, vol. 15.

Sillman FH, Sedlis A, Boyce JG. 1985. A review of lower genital intraepithelial neoplasia and the use of topical 5-fluorouracil. *Obstet Gynecol Surv* 40:190–220.

Stafl A. 1975. Colposcopy. *Clin Obstet Gynecol* 18:195–213.

Stafl A. 1983. Cervicography. *Clin Obstet Gynecol* 26:1007–1016.

Stafl A, Mattingly RF. 1973. Colposcopic diagnosis of cervical neoplasia. *Obstet Gynecol* 41:168–176.

Stafl A, Wilkinson EJ, Mattingly RF. 1977. Laser treatment of cervical and vaginal neoplasia. *Am J Obstet Gynecol* 128:128–136.

Topek NH. 1967. Surgical treatment of carcinoma in situ of the cervix. *Clin Obstet Gynecol* 10:853–870.

Townsend DE. 1977. Detection and management of preinvasive cervical neoplasia. *Current Problems in Obstetrics and Gynecology* 1:3–31.

Townsend DE, Ostergard DR, Mishell D, Hirose FM. 1970. Abnormal Papanicolaou smear. *Am J Obstet Gynecol* 108:429–436.

Townsend DE, Richart RM. 1981. Diagnostic errors in colposcopy. *Gynecol Oncol* 12: S259–S264.

Townsend DE, Richart RM. 1983. Cryotherapy and carbon dioxide laser management of cervical intraepithelial neoplasia: A controlled comparison. *Obstet Gynecol* 61:75–78.

Trimbos JB, Heintz APM, van Hall EV. 1983. Reliability of cytological follow-up after conization of the cervix: A comparison of three surgical techniques. *Br J Obstet Gynaecol* 90:1141–1146.

Veridiano NP, Delke I, Tancer ML. 1981. Accuracy of colposcopically directed biopsy in patients with cervical dysplasia. *Obstet Gynecol* 58:185–191.

Walton RJ, chmn. 1976. Canadian Task Force on Cervical Screening Programs. *Can Med Assoc J* 114:1003–1033.

Walton RJ, chmn. 1982. Reconvened Task Force on Cervical Screening Programs. *Can Med Assoc J* 130:1–31.

Welch WR, Robboy SJ, Townsend DE, Barnes AB, Scully RE, Herbst AL. 1978. Comparison of histologic and colposcopic findings in DES-exposed females. *Obstet Gynecol* 52:457–461.

Wright VC, Davies EM. 1981. The conservative management of cervical intraepithelial neoplasia: The use of cryosurgery and the carbon dioxide laser. *Br J Obstet Gynaecol* 88: 663–669.

Wright VC, Davies EM, Riopelle MA. 1983. Laser surgery for cervical intraepithelial neoplasia: Principles and results. *Am J Obstet Gynecol* 145:181–184.

Wright VC, Riopelle MA. 1982. Age at time of first intercourse v. chronologic age as a basis for Pap smear screening. *Can Med Assoc J* 127:127–131.

Annual Clinical Conference on Cancer, Vol. 29
Gynecologic Cancer: Diagnosis and Treatment Strategies
© 1987 by The University of Texas System Cancer Center

16. Stage I Adenocarcinoma of the Cervix

C. Allen Stringer

Adenocarcinoma of the cervix is an uncommon neoplasm. The generally reported incidence is 5% to 8% of all primary malignancies arising in the cervix. Over the past decade, however, the incidence appears to have increased (Davis and Moon 1975; Gallup and Abell 1977; Shingleton et al. 1981). The reason for this increase is not clear. One possible explanation is that the incidence of squamous carcinoma of the cervix has declined, resulting in a relative increase in the incidence of adenocarcinoma. Alternatively, the true incidence of adenocarcinoma may be increasing. This is the more likely explanation (Shingleton et al. 1981).

The association between human papilloma virus (HPV) infection, cervical dysplasia, and squamous carcinoma is becoming increasingly evident. Several facts also suggest a possible relationship between HPV and adenocarcinoma of the cervix. Human papilloma virus has been identified in some cases of pure adenocarcinoma of the cervix (Smotkin, Berek, and Fu 1985). Adenocarcinoma in situ and invasive adenocarcinoma frequently coexist with squamous carcinoma in situ (Gloor and Ruzicka 1982; Maier and Norris 1980), and a report by Teshima and his colleagues (1985) suggests that adenocarcinomas of the cervix originate from endocervical glands adjoining the transformation zone. Although these data indirectly support a relationship between HPV and adenocarcinoma of the cervix, they are not as convincing as the data regarding squamous carcinoma, and they do not explain the increasing incidence. The apparent increase in HPV infection of the cervix is most likely due to increased recognition of the entity histologically rather than a true increase in incidence (Bernstein, Woet, and Guzick 1985).

The majority of patients with adenocarcinoma of the cervix have stage I disease. Despite the increasing incidence of the disease and the preponderance of stage I lesions, the management remains controversial. Two unanswered questions of fundamental importance contribute to the persisting controversy. Both deal with the inherent biologic behavior of adenocarcinoma of the cervix. The first question regards the risk of lymph node metastasis for a given stage of disease, and the second concerns the radiosensitivity of adenocarcinoma relative to squamous carcinoma. Extrapolation of the considerable experience with squamous carcinoma to patients with adenocarcinoma requires a comparable risk of nodal metastasis and equivalent radiosensitivity for a given stage and volume of tumor. Few reports in the literature contain patient numbers of sufficient size to address these important questions. The University of Texas M. D. Anderson Hospital and Tumor Institute experience with adenocarcinoma of the cervix between 1947 and 1971 has been previously reported (Rutledge et al. 1975). Of the 219 patients reported, 95 had stage I disease but only

9 were treated by radical hysterectomy. It was difficult, therefore, from those data to assess the role of radical surgery in the management of early stage disease. Between 1962 and 1981, 164 patients with stage I adenocarcinoma were evaluated and managed at U.T. M. D. Anderson Hospital. A pathology review resulted in the exclusion of 10 patients, leaving 154 evaluable patients. Of these, 33 were treated by radical hysterectomy, 74 by radiation therapy, and 47 by a combination of radiation therapy and extrafascial hysterectomy.

Treatment with Radical Hysterectomy

The role of radical hysterectomy in the management of small volume (< 3 cm diameter) stage I adenocarcinoma of the cervix is well established (Shingleton et al. 1981; Berek et al. 1981). All 33 patients in the current U.T. M. D. Anderson Hospital series had lesions of less than 3 cm in diameter. Nine patients had received prior radiation therapy. This proved to be a significant complicating factor. Patients who had received prior radiation therapy had significantly greater blood loss ($p < 0.01$). There was one case of postoperative ureteral obstruction and one case of postoperative vesicovaginal fistula. Both of these patients had also received prior radiation therapy.

Vascular or lymphatic space involvement was present in eight patients (24%), and unilateral pelvic node metastases were present in two patients (6%) treated by radical hysterectomy. Of the two patients with positive nodes, one received adjuvant radiation therapy and is alive without disease. The other received no adjuvant therapy, had a subsequent recurrence, and is dead of disease. Parametrial and vaginal margins were negative in all cases.

Five patients (15%) developed recurrent disease. Two of these patients have been salvaged. One underwent resection for an isolated pulmonary tumor recurrence. The other was treated with radiation therapy for a central recurrence. She developed liver metastases, which were treated by intraarterial chemotherapy followed by hepatic resection. No viable tumor remained in the specimen. The resulting two- and five-year uncorrected survival rates were 86% and 79%, respectively. Survival was significantly worse in patients with vascular space involvement ($p = 0.02$). No significant relationship was observed when survival was compared on the basis of age, histological grade, nuclear grade, number of mitoses, or depth of invasion. Although there was a trend toward poor survival for patients with adenosquamous or glassy cell tumors, the difference did not achieve statistical significance.

The role of radical hysterectomy in the management of larger lesions is less clear. In the series reported by Shingleton and associates, 14 of 22 patients with lesions larger than 3 cm in diameter underwent radical hysterectomy, and 8 have experienced disease recurrence (Shingleton et al. 1981). Of the eight patients treated by radiation therapy, however, only one has had recurrence. By contrast, in the series reported by Berek and colleagues (1981), survival in cases with lesions larger than 2 cm was poorer when patients were treated by radiation alone compared with radical hysterectomy or surgery plus radiation therapy.

Treatment with Radiation and Combination Therapy

The role of adjunctive hysterectomy is perhaps the most controversial issue regarding the management of stage I adenocarcinoma of the cervix. Several authors have reported improved survival for patients treated by radiation followed by an extrafascial hysterectomy (Gallup and Abell 1977; Berek et al. 1981; Kagan et al. 1973). Others have observed equivalent survivals (Cuccia, Bloedorn, and Onal 1967; Mayer et al. 1976), and one study not only reports no improvement in survival with combination therapy but also an increased complication rate (Weiner and Witzenberg 1975). There have been no prospective, randomized studies performed to evaluate this issue. An obvious source of bias in these retrospective studies is the overall medical status of the patient, which favors the adjunctive surgery group. The published data from U.T. M. D. Anderson Hospital (Rutledge et al. 1975) have been quoted by many authors who advocate an adjuvant hysterectomy. The data, however, show no statistically significant difference in survival between patients treated by radiation alone and those treated by radiation followed by hysterectomy. However, they did observe a trend toward poor survival in patients with bulky lesions and a fourfold higher central recurrence rate in patients with stage II disease treated by radiation alone.

In the present series, of 121 patients treated by radiation therapy, 47 had an adjunctive extrafascial hysterectomy. Twelve patients had lesions greater than 6 cm in diameter. The incidence of morbidity related to the radiation therapy was 18%. In 7%, the complication required surgical management. The complication rate associated with adjunctive hysterectomy was 23%.

Eight patients (6%) had progression of disease during therapy, and all are dead of disease. An additional 19 patients (16%) developed recurrent disease. Two patients have been salvaged and remain free of disease 3 and 12 years following disease recurrence. The resulting uncorrected two- and five-year survivals were 81% and 73%, respectively. The five-year survival was 69% in the 74 patients treated by radiation alone and 80% in the 47 patients who had an adjunctive hysterectomy. This difference was not statistically significant. Seven of the 12 patients with lesions greater than 6 cm in diameter underwent an adjunctive hysterectomy. As with the overall group, no significant survival advantage resulted from the use of adjuvant surgery. The two- and five-year survivals in the patients with bulky lesions were 83% and 61%, respectively. Although the numbers are small, this was not significantly different from those with lesions that were less than 6 cm in diameter. Thus, although radical hysterectomy was used only in patients with small lesions, comparable survivals were observed in patients treated by radiation therapy alone or in combination with adjunctive hysterectomy (fig. 16.1).

Fifty-one patients had a pretreatment lymphangiogram. The incidence of lymph node metastases in these patients was 20%. Survival in patients with unilaterally positive pelvic nodes as determined by lymphangiography was not significantly different from that in patients with negative nodes, but survival was significantly worse in those with bilaterally positive pelvic or positive common iliac nodes (table 16.1). As was observed in the radical hysterectomy group, survival was significantly worse

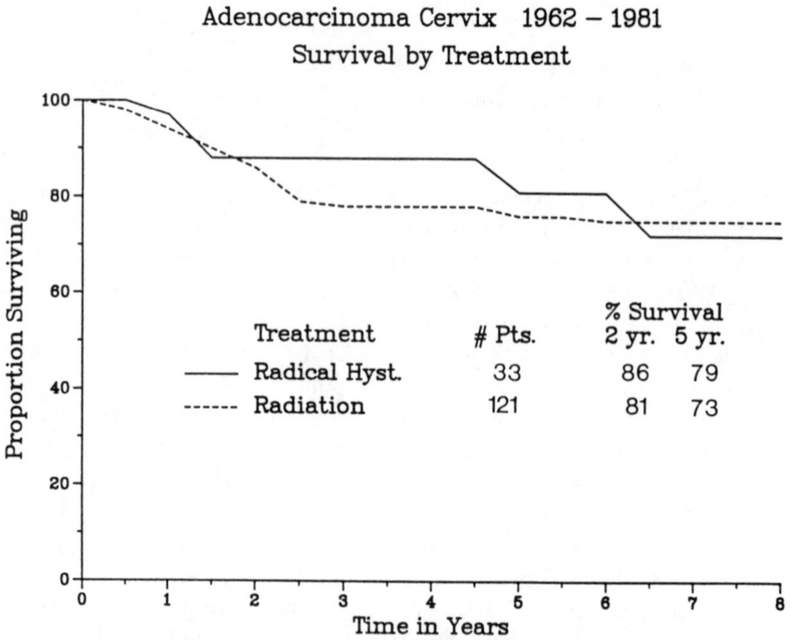

Fig. 16.1. Survival by treatment modality in 154 patients with adenocarcinoma of the cervix.

in patients with vascular or lymphatic space involvement by the tumor ($p < 0.01$). Patients with grade 1 tumors had significantly better survival than those with grade 2 or 3 tumors ($p < 0.01$). This difference was not observed in the radical hysterectomy group. No difference in survival was observed in the radiation therapy group when compared on the basis of age, histological subtype, nuclear grade, or number of mitoses.

Nodal Metastases

It has been suggested that the incidence of nodal metastases is higher in patients with adenocarcinoma of the cervix than in patients in a similar stage with squamous

Table 16.1. *Lymphangiography Results and Survival Rates in 51 Patients with Adenocarcinoma of the Cervix*

Lymphangiography Results	No. of Patients	Percentage of Survival		Tumor Grade	*p* Value
		Two Year	Five Year		
Negative	41	87	76	1 vs. 2	0.36
Unilateral	6	62	62	2 vs. 3	0.24
Bilateral or common	4	25	25	1 vs. 3	0.01

carcinoma (Nogales and Botella-Llusia 1965). More recent studies have failed to confirm this finding (Shingleton et al. 1981; Webb and Symmonds 1979). Our findings of 6% nodal disease in patients treated by radical hysterectomy and 20% in those treated by radiation who underwent a lymphangiogram are similar to these latter studies and are consistent with the generally reported incidence for stage I squamous carcinoma. The poor prognosis associated with capillary space involvement that was suggested by Tamimi and Figge was confirmed by the U.T. M. D. Anderson Hospital data (Tamimi and Figge 1982).

Conclusion

Our data support the conclusions of Shingleton and Korhonen that survival is not influenced by the various histological subtypes of adenocarcinoma (Shingleton et al. 1981; Korhonen 1984). Milsom found tumor grade to be of little prognostic value (Milsom and Friberg 1983), whereas other authors have found grade to be an important prognostic factor (Korhonen 1984; Berek et al. 1985; Prempree, Amornmarn, and Wizenberg 1985). In our series, grade did not influence survival in patients with small tumor volume treated by radical hysterectomy but was of prognostic significance in the radiation group in which those with grade 1 tumors had significantly better survival than those with grade 2 or 3 tumors.

In conclusion, radical hysterectomy is acceptable therapy for small volume disease. The role of radical hysterectomy for larger volume disease and the role of extrafascial hysterectomy as an adjunct to radiation therapy remain controversial. The U.T. M. D. Anderson Hospital data failed to demonstrate a survival advantage for adjuvant surgery, which was associated with a significant complication rate. If adjunctive hysterectomy has a role, it would appear to be in treating patients with bulky lesions. This controversy, which also pertains to squamous carcinoma, will persist until a prospective, randomized trial is conducted. Of the histological variables evaluated, only nodal metastases, capillary space involvement, and tumor grade were found to have prognostic value.

References

Berek JS, Castaldo TW, Hacker NF, Petrilli ES, Lagasse LD, Moore JG. 1981. Adenocarcinoma of the uterine cervix. *Cancer* 48:2734–2741.

Berek JS, Hacker NF, Fu YS, Sokale JR, Leuchter RC, Lagasse LD. 1985. Adenocarcinoma of the uterine cervix: Histologic variables associated with lymph node metastasis and survival. *Obstet Gynecol* 65:46–52.

Bernstein SG, Woet RC, Guzick DS. 1985. Prevalence of papillomavirus infection in colposcopically directed cervical biopsy specimens in 1972 and 1982. *Am J Obstet Gynecol* 151:577–581.

Cuccia CA, Bloedorn FG, Onal M. 1967. Treatment of primary adenocarcinoma of the cervix. *American Journal of Roentgenology, Radium Therapy, and Nuclear Medicine* 99: 371–375.

Davis JR, Moon LB. 1975. Increased incidence of adenocarcinoma of uterine cervix. *Obstet Gynecol* 45:79–83.

Gallup DG, Abell MR. 1977. Invasive adenocarcinoma of the uterine cervix. *Obstet Gynecol* 49:596–603.

Gloor E, Ruzicka J. 1982. Morphology of adenocarcinoma in situ of the uterine cervix: A study of 14 cases. *Cancer* 49:294–302.

Grundsell H, Henriksson H, Johnsson JG, Troupe C. 1979. Prognosis of adenocarcinoma of the uterine cervix. *Gynecol Oncol* 8:204–208.

Kagan AR, Nussbaum H, Chan PYM, Ziel HK. 1973. Adenocarcinoma of the uterine cervix. *Am J Obstet Gynecol* 117:464–468.

Kjorstad KE. 1977. Adenocarcinoma of the uterine cervix. *Gynecol Oncol* 5:219–223.

Korhonen MO. 1984. Adenocarcinoma of the uterine cervix: Prognosis and prognostic significance of histology. *Cancer* 53:1760–1763.

Maier RC, Norris HJ. 1980. Coexistence of cervical intra-epithelial neoplasia with primary adenocarcinoma of the endocervix. *Obstet Gynecol* 56:361–364.

Mayer EG, Galindo J, Davis J, Aristizabul S. 1976. Adenocarcinoma of the uterine cervix: Incidence and the role of radiation therapy. *Radiology* 121:725–729.

Milsom I, Friberg LG. 1983. Primary adenocarcinoma of the uterine cervix: A clinical study. *Cancer* 52:942–947.

Nogales F, Botella-Llusia J. 1965. The frequency of invasion of the lymph nodes in cancer of the uterine cervix. *Am J Obstet Gynecol* 93:91–94.

Prempree T, Amornmarn R, Wizenberg MJ. 1985. A therapeutic approach to primary adenocarcinoma of the cervix. *Cancer* 56:1264–1268.

Rutledge FN, Galakatos AE, Wharton JT, Smith JP. 1975. Adenocarcinoma of the uterine cervix. *Am J Obstet Gynecol* 122:236–245.

Shingleton HM, Gore H, Bradley DH, Soong SJ. 1981. Adenocarcinoma of the cervix: I. Clinical evaluation and pathologic features. *Am J Obstet Gynecol* 139:799–814.

Smotkin D, Berek JS, Fu YS. 1985. Human papillomavirus DNA in adenocarcinomas and adenosquamous carcinoma of the uterine cervix. Paper presented at the annual meeting of the Western Association of Gynecologic Oncology, 6 June, at San Diego.

Tamimi HK, Figge DC. 1982. Adenocarcinoma of the uterine cervix. *Gynecol Oncol* 13: 335–344.

Teshima H, Shimosato Y, Kishi K, Kasamatsu T, Ohmi K, Uei Y. 1985. Early stage adenocarcinoma of the uterine cervix. Histopathologic analysis with consideration of histogenesis. *Cancer* 56:167–172.

Webb MJ, Symmonds RE. 1979. Wertheim hysterectomy: A reappraisal. *Obstet Gynecol* 54:140–145.

Weiner S, Witzenberg MJ. 1975. Treatment of primary adenocarcinoma of the cervix. *Cancer* 35:1514–1516.

Annual Clinical Conference on Cancer, Vol. 29
Gynecologic Cancer: Diagnosis and Treatment Strategies
© 1987 by The University of Texas System Cancer Center

17. Small Cell Carcinoma of the Cervix Uteri: A Review of the Pathology of 33 Cases

Elvio G. Silva

There have been a number of reports in the literature of small cell carcinoma of the cervix uteri, although it does not at first seem so because of the different terms used to describe this tumor. The variety in terminology reflects an absence of diagnostic criteria in this disease. Diagnosis has been based on the subjective evaluation of tumor cell size without specific parameters. In an attempt to identify pathology parameters useful in the prognosis of small cell carcinoma of the cervix, I review the pathology of 33 cases.

Materials and Methods

All cases diagnosed as poorly differentiated carcinoma of the cervix at The University of Texas M. D. Anderson Hospital and Tumor Institute at Houston between 1965 and 1985 were reviewed. In most cases, light-microscopy slides stained with hematoxylin and eosin were available. Only those cases in which the nuclei of the tumor cells measured less than 21 μm were included in this study. In accordance with this criterion, 33 cases were classified as small cell carcinoma. When areas of squamous cell carcinoma or adenocarcinoma were also present, the case was included only if more than 50% of the tumor was characterized by the small cell component. Grimelius staining (argyrophilia), immunohistochemistry, and electron microscopy were used to determine whether there was neuroendocrine differentiation. Immunohistochemical studies were performed on formalin-fixed, paraffin-embedded tissue sections, using the peroxidase-antiperoxidase method described by Sternberger et al. (1982). The antigen neuron-specific enolase was searched for with rabbit anti-bovine antibody at a 1:700 dilution (Dakopatt, Accurate Chemical & Scientific Corporation, Westbury, New York). The slides were stained by the avidin-biotin complex method. Material for electron microscopy was available in 21 cases. These specimens were fixed in 2% glutaraldehyde in phosphate buffer, postfixed in osmium tetroxide, and embedded in epoxy resin.

Neuroendocrine differentiation was diagnosed in electron microscopy when dense-core, membrane-bound granules, 120 to 180 MM in diameter, were found in the cytoplasm of the tumor cells. These granules often formed groups of four or five, and in some cases they were found within small, short cell processes.

Results

Pathology Examination

Light microscopy showed the tumor cells to be most often arranged in solid sheets. In some cases, the tumor cells formed nests separated by fibrous stroma.

In all the cases, the small cells were round or oval and had scant cytoplasm, hyperchromatic nuclei, and inconspicuous nucleoli; spindle cells were focally present in some cases. Molding was commonly seen.

Based on the presence or absence of glandular or squamous differentiation/association by light microscopy, the cases were divided into three groups: those of pure small cell carcinoma (11 cases), those with associated adenocarcinoma (13), and those with associated squamous carcinoma (9). The number of cervical quadrants involved by tumor, occurrence of carcinoma in situ, number of mitotic figures per 10 high-power fields (HPF), presence of neuroendocrine differentiation, and finding of vascular invasion are outlined by group in table 17.1. The thickness of all the tumors was more than 3 mm. In several cases, the tumor infiltrated the entire thickness of the biopsy, which varied between 3 mm and 7 mm.

Pure Small Cell Carcinoma

In the ten cases in which carcinoma in situ was not found, the tumor destroyed the epithelium, producing ulcers with a necrotic base.

Neuroendocrine differentiation was detected by electron microscopy in all six cases so described; Grimelius staining was positive in three of these six cases.

Small Cell Carcinoma Associated with Adenocarcinoma

Eight tumors in the study were composed of small cells forming glands, which sometimes were difficult to see because of their small size. In five other cases, there was adenocarcinoma of medium cell size in some parts of the biopsy material, with the rest of the tumor made up of small cell carcinoma.

Carcinoma in situ was exclusively found in the adenocarcinoma component.

Electron microscopy and Grimelius staining detected neuroendocrine differentiation in four cases. Immunoperoxidase staining for neuron-specific enolase was positive for such differentiation in a fifth case. In this last case, Grimelius staining was negative, and no membrane-bound granules were seen by electron microscopy.

Small Cell Carcinoma Associated with Squamous Carcinoma

In eight cases, small cell carcinoma was admixed with squamous carcinoma; in a ninth case, small cell carcinoma was preceded by squamous carcinoma by eight months.

Prognosis

Of the 33 patients, 19 died of disease, 2 died of unrelated causes, 1 is alive with metastases, and 11 are alive with no evidence of disease. The most significant prog-

Table 17.1. *Tumor Characteristics by Light-Microscopy Diagnosis*

	N	No. of Cervical Quadrants Involved by Tumor				Carcinoma In Situ	No. of Mitoses/ 10 High-Power Fields		Neuroendocrine Differentiation	Vascular Invasion
		4	3	2	Unknown		20–49	50–90		
Pure SCC	11	5	3		1[a]	1	7	4	6	1
SCC + adenocarcinoma	13	9	2		2	5[b]	7	6	5	3
SCC + squamous carcinoma	9	5	1	1	2	8	8	1	4	2

Note: SCC, small cell carcinoma.
[a] Additionally, in two other cases, there was a single mass (barrel type) larger than 4 cm in diameter.
[b] Exclusively adenocarcinoma.

nostic indicator was staging. Of 13 patients with stage I or II disease, 56% are without evidence of disease, at an average follow-up of 4.5 years; another 2 of these 13 are the 2 who died of unrelated causes (at one and two years). Of 20 patients with stage III or IV disease, 90% died of disease within two years (average, 11 months), 1 is alive with metastasis at two years, and 1 is without evidence of disease at three years.

Pure small cell carcinoma entailed a worse prognosis (82% died of disease) than did small cell carcinoma associated with adenocarcinoma or squamous carcinoma (52% died of disease).

There was no correlation between prognosis and number of mitoses, vascular invasion, neuroendocrine differentiation, or quadrants involved.

Discussion

Small cell carcinoma of the cervix has been reported in the literature under a variety of terms, including carcinoid tumors (Albores-Saavedra et al. 1976; Albores-Saavedra, Rodríguez-Martínez, and Larraza-Hernández 1979), argyrophil cell carcinoma (Matsuyama et al. 1979; Stassart et al. 1982; Tateishi et al. 1975), neuroendocrine carcinoma (Pazdur et al. 1980), small cell tumor with neuroepithelial features (Mackay, Osborne, and Wharton 1979), oat cell carcinoma (Jacobs et al. 1980), endocrine cell carcinoma (Johannessen et al. 1980), and small cell carcinoma (van Nagell et al. 1977; Jones et al. 1976; Lojek et al. 1980; Groben, Reddick, and Askin 1985).

We prefer to refer to this tumor as "small cell carcinoma" because this is a less controversial term and allows for classification by these tumors by standard hematoxylin-and-eosin staining and light microscopy. "Carcinoid tumors" (Albores-Saavedra et al. 1976; Albores-Saavedra, Rodríguez-Martínez, and Larraza-Hernández 1979) should not be used for this type of carcinoma because "carcinoid" is a term created to designate a tumor morphologically similar to but less aggressive than carcinoma (Obendorfer 1907). In some organs, such as the lung, carcinoid tumors and small cell carcinomas can be distinguished by differences in morphology, clinical characteristics, and prognosis, owing to the large number of cases available for review. My coworkers and I believe that these two tumor types should be similarly designated by different terms when occurrence is in the cervix. Terms such as "argyrophil," "neuroendocrine," and "neuroepithelial" should also not be used: many of the small cell carcinomas do not show an argyrophil reaction or endocrine substance on staining procedures, nor do they show neuroepithelial features.

Terminology and methodology need to be clarified to define the characteristics of small cell carcinoma. Previous reports found that the incidence of small cell carcinoma of the cervix varied between 4% of all cases of cervical carcinoma (van Nagell et al. 1977) and 19.5% of all cases of squamous carcinoma (Field, Dockerty, and Symmonds 1964). However, in neither of these reports is there a description of the precise boundaries of size that will separate small cell carcinoma from non–small cell carcinoma.

In our study, small cell carcinoma of the cervix was characterized either by extensive cervical involvement or by the large size of the tumor. This information was available in 28 of 33 cases. The tumor involved four quadrants of the cervix in 19 cases, three quadrants in 6 cases, and two quadrants in only 1 case. In two cases, the tumor was larger than 4 cm and of barrel type. The histological appearance of the small cell carcinoma was similar in all cases associated with glands, whether of squamous or pure small cell composition. All tumors were composed of round-to-oval cells, and in some cases spindle cells were also present. Carcinoma in situ was present in 38% of the group associated with adenocarcinoma and in 89% of the group associated with squamous carcinoma, but in only 1 of 11 pure small cell carcinomas. All tumors were invasive to a depth of more than 3 mm. All tumors had more than 20 mitotic figures per 10 HPF, and 15 cases had more than 40 mitoses per 10 HPF.

The prognosis of small cell carcinoma has been debated in previous studies. Wentz and Reagan in 1959 and Wentz in 1961 found that small cell squamous carcinoma had a 10% five-year survival, very different from the 65% and 45% five-year survivals seen in large cell and intermediate cell carcinomas, respectively. These figures were challenged by Sidhu, Koss, and Barber in 1970, who found no survival difference between the three histological cell types when same-stage tumors were analyzed. Goellner in 1976 also found no correlation between cell type and survival for same-stage tumors.

Our study shows that stage is the most important parameter in the evaluation of the prognosis of small cell carcinoma. There was no evidence of disease at five years in 56% of stage I and II cases, whereas 90% of patients with stage III or IV cancer died of disease within two years. It needs to be recognized that small cell carcinoma is a tumor that more often than not is a high-stage lesion. Over 60% of the patients in our study had stage III or IV disease. This percentage contrasts with the 10% or 20% for similar stages in large series of squamous carcinoma or adenocarcinoma (Goellner 1976; Shingleton et al. 1981; Rutledge et al. 1975). The only pathology that we found a useful prognostic indicator was the presence of adenocarcinoma or squamous carcinoma in areas of the small cell carcinoma. Although our series is a small one, small cell carcinomas with foci of adenocarcinoma or squamous carcinoma yielded better survival (52% died of disease) than did small cell carcinomas without these involvements (82% died of disease). Other pathology features are not important in the prognosis of these tumors; in particular, the presence or absence of neuroendocrine differentiation has no prognostic significance. Of 15 patients in whose cases neuroendocrine differentiation was detected, 10 died of disease. Of 18 with no indication of neuroendocrine differentiation, 9 died of disease.

The cell of origin of this tumor is most probably the undifferentiated basal cell of the cervical epithelium; this cell has the potential to proliferate to neoplasm composed of small cells, glands, or squamous components.

The differential diagnosis of small cell carcinoma of the cervix includes other small cell tumors of the cervix. Of the sarcomas, the botryoid type of rhabdomyosarcoma (Copeland et al. 1985; Daya and Scully 1985) is probably the entity most likely to be confused with small cell carcinoma. This differential diagnosis should be based on the younger age of the patient, on the finding of polypoid tumor, and histologically on the presence of cambium layer and muscle differentiation. Probably the most difficult tumor to differentiate from small cell carcinoma is lymphoma. Primary lymphoma of the cervix is unusual (Komaki et al. 1984; Harris and Scully 1984), but when it infiltrates the cervix diffusely it can be impossible to differentiate by light microscopy alone from small cell carcinoma. In this situation, positive immunoperoxidase staining for keratin, testing for neuron-specific enolase reaction, and identification of cell junctions by electron microscopy are the most helpful approaches to diagnosing carcinoma.

Thus, small cell carcinoma of the cervix can include areas of squamous carcinoma or adenocarcinoma, and this differential diagnosis is important in the prognosis. However, the most important prognostic indicator is stage. In addition, small cell carcinomas are aggressive tumors: more than 60% of the patients reported here presented with high-stage disease.

References

Albores-Saavedra J, Larraza O, Poucell S, Rodríguez-Martínez HA. 1976. Carcinoid of the uterine cervix: Additional observations on a new tumor entity. *Cancer* 38:2328–2342.

Albores-Saavedra J, Rodríguez-Martínez HA, Larraza-Hernández O. 1979. Carcinoid tumors of the cervix. *Pathol Annu* 14:273–291.

Copeland LJ, Gershenson DM, Saul PB, Sneige N, Stringer CA, Edwards CL. 1985. Sarcoma botryoides of the female genital tract. *Obstet Gynecol* 66:262–266.

Daya D, Scully RE. 1985. Sarcoma botryoides of the cervix: A clinicopathologic study of 16 cases (abstract). *Lab Invest* 52:17A.

Field CA, Dockerty M, Symmonds RE. 1964. Small cell carcinoma of the cervix. *Am J Obstet Gynecol* 88:447–451.

Goellner JR. 1976. Carcinoma of the cervix. Clinicopathologic correlation of 196 cases. *Am J Clin Pathol* 66:775–785.

Groben P, Reddick R, Askin F. 1985. The pathologic spectrum of small cell carcinoma of the cervix. *Int J Gynecol Pathol* 4:42–57.

Harris NL, Scully RE. 1984. Malignant lymphoma and granulocytic sarcoma of the uterus and vagina. A clinicopathologic analysis of 27 cases. *Cancer* 53:2530–2545.

Jacobs AJ, Marchevsky A, Gordon RE, Deppe G, Cohen CJ. 1980. Oat cell carcinoma of the uterine cervix in a pregnant woman treated with *cis*-diamminedichloroplatinum. *Gynecol Oncol* 9:405–410.

Johannessen JV, Capella C, Solcia E, Davy M, Sobrinho-Simöes M. 1980. Endocrine cell carcinoma of the uterine cervix. *Diagn Gynecol Obstet* 2:127–134.

Jones HW III, Plymate S, Gluck FB, Miles PA, Greene JF Jr. 1976. Small cell nonkeratinizing carcinoma of the cervix associated with ACTH production. *Cancer* 38:1629–1635.

Komaki R, Cox JD, Hansen RM, Gunn WG, Greenberg M. 1984. Malignant lymphoma of the uterine cervix. *Cancer* 54:1699–1704.

Lojek MA, Fer MF, Kasselberg AG, Glick AD, Burnett LS, Julian CG, Greco FA, Oldham RK. 1980. Cushing's syndrome with small cell carcinoma of the uterine cervix. *Am J Med* 69:140–144.

Mackay B, Osborne BM, Wharton JT. 1979. Small cell tumor of cervix with neuroepithelial features. *Cancer* 43:1138–1145.

Matsuyama M, Inoue T, Ariyoshi Y, Doi M, Suchi T, Sato T, Tashiro K, Chihara T. 1979. Argyrophil cell carcinoma of the uterine cervix with ectopic production of ACTH, β-MSH, serotonin, histamine, and amylase. *Cancer* 44:1813–1823.

Obendorfer S. 1907. Karzinoide Tumoren des DunnDarms. *Frankfurter Zeitschrift fuer Pathologie* 1:426–433.

Pazdur R, Bonomi P, Slayton R, Gould VE, Miller A, Jao W, Dolan T, Wilbanks G. 1980. Neuroendocrine carcinoma of the cervix: Implications for staging and therapy. *Gynecol Oncol* 12:120–128.

Rutledge FN, Galakatos AE, Wharton JT, Smith JP. 1975. Adenocarcinoma of the uterine cervix. *Am J Obstet Gynecol* 122:236–245.

Shingleton HM, Gore H, Bradley DH, Soong S-J. 1981. Adenocarcinoma of the cervix. *Am J Obstet Gynecol* 139:799–814.

Sidhu GS, Koss LG, Barber HRK. 1970. Relation of histologic factors to the response of stage I epidermoid carcinoma of the cervix to surgical treatment. Analysis of 115 patients. *Obstet Gynecol* 35:329–338.

Stassart J, Crum CP, Yordan EL, Fenoglio CM, Richart RM. 1982. Argyrophilic carcinoma of the cervix: A report of a case with coexisting cervical intraepithelial neoplasia. *Gynecol Oncol* 13:247–251.

Sternberger LA, Hardy PHJ, Cuculis JJ, Meyer HG. 1982. The unlabeled antibody enzyme method of immunohistochemistry preparation and properties of soluble antigen: Antibody complex (horseradish peroxidase–anti–horseradish peroxidase) and its use in the identification of spirochetes. *J Histochem Cytochem* 18:315–323.

Tateishi R, Wada A, Hayakawa K, Hongo J, Ishii S, Terakawa N. 1975. Argyrophil cell carcinoma (apudomas) of the uterine cervix. Light and electron microscopic observations of 5 cases. *Virchows Arch [A]* 366:257–274.

van Nagell JR Jr, Donaldson ES, Wood EG, Maruyama Y, Utley J. 1977. Small cell cancer of the uterine cervix. *Cancer* 40:2243–2249.

Wentz WB. 1961. Histologic grade and survival in cervical cancer. *Obstet Gynecol* 18: 412–416.

Wentz WB, Reagan JW. 1959. Survival in cervical cancer with respect to cell type. *Cancer* 12:384–388.

Annual Clinical Conference on Cancer, Vol. 29
Gynecologic Cancer: Diagnosis and Treatment Strategies
© 1987 by The University of Texas System Cancer Center

18. The Clinical Management of Small Cell Carcinoma of the Cervix

Patton B. Saul

Investigators have attempted to identify certain characteristics of tumors that would be helpful in predicting their response to treatment. This would allow individualization of therapy and, hopefully, improve survival.

Wentz and Reagan (1959) proposed a histological classification of squamous cell carcinoma of the cervix based on the histopathologic structure of the tumor cells. Three cell types were described: large cell nonkeratinizing, large cell keratinizing, and small cell. Subsequently, a definite correlation was shown between the tumor cell type and patient survival (Swan and Roddick 1973).

The etiology and clinical behavior of the small cell tumors described by Wentz and Reagan have been the subject of much controversy. Some believe that these tumors are carcinoids and are not of epithelial origin (Albores-Saavedra, Rodríguez-Martínez, and Larraza-Hernández 1979). Others have described these tumors as argyrophil cell carcinomas (Matsuyama et al. 1979; Stassart et al. 1982; Tateishi et al. 1975), endocrine cell carcinomas (Johannessen et al. 1980), small cell tumors with neuroepithelial features (Mackay, Osborne, and Wharton 1979), and small cell carcinomas (van Nagell et al. 1977; Jones et al. 1976). The many names for the tumor reflect the lack of universally accepted criteria for diagnosis. A review of our cases of small cell carcinoma (for details, see Silva in this volume) has led to the establishment of precise criteria using light microscopy for the diagnosis of this tumor. The purpose of this report is to examine the clinical presentation, behavior, and treatment of these tumors in an effort to detect features that would be helpful in predicting a favorable response to therapy and improved overall survival.

Materials and Methods

All cases of small cell carcinoma of the cervix diagnosed at U.T. M. D. Anderson Hospital and Tumor Institute at Houston were reviewed. Silva has described the pathological parameters that were found to be useful in the prognosis of these tumors (see Silva in this volume).

The clinical parameters believed to be useful in predicting prognosis were studied. They included patient age, presenting symptoms, stage of disease, nodal status at presentation, histology of the small cell tumor, and treatment.

Results

The diagnosis of small cell carcinoma of the cervix has been employed at U.T. M. D. Anderson Hospital since 1978. From 1978 through November 1985, 2,932 cases of squamous cell carcinoma of the cervix were diagnosed and treated. Thirty-three (1%) of these cases met the criteria for designation as small cell carcinomas.

The average age of these patients was 55 years, with a range of 24 to 86 years. When analyzed by stage, the patient age was not different from that found in all patients with squamous cell cancers of the cervix.

Twenty-five of the 33 patients (75%) presented with some form of abnormal vaginal bleeding. Fifty-five percent experienced postmenopausal bleeding for two or more months. The remainder had either intermenstrual or postcoital bleeding. Three patients (9%) presented with back and abdominal pain. The remaining five patients (15%) were asymptomatic. Symptoms of endocrine origin were absent. Specific tests for serum adrenocorticotropic hormone (ACTH), insulin, and cortisol were not performed.

All patients were staged according to the criteria set forth by the International Federation of Gynecology and Obstetrics (FIGO) (table 18.1). Eighteen patients (55%) presented with early stages of disease, stages I and II, whereas 15 patients (45%) had advanced disease, stages III or IV.

Lymph node status was evaluated at the time of presentation by either lymphangiogram, radiographic examination (chest X ray, computerized tomography scan), or needle aspiration in 18 of the 33 patients (55%). Of these 18, 12 (67%)

Table 18.1. *Stage of Disease in Study Group*

Stage	No. of Patients	(%)
IB	15	(46)
IIA	1	(3)
IIB	2	(6)
IIIA	1	(3)
IIIB	8	(24)
IVB	6	(18)
Total	33	(100)

Table 18.2. *Nodal Status at Diagnosis*

Stage	No. of Patients	No. of Patients in Whom Nodal Status Known	No. of Patients with Positive Nodes	(%)
I	15	6	3	(50)
II	3	3	0	(0)
III	9	6	6	(100)
IV	6	3	3	(100)
Total	33	18	12	(36)

Table 18.3. *Tumor Histology Related to Stage of Disease*

Stage	Pure (%)	Squamous Differentiation (%)	Adenomatous Differentiation (%)
I	4 (27)	2 (13)	9 (60)
II	1 (33)	2 (67)	0 (0)
III	5 (56)	3 (33)	1 (11)
IV	1 (17)	2 (33)	3 (50)
Total	11 (33)	9 (27)	13 (39)

Table 18.4. *Summary of Treatments*

Treatment	Stage I	Stage II	Stage III	Stage IV
Surgery alone	1			
Irradiation alone	8	2	2	1
Chemotherapy alone			1	1
Irradiation + surgery		1		
Irradiation + chemotherapy	4		3	1
Irradiation + tamoxifen + megestrol	1			
Intraarterial chemotherapy + surgery + systemic chemotherapy			2	
Intraarterial chemotherapy + irradiation + chemotherapy			1	1
No treatment	1			2

had positive nodes at diagnosis. Therefore, 12 of the 33 patients (36%) with small cell cancer of the cervix presented with positive nodes (table 18.2).

Based on the presence or absence of glandular or squamous differentiation, the small cell tumors were divided into three categories: pure small cell tumors showing no further differentiation, small cell carcinoma associated with adenocarcinoma, and small cell carcinoma associated with squamous carcinoma (table 18.3). There was no predominant histological type in our series.

Thirty patients were treated with a total of eight different treatment regimens (table 18.4). Three patients were in such poor medical condition at the time of presentation that they could not undergo therapy. Surgery, in the form of a radical hysterectomy and bilateral pelvic lymphadenectomy, was employed in only one patient. All other patients were believed to be unsuitable for surgical therapy, either because of the presence of a cervical lesion greater than 3 cm in diameter or evidence suggesting the presence of nodal disease. Thirteen patients (39%) were treated exclusively with irradiation. An additional 12 patients (36%) received radiation in combination with some other form of therapy; therefore, irradiation was included in the treatment plan for 25 patients (76%). The "standard" radiation therapy administered consisted of 4,000 rad to the whole pelvis in 20 fractions over four weeks, followed by two intracavitary radium insertions of approximately 48 hours each, two weeks apart, delivering a total of 6,000 mg-hr. Many chemotherapeutic agents were employed, both as single drugs and in combination. They included such agents

Table 18.5. *Survival by Stage*

Stage	No. of Patients	Median Survival (Months)
I	15	66.6
II	3	42.0
III	9	12.2
IV	6	3.0
Total	33	14.2

Table 18.6. *Survival Related to Histology*

Histology	No. of Patients	Alive Without Disease (%)	Died of Disease (%)	Median Survival (Months)
Pure	11	2 (18)	9 (82)	13
Squamous	9	5 (56)	4 (44)	45
Adenomatous	13	4 (31)	9 (69)	28
Total	33	11 (33)	22 (67)	

as cisplatin, cyclophosphamide, bleomycin, VP-16-213, doxorubicin HCl, vincristine, vindesine, and mitomycin C. Because of the large number of different drugs and different combinations of drugs used in treatment and the small number of patients receiving each, a detailed analysis of this aspect of therapy has little meaning.

Survival was evaluated in relation to age, presenting symptoms, stage of disease, status of nodes at time of diagnosis, histological type of small cell tumor, and treatment. The sample size was too small and the variables too numerous to allow statistically significant conclusions to be drawn. Several general statements can be made, however, and certain trends can be identified.

The overall survival rate of patients with small cell carcinoma of the cervix is extremely poor, 56%, at five years in patients with stage I disease; for all other stages, the five-year survival was zero. The median survival time of the entire group of 33 patients was 14.2 months (table 18.5).

Aside from stage, the only other factors appearing to influence survival were that of nodal status and tumor histology (table 18.6). As with other squamous cell cancers, patients presenting with positive nodes have a very poor prognosis. Of the 12 patients with known positive nodes at diagnosis, only 2 (17%) were salvaged: 1 with irradiation and 1 with intraarterial chemotherapy and irradiation. Again, our number of cases is too small to make definitive statements. There appears to be a trend toward decreased survival in patients with the pure small cell tumor. Their median survival was 13 months. In patients having tumors with squamous and adenomatous differentiation, survival times were 45 and 28 months, respectively.

Recurrent disease was noted in six (18%) patients, two locally and four at sites distant from the original tumor. All but one were treated with chemotherapy. The remaining patient was found to have a positive supraclavicular node and received radiation to that area. All died of the disease.

Discussion

Despite the multiple histological staging classifications proposed for squamous cell carcinoma, no system has been uniformly adopted. The lack of precise criteria for defining the small cell carcinoma has led to the adoption of a variety of terms for this tumor. Silva has identified specific criteria for the small cell carcinoma that allow its recognition using standard light microscopy and routine hematoxylin and eosin stains. Hopefully, this will improve the diagnosis of this tumor and allow us to gain more knowledge of its behavior and treatment.

This tumor represents only a small fraction of squamous cell cancers of the cervix, but is very important because of its extremely malignant nature and the high mortality associated with it. In our series, 45% of the patients had advanced disease (stage III or IV) at the time of initial presentation. This contrasts with other histological types of squamous cell carcinoma, where only 10% to 20% of patients present in stages III and IV of the disease. Stage for stage, in those patients in whom nodal status was known, positive nodes were found much more frequently with this tumor than with other squamous cancers. Sites of recurrence were similar to those of other histological types of this disease. It is possible, then, that small cell carcinomas of the cervix may actually represent disseminated disease even when detected at an early stage. This may explain the failure of irradiation to control a disease that has traditionally been responsive to such measures. Future treatments may include chemotherapy and conventional radiation therapy, especially in the "pure" small cell squamous carcinomas. Unfortunately, the large variety of treatment schemes used in the therapy of such small numbers of patients did not allow an analysis of their effectiveness in controlling the disease in our series.

References

Albores-Saavedra J, Rodríguez-Martínez HA, Larraza-Hernández O. 1979. In *Pathology Annual*, part 1, vol. 14, pp. 273–291. New York: Appleton-Century-Crofts.

Johannessen JV, Capella C, Solcia E, Davy M, Sobrinho-Simöes M. 1980. Endocrine cell carcinoma of the uterine cervix. *Diagn Gynecol Obstet* 2:127–134.

Jones HW III, Plymate S, Gluck FB, Miles PA, Green JF Jr. 1976. Small cell nonkeratinizing carcinoma of the cervix associated with ACTH production. *Cancer* 38:1629–1635.

Mackay B, Osborne BM, Wharton JT. 1979. Small cell tumor of the cervix with neuroepithelial features. *Cancer* 43:1138–1145.

Matsuyama M, Inoue T, Ariyosii Y, Doi M, Suchi T, Sato T, Tashiro K, Chihara T. 1979. Argyrophil cell carcinoma of the uterine cervix with ectopic production of ACTH, β-MSH, serotonin histamine, and amylase. *Cancer* 44:1813–1823.

Stassart J, Crum CP, Yordan EL, Fenoglio CM, Richart RM. 1982. Argyrophilic carcinoma of the cervix: A report of a case with coexisting cervical intraepithelial neoplasia. *Gynecol Oncol* 13:247–251.

Swan DS, Roddick JW. 1973. A clinical-pathological correlation of cell type classification of cervical cancer. *Am J Obstet Gynecol* 116:666–670.

Tateishi R, Wade A, Hayakawa K, Hongo J, Ishii S, Terakawa N. 1975. Argyrophil cell carcinoma (apudomas) of the uterine cervix. Light and electron microscopic observations of 5 cases. *Virchows Arch [A]* 366:257–274.

van Nagell JR Jr, Donaldson ES, Wood EG, Marvyama Y, Utley J. 1977. Small cell cancer of the uterine cervix. *Cancer* 40:2243–2249.

Wentz WB, Reagan JW. 1959. Survival in cervical cancer with respect to cell type. *Cancer* 12:384–388.

Annual Clinical Conference on Cancer, Vol. 29
Gynecologic Cancer: Diagnosis and Treatment Strategies
© 1987 by The University of Texas System Cancer Center

19. Current Management of Lymph Node Metastasis in Early and Locally Advanced Cervical Cancer

M. Steven Piver

Lymph node metastasis in early and locally advanced cervical cancer remains the main deterrent to improved survival for most women with carcinoma of the uterine cervix. This chapter considers two major subgroups of patients—those with stage IB disease and those with stage II and stage III disease—and how management of the disease is affected by lymph node metastasis.

For lymph node metastasis in stage IB, the following will be reviewed: (1) incidence of pelvic lymph node metastasis and its relation to the size of the primary tumor, (2) five-year survival rate and its relation to the incidence of pelvic lymph node metastasis, (3) incidence of paraaortic lymph node metastasis, (4) five-year survival rate and its relation to surgery and pelvic lymph node metastasis, (5) survival rate and the number of pelvic lymph nodes remaining after radical hysterectomy and pelvic lymphadenectomy, (6) recurrence rate and its relation to the number of pelvic lymph nodes remaining after pelvic lymphadenectomy, (7) five-year survival rate of patients with known pelvic lymph node metastases treated with radical hysterectomy and pelvic lymphadenectomy who do or do not undergo postoperative pelvic irradiation, (8) survival and how it is affected by the number of pelvic lymph node metastases and whether the patient received postoperative irradiation or no radiation therapy, (9) survival rate of patients with known paraaortic lymph node metastases treated by pelvic and paraaortic radiation.

The second part of this chapter will discuss the management of lymph node metastasis in stages II, III, and IV, including the following categories: (1) incidence of pretherapy paraaortic lymph node metastasis, (2) non–lymph node metastasis documented at the time of pretherapy surgical staging, (3) results of paraaortic and pelvic irradiation in patients with histologically documented paraaortic lymph node metastasis, (4) use of elective pelvic and paraaortic irradiation without biopsy documentation of disease in the paraaortic lymph nodes, (5) five-year survival rates of patients with stage IIB cervical cancer without histological evidence of paraaortic lymph node metastasis who undergo pelvic irradiation plus treatment with the radiation sensitizer hydroxyurea, (6) five-year survival rates in patients with stage IIB cervical cancer with negative results on pretherapy lymphangiograms who did not undergo paraaortic lymph node biopsy and were treated with hydroxyurea and pelvic irradiation, (7) five-year survival rates after pelvic irradiation and treatment with hydroxyurea for stage IIIB carcinoma of the cervix in patients with negative findings at a pretherapy paraaortic lymphadenectomy, and (8) a preliminary report on using chemotherapy and pelvic irradiation in patients with extensive paraaortic node metastases.

Stage IB Cervical Cancer

Chung and I (1975) evaluated the incidence of pelvic lymph node metastasis in 145 women with stage IB cervical cancer who underwent radical hysterectomy and bilateral pelvic lymphadenectomy. Of 145 patients, 39 (26.9%) had pelvic lymph node metastasis. The incidence of pelvic lymph node metastasis in stage IB carcinoma of the cervix was 21.1% for patients with cervical cancer lesions ≤ 3 cm, and this increased to 35.2% for those lesions > 3 cm (table 19.1). Moreover, the survival rate was 90.1% for patients with 2- to 3-cm tumors and 84% for patients with lesions ≤ 1 cm, but this decreased to between 60% and 65% for tumors > 3 cm (table 19.2). It was clear, therefore, that patients whose stage IB cervical tumors were ≥ 3 cm in greatest diameter had an unacceptably low survival rate for cancer clinically limited to the cervix and that this was due to the inordinately high rate of pelvic lymph node metastasis as the size of the cervical tumor increased.

Thus, the inability to cure a significant number of patients with pelvic lymph node metastasis by surgical resection became the management problem. Low survival rates for patients with known pelvic lymph node metastases were not ac-

Table 19.1. *Size of Cervical Lesion and Lymph Node Metastasis in Stage IB Cervical Cancer*

Lesion Size (cm)	No. of Patients	Patients with Metastasis	%	
≤1	22	4	18.1	21.1
2–3	72	16	22.2	
4–5	45	16	35.6	35.2
≥6	6	3	50.0	
Total	145	39	26.9	

Source: Adapted from Piver and Chung 1975.

Table 19.2. *Size of Cervical Lesion and Five-Year Survival Rate in Stage IB Cervical Cancer*

Lesion Size (cm)	No. of Patients	NED[a]	Dead of Cancer	Dead ID[b]	Survival (%)
≤1	28	21	4	3	84.0
2–3	74	64	7	3	90.1
4–5	49	31	16	2	65.9
≥6	6	3	2	1	60.0

Source: Adapted from Piver and Chung 1975.

[a] NED, no evidence of disease.

[b] ID, intercurrent disease with no evidence of recurrent disease. These patients were excluded from survival calculations.

Table 19.3. *Paraaortic Node Metastasis in Stage I Cervical Cancer*

Study	No. of Patients	Patients with Paraaortic Metastasis	%
Berman et al. 1984[a]	158	8	5.0
Hughes et al. 1980	140	6	4.3
Sudarsanam et al. 1978	155	11	7.0
Ballon et al. 1981	22	5	23.0
Rutledge[b]	21	0	0.0
Delgado, Caglar, and Walker 1978	18[c]	0	0.0
Buchsbaum 1979	16	4	25.0
Total	530	34	6.4

[a] For the Gynecologic Oncology Group.
[b] Rutledge as quoted by Lewis 1975.
[c] ≤3 cm cervical tumor.

counted for in great part by a high incidence of concomitant paraaortic lymph node metastasis in stage IB carcinoma of the cervix (table 19.3). In seven series of patients with stage IB carcinoma of the cervix (table 19.3), 530 patients underwent pretherapy staging paraaortic lymphadenectomy or paraaortic lymph node biopsy; only 34 (6.4%) had paraaortic node metastasis. It is significant that this 6.4% rate includes stage IB tumors of all sizes; however, in their study that related the size of the cervical tumor to the incidence of paraaortic lymph node metastasis, Delgado, Caglar, and Walker (1978) reported 18 patients with cervical tumors ≤ 3 cm in diameter, none of whom had paraaortic lymph node metastasis. It would seem, therefore, that patients with cervical lesions ≤ 3 cm would have an incidence of disease outside of the pelvis near zero and a significantly low incidence of pelvic lymph node metastasis. Therefore, radical hysterectomy and pelvic lymphadenectomy in patients with cervical tumors ≤ 3 cm in diameter should be associated with a significantly high cure rate. In the young patient such surgery has the added advantage of preserving ovarian and vaginal function.

Unfortunately, pelvic lymphadenectomy does not remove all of the pelvic lymph nodes (Kjorstad, Kolbenstvedt, and Strickert 1984). Kjorstad and coworkers (1984) reported 258 women who underwent radical hysterectomy and pelvic lymphadenectomy; all had pretherapy lymphangiograms. Postoperative radiographs were taken to document the completeness of the lymph node dissection, including the number of remaining pelvic nodes and their location. As seen in table 19.4, 66 patients had no remaining pelvic lymph nodes seen on postoperative radiographs; the five-year survival rate was 83%. For 131 patients who had one to three remaining lymph nodes, the five-year survival rate was 92%, but for the 61 patients who had four or more remaining lymph nodes, the five-year survival was only 77%. It is of special importance that in those patients with no remaining pelvic lymph nodes, the incidence of pelvic recurrence was 8%, but it increased to 18% for patients with four or more remaining lymph nodes, thus leading us to infer that the recurrences were in the nonresected pelvic lymph nodes.

Table 19.4. *Stage IB Carcinoma of the Cervix*
Survival Versus Number of Remaining Pelvic Nodes after Surgery

Remaining Nodes	No. of Patients	Metastases (%)	Survival (%) 5 Year	10 Year
None	66	24	83	83
1–3	131	21	92	89
4+	61	31	77	74

Source: Kjorstad, Kolbenstevdt, and Strickert 1984.

In order to prevent recurrences in patients found to have pelvic lymph node metastasis at the time of radical hysterectomy and pelvic lymphadenectomy for stage IB cervical cancer, two factors are important: (1) no histological evidence of metastasis above the pelvis in the paraaortic lymph nodes and (2) the amount of radiation needed to control residual, subclinical, or macroscopic cancer in the pelvis. According to Wharton et al. (1977), to control 90% of subclinical disease within the pelvis, 5,000 rad over five to five and one-half weeks is required. For a 2-cm residual cancer, 90% local control requires 6,000 rad over six to six and one-half weeks. For tumors greater than 2 cm, it requires 7,000 rad over seven to seven and one-half weeks. Very few patients receive this amount of radiation; therefore, for a 90% local pelvic control rate, there must be no metastases above the field of planned pelvic irradiation and patients should be treated with a minimum of 5,000 to 6,000 rad whole-pelvis radiation. Verification of this minimum has recently been reported (Himmelmann et al. 1985). Of 52 women with pelvic lymph node metastases (stages IB and IIA), the five-year survival rate was 49% for those receiving no postoperative radiation and 53% for those receiving 4,000 rad postoperatively, but it increased to 85% for those women treated with 5,500 to 6,000 rad.

The five-year survival rates collated from five institutions for patients with stage IB cervical cancer who were treated by radical hysterectomy and pelvic lymphadenectomy with or without postoperative radiation are shown in table 19.5 (Morrow 1980). Of these patients, 14% received less than 4,500 rad, 55%, 4,500 to 5,500 rad, and 28%, > 5,500 rad. For the 30 women with known pelvic lymph node metastases after surgery, the five-year survival rate was 60%. However, for the 144 patients who did not receive postoperative pelvic irradiation, the five-year survival rate was nearly identical (59%). Thus, the authors concluded from this retrospective collated analysis that postoperative irradiation was of no value except possibly in patients who had four or more positive nodes. There were only seven patients who had four or more positive nodes who received radiation, so no conclusion can be drawn. For 139 patients reported in the literature who received postoperative irradiation for metastasis to the pelvic lymph nodes after radical hysterectomy and pelvic lymphadenectomy for stage IB cervical cancer, the five-year survival rate with no evidence of disease was 61% (Masubuchi et al. 1969; Kelso and Funnell 1973; Rampone, Klem, and Kolstad 1973; Morrow 1980) compared with 55% for 243 patients who did not receive postoperative radiation (Burch and Chalfant 1970; Hsu, Cheng, and Su 1972; Piver and Chung 1975; Morrow 1980).

In a much larger series reported from the Norwegian Radium Hospital, 442 patients with stage IB cervical cancer treated by radical hysterectomy and pelvic lymphadenectomy whose pelvic lymph nodes were found to be negative for metastasis had a five-year survival rate of 92% compared with only 53% for 120 patients with known pelvic lymph node metastasis treated by radical hysterectomy, pelvic lymphadenectomy, and postoperative pelvic radiation (4,000 to 5,000 rad) (Martinbeau, Kjorstad, and Iversen 1982). All 562 patients except 20 with tumors < 2 cm had radium treatment before surgery. It is probable that the 53% five-year survival rate achieved by postoperative irradiation in this series is not significantly different from that which would have been achieved by no postoperative therapy. All of these studies suffer from lack of knowledge of the status of the paraaortic lymph nodes, and most patients received amounts of radiation (≤ 4,500 rad) insufficient to achieve a 90% or greater control rate.

Of special interest is the report by Rubin et al. (1984) of 14 patients with clinically staged early cervical cancer (13, stage IB; 1, stage II) with histologically documented paraaortic lymph node metastasis treated with 4,000 to 6,000 rad of whole-pelvis irradiation, 3,000 rad intracavitary radium (one patient underwent hysterectomy and received no radium), and 4,000 to 5,000 rad paraaortic irradiation. The five-year survival rate with no evidence of disease was 43% (six patients), which was not significantly lower than that reported for patients with stage IB carcinoma of the cervix treated with postoperative pelvic radiation for known pelvic lymph node metastasis. (This five-year survival rate includes one patient alive with no evidence of disease for only three years.) Of the remaining eight patients, two (14%) are alive after recurrence, five (36%) died of cervical cancer, and one (7%) patient died of complications with no evidence of disease. In a contrasting report from the Norwegian Radium Hospital, 6 of 562 (1.1%) patients with stage IB carcinoma of the cervix had paraaortic lymph node metastasis documented at the time of radical hysterectomy and pelvic lymphadenectomy. These six patients were treated with 5,000 rad of pelvic and paraaortic radiation but did not have the advantage of

Table 19.5. *Stage IB Cervical Cancer Pelvic Nodal Metastasis*

Positive Nodes	Five-Year Survival NED			
	Radiation		No Radiation	
	N	%	*N*	%
1	14	50	42	69
2–3	9	67	58	71
4–5	1	0	25	32
>5	6	83	19	37
Total	30	60	144	59

Source: Adapted from Morrow (for the Society of Gynecologic Oncologists) 1980.

intracavitary radium. All six developed a recurrence, and five died (Martinbeau, Kjorstad, and Iversen 1982).

Stage II, III, and IV Cervical Cancer

Nine studies reported 1,339 women with stage II, III, and IV cervical cancer who underwent surgical staging by paraaortic lymphadenectomy before radiation therapy (table 19.6). Of the 675 women with stage II cervical cancer, 16% had documented paraaortic lymph node metastasis. This percentage increased to 28% for the 589 stage III patients and to 33% for the stage IV patients. It is clear, therefore, that with increasing stage there is increasing incidence of metastasis, not only to the pelvic lymph nodes but also to the paraaortic lymph nodes.

In almost all instances, cervical cancer spreads orderly and predictably from the cervix to the pelvic lymph nodes to the paraaortic lymph nodes and finally to non–lymph node distant sites. Only rarely are the paraaortic lymph node metastases associated with non–lymph node metastases. Of 100 patients who underwent paraaortic lymphadenectomy for cervical cancer (Piver 1977), 28 had metastasis to the paraaortic lymph nodes and only 3 had systemic spread of their disease, 2 to the liver and 1 to the omentum. All patients had metastasis to the paraaortic lymph nodes. Thus, no patient had systemic spread without concomitant paraaortic lymph node metastasis. In a similar study, Wharton et al. (1977) performed paraaortic lymphadenectomy staging on 120 women with cervical cancer, and only 4 (3.3%) had disease that had spread outside of the lymph nodes. Sites of metastases were the ovary (1), terminal ileum (1), omentum (1), and sigmoid colon (1).

Unfortunately, the results of radiation treatment in patients documented as having paraaortic lymph node metastases from cervical cancer have been disappointing. My colleagues and I (1981) reported 31 women with biopsy-confirmed aortic lymph

Table 19.6. *Paraaortic Node Metastasis in Stage II, III, and IV Cervical Cancer*

	Stage					
	II		III		IV	
Study	*N*	%+	*N*	%+	*N*	%+
Sudarsanam et al. 1978	43	16	19	15	3	0
Buchsbaum 1979	19	5	104	32	10	40
Nelson et al. 1977	63	14	39	38	2	0
Rutledge[a]	50	14	41	34	1	0
Piver 1977	44	13	49	36	7	57
Hughes et al. 1980	80	17	96	23	23	43
Berman et al. 1984[b]	265	16	180	25	17	17
Ballon et al. 1981	48	18	23	17	—	—
Welander et al. 1981	63	20	38	26	12	13
Total	675	16	589	28	75	33

Note: + = positive.
[a] Rutledge as quoted by Lewis 1975.
[b] For the Gynecologic Oncology Group.

node metastasis from carcinoma of the uterine cervix treated with pelvic and paraaortic radiation. Of the 31 patients, the initial patients received radium plus 6,000 rad split-course irradiation to the pelvis and paraaortic area. Because the complication rate was so high in this series, subsequent patients received 4,400 to 5,000 rad paraaortic radiation and 5,000 to 6,000 rad pelvic radiation and intracavitary radium. The intestinal complication rate in those patients who received 6,000 rad split-course radiation in eight weeks was 59.2% but only 10% for the patients treated by 4,400 to 5,000 rad in four and one-half to five weeks.

The five-year survival rate for the 31 patients with no evidence of disease was only 9.6%. A death rate of 16.1% was owed to complications of treatment (with no evidence of recurrent cervical cancer) and one of 74.1% to cervical cancer. Survival was related to the status of the tumor within the paraaortic lymph node metastasis. Of the nine women with microscopic evidence of aortic node metastasis in clinically negative aortic nodes, two are surviving with no evidence of disease after five years, but seven have died of cervical cancer. Six women had a single, clinically positive aortic lymph node metastasis, and only one of them is alive with no evidence of disease after five years. Thus, 3 of 15 patients with microscopic metastasis or a single known metastasis are alive with no evidence of disease at five years compared with none of 16 with multiple paraaortic lymph node metastases. All 16 women with multiple lymph node metastases died of cervical cancer, including 6 patients who had 100% resection of the multiple paraaortic lymph node metastases before receiving radiation.

Wharton and coauthors (1977) reported 24 patients with biopsy-proven aortic lymph node metastasis treated with pelvic radiation and paraaortic radiation delivering 5,500 rad (850 rad/day) to T12. Only 3 (13%) are alive without disease; 13 (54%) are dead or alive with cervical cancer and 8 (33%) are dead of complications—percentages not dissimilar to those I reported with Barlow and Krishnamsetty (1981).

Finally, in a series of 23 women with cervical cancer with biopsy-proven aortic node metastasis, Tewfik et al. (1982) reported a 23% life-table survival rate, 65% dead of cervical cancer, 4% dead of complications but no evidence of disease, and 8% dead of intercurrent disease with no evidence of disease. Of note, however, is that the authors had another 20 patients who had biopsy-confirmed aortic node metastasis but apparently were not treated with paraaortic radiation. Thus, of their 43 women with paraaortic lymph node metastases, only 11% are known to have survived five years, a percentage nearly equal to that we (Piver, Barlow, and Krishnamsetty 1981) and Wharton and coauthors (1977) found.

Most probably, those patients with paraaortic lymph node metastasis that can be cured by extended field irradiation are those with minimal metastasis to the paraaortic lymph nodes and those with a limited volume of pelvic tumor. Relevant to the latter is the recent report of Nori, Valentine, and Hilaris (1985). They treated 27 patients with 4,400 rad of paraaortic radiation plus a 600 to 800 rad boost to the area of known paraaortic lymph node metastasis. Although they reported a 29% five-year survival rate, all eight survivors had stage I and II cervical cancer (International Federation of Gynecology and Obstetrics staging), whereas none of the stage III or IV patients survived five years, findings similar to those reported by Rubin et al. (1984).

It is clear that intraperitoneal surgical staging by paraaortic lymph node biopsy followed by high-dose (5,500–6,000 rad) paraaortic radiation results in a postoperative complication rate and mortality that are too high and survival rates that are too low. Whether doses in the range of 4,500 rad over five weeks will result in a decreased complication rate and a concomitant increase in survival rates is still problematic. Those with numerous paraaortic lymph node metastases probably have systemic spread of the disease undetected at the time of surgical staging that will require systemic therapy (chemotherapy), and none is known at this time.

In an interesting study of 71 patients with stage IIB, 69 patients with stage III, and 11 patients with stage IV cervical cancer treated at the Norwegian Radium Hospital 1975–1977 without pretherapy paraaortic lymph node biopsy, all received paraaortic radiation in addition to pelvic radiation (Kolstad 1983). The three- to five-year survival rate for those patients treated by radium and pelvic and paraaortic radiation was 54% compared with only 0% to 18% for those treated with pelvic and paraaortic radiation without intracavitary radium (table 19.7). The intestinal complication rate was extremely low: seven (4.6%) developed gastric ulcers and only two (1.3%) developed intestinal obstruction and perforation, probably related to the nonperformance of pretherapy surgical staging by paraaortic lymphadenectomy. This complication rate was comparable to the 45.1% my coworkers and I reported (Piver, Barlow, and Krishnamsetty 1981) and the 33.0% reported by Wharton and coauthors (1977).

For stage IIB and IIIB cervical cancer the mean incidence of pelvic lymph node metastasis is 30% and 50%, respectively. My colleagues and I found that these occurrences can be controlled in over 90% of the cases by utilizing hydroxyurea and pelvic irradiation in patients whose pelvic lymph nodes are found to be negative either by pretherapy surgical staging or pretherapy lymphangiography (Piver et al. 1983; Piver, Krishnamsetty, and Emrich 1985; Piver, Vongtama, and Emrich, in press).

Table 19.7. *Elective Paraaortic Radiation for Stage IIB, III, and IV Cervical Cancer at the Norwegian Radium Hospital*

Treatment	No. of Patients	Three- to Five-Year Survival *N*	Three- to Five-Year Survival (%)
5,000 pelvic and paraaortic radiation plus radium	121	65	(54)
5,000 pelvic and paraaortic radiation	22	4	(18)
6,000 pelvic and 5,000 paraaortic radiation	8	0	(0)
Total	151	69	(46)

Source: Kolstad 1983.

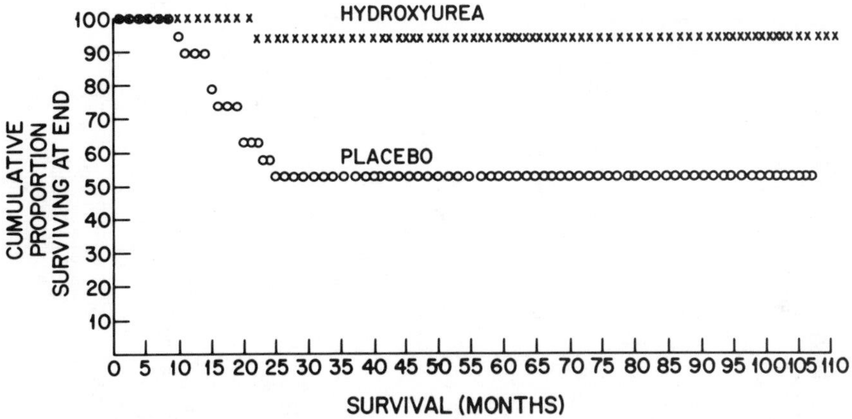

Fig. 19.1. Duration of survival of 40 patients with stage IIB cervical cancer. Reprinted, by permission, from *Am J Obstet Gynecol* 1983; 147:803–808.

Our first study, performed from June 1972 to December 1976, included 40 patients with FIGO stage IIB carcinoma of the uterine cervix in a prospective double-blind randomized evaluation of possible radiation-potentiating properties (i.e., those of the S-phase cell cycle–specific inhibitor of DNA synthesis) of hydroxyurea (Piver et al. 1983). All patients were documented to be without aortic lymph node metastasis by pretherapy paraaortic lymphadenectomy. All patients were followed for longer than five years (5.2–9.2 years) or until death.

The double-blind code was not broken until all patients had been followed for a minimum of two years. Patients received 5,000 rad pelvic radiation over five weeks plus intracavitary radium. During irradiation and for 12 weeks, patients received hydroxyurea (80 mg/kg body weight) every 3 days. The life-table survival rate of patients given hydroxyurea was 94%, compared with 53% for patients given a placebo ($p = .006$) (fig. 19.1). Only one patient (5%) given hydroxyurea died of cervical cancer. All other patients receiving hydroxyurea who died were confirmed by postmortem examination to be without recurrent cervical cancer. In contrast, nine (45%) of the patients given placebo plus pelvic irradiation died of cervical cancer.

In our second study, 20 patients with stage IIB carcinoma of the cervix did not undergo pretherapy paraaortic lymphadenectomy but had negative results on preirradiation lymphangiograms (Piver, Krishnamsetty, and Emrich 1985). All patients were treated with pelvic radiation and hydroxyurea. Patients received a median of 5,020 rad of pelvic radiation and 4,000 rad of radium to point A.

The estimated five-year survival rate was 92% (fig. 19.2). Seventeen patients are alive with no evidence of disease, one is alive with no evidence of disease after recurrence, one died of intercurrent disease with no evidence of disease, and one died of cervical cancer at 22 months. Thus, the survival rate of patients who were nonsurgically staged and had negative results on pretherapy lymphangiograms and had

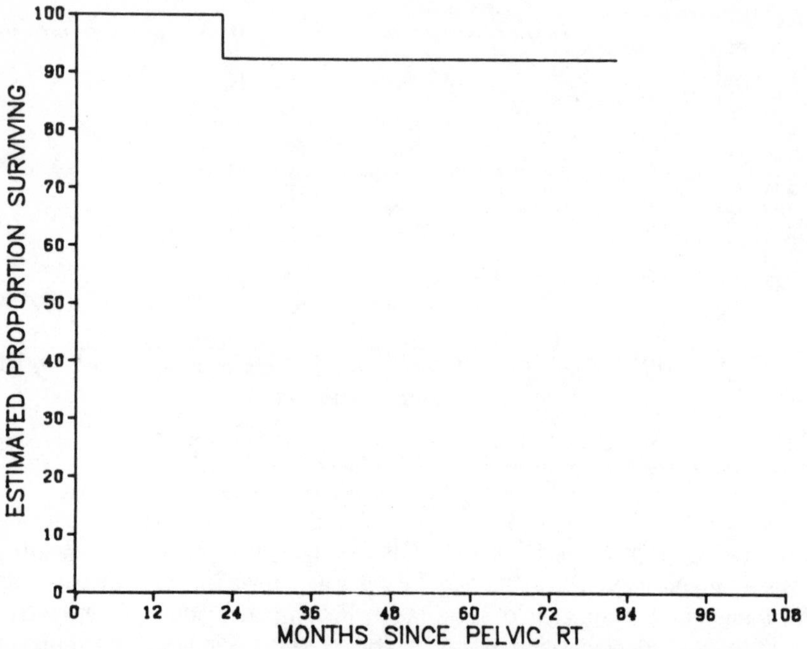

Fig. 19.2. Disease-free survival rate in 20 nonsurgically staged patients with negative results on lymphangiograms who had stage IIB carcinoma of the cervix treated by pelvic radiation and hydroxyurea. Reprinted, by permission, from *Am J Obstet Gynecol* 1985; 151:1006–1008.

stage IIB cervical cancer treated by pelvic radiation and hydroxyurea approximated the improved survival rate for patients with negative pretherapy paraaortic lymphadenectomy who were treated with paraaortic radiation and hydroxyurea. Moreover, no patient developed a recurrence within the treated field.

The third study included patients with FIGO stage IIIB cervical cancer, all of whom had surgically established negative paraaortic lymph nodes before radiation and were randomized to hydroxyurea and 6,000 rad of radiation over six weeks or placebo plus 6,000 rad of radiation in six weeks (Piver et al. 1985). The five-year disease-free survival rate was 91% for the group receiving hydroxyurea plus radiation therapy compared with 60% for the group receiving placebo and radiation therapy (fig. 19.3). Of the 52 patients in these trials who received pelvic radiation and hydroxyurea, only 1 patient (1.9%) developed a central pelvic recurrence (table 19.8).

To date there are no known trials using chemotherapy in an attempt to control large paraaortic lymph node metastases from cervical cancer. My colleagues and I (Piver, Lele, and Malfetano in press) treated nine patients with known large metastases to the paraaortic lymph nodes discovered at the time of surgical staging in the following protocol: patients underwent pretherapy surgical staging and were found to have large metastases to the paraaortic lymph nodes. Postoperatively, patients received 5,040 rad of pelvic radiation plus cisplatin at a dose of 1 mg/kg/wk during

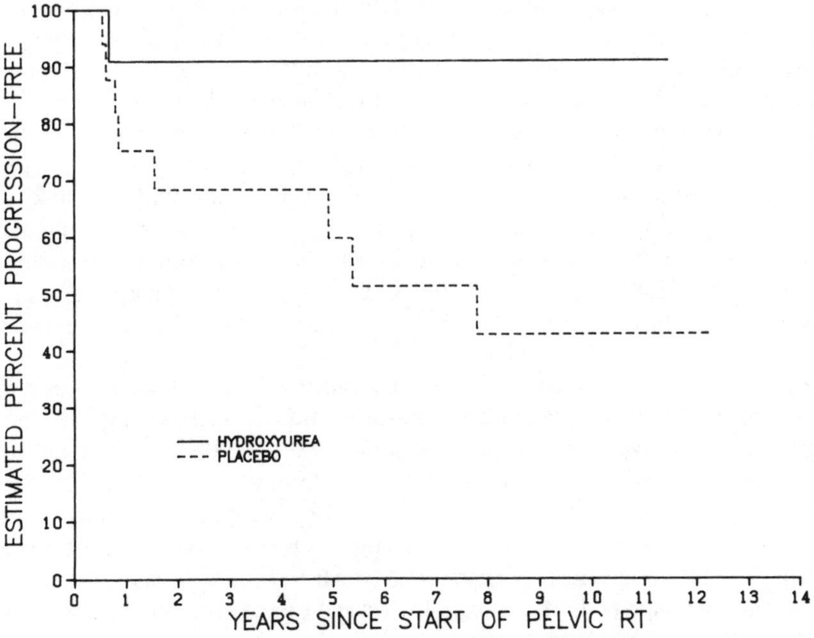

Fig. 19.3. Duration of progression-free survival for 29 patients with stage IIIB cervical cancer treated by continuous-course pelvic radiation. Reprinted, by permission, from *J Surg Oncol* (in press).

Table 19.8. *Pelvic Recurrence Rate in Cervical Cancer after Pelvic Radiation and Hydroxyurea Treatment*

Stage	Paraaortic Nodes	No. of Patients	Pelvic Recurrence
IIB	Negative lymphadenectomy	20	1[a]
IIB	Negative lymphangiogram	20	0
IIIB	Negative lymphadenectomy	12[b]	0
Total		52	1 (1.9%)

[a] Recurrence rectosigmoid.
[b] Recurrence breast.

radiation therapy. Cisplatin was to act as a radiation sensitizer and systemic chemotherapy agent to control paraaortic lymph node metastasis. Radiation was followed by monthly cisplatin, doxorubicin HCl, and cyclophosphamide. Seventy-eight percent of the patients had complete remission of central disease, but only 22% remain alive with no evidence of disease; the remainder have uncontrolled distant metastases (Piver, Malfetano, and Lele in press).

Based on the data presented, preventing recurrence in patients with pelvic lymph node metastasis discovered at the time of planned radical hysterectomy would entail the following: If clinically positive pelvic lymph nodes are present, they should be excised and documented to be positive by frozen section. If positive, a staging paraaortic lymphadenectomy should be carried out and the uterus left in situ for intracavitary treatment with radium or cesium. If the paraaortic lymph nodes are negative, patients should undergo pelvic irradiation ≥ 5,000 rad over five weeks plus radium with or without a radiation sensitizer (hydroxyurea). If the pelvic lymph nodes are found to be microscopically positive only after radical hysterectomy and bilateral pelvic lymphadenectomy (i.e., microscopic metastasis), then a minimum of 5,500 rad in five and one-half to six weeks with or without hydroxyurea should be delivered. In an ideal situation, reoperation by retroperitoneal paraaortic lymphadenectomy should be carried out to be certain that there is no disease above the pelvis.

For patients with stage IIB or IIIB cervical cancer who have no evidence of metastasis to the paraaortic lymph nodes by paraaortic lymphadenectomy or lymphangiography, the five-year survival rates with 5,000 to 6,000 rad pelvic radiation and intracavitary radium and hydroxyurea ranged from 91% to 94%, and local pelvic control was achieved in 98.1%. These results highly suggest that control of central pelvic tumor and pelvic lymph node metastasis by this treatment is nearly universal. Patients with microscopic paraaortic lymph node metastasis or metastasis to the paraaortic lymph nodes from stage IB cervical cancer discovered at the time of pretherapy surgical staging by paraaortic lymphadenectomy may have their disease controlled in a small but not insignificant number of cases by pelvic and paraaortic irradiation. However, patients with large or several paraaortic lymph node metastases most likely have systemic metastases at the time of pretherapy staging paraaortic lymphadenectomy and require systemic chemotherapy, a method of therapy still being evaluated.

References

Ballon SC, Berman ML, Lagasse LD, Petrilli ES, Castaldo TW. 1981. Survival after extraperitoneal pelvic and paraaortic lymphadenectomy and radiation therapy in cervical carcinoma. *Obstet Gynecol* 57:90–95.

Berman ML, Keys H, Creasman W, DiSaia P, Bundy B, Blessing J. 1984. Survival and patterns of recurrence in cervical cancer metastatic to periaortic lymph nodes. *Gynecol Oncol* 19:8–16.

Buchsbaum HJ. 1979. Extrapelvic lymph node metastases in cervical carcinoma. *Am J Obstet Gynecol* 133:814–824.

Burch JC, Chalfant RL. 1970. Preoperative radium, irradiation and radical hysterectomy in the treatment of cancer of the cervix. *Am J Obstet Gynecol* 106:1054–1064.

Delgado G, Caglar H, Walker P. 1978. Survival and complications in cervical cancer treated by pelvic and extended field radiation after paraaortic lymphadenectomy. *Am J Roentgenol* 130:141–143.

Himmelmann A, Holmberg E, Jansson I, Odén A, Skogsberg K. 1985. The effect of postoperative external radiotherapy on cervical carcinoma stage IB and IIA. *Gynecol Oncol* 22:73–84.

Hsu CT, Cheng YS, Su SC. 1972. Prognosis of uterine cervical cancer with extensive lymph node metastasis. *Am J Obstet Gynecol* 114:954–962.

Hughes RR, Brewington KC, Hanjani P, Photopulous G, Dick D, Votava C, Moran M, Coleman S. 1980. Extended field irradiation for cervical cancer based on surgical staging. *Gynecol Oncol* 9:153–161.

Kelso JW, Funnell JD. 1973. Combined surgical radiation treatment of invasive carcinoma of the cervix. *Am J Obstet Gynecol* 116:205–213.

Kjorstad KE, Kolbenstvedt ALF, Strickert T. The value of complete lymphadenectomy in radical treatment of cancer of the cervix, stage IB. *Cancer* 54:2215–2219.

Kolstad P. 1983. Value and complications of periaortic irradiation in advanced cervical cancer. In *Recent Clinical Developments in Gynecologic Oncology*, ed. C. Paul Morrow. New York: Raven Press.

Lewis JL. 1975. Cancer of the cervix: Prognostic factors in the response to therapy. In *Cancer Therapy: Prognostic Factors and Criteria of Response*, ed. MJ Staquet. New York: Raven Press.

Martimbeau PW, Kjorstad KE, Iversen T. 1982. Stage IB carcinoma of the cervix. The Norwegian Radium Hospital: II. Results when pelvic nodes are involved. *Obstet Gynecol* 60:215–218.

Masubuchi K, Tenjin Y, Kubo H, Kimura M. 1969. Five-year cure rate for carcinoma of the cervix uteri. *Am J Obstet Gynecol* 103:566–573.

Morrow CP. 1980. Panel report: Is pelvic radiation beneficial in the postoperative management of stage IB squamous cell carcinoma of the cervix with pelvic node metastasis treated by radical hysterectomy and pelvic lymphadenectomy? *Gynecol Oncol* 10:105–110.

Nelson JH, Boyce J, Macasaet M, Lu T, Bohorquez JF, Nicastri AD, Fruchter R. 1977. Incidence, significance, and follow-up of paraaortic lymph node metastases in late invasive carcinoma of the cervix. *Am J Obstet Gynecol* 128:336–340.

Nori D, Valentine E, Hilaris BS. 1985. The role of paraaortic node irradiation in the treatment of cancer of the cervix. *Int J Radiat Oncol Biol Phys* 11:1469–1473.

Piver MS. 1977. The value of pretherapy paraaortic lymphadenectomy for carcinoma of the cervix uteri. *Surg Gynecol Obstet* 145:17–18.

Piver MS, Barlow JJ, Krishnamsetty R. 1981. Five-year survival (NED) in patients with biopsy confirmed aortic node metastasis from cervical carcinoma. *Am J Obstet Gynecol* 139:474–478.

Piver MS, Barlow JJ, Vongtama V, Blumenson L. 1983. Hydroxyurea: A radiation potentiator in carcinoma of the uterine cervix. *Am J Obstet Gynecol* 147:803–808.

Piver MS, Chung WS. 1975. Prognostic significance of cervical lesion size and pelvic node metastasis in cervical carcinoma. *Obstet Gynecol* 46:507–510.

Piver MS, Krishnamsetty RM, Emrich LJ. 1985. Survival of non-surgically staged patients with negative lymphangiograms who had stage IIB carcinoma of the cervix treated by pelvic radiation plus hydroxyurea. *Am J Obstet Gynecol* 151:1006–1008.

Piver MS, Lele SB, Malfetano J. In press. *Cis*-diamminedichloroplatinum II-based combination chemotherapy for control of extensive paraaortic lymph node metastases in cervical cancer. *Gynecol Oncol.*

Piver MS, Vongtama V, Emrich LJ. In press. Hydroxyurea plus pelvic radiation versus placebo plus pelvic radiation in surgically staged stage IIIB cervical cancer. *J Surg Oncol.*

Rampone JF, Klem V, Kolstad P. 1973. Combined treatment of stage IB carcinoma of the cervix. *Obstet Gynecol* 41:163–167.

Rubin SC, Brookland R, Mikuta JJ, Mangan C, Sutton G, Danoff B. 1984. Paraaortic nodal metastases in early cervical carcinoma: Long-term survival following extended field radiotherapy. *Gynecol Oncol* 18:213–217.

Sudarsanam A, Charyulu K, Belinson J, Averette H, Goldberg M, Hintz B, Thirumala M, Ford J. 1978. Influence of exploratory celiotomy on the management of carcinoma of the cervix. *Cancer* 41:1049–1053.

Tewfik HH, Buchsbaum HJ, Latourette HB, Lifshitz SG, Tewfik FA. 1981. Para-aortic lymph node irradiation in carcinoma of the cervix after exploratory laparotomy and biopsy-proven positive aortic nodes. *Int J Radiat Oncol Biol Phys* 8:13–18.

Welander CE, Pierce VK, Nori D, Hilaris BS, Kosloff C, Clark DG, Jones WB, Kim WS, Lewis JL Jr. 1981. Pretreatment laparotomy in carcinoma of the cervix. *Gynecol Oncol* 12:336–347.

Wharton JT, Jones HW III, Day TG Jr. 1977. Preirradiation celiotomy and extended field irradiation for invasive carcinoma of the cervix. *Obstet Gynecol* 49:333–338.

Annual Clinical Conference on Cancer, Vol. 29
Gynecologic Cancer: Diagnosis and Treatment Strategies
© 1987 by The University of Texas System Cancer Center

20. Intraoperative Irradiation in Advanced Cervical Cancer

Gregorio Delgado, Alfred L. Goldson, Ebrahim Ashayeri, and Edmund S. Petrilli

The incidence of invasive cancer of the cervix uteri has steadily decreased in North America since the turn of the century, primarily as a result of screening procedures (National Cancer Institute 1972). In underdeveloped countries, however, this cancer remains a primary medical problem. In Latin America, for example, the mortality is very high (Olivares 1981). Further, the impact of cervical cancer on individual lives is greater than statistics would indicate, particularly since cervical cancer occurs at a young age and appears more frequently in women with many children (Castellano 1975).

Conventional treatment of cervical cancer, such as radical hysterectomy with lymphadenectomy or pelvic exenteration, is limited to the pelvis. Standard radiotherapeutic treatment is a combination of external-beam radiotherapy to the pelvis and intracavitary applications. However, there is a group of patients for whom external radiotherapy alone has limitations. This group consists primarily of patients with large pelvic lymph nodes containing metastatic cancer, metastatically involved paraaortic lymph nodes outside the usual pelvic radiation field, or large central tumors with parametrial involvement (Buchsbaum 1972; Wharton et al. 1977).

In patients with cancer of the cervix, the incidence of metastasis to paraaortic lymph nodes is high (Delgado, Smith, and Ballantyne 1975; Delgado, Caglar, and Walter 1978). Attempts to treat paraaortic nodes with external radiotherapy have resulted in high complication rates because the treatment field includes the highly sensitive gastrointestinal tract (Delgado, Caglar, and Walter 1978; Wharton et al. 1977; Fletcher and Rutledge 1972; Lepanto et al. 1975). External radiation therapy after retroperitoneal exploration of lymph nodes does not seem to improve survival.

In an attempt to circumvent the morbidity and mortality associated with conventional external-beam irradiation, we initiated a pilot study of intraoperative electron-beam irradiation of the paraaortic nodes and of the large metastatic lymph nodes in the pelvis (Goldson, Delgado, and Hill 1978; Delgado et al. 1984). The intraoperative boost was followed by conventional fractionated external-beam irradiation. The theoretical advantages of this procedure include a higher radiation tumor dose without a concomitant increase in treatment morbidity and mortality.

Intraoperative radiotherapy (IORT) was used in the earliest days of radiotherapy in Europe and the United States (Finsterer 1915; Henschke and Henschke 1944; Barth 1959; Fuchs and Ueberal 1969; Beck 1919; Eloesser 1937; Pack and Livingston 1940), but small fields and low penetration of the beam from the ultravoltage therapy units in use at that time restricted its application. Consequently, no significant clinical series were accumulated. The current revival of IORT was initiated with the work of Abe (Abe et al. 1975, 1980) in Japan and with our work in Washington, D.C., at Howard University Hospital and Georgetown University Hospital (Delgado et al. 1984; Goldson, Delgado, and Hill 1978).

In IORT, or direct-view irradiation, radiosensitive structures are mobilized and retracted away from the radiation field, so that the procedure is performed by a surgery-radiotherapy team. An external beam of radiation with electrons that have a sharp and rapid falloff in depth doses is delivered during the operation to the surgically exposed tumor (Delgado et al. 1984). Because the tumor area is visualized directly, an accurate treatment determination can be made. Sufficiently high doses of radiation can be delivered to the parametrium and paraaortic and pelvic nodes without affecting other tissues and organs, such as the bowel, bladder, and rectum.

Methods

Nineteen patients with advanced cervical cancer underwent IORT after a staging laparotomy. Sixteen of these patients had primary cancer and three had recurrent cancer. Only patients with stage II, III, or IV disease or recurrent cancer were selected for the study.

All patients underwent a clinical staging procedure that included physical examination, chest X ray, intravenous pyelography, cystoscopy, colon X ray (barium enema), proctoscopy, lymphangiography, and computed tomography when clinically indicated. When the lymphangiogram was positive for disease in nodes, needle biopsies of the paraaortic nodes were attempted.

All 16 patients with primary cancer received IORT to one or more of the following areas: pelvic nodes, parametrium, and pelvic sidewall. When this intraoperative protocol was first initiated, only the paraaortic node area was treated.

Three patients presented with pelvic and leg pain as a result of the recurrence, confirmed histologically by surgery, of cervical carcinoma to the pelvic sidewall. Two years before, these three patients had been treated for stage II or III cervical carcinoma with external irradiation and intracavitary radium. For palliation, irradiation was now given intraoperatively at the sites of recurrence.

After clinical staging, the patients were taken to the IORT facility for surgery.

The Surgical-Radiotherapeutic Suite

Radiotherapy Equipment

At Howard University, a radiotherapy suite with supervoltage capacity was converted into an operating facility (fig. 20.1). A modified surgical suite includes the radiation shielding required to accommodate a Varian Clinac 18-MeV linear accelerator, which was chosen because it has electron-beam capabilities of 6, 9, 12, 15, and 18 MeV.

The electron beam has the ideal characteristics for IORT. The sharp and rapid

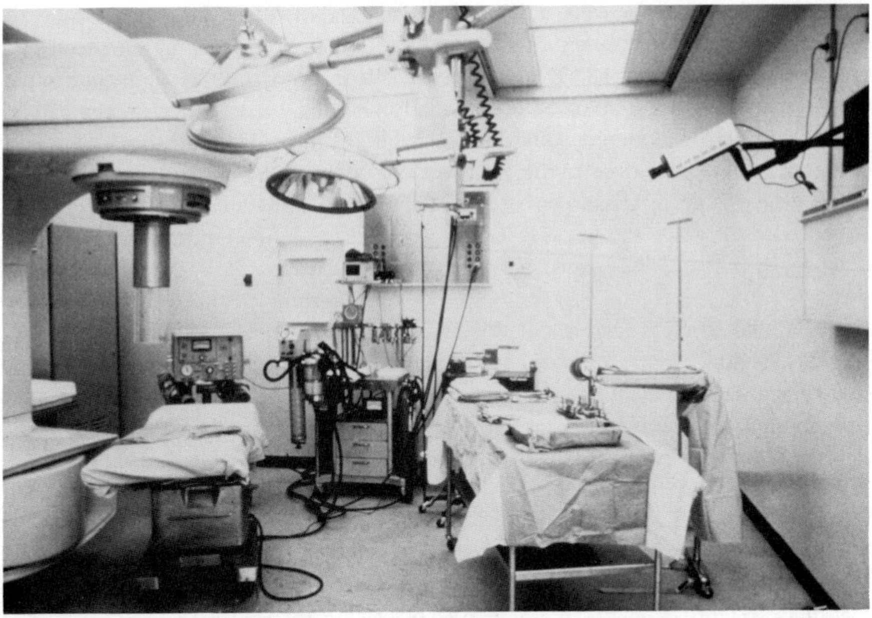

Fig. 20.1. Intraoperative radiation therapy suite equipped for any type of major surgery. Note the 18-MeV linear accelerator. Reprinted with permission from the American College of Obstetricians and Gynecologists (*Obstet Gynecol* 1978; 52 [6]:714).

falloff in depth doses protects the tissue behind the tumor. Loss of skin sparing is not a problem with IORT, because the skin is retracted out of the path of the electron beam. Treatment times are short, on the order of a few minutes.

Specially designed intraoperative treatment collimators (or "beam-sharpers") were fabricated for this unique treatment procedure. The electron collimator consists of an anodized or hard-coated outer aluminum collimator and a telescoping inner Lucite collimator; both components are 30 cm long and have walls that are one fourth of an inch thick. The two collimators overlap by 10 cm. The Lucite collimator is constructed so that it provides clear visualization of the tumor and confirmation that normal tissue has not drifted into the treatment field. The Lucite collimator also acts as a secondary retractor device by providing a physical barrier between surrounding normal tissue and the treatment field. The inner Lucite portion can telescope into the aluminum section for a distance of 20 cm before stopping. This characteristic prevents undue static pressure against structures that the collimator may rest upon during the IORT procedure. The treatment collimators come in various circular diameters and are also made in rectangular and square shapes. The aluminum portion of the collimator is autoclaved and the Lucite portion is gas sterilized. Both segments are numbered and stored in cabinets in the IORT suite. The anticrush, gravity-oriented aluminum and Lucite applicators have been fabricated with three different field sites (10 x 6, 15 x 6, and 8 x 4 cm^2).

The electron beam delivers its effective dose in a few centimeters of tissue, with a rapid dose falloff beyond this critical distance. The effective dose range in centimeters of tissue is determined by the amount of energy delivered by the electrons, which is 6, 9, 12, 15, or 18 MeV in this case. By applying this physical value to the known thickness of the involved nodes, the lowest possible effective energy can be selected to give a homogeneous dose distribution throughout the treatment area while minimizing the dose to the great vessels in the spinal cord. A homogeneous tumor dose of single exposure is calculated at an 80% isodose curve and is delivered at approximately 500 rad per minute.

Surgical Equipment

Conventional surgical instrumentation is used in carrying out retroperitoneal dissection around the paraaortic and pelvic areas that are predicted by the primary tumor's histology and anatomic location. The standard metal retractors, Metzenbaum scissors, and tissue and hemostatic forceps are used during both the surgical procedure and the intraoperative phase of the operation.

Anesthesia Equipment

Standard anesthesia equipment and procedures are followed during surgery and IORT. However, during the short interval during which radiation is administered to the tumor, the anesthesia team, as well as the rest of the surgical team, must leave the room. Additional anesthesia equipment has been installed in the specialized surgical unit at Howard: a second multichannel oscilloscope capable of remotely monitoring arterial blood pressure, respirations, electrocardiogram, and pulse rate. Beyond this, no extraordinary anesthesia equipment is required.

Procedures and Techniques

A surgical-radiotherapeutic team approach is essential for a favorable outcome with the procedure. Preoperative consultation among the team members provides an invaluable exchange of ideas, plans of therapy, surgical approaches, and suggestions for positioning the patient and for the optimum site of placement and extent of the surgical incision. The surgeon must understand clearly all the capabilities of the intraoperative equipment; his determination of the base exposure upon which the radiotherapist will perform the IORT is dependent on his knowledge of the size and flexibility of the intraoperative cones.

Intraoperative Irradiation of Paraaortic Areas

A paraaortic lymphadenectomy or paraaortic node biopsies were performed in this series as follows: The peritoneum was opened at the level of the bifurcation of the aorta and extended cephalad for 5 cm. The mesentery of the small bowel was retracted and the aorta and vena cava visualized. After the right ureter and the ovarian blood vessels were identified and retracted laterally, the fatty tissue containing the lymph nodes anterior and lateral to the vena cava was carefully dissected and removed. A similar dissection was performed on the left side, anterior and lateral to the aorta. The dissection was performed about 5 to 8 cm above the bifurcation of the

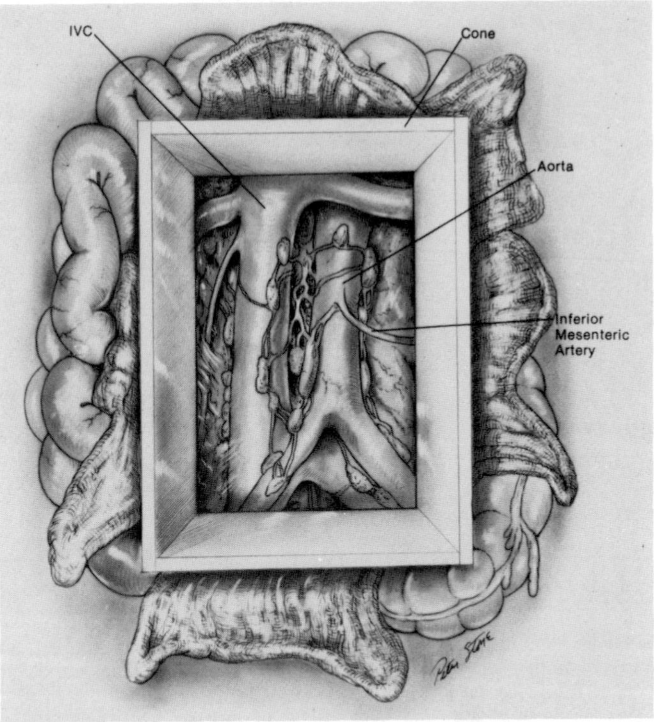

Fig. 20.2. The rectangular cone covering the lymph nodes in the aortic area. Reprinted with permission from the American College of Obstetricians and Gynecologists (*Obstet Gynecol* 1984; 63 [2]:247).

aorta. Metallic clips were placed at the highest area of dissection. When the lymph nodes were large and fixed to the vena cava, only biopsies were performed.

The peritoneum parallel and lateral to the descending colon was opened, and pulled medially for better exposure. After the aorta was exposed, biopsy was performed on lymph nodes suggesting metastatic tumor and the area marked with hemoclips (Piver and Barlow 1973; Delgado et al. 1977; Ucmakli and Bonney 1972).

Before IORT was administered, the skin, small bowel, and uninvolved visceral structures were retracted out of the field. After the surface area of the region to be irradiated was determined, a collimator of the appropriate size and shape was selected so that it would encompass the area with a 1- to 2-cm margin of normal tissue (fig. 20.2).

After the patient was positioned under the linear accelerator unit, the clear Lucite section of the treatment applicator was connected to the anodized aluminum portion of the applicator that had been attached to the collimator head of the accelerator (10 x 4 cm) (fig. 20.3). A maximum dose of 2,500 rad was delivered in four minutes with an electron-beam source of 9 to 12 MeV. Before leaving the treatment room, the anesthesiologist checked the patient's vital signs and the surgeon assessed the pa-

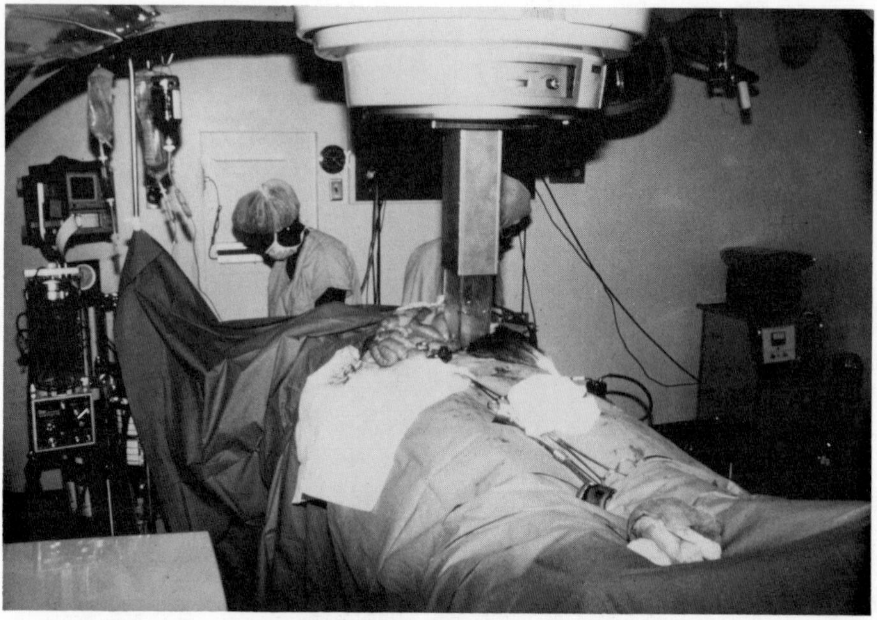

Fig. 20.3. The Lucite cone is attached to the 18-MeV linear accelerator and is ready for treatment. Reprinted with permission from the American College of Obstetricians and Gynecologists (*Obstet Gynecol* 1978; 52 [6]:715).

tient's hemostatic status. After confirming the patient's stability, all members of the team left the IORT suite. The anesthesiologist monitored the patient's vital signs with an oscilloscope mounted inside the treatment control area. If, during the delivery of the intraoperative dose, any abnormalities are noted in the patient's vital signs, the accelerator can be turned off by the anesthesiologist by simply opening the door, allowing immediate entry into the room to assist the patient.

Intraoperative Pelvic Irradiation

After the paraaortic nodes were treated, the bowels were packed upwards and the pelvis was carefully explored. On the left side, the retroperitoneal spaces were entered on top of the psoas muscle and the sigmoid colon was retracted medially, pulled up from its retroperitoneal insertion (fig. 20.4). The ureter was identified and retracted medially. The blood vessels—including the common, external, and internal iliac arteries and veins—were identified. With blunt dissection, the pararectal space was entered medial to the internal iliac artery. The rectum and the rectosigmoid were retracted medially. The vascular space lateral to the bladder was then identified and bluntly dissected medial to the pelvic blood vessels, and the paravesical space was identified. The bladder was then retracted medially. To retract the rectosigmoid, the bladder, and all related tissue, two fingers were used, one placed in the pararectal space and the other in the paravesical space (fig. 20.5). At the same time, the ureter from the pelvic brim to the ureteral vesicle junction was also retracted medially to be sure that it was not included in the IORT field.

Large pelvic nodes were removed for confirmation of metastatic tumor. Dissection of the bladder was performed from the suprapubic space (space of Retzius). The bladder was then detached from the pubic area, bladder pillars were transected, and the bladder was dropped and medially retracted. At this time, the rest of the abdominal viscera were retracted and the treatment cone (6 x 10 or 6 x 15 cm) was introduced after it was ascertained that the previous paraaortic intraoperative field was not overlapped. The field size was selected to cover all of the pelvic nodes from the distal end of the external iliac artery to the bifurcation of the aorta (fig. 20.6). With the rectosigmoid and the bladder retracted medially, the parametrium was included in the radiation field. However, when the viscera to be retracted are very

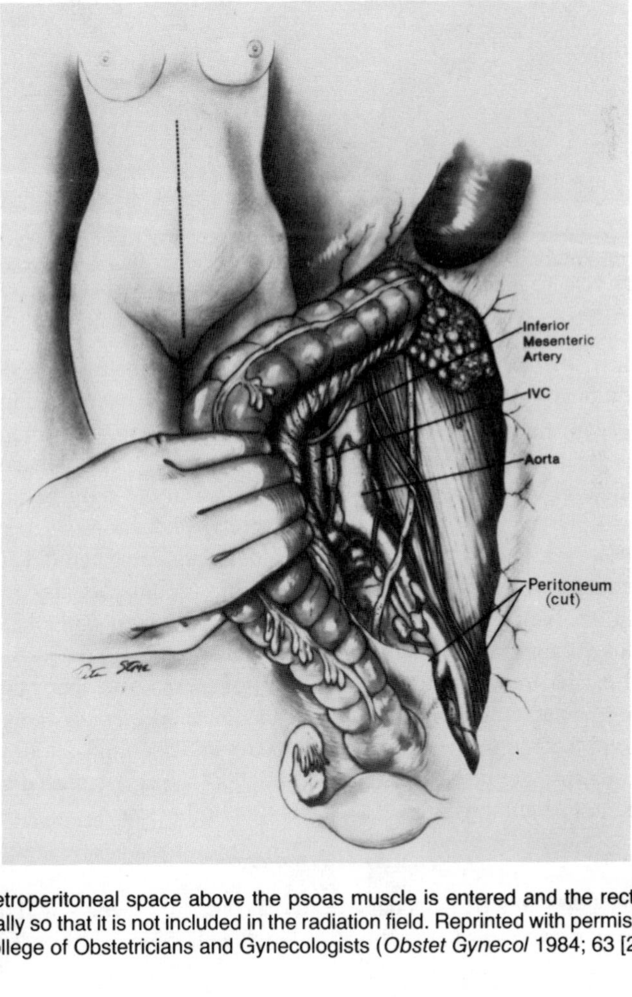

Fig. 20.4. Retroperitoneal space above the psoas muscle is entered and the rectosigmoid retracted medially so that it is not included in the radiation field. Reprinted with permission from the American College of Obstetricians and Gynecologists (*Obstet Gynecol* 1984; 63 [2]:248).

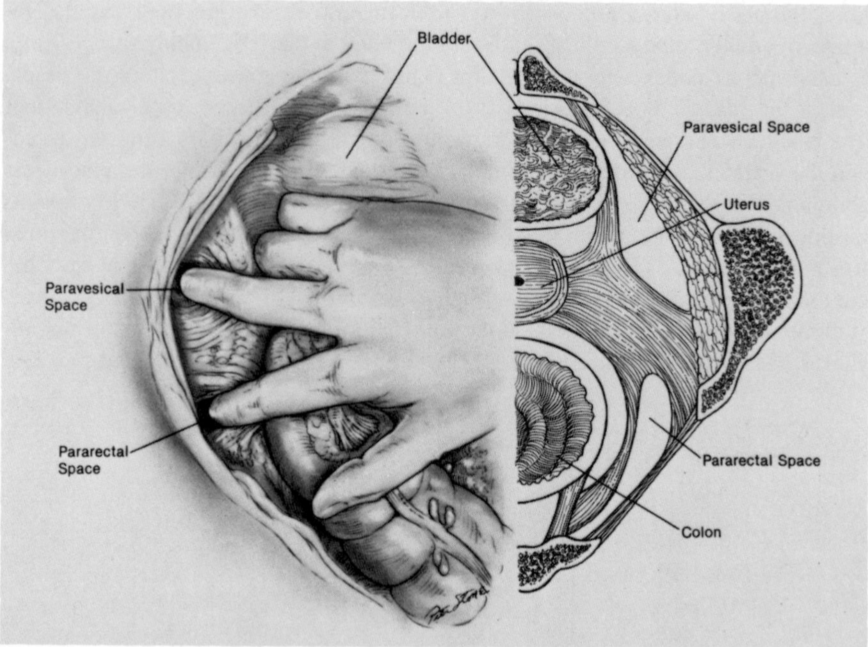

Fig. 20.5. The pararectal and paravesical spaces and the space of Retzius are opened, and the abdominal viscera retracted medially so that they are not included in the radiation field. Reprinted with permission from the American College of Obstetricians and Gynecologists (*Obstet Gynecol* 1984; 63 [2]: 248).

bulky and only a small part of the parametrium can be included in the radiation field, an additional area may be irradiated separately. After the cone had been secured, the patient was again left alone, and an application of a maximum 2,500 rad of IORT was given with a 9- to 12-MeV linear accelerator electron beam.

After irradiation was completed, dissection began in the right pelvic wall. The retroperitoneal spaces were opened, the pararectal and paravesical spaces were opened as described, and all the structures, including the rectosigmoid and the bladder, were retracted (fig. 20.7). In some cases, the cecum was also retracted upwards. Again, the lymph nodes, pelvic wall, and parametrium were placed in a field that would cover the pelvic nodes but not overlap the field from the paraaortic IORT area marked earlier by metallic clips. After all of these structures were separated and retracted, the patient was again put under the linear accelerator and given IORT, monitored from the control room. The peritoneum and abdominal wall were closed by retention sutures. At present, a small lead shield (4 x 6 cm) is placed on top of the psoas muscle to prevent any irradiation of the femoral nerve.

External Irradiation

Ten days after IORT, the patients began external radiation therapy with an 18-MeV linear accelerator; two weeks after this was concluded, they underwent intracavitary cesium applications. In two patients in whom gross examination revealed metastasis in the paraaortic nodes, 2,500 rad of external irradiation was directed toward the area of disease defined at the time of surgery by surgical markers. The radiation portals covered the upper border of the pelvic field with adequate gap and a matchline above the interspace of T12, L1.

A minimum total dose of 4,500 rad was delivered homogeneously to the pelvis in daily doses of 180 to 200 rad (midplane calculation). Four to five fractions were given per week for four to five weeks. Standard anterior and posterior opposing-field arrangements were used unless the clinical situation dictated the need for four-field rotational modification techniques (Fletcher and Rutledge 1972).

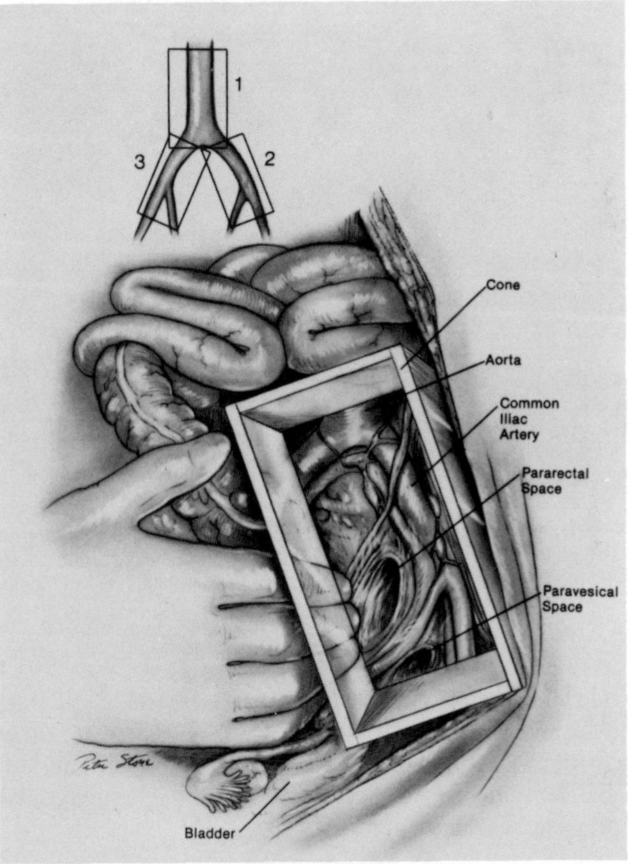

Fig. 20.6. A view (*upper left*) of the three fields covering the lymphatics, the parametrium, and pelvic and paraaortic area (*lower right*). The cone, in this case a rectangular one, is placed so that the parametrium and the lymph nodes will be irradiated after the retroperitoneal spaces have been opened and the rectum, sigmoid, and bladder have been retracted so as not to be included in the radiation field. Reprinted with permission from the American College of Obstetricians and Gynecologists (*Obstet Gynecol* 1984; 63 [2]:249).

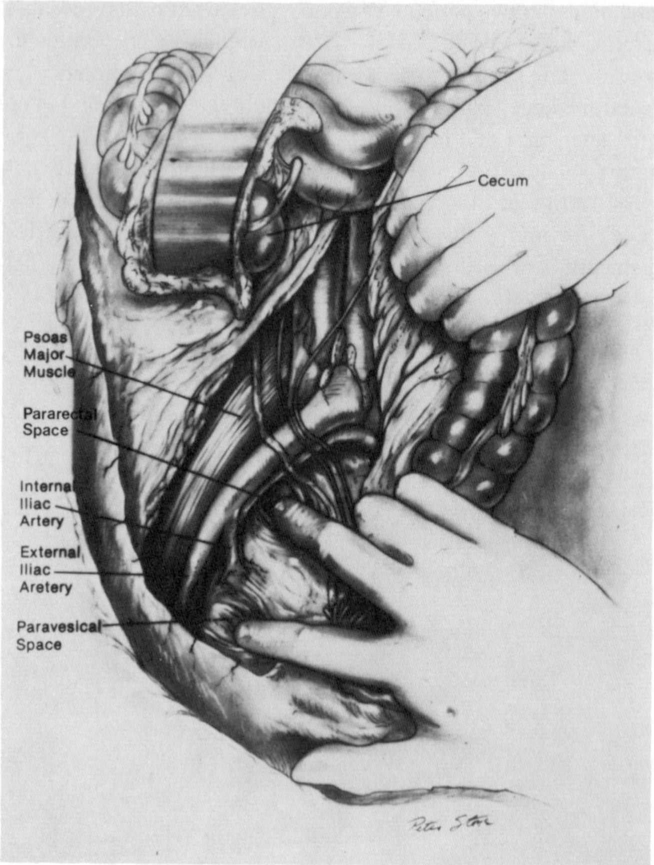

Fig. 20.7. The right pelvic sidewall is exposed and the rectosigmoid and bladder retracted in the opposite direction so that they are not included in the radiation field. Reprinted with permission from the American College of Obstetricians and Gynecologists (*Obstet Gynecol* 1984; 63 [2]:250).

External irradiation portals, designed to match the extent of the disease, covered the external iliac, hypogastric, and obturator lymph nodes. Treatment was based on the following boundaries: superiorly, the interspace of L4, L5; inferiorly, the upper third of the obturator foramen; and laterally, at least 1 cm beyond the lateral margin of the bony pelvis at its widest point.

Intracavitary Irradiation

Fourteen patients received intracavitary cesium treatment by an after–loading Fletcher-Suit intrauterine applicator. Intracavitary treatment began approximately two weeks after completion of external pelvic or paraaortic irradiation. Two intracavitary treatments were given, the second performed one to two weeks after the

Table 20.1. *Radiation Therapy for Patients with Advanced Cervical Cancer Receiving Intraoperative Irradiation: Protocol of the Howard and Georgetown University Hospitals*

Type of Irradiation[a]	Maximum Dose (rad)	Energy (MeV)
Intraoperative irradiation		
Paraaortic area[b]		
Negative nodes	1,500	9–12
Positive nodes		
Microscopic metastasis (surgically removed)	2,000	9–12
Grossly positive (biopsy only)	2,500	
Pelvic area: lymph nodes		
Microscopic metastasis	1,500	9–12
Grossly positive nodes	2,500	12
Parametrium	2,500	
External irradiation		
Paraaortic area (enlarged node)	2,500	12
Positive pelvic area	4,500–5,000	

[a]The third type of irradiation given consists of intracavity applications to the pelvic area, administered in two Fletcher–Suit applications of 48 hours each.
[b]Administered to all patients with primary cancer.

first; in each application, 2,000 to 3,000 mg-hr was delivered over 48 hours. The dose to point A ranged from 4,500 to 6,500 rad.

Treatment Protocol

The treatment protocol of the Howard/Georgetown pilot study is illustrated in table 20.1.

Preclinical Radiation Biology

Preclinical animal studies conducted at several institutions in the United States provided fundamental data on normal tissue tolerances to single high doses of intraoperative electrons. At Howard University, irradiation was used in dogs. The retroperitoneal space, including the aorta and vena cava, was given single electron doses of 2,000, 3,000 and 4,000 rad (Goldson et al. 1984). After 16 months, the animals were killed. Upon gross examination, the aorta and vena cava appeared normal. Microscopically, there was some degree of intimal thickening of the vessels, but the overall integrity of the great vessels was maintained.

In contrast, the small intestine tolerated the intraoperative electrons poorly, with progressive ulceration and gangrenous bowel developing when single doses exceeded 2,000 rad. Radiobiological studies carried out at the National Cancer Institute by Sindelar, Tepper, and associates (Sindelar et al. 1982) demonstrated that dog aortas subjected to single doses of up to 5,000 rad of electron-beam irradiation maintained structural integrity (Sindelar et al. 1982, 1983; Tepper et al. 1983). Microscopically, there was subintimal and medial fibrosis in the canine aortic wall at dose levels of 3,000 rad.

The ability of the great vessels to tolerate single high-dose IORT was significant because these structures are routinely irradiated in the treatment of the paraaortic nodes.

The ability of the kidneys and ureters to tolerate irradiation had to be established to further understand the radiation biology of the retroperitoneum. In animal studies (Gunderson et al. 1983), renal sensitivity was found with high-dose IORT to the kidneys; at doses as low as 2,000 rad, parenchymal atrophy and hyalinization necrosis occurred. The ureter was also shown to be radiosensitive, with ureteral fibrosis and secondary obstruction at doses of 3,000 rad. Clinically, these effects can be avoided by surgically dissecting the ureters and retracting them out of the treatment field.

Additional canine studies indicated that the maximum tolerated doses are 1,500 rad for the colon, 2,500 rad for the small intestine, and 3,000 rad for the bladder (Gunderson et al. 1983).

Results

The tumor stage and cell type and the status of the paraaortic nodes of the 19 patients in the study are shown in table 20.2. The types of therapy the patients received are shown in table 20.3. As mentioned before, when IORT first began to be used, only the paraaortic area was treated. All 16 patients with primary cancer in this series received IORT to the paraaortic area. Eleven of these patients had positive paraaortic nodes; five did not. Six of the patients with positive paraaortic nodes and two with negative nodes also received IORT to one or more of the following structures: pelvic nodes, iliac nodes, parametrium, and pelvic sidewalls. The three patients with recurrent pelvic sidewall disease after radiation therapy of their primary cervical cancer received IORT to the pelvic area only.

After IORT, 16 patients received external irradiation to the pelvis. The other three patients had received external irradiation and intracavitary radium treatment of the cervical cancer two years before. Patients with recurrent pelvic sidewall disease had

Table 20.2. *Number of Patients with Advanced Cervical Cancer Receiving Intraoperative Irradiation by Cancer Stage, Cell Type, and Status of Paraaortic Nodes*

Stage	Cell Type		Paraaortic Node Status[a]		Total
	Squamous	Adeno-carcinoma	Positive	Negative	
II	3	2	2	3	5
III–IV	10	1	9	2	11
Recurrent[b]	3	0	0	3	3
Total	16	3	11	8	19

[a]Three patients had therapy to site of recurrence only. Five patients with paraaortic nodes had 1,500 rad to the paraaortic area as per table 20.1.

[b]Patients had prior radiation therapy for cervical cancer treatment given to recurrence in the pelvic sidewall.

Table 20.3. *Number of Patients with Advanced Cervical Cancer Receiving Intraoperative, External, or Intracavitary Radiation Therapy and Paraaortic Node Status*

	Disease Status of Paraaortic Nodes		
	Positive	Negative	Total
Total number of patients	11	8	19
Intraoperative irradiation			
Paraaortic nodes	11	5	16
Pelvic nodes/iliac nodes/parametrium	6	2	8
Pelvic sidewall[a]	0	3	3
External irradiation			
Before intraoperative irradiation	0	3	3
After intraoperative irradiation	10	6	16
Intracavitary application[b]			
Single	2	0	2
Double	5	7	12

[a]Three patients with tumor recurrence in the pelvic wall after radiation therapy for cervical cancer had intraoperative irradiation in only pelvic sites.
[b]The three patients with recurrence had received prior treatment with intracavitary radium. Two other patients refused intracavitary cesium.

IORT to the pelvic sites only. In addition, two patients were treated with an additional 2,500 rad of external-beam therapy to the paraaortic area. After external irradiation, 14 patients had intracavitary applications: 12 with double, 2 with single. Of the remaining patients, two refused the intracavitary applications and three others with tumor recurrence had received intracavitary application as part of their primary treatment.

The 11 patients with positive paraaortic nodes are dead, one from causes other than cancer. The survival range was 10 to 36 months, with a median of 17 months.

Of the five patients with negative paraaortic nodes, primarily treated, two are alive and free of disease. Two patients died of disease, the third from other causes. The median survival for this group was 33.3 months, with a range of 17 to 71 months. The three patients with recurrent disease died from cancer after therapy was complete. In two patients, reexploration was done to rule out recurrence. In one of them, the irradiated lymph nodes were negative; in the other, the irradiated pelvic mass recurrence was also negative. In both cases, the therapy was IORT alone.

Treatment-Related Toxicity

The complications related to the surgical procedure itself included (1) ileus lasting more than five days, corrected with nasogastric suction and intravenous fluids, and (2) vena cava bleeding (in two cases), requiring suture at the time of surgery.

Toxicity related to the radiation therapy was confined to the pelvis and was seen when intraoperative irradiation plus external irradiation and intracavitary radium was used (fig. 20.8). Two patients developed motor weakness related to femoral nerve damage. In view of this complication, a lead shield was placed on top of the psoas muscle to cover the femoral nerve; this technique adequately protected the nerve. Two patients developed significant vascular problems, with rupture of the

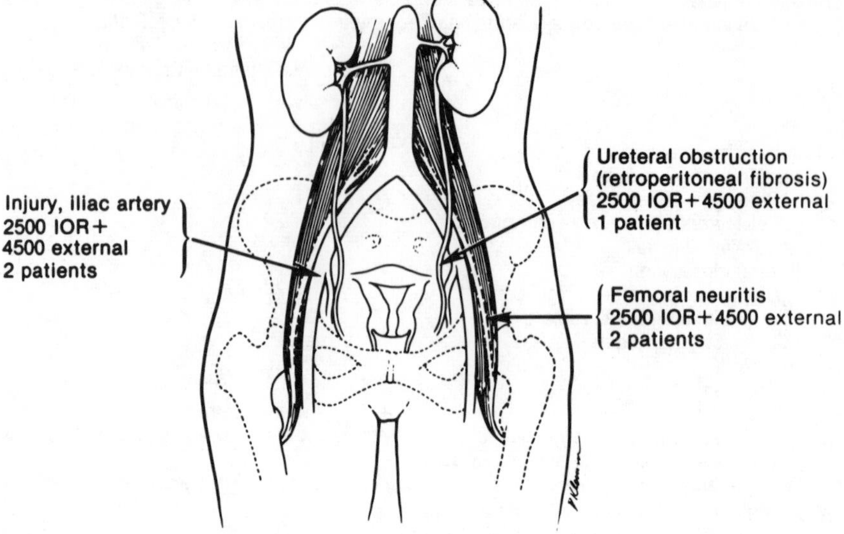

Fig. 20.8. Complications of intraoperative, external, and intracavitary irradiation.

arteries from the internal iliac system. Both patients had persistent disease and, after several arterial ligations and embolizations, eventually died. One of these patients also developed ureteral obstruction from retroperitoneal fibrosis that was confirmed at the time of reexploration. The obstruction was corrected by a ureteroileoneocystotomy. There were no complications related to the paraaortic irradiation.

Discussion

Conventional radiation therapy has limitations: it does not necessarily enhance survival, and it frequently results in complications to the gastrointestinal tract. The use of IORT with an electron-beam linear accelerator permits irradiation of affected areas without including sensitive areas. With the dissection of the retroperitoneal spaces in the paraaortic area, the intestines are retracted from the radiation field. The peritoneum lateral to the sigmoid is entered, and the paravesical, pararectal, and suprapubic spaces identified and developed. The sigmoid, rectum, and bladder can be retracted away from the radiation field separately in each pelvic sidewall. Thus, the pelvic organs are not irradiated intraoperatively and external irradiation and intracavitary cesium can be added to the treatment regimen (fig. 20.5). In this way, areas of frequent failure, such as the lymph nodes and parametrium, receive additional radiation without affecting the rectosigmoid or bladder.

All of the complications of IORT were related to the pelvic area where external radiation therapy was given before or after IORT. In these cases, significant complications developed, related to (1) the femoral nerve (this complication has since been avoided by placing a lead shield on top of the psoas muscle); (2) ureteral obstruction from retroperitoneal fibrosis and encasement of the ureter (one of the patients required a ureteroileoneocystotomy); or (3) the hypogastric arterial system (e.g., severe bleeding). The second problem can be prevented by retracting the ureters from the radiation field. Both of the patients with the third complication required several embolizations and ligations to control the bleeding temporarily; the complication can be avoided by decreasing the amount of irradiation given intraoperatively to the pelvic area in patients who will also receive external irradiation. These changes have all been incorporated into the protocol we now use.

Summary

We performed IORT of the pelvic and paraaortic lymph nodes using three separate fields. Areas of high risk, such as the paraaortic nodes and parametrium, received intraoperative application. Patients tolerated the intraoperative treatment of the paraaortic area very well. However, when IORT was combined with external radiation therapy to the pelvis, significant complications arose. We have discussed ways to avoid these complications. We conclude that IORT in combination with external radiation therapy needs further controlled studies.

References

Abe M, Takahashi M, Yabumoto E, Adachi H, Yoshii M, Mori K. 1980. Clinical experiences with intraoperative radiotherapy of locally advanced cancers. *Cancer* 45:40–48.

Abe M, Takahashi M, Yabumoto E, Onoyama Y, Torizuka K, Tobe T, Mori K. 1975. Techniques, indications and results of intraoperative radiotherapy of advanced cancers. *Radiology* 116:693–702.

Barth G. 1953. Erhahrungen und Ergebnisse mit der Nahbestrahlung operative freigelegter Tumoren. *Strahlentherapie* 91:481–527.

Beck C. 1919. On external roentgen treatment of internal structures (eventration treatment). *NY State J Med* 89:621–622.

Buchsbaum HJ. 1972. Paraaortic lymph node involvement in cervical carcinoma. *Am J Obstet Gynecol* 113:942–947.

Castellano CJ. 1975. Carcinoma de cuello uterino. *Libro de Oncologia del Instituto Nacional Efermedades Neoplasicas.*

Delgado G, Caglar H, Walter P. 1978. Survival and complications in cervical cancer treated by pelvic and extended-field radiation after paraaortic lymphadenectomy. *AJR* 130: 141–143.

Delgado G, Chun B, Caglar H, Bepko F. 1977. Paraaortic lymphadenectomy in gynecologic malignancies confined to the pelvis. *Obstet Gynecol* 50:418–423.

Delgado G, Goldson AL, Ashayeri E, Hill LT, Petrilli ES, Hatch KD. 1984. Intraoperative radiation in the treatment of advanced cervical cancer. *Obstet Gynecol* 63:246–252.

Delgado G, Smith JP, Ballantyne AJ. 1975. Scalene node biopsy in carcinoma of the cervix: Pelvic and paraaortic lymphadenectomy. *Cancer* 35:784–786.

Eloesser L. 1937. The treatment of some abdominal cancers by irradiation through the open abdomen combined with cautery excision. *Ann Surg* 106:645–652.

Finsterer H. 1915. Zur Therapie inoperabler Magen und Darmkarzinome mit Freilegung und Nachfolgen der Rontgenbestrahlung. *Strahlentherapie* 6:205–213.

Fletcher GH, Rutledge FN. 1972. Extended-field technique in the management of the cancers of the uterine cervix. *AJR* 114:116–122.

Fuchs G, Ueberal R. 1969. Die intraoperative Roentgentherapie des Blasenkarzinoms. *Strahlentherapie* 135:280–284.

Goldson AL, Ashayeri E, Jacobs M, Nibhanupuduy JR, Manning J, Streeter DE Jr. 1984. Intraoperative radiotherapy. In *Proceedings of Varian's Fourth European Clinac Users Meeting, Malta*, pp. 99–103.

Goldson AL, Delgado G, Hill LT. 1978. Intraoperative radiation of paraaortic nodes in carcinoma of the uterine cervix. *Obstet Gynecol* 52:713–717.

Gunderson LL, Tepper JE, Biggs PJ, Goldson A, Martin JK, McCullough EC, Rich TA, Shipley WU, Sindelar WF, Wood WC. 1983. Intraoperative +/- external beam irradiation. *Curr Probl Cancer* 7:1–69.

Henschke U, Henschke G. 1944. Zur Technik der Operation-strahlung. *Strahlentherapie* 74:223–239.

Lepanto P, Littman P, Mikuta J, Davis L, Celebre J. 1975. Treatment of paraaortic nodes in carcinoma of the cervix. *Cancer* 35:1510–1513.

National Cancer Institute. 1972. *End Results in Cancer*. Report no. 4. DHEW publication no. (NIH) 73–272. Bethesda, Md.: U.S. Department of Health, Education, and Welfare, p. 104.

Olivares L. 1981. Cancer incidence in Peru. In *Proceedings of the First UICC Conference of Cancer Prevention in the Developing Countries*. Nagoya: University of Nagoya Press.

Pack GT, Livingston BM. 1940. Palliative irradiation of gastric cancer. In *Treatment of Cancer and Allied Diseases*, ed. GT Pack, BM Livingston, vol. 2, pp. 1100–1102. New York: P. B. Hoeber.

Piver MS, Barlow JJ. 1973. Paraaortic lymphadenectomy, aortic node biopsy, and aortic lymphangiography in staging patients with advanced cervical cancer. *Cancer* 32:367–370.

Sindelar WF, Morrow BM, Travis EL, Tepper J, Merkel AB, Kranda K, Terrill R. 1983. Effects of intraoperative electron irradiation in the dog on cell turnover in intact and surgically anastomosed aorta and intestine. *Int J Radiat Oncol Biol Phys* 9:523–532.

Sindelar WF, Tepper J, Travis EL, Terrill R. 1982. Tolerance of retroperitoneal structures to intraoperative radiation. *Ann Surg* 196:601–608.

Tepper JE, Sindelar W, Travis EL, Terrill R, Padikal T. 1983. Tolerance of canine anastomoses to intraoperative radiation therapy. *Int J Radiat Oncol Biol Phys* 9:987–992.

Ucmakli A, Bonney WA Jr. 1972. Exploratory laparotomy as routine pretreatment investigation in cancer of the cervix. *Radiology* 104:371–377.

Wharton JT, Jones HW, Day TG, Rutledge FN, Fletcher GH. 1977. Pre-irradiation celiotomy and extended-field irradiation for invasive carcinoma of the cervix. *Obstet Gynecol* 49: 333–338.

Annual Clinical Conference on Cancer, Vol. 29
Gynecologic Cancer: Diagnosis and Treatment Strategies
© 1987 by The University of Texas System Cancer Center

21. Arterial Chemotherapy Prior to Radiotherapy in Advanced Gynecologic Cancer

John J. Kavanagh, Luis Delclos, and Sidney Wallace

Localized carcinomas of the gynecologic system are usually amenable to radiotherapy. However, in advanced disease such as International Federation of Gynecology and Obstetrics (FIGO) stage III and IV carcinomas of the cervix and vagina, there is a high rate of relapse in both distant and local sites. The local failures are considered to be secondary to the bulk of tumor at the beginning of radiotherapy (Fletcher 1980). If such bulk were lessened, then perhaps local relapse and subsequent survival would be improved. Arterial chemotherapy has been used previously and consistently produces an objective response rate of 10% to 40% in patients in whom radiotherapy has failed as disease treatment (Cromer et al. 1952; Krakoff and Sullivan 1958; Bateman 1965; Stephens, Harker, and Crea 1980; Hulka and Bisel 1965; Sullivan, Miller, and Sikes 1959; Swenerton et al. 1979; Morrow et al. 1977; Carlson, Freedman, and Wallace 1981). In an attempt to reduce tumor volume, arterial chemotherapy was given prior to radiation treatment in patients with advanced localized gynecologic malignancies.

Materials and Methods

All patients entered in the treatment program were classified upon examination by gynecologic and radiation oncologists as having bulky malignancy of poor prognosis. All patients underwent tumor staging consisting of a chest X ray, barium enema, intravenous pyelogram, cystoscopy, and proctoscopy. Lymphangiograms were usually done unless the performance status or medical conditions were contraindications. Patients with metastatic disease outside the pelvis were excluded from the program. Surgical staging was not performed in any patient.

Arteriography was performed through the femoral approach and catheters placed bilaterally in the internal iliac arteries or divisions thereof. After chemotherapy was completed, the catheters were removed. Patients received modest anticoagulation treatment while the catheters were in place.

The treatment program consisted of three courses of chemotherapy three weeks apart. A course consisted of the following sequentially used drugs: mitomycin C at 10 mg/m^2 (courses 1 and 3 only) over 4 hours, bleomycin at 35 mg/m^2 over 24 hours, and cisplatin at 100 mg/m^2 over 24 hours. The drugs were divided in the pelvis depending on the results of the pelvic examination and a nuclear medicine flow study. The latter consisted of macroaggregated technetium-labeled albumin injected into the arterial catheters. Distribution of the material into the buttocks, pelvis, and genitalia was evaluated. The aim was to maximally concentrate the chemotherapy in the pelvis and genitalia ipsilateral to the dominant side of the bulk of tumor (Kim et al. 1984).

Four weeks after chemotherapy, patients were examined to determine response. A partial response was defined as a 50% reduction of volume of disease with clinically significant improvement in disease. Radiotherapy was then started. This consisted of four to six weeks of external-beam therapy (4,000–5,000 rad) followed by application of two intracavitary systems.

Results

Forty-six patients have entered this treatment program. Forty have completed therapy. Three are under treatment and three are unevaluable (one was lost to follow-up, one refused radiation therapy, and one refused further chemotherapy after one course).

Patient characteristics are shown in table 21.1. Nineteen (44%) of the 43 evaluable patients had obstructive uropathy, which was usually unilateral. Lymphangiograms were done on 36 patients (84%); 16 (37%) were positive for disease. Four patients (9%) had common iliac lymph node disease and two (5%) had bilateral involvement. Usually the patients had squamous cell carcinoma. However, three had small cell carcinoma, one had papillary carcinoma, and one had spindle cell carcinoma.

Thirty-two (74%) of the patients responded to arterial chemotherapy. Nine patients (21%) had stable disease and two (5%) had progression. During treatment there were three deaths from renal failure, a probable pulmonary embolus, and an interstitial pneumonitis secondary to bleomycin.

Hematologic toxicity was moderate, with a median nadir granulocyte count of 1.8 x 10^3 cells/mm^3 and platelet count of 120,000 cells/mm^3. Nadir granulocyte counts were 1.0 x 10^3 cells/mm^3 or less in 27 (32%) of 85 evaluable courses.

Table 21.1. *Characteristics of Evaluable Patients*

	No. of patients (%)
Total	43
Median age in years (range): 54 (35–79)	
Zubrod performance status	
0	2 (5)
1	29 (67)
2	5 (12)
3	7 (16)
FIGO stage—cervix	
IIIA	1 (2)
IIIB	30 (70)
IVA	6 (14)
FIGO stage—vagina	
III	3 (7)

Note: FIGO, International Federation of Gynecology and Obstetrics.

A chemodermatitis/neuropathy developed in 16 patients (37%). In three (7%), it was severe and temporarily affected the gait. Usually there were slight areas of hypopigmentation or hyperpigmentation on the buttocks area, accompanied by mild leg paresthesia. These changes were slowly self-resolving.

Complications of arteriography and the indwelling catheters were minimal. Four patients who, between them, underwent six courses of therapy had such problems. One had an internal dissection of a major artery. Thrombosis occurred in five vessels (three, internal iliac; two, common iliac). One patient required elective placement of a vascular graft. Emergency intervention was not required in any of the patients.

Radiotherapy following chemotherapy was well tolerated. No interruptions of therapy resulted from myelosuppression. Two patients required laparotomy for radiation enteritis; one of them died postoperatively.

As of this report, 17 (39%) of the original 43 evaluable patients remain disease free. Relapses have occurred in 21 (49%). Three patients (7%) died as a result of therapy. There was disease progression during treatment in two (5%).

The median time to relapse following completion of therapy was six months. Treatment failed in all four patients with lymphangiographically demonstrated common iliac nodal involvement, as it did in six of seven patients unable to have the study performed. Also, treatment failed in all patients with histological patterns other than squamous cell carcinoma. The location of relapse was local in 14 (67%), distant in 3 (14%), and both local and distant in 4 (19%). Survival was generally short following relapse.

Conclusions

Arterial combination chemotherapy with mitomycin C, bleomycin, and cisplatin in advanced localized carcinomas of the gynecologic tract may induce, as determined by the pelvic examination, a satisfactory bulk reduction of tumor. Standard radiotherapy may be given sequentially without undue interruption or complication. However, both local and distant relapses remain a significant problem. A randomized trial with consideration of appropriate prognostic factors is needed.

References

Bateman JC. 1965. Can chemotherapeutic perfusion of pelvic viscera palliate patients with advanced or recurrent cervical cancer? *JAMA* 194:163–164.

Carlson JA Jr, Freedman RS, Wallace S, Chuang VP, Wharton JT, Rutledge FN. 1981. Intra-arterial *cis*-platinum in the management of squamous cell carcinoma of the uterine cervix. *Gynecol Oncol* 12:92–98.

Cromer JK, Bateman JC, Berry GN, Kennelly JM, Klopp CT, Platt LI. 1952. Use of intra-arterial nitrogen mustard therapy in the treatment of cervical and vaginal cancer. *Am J Obstet Gynecol* 63:538–548.

Fletcher GH. 1980. *Textbook of Radiotherapy*, Philadelphia: Lea & Febiger, p. 418.

Hulka JF, Bisel HF. 1965. Combined intra-arterial chemotherapy and radiation treatment for advanced cervical carcinoma. *Am J Obstet Gynecol* 91:486–490.

Kim EE, Bledin AG, Kavanagh J, Haynie TP, Chuang VP. 1984. Chemotherapy of cervical carcinoma: Use of Tc-99m-MAA infusion to predict drug distribution. *Radiology* 150: 677–681.

Krakoff IH, Sullivan RD. 1958. Intra-arterial nitrogen mustard in the treatment of pelvic cancer. *Ann Intern Med* 48:839–850.

Morrow CP, DiSaia PJ, Mangan CF, Lagasse LD. 1977. Continuous pelvic arterial infusion with bleomycin for squamous carcinoma of the cervix recurrent after irradiation therapy. *Cancer Treat Rep* 61:1403–1405.

Stephens FO, Harker GJ, Crea P. 1980. The intra-arterial infusion of chemotherapeutic agents as basal treatment of cancer: Evidence of increased drug activity in regionally infused tissues. *Aust NZ J Surg* 50:597–602.

Sullivan RD, Miller E, Sikes MP. 1959. Antimetabolite-metabolite combination cancer chemotherapy: Effects of intra-arterial methotrexate intramuscular citrovorum factor therapy in human cancers. *Cancer* 12:1248–1262.

Swenerton KD, Evers JA, White GW, Boyes DA. 1979. Intermittent pelvic infusion with vincristine, bleomycin, and mitomycin C for advanced recurrent carcinoma of the cervix. *Cancer Treat Rep* 63:1379–1381.

Annual Clinical Conference on Cancer, Vol. 29
Gynecologic Cancer: Diagnosis and Treatment Strategies
© 1987 by The University of Texas System Cancer Center

22. Management of Early Stage Carcinoma of the Vulva

Creighton L. Edwards and C. Allen Stringer

The foundation for the modern management of invasive carcinoma of the vulva first appeared in a monograph published in 1912 by Antoine Basset on the management of squamous carcinoma of the clitoris. He recommended a radical anterior resection of the vulva and en bloc resection of the regional lymph nodes. Despite this recommendation, standard therapy prior to 1940 consisted of a wide local excision with or without inguinal node sampling. The resulting survival rate was approximately 20%.

In the early 1940s Taussig and Way implemented the recommendation outlined by Basset. Based on their work, standard therapy became radical vulvectomy and bilateral inguinal and pelvic lymphadenectomy (Taussig 1940; Way 1948). The survival rate promptly increased to 55%–65% and has remained essentially unchanged since that time. There have been few basic changes in the standard management. As early as the 1950s, Way recognized the increased morbidity of a concomitant pelvic lymphadenectomy and deleted it in patients with negative inguinal lymph nodes (Way 1960). The only other change in standard management, although not universally accepted, has been the recognition that one can decrease the morbidity without adversely affecting recurrence rate or survival by performing the inguinal lymphadenectomies through separate groin incisions rather than en bloc with the radical vulvectomy (Ballon and Lamb 1975).

The morbidity associated with radical vulvectomy and bilateral inguinal lymphadenectomy remains high. Despite improvements in anesthesia and perioperative care, operative mortality remains in the 2% to 5% range (Podratz et al. 1983). Early and late complications are listed in table 22.1. A late complication that has received little attention is that of sexual dysfunction. In a recent paper, Andersen and Hacker report levels of sexual arousal at the eighth percentile and body image scores in the fourth percentile for those who have undergone vulvectomy (Andersen and Hacker 1983).

Interest in identifying a group of women with early disease who could be treated more conservatively than by radical vulvectomy and bilateral inguinal lymphadenectomy has been spurred by a number of observations: (1) the stability in survival rates over the past four decades, (2) the considerable morbidity associated with standard therapy, (3) the increasing frequency of early stage disease, (4) the increasing incidence of invasive vulvar cancer in young women, and (5) the identification of a subset of patients with early cervical cancer who can safely be treated by a more conservative approach. For these reasons, since the 1970s a number of papers

Table 22.1. *Complications of Radical Vulvectomy and Inguinal Lymphadenectomy*

Early complications
Wound breakdown
Lymphocyst
Thrombophlebitis
Hemorrhage
Late complications
Lymphedema
Lymphangitis
Urinary incontinence
Genital prolapse
Sexual dysfunction

have addressed the issue of "microinvasive carcinoma of the vulva." The histopathologic parameters that have been identified (by one or more authors) to be important prognostic factors in patients with stage I disease include depth of invasion, lesion size, tumor confluency, vascular or lymphatic space involvement, histological grade, and coexisting squamous carcinoma in situ (Zucker and Berkowitz 1985). Early reports showed an excellent prognosis in patients with less than 5 mm of invasion, irrespective of the other prognostic factors (Wharton, Gallager, and Rutledge 1974; Dean et al. 1974). As data accumulated, however, it became clear that the risk of nodal metastasis is significant with depth of invasion greater than 1 mm below the basement membrane (Wilkinson 1985). The additional prognostic variables listed above were then utilized in an effort to identify subsets of patients with invasion greater than 1 mm who had a negligible risk of nodal metastases. It is clear, however, that for any individual patient with invasion greater than 1 mm from the basement membrane, there are no combinations of these prognostic variables that result in a negligible risk of nodal metastases (Zucker and Berkowitz 1985). This fact was emphasized in the report by Hacker and associates of seven patients with superficially invasive stage I squamous carcinoma of the vulva, all of whom had nodal metastases (Hacker et al. 1983b). Two patients had invasion less than 2 mm, six had grade 1 or 2 tumors, five had associated carcinoma in situ, and four patients had no evidence of vascular space involvement. Of the seven patients, four received standard therapy consisting of radical vulvectomy and bilateral inguinal lymphadenectomy, and one has subsequently died of disease. In the three patients who did not undergo a bilateral inguinal lymphadenectomy, all had recurrence in the inguinal nodes, and all are dead of disease. This highlights the importance of a timely diagnosis of inguinal node metastasis when it exists.

In 1979, DiSaia and associates reported a series of 18 patients with squamous carcinomas of the vulva less than 1 cm in diameter and invasive to a depth less than 5 mm. These patients were treated by bilateral superficial inguinal lymphadenectomy with frozen section followed by wide local excision of the vulvar lesion when results of the frozen section proved negative (DiSaia, Creasman, and Rich 1979). With a median follow-up of 32 months, no recurrences were observed. They recommended, however, that patients with positive superficial inguinal nodes continue to be treated by radical vulvectomy and inguinal and femoral lymphadenectomy. This novel approach acknowledges that the presence or absence of nodal metastases is the single most important prognostic variable. Irrespective of stage, the five-year survival is 80% to 95% in patients with negative inguinal lymph nodes and 30% to 40% in patients with positive inguinal lymph nodes (Morley 1981). This approach, however, implies that control of local disease in patients with positive superficial inguinal lymph nodes requires radical vulvectomy. This premise is refuted in a paper by Hacker and associates in which patients with stage I disease treated by wide local excision or partial radical vulvectomy had an incidence of local recurrence identical to those treated by standard radical vulvectomy, despite the fact that they had a slightly higher incidence of positive inguinal lymph nodes (Hacker et al. 1984). The approach outlined by DiSaia and colleagues also implies that the deep femoral nodes are not at risk when the superficial inguinal nodes are negative. There have been at least three reports, however, of positive femoral nodes with negative inguinal nodes (Hacker et al. 1983b). Any modification of the standard operative approach to the regional lymph nodes must take into account the therapeutic value of a bilateral inguinal lymphadenectomy. Hacker and colleagues have reported a five-year survival rate of 80% in patients with two positive inguinal nodes treated by bilateral inguinal lymphadenectomy alone (Hacker et al. 1983a), and Rutledge and associates report a 68% five-year survival rate with surgery alone for patients with three or fewer positive inguinal lymph nodes (Rutledge, Smith, and Franklin 1970). The use of bilateral inguinal lymphadenectomy should be individualized, however. Multiple studies have demonstrated that the risk of contralateral inguinal nodal metastases is negligible when the ipsilateral nodes are negative in patients with well-lateralized lesions. The indications and therapeutic value of pelvic lymphadenectomy are controversial. Morley states in his review article that pelvic lymphadenectomy is appropriate when one or more inguinal nodes are positive (Morley 1981). Hacker and associates, on the other hand, concluded that pelvic lymphadenectomy was not justified with fewer than three positive inguinal nodes. Furthermore, in their series no patient with positive pelvic nodes was cured despite the use of pelvic lymphadenectomy (Hacker et al. 1983a).

Reports to date have restricted consideration for a modification of standard therapy to those patients with stage I disease. Although lesion size is certainly an important prognostic variable with regard to risk of nodal metastases, size alone does not preclude the necessity for surgical assessment of the regional nodes. In the series reported by Donaldson and coworkers, the incidence of nodal metastases was 19% in patients with lesions 3 cm or less in diameter and 72% in patients with lesions greater than 3 cm in diameter (Donaldson et al. 1980). Based on these data, a more appropriate cutoff for consideration for conservative management may be 3 cm rather than 2 cm.

A number of conclusions can be drawn from the data presented. Patients having lesions with invasion less than 1 mm below the basement membrane have a negligible risk of nodal metastases and can be adequately managed by wide local exci-

Table 22.2. *Complications in Patients with Stages I and II Disease Based on Surgical Procedure*

Procedure	No. of Patients	Complications Early	(%)	Late	(%)
Modified	41	8	(19.5)	9	(21.9)
Standard	163	104	(63.8)	95	(58.2)

sion. Patients having lesions with invasion greater than 1 mm below the basement membrane require surgical evaluation of the regional nodes. The surgical treatment of the vulvar lesion and the regional nodes should be independent of each other. Surgical treatment of the local disease should be individualized to secure ample free margins. This may require a procedure ranging from a wide local excision to hemivulvectomy for lateralized lesions to a radical vulvectomy for extensive midline lesions. Patients with lateralized lesions should have an ipsilateral inguinal lymphadenectomy with frozen section. Positive ipsilateral lymph nodes mandate a contralateral inguinal lymphadenectomy. Patients with midline lesions should undergo a bilateral inguinal lymphadenectomy. This should be performed through separate incisions except in patients with periclitoral lesions in whom an en bloc resection of the local lesion and the regional nodes may be required to secure ample margins. Patients with more than two positive inguinal lymph nodes should undergo postoperative radiation therapy to include both the inguinal and pelvic lymph nodes.

Although many reports have dealt with the topic of a conservative approach to the

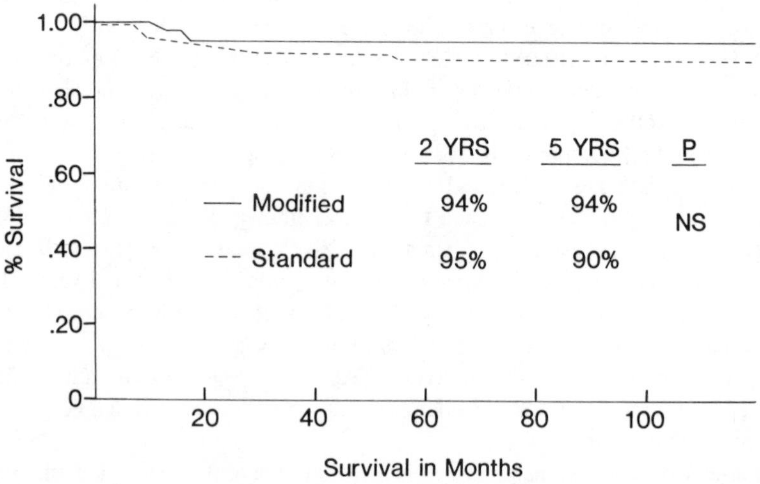

Fig. 22.1. Corrected actuarial survival for patients with stage I and II vulvar cancer. The solid line represents modified and broken line represents standard surgical technique.

management of patients with early vulvar cancer and its effect on risk of recurrence, little information is available regarding its impact on morbidity or hospital costs. At U.T. M. D. Anderson Hospital, a retrospective review of patients with stages I and II carcinoma of the vulva identified 41 patients treated with a conservative surgical procedure. Surgical management of the vulvar disease ranged from wide local excision to hemivulvectomy, and management of the regional nodes ranged from ipsilateral node sampling to ipsilateral inguinal lymphadenectomy and contralateral node sampling. The incidences of early and late complications for patients treated by a conservative or modified procedure compared with patients treated in a standard fashion are shown in table 22.2. The differences for both early and late complications are statistically significant ($p < 0.0001$). This resulted in significantly longer hospitalizations for those treated in a standard fashion ($p < 0.0001$). The incidences of local recurrence and survival, however, were not significantly different (fig. 22.1). By adopting an individualized approach using the guidelines presented above, the morbidity, hospital stay, and cost can be significantly reduced without compromising risk of recurrence or survival.

References

Andersen BL, Hacker NF. 1983. Psychosocial adjustment after vulvar surgery. *Obstet Gynecol* 62:457–462.

Ballon SC, Lamb EJ. 1975. Separate incisions in the treatment of carcinoma of the vulva. *Surg Gynecol Obstet* 140:81–84.

Basset A. 1912. Traitement chirurgical operatoire de l'epithelioma primitif du clitoris indications-technique-resultats. *Rev Chir Orthop* 46:546–570.

Dean RE, Taylor ES, Weisbroel DM, Martin JW. 1974. The treatment of premalignant and malignant lesions of the vulva. *Am J Obstet Gynecol* 119:59–68.

DiSaia PJ, Creasman WT, Rich WM. 1979. An alternate approach to early cancer of the vulva. *Am J Obstet Gynecol* 133:825–832.

Donaldson ES, Powell DE, Hanson MB, van Nagell JR. 1980. Prognostic parameters in invasive vulvar cancer. *Gynecol Oncol* 11:184–190.

Hacker NF, Berek JS, Lagasse LD, Leuchter RS, Moore JG. 1983a. Management of regional lymph nodes and their prognostic influence in vulvar cancer. *Obstet Gynecol* 61:408–412.

Hacker NF, Berek JS, Lagasse LD, Nieberg RK, Leuchter RS. 1984. Individualization of treatment for stage I squamous cell vulvar carcinoma. *Obstet Gynecol* 63:155–162.

Hacker NF, Nieberg RK, Berek JS, Leuchter RS, Lucas WE, Tamimi HK, Nolan JF, Moore JG, Lagasse LD. 1983b. Superficially invasive vulvar cancer with nodal metastases. *Gynecol Oncol* 15:65–77.

Morley GW. 1981. Cancer of the vulva: A review. *Cancer* 48:597–601.

Podratz KC, Symmonds RE, Taylor WF, Williams TJ. 1983. Carcinoma of the vulva: Analysis of treatment and survival. *Obstet Gynecol* 61:63–74.

Rutledge FN, Smith JP, Franklin EW. 1970. Carcinoma of the vulva. *Am J Obstet Gynecol* 106:1117–1130.

Taussig FJ. 1940. Cancer of the vulva. An analysis of 155 cases. *Am J Obstet Gynecol* 40:764–779.

Way S. 1948. The anatomy of the lymphatic drainage of the vulva and its influence on the radical operation for carcinoma. *Ann R Coll Surg Engl* 3:187.

Way S. 1960. Carcinoma of the vulva. *Am J Obstet Gynecol* 79:692–697.

Wharton JT, Gallager S, Rutledge FN. 1974. Microinvasive carcinoma of the vulva. *Am J Obstet Gynecol* 118:159–162.

Wilkinson EJ. 1985. Superficial invasive carcinoma of the vulva. *Clin Obstet Gynecol* 28:188–195.

Zucker PK, Berkowitz RS. 1985. The issue of microinvasive squamous cell carcinoma of the vulva: An evaluation of the criteria of diagnosis and methods of therapy. *Obstet Gynecol Surv* 40:136–143.

ENDOMETRIAL CANCER

Annual Clinical Conference on Cancer, Vol. 29
Gynecologic Cancer: Diagnosis and Treatment Strategies
© 1987 by The University of Texas System Cancer Center

23. Melville Cody Memorial Lecture: Prognostic Factors in Endometrial Carcinoma

C. Paul Morrow

Prognostic factors, known also as risk factors or prognostic variables, encompass the patient's and the cancer's clinical-pathological characteristics that correlate with the probability of cure. More precisely, prognostic variables correlate with the probability of local extension or metastasis, recurrence, and survival. More than 15 prognostic variables for endometrial cancer have been reported in the literature. These can be divided roughly into patient factors, tumor extent, histological factors, and treatment. Included in patient factors are age, ethnic origin, health, previous radiation exposure, and symptoms. Among the prognostic variables of tumor extent are the spread of disease as determined by clinical and surgical-pathological investigations (cervix invasion, node metastasis, adnexal involvement, and peritoneal cytological findings), uterine size, and length of the uterine cavity. Histological type and grade, nuclear grade, myometrial invasion, vascular space invasion, and hormone receptor content constitute the histological risk factors. Treatment factors involve the quality of surgical and radiation therapy.

From a practical point of view, prognostic variables are important and useful to the degree that they provide precise, accurate, and quantifiable information about tumor behavior and patient outcome. Reliable data about tumor status are essential if the clinician is to devise the best possible individualized treatment plan that will minimize over- as well as undertreatment. Furthermore, the information permits the clinician to give the patient and her family a realistic appraisal of her chances for cure. Accurate knowledge of prognostic variables is also a prerequisite for the development of investigational treatment protocols and, ultimately, improved patient care. The purpose of this paper is to provide a critical assessment of the prognostic variables in endometrial cancer with respect to their importance and utility. In reviewing the relevant literature, it was interesting to find that very little was added to our understanding of endometrial carcinoma from 1955 to 1975, a time in which the focus of publications was the methodology of radiation therapy.

Uterine Size

Uterine size was among the earliest clinical features of endometrial carcinoma that were recognized as having prognostic significance and were incorporated into a staging system. In 1939, Healy and Brown reported a five-year survival rate of 60% of patients with endometrial cancer in whom the uterus was not larger than two and

Table 23.1. *Survival Rates of Endometrial Carcinoma Patients in Relation to Uterine Size and Cavity Length*

Study	Uterine Gestational Size or Length[a] and Five-Year Survival Rate	
Healy and Brown 1939	≤2-1/2 months 59.7%	>2-1/2 months 35.0%
Arneson 1953	≤12 cm 87.0%	>12 cm 52.0%
Recent series combined[b]	≤8 cm 86.4%	>8 cm 75.3%

[a] No extrauterine extension.
[b] Frick et al. 1973; De Palo et al. 1982; Kauppila, Gronroos, and Nieminen 1982a.

one-half months gestational size, compared with 35% of patients in whom the uterus was larger (table 23.1). In 1940, Miller incorporated the measured length of the uterine cavity in his clinical stage grouping but combined it with uterine size, and Arneson in 1953 reported his results based on cavity length alone (table 23.1). More contemporary series have produced inconsistent results, partly because uterine enlargement often reflects the presence of fibroids or of muscular hypertrophy rather than tumor volume. Javert (1958) observed that only 8% of his patients had a uterus enlarged by tumor. Nevertheless, the combined results of Frick et al. (1973), De Palo et al. (1982), and Kauppila et al. (1982a) showed the five-year survival rate for FIGO (International Federation of Gynecology and Obstetrics) stage IA patients to be 86.4% (591/684) compared with 75.3% (530/704) for stage IB patients. Others have reported no significant survival difference for these substages (Aalders et al. 1980; Lotocki et al. 1983).

Histological Type

Adenosquamous Carcinoma

The endometrium gives rise to a surprising variety of malignant tumors that exhibit a wide range of biologic behavior (table 23.2). Adenocarcinoma (AC) of the tubular type, the predominant form, when poorly differentiated, is composed of solid cellular masses. Although the frequency with which the less common types are reported varies widely, as many as 20% of cases are adenosquamous, clear cell, papillary serous, mucinous, secretory, pure squamous, and other rarer forms of cancer. Historically, the term adenoacanthoma was applied to all endometrial cancers composed of squamous and glandular components whether the squamous component was malignant or not. This led to extreme differences in assessing its relative degree of malignancy. The recommendation of Ng and associates (Ng 1968; Ng et al. 1973) that adenocarcinomas with malignant squamous components, referred to as adenosquamous carcinoma (AS), and those with benign squamous components, adenoacanthomas (AA), be considered as separate histological entities has been widely accepted. Although in the initial report (1968) and again in the 1973 follow-up study, the Ng group's data indicated that AS is increasing in frequency (from 7.5% to 32.8% between 1956 and 1971), that it occurs in older women (mean age, 59 years for AA compared with 68 years for AS), and that it is more malignant than the more common AC (five-year survival, 19.2% for AS compared with 72% for AC patients), other centers have reported mixed results (table 23.3). For example, during a similar time period, Salazar et al. (1977) noted a fairly constant fraction (20%–25%) of AS lesions among their endometrial cancer patients and no difference in mean age or survival.

On the other hand, Alberhasky et al. (1982) and Christopherson et al. (1983), in a registry study of 595 patients, observed that 32.7% of patients with stage I AS died of disease by five years compared with 6.2% patients with AC. They also noted that the AS patients were an average of five years older than the AC patients, but the proportion of AS cases was fairly constant (6%–8%) during the study period (1953–1976).

Consonant with reports that the prognosis for AS is worse than for AC are the findings of some investigators that the AS lesions are more often associated with advanced stage at presentation (Underwood et al. 1977; Julian et al. 1977), deep

Table 23.2. *Five-Year Status of Patients with Endometrial Cancer Subtypes, Stage I*

Histological Subtype	Patients Alive (%)	Patients Dead of Cancer (%)
Adenoacanthoma	87.5	6.3
Adenocarcinoma	79.8	6.3
Papillary carcinoma	69.7	21.2
Adenosquamous carcinoma	53.1	32.7
Clear cell carcinoma	44.2	51.2

Source: Christopherson et al. 1983.

Table 23.3. *Clinical Features of Patients with Adenosquamous Carcinoma and Adenocarcinoma of the Endometrium*

	Five-Year Survival (%)		Mean Age (Yr.)		Stage I (%)		G3 Glandular Component (%)	
Study	AS	AC	AS	AC	AS	AC	AS	AC
Silverberg, Bolin, and DeGiorgi 1972	35.3	66.0	63.0	60.0	—	—	96.2	14.8
Ng et al. 1973	19.2	72.0	68.0	59.0	—	—	24.7	28.0
Salazar et al. 1977	85.0[a]	85.0[a]	62.0	61.0	82.8	84.0	26.0	12.0
Alberhasky, Connelly, and Christopherson 1982	53.1[a]	79.8[a]	64.7	60.0	81.7	—	62.7	—

Note: AS, adenosquamous carcinoma; AC, adenocarcinoma; G3, grade 3.
[a] Stage I patients.

myometrial invasion (Burrell et al. 1982; Julian et al. 1977; Silverberg et al. 1972), pelvic node metastasis (Boronow et al. 1984), vascular space invasion (VSI) (Ng et al. 1973; Alberhasky et al. 1982; Hanson et al. 1985), and postirradiation residual tumor (Silverberg et al. 1972). Furthermore, in the series of Silverberg et al. and Julian et al., more than 90% of the AS lesions had a poorly differentiated AC component, and the patients' survival was the same as for those who had poorly differentiated AC with no squamous component. Thus, the adverse prognostic significance of the AS histology seems to reflect to a high degree the differentiation of the glandular part of the lesion.

Papillary Serous Carcinoma

Papillary serous carcinoma (PSC), a recently described variant of endometrial carcinoma (Lauchlan 1981; Hendrickson et al. 1982), is characterized histologically by features resembling PSC of the ovary, often with psammoma bodies. Frequently, areas of clear cell carcinoma are seen. Papillary serous carcinoma is reported to have a poorer prognosis and to be more invasive and less well differentiated than AC (table 23.4).

In the Hendrickson group's series, 26 of 256 patients with endometrial cancer had PSC; 20 of these had stage I PSC, the same stage ratio as that of other histological types. Forty percent of the patients with PSC had deep myometrial invasion, however, compared with 11.6% of patients with AC. The relapse rate for patients with stage I PSC was 40% compared with 5% for those with all other stage I histological subtypes combined. In other words, PSC accounted for 47% of the recurrences but only 10.2% of the stage I cases. Hendrickson and associates also noted that 6 of 22 evaluable patients with PSC had evidence of VSI, and five of those died of the cancer. Almost all cases of PSC were considered to be high grade. Even patients with stage I, deeply invasive PSC had a higher relapse rate (5 of 8) than did the non-PSC patients with deep invasion (6 of 20). Another interesting observation by Hendrickson et al. was that 6 of 13 PSC recurrences were in the upper abdomen compared with only 1 of 13 for the other histological categories. All their patients with clear

Table 23.4. *Clinical-Pathological Features of Papillary (Serous) Carcinoma of the Endometrium*

	PSC	Patients Dead of Cancer or Relapses (%)		Patients with Deep Invasion (%)	
Study	% of All Cases	PSC	AC	PSC	AC
Hendrickson et al. 1982	10.2	40.0	5.0	40.0	11.6
Christopherson, Alberhasky, and Connelly 1982b	4.6	21.2	6.2	—	—
Burrell, Franklin, and Powell 1982	9.2[a]	37.5	2.2	12.5	22.4

Note: PSC, papillary serous carcinoma; AC, adenocarcinoma.
[a]Stage I and II cases.

cell carcinoma had PSC areas, and these mixed neoplasms had as poor a prognosis as the pure PSC cases.

Christopherson et al. (1982b) reported that among 46 patients with papillary carcinoma of the endometrium, the five-year survival rate was 69.7% for patients with stage I disease compared with 79.8% for those who had typical adenocarcinomas. At five years, 21.2% of the former and 6.2% of the latter patients had died of the disease. None of the Christopherson group's patients with papillary carcinoma more advanced than stage I survived five years, although only 63.6% were known to have died of the malignancy. In contrast to the study by Hendrickson et al. (1982), only 2 of 46 patients in this study had a clear cell component. Although Christopherson and associates did not use the term "serous," the description and photomicrographs in the report suggest the 46 patients were similar to those discussed by Hendrickson et al.

Burrell et al. (1982) classified 9.2% of 172 patients with stage I endometrial cancers as having PSC. The proportion who had grade 3 differentiation was the same as among the AC patients, but deep myometrial invasion (after radium treatment) occurred in half as many AC patients (12.5% vs. 22.4%). Nevertheless, the 16 patients with PSC in the Burrell study had a cancer death rate of 37.5% compared with 2.2% for those with AC.

Clear Cell Carcinoma

The clear cell carcinoma (CC) type of endometrial cancer represents 1% to 5% of cases studied in recent series. Most investigators have concluded that the prognosis, stage for stage, is worse for this than for the common variety of endometrial carcinoma. They generally agree that women with CC are an average of six to seven years older than women with AC. The stage distribution for CC is probably not significantly different than for AC, stage I representing about 75% of cases and stage II, 15%. In the largest series (Christopherson et al. 1982a), 49% of 45 patients with stage I CC had died of disease at five years. All 11 patients with more advanced disease died of cancer. In the series of Kurman and Scully (1976), 3 of 14 women with stage I disease who were followed up for at least two years died without evidence of cancer before five years, whereas three died of recurrent cancer. Four of the five evaluable patients with stage II disease died of cancer. Although Photopulos et al. (1979) followed up only one of their 22 patients longer than 36 months, one of five patients with stage I disease had experienced disease recurrence, five of ten patients with stage II disease were dead of cancer, and all six women who had stage III and IV disease had died of cancer.

Histological Grade and Myometrial Invasion

A strong interrelationship between histological grade, depth of myometrial invasion, and prognosis has been demonstrated repeatedly since the reports by Mahle (1923) and Norris and Vogt (1924). Jones (1975) and Morrow et al. (1973) summarized the data accumulated on these prognostic indicators. More recent studies have continued to confirm these relationships. The combined data from the series of Mal-

Table 23.5. *Relationship of Histological Grade and Myometrial Invasion in Endometrial Carcinoma Stage I*

Histo-logical Grade	Myometrial invasion ≤1/3 *N* (%)	Mid 1/3 *N* (%)	Outer 1/3 *N* (%)	All Patients *N* (%)
1	328 (89.4)	22 (6.0)	17 (4.6)	367 (47.5)
2	212 (69.7)	50 (16.4)	42 (13.8)	304 (39.4)
3	54 (54.4)	15 (14.8)	32 (31.7)	101 (13.1)
Total	594 (76.9)	87 (11.3)	91 (11.8)	772 (100.0)

Source: Malkasian, Annegers, and Fountain 1980; Boronow et al. 1984.

Table 23.6. *Relationship of Five-Year Survival, Histological Grade, and Myometrial Invasion in Stage I Endometrial Carcinoma*

Grade	Myometrial Invasion ≤1/3 *N* (%)	Mid 1/3 *N* (%)	Outer 1/3 *N* (%)
1	243 (93.7)	18 (83.3)	13 (92.3)
2	145 (88.7)	42 (81.0)	29 (71.9)
3	34 (76.3)	10 (60.0)	16 (56.3)

Source: Malkasian, Annegers, and Fountain 1980.

Table 23.7. *Comparison of Histological Grade Based on Curettage and Hysterectomy in Endometrial Carcinoma*

Grade on Curettings	Total Patients	Higher Grade at Hysterectomy *N*	(% total)
1	66	7	(10.6)
2	40	12	(30.0)

Source: Macasaet et al. 1980; Cowles et al. 1985.

kasian et al. (1980) with those of Boronow et al. (1984) show that among 367 patients with grade 1 carcinoma, 89% had one third or less myometrial invasion, and less than 5% had greater than two-thirds invasion (table 23.5). In contrast, among the 101 patients with grade 3 invasive cancer, 54% had one-third or less and 32% had greater than two-thirds myometrial invasion. In terms of survival, the data of Malkasian et al. (1980) show that among the patients with grade 1 disease and one-third or less invasion, the five-year survival rate was 93.7%, whereas for patients with grade 3 outer one-third invasion, it was only 56.3% (table 23.6).

Less well appreciated is the probability of undergrading or missing the least differentiated part of the tumor during dilatation and currettage (D&C) or endometrial biopsy (table 23.7). According to the data of Macasaet et al. (1980) and Cowles et al. (1985), 11% of patients diagnosed as having grade 1 cancer at curettage were found to have grade 2 or 3 disease at hysterectomy, and in 30% (12 of 40) of patients diagnosed as having grade 2 cancer, the grade was raised. Silverberg and DeGiorgi (1974) also noted a significant rate of upgrading (15.4%) based on hysterectomy specimens.

Age of Patients

Variously defined age groups have often been reported to have significantly different prognoses. A better outcome is expected for premenopausal women, the great majority of whom have well-differentiated cancers. Only 4 of 114 premenopausal women in the series of Malkasian et al. (1980) had grade 3 lesions compared with 62 of 463 postmenopausal women. But, as the information in table 23.8 shows, a prognostic differential is not limited to comparisons of pre- with postmenopausal women. (In the Malkasian group's series, only 6.8% of women aged 45 to 64 had grade 3 lesions, whereas 16.7% of women older than 64 had grade 3 lesions.) Aalders et al. (1980) also observed in their study of endometrial cancer at the Norwegian Radium Hospital that the risk of treatment failure was influenced by age (table 23.8). Among 294 stage I patients younger than 60 years of age, there was an 8.5% recurrence rate compared with a 17.5% recurrence rate among 246 women 60 years of age or older. Although the frequency of grade 3 lesions was similar in the two age groups, the proportion with deep invasion in the older group was double that of the younger group (46.3% vs. 24.1%). Thus, the adverse effect of age seems to result from greater invasiveness, less differentiation, and perhaps a higher proportion of the AS and CC types of endometrial cancer.

Isthmus or Cervical Extension

Cervical extension of endometrial cancer detected by clinical examination, biopsy, or fractional curettage is a stage II growth according to the FIGO system, acknowledging the long-recognized fact that survival of patients who have cervical extension of the cancer is lower than that in patients in whom the carcinoma is confined to the fundus. Nevertheless, the FIGO system predecessor, the League of Nations stage grouping, did not separate cases involving the cervix from those confined to

Table 23.8. *Frequency of Tumor Grade and Recurrence in Endometrial Carcinoma Related to Age and Menopausal Status*

Age Group	All Cases	Grade 3 *N* (%)	Recurrence (%)
Premenopausal[a]	114	4 (3.5)	—
Postmenopausal	463	58 (12.5)	—
Age 45–64 years[a]	337	23 (6.8)	—
>64 years	215	36 (16.7)	—
<60 years[b]	294	—	(8.5)
>60 years	246	—	(17.5)

[a]Malkasian, Annegers, and Fountain 1980.
[b]Aalders et al. 1980—stage I cases only.

Table 23.9. *Comparison of Five-Year Survival of Stage II Endometrial Carcinoma Patients with Clinically Occult or Gross Involvement*

	Occult		Gross	
Study	*N*	Survival (%)	*N*	Survival (%)
Kinsella et al. 1980	37	(95)	18	(44)
Homesley, Boronow, and Lewis 1977	61	(61)	23	(48)
Onsrud et al. 1982	86	(82)	10	(60)
Bruckman et al. 1978	28	(93)	12	(66)
Boronow 1973	14	(61)	19	(58)

Table 23.10. *Survival in Stage II Endometrial Carcinoma Related to Cervical Stromal Invasion as Shown at Endocervical Curettage or Hysterectomy*

	Stromal Invasion	
Study	Present *N* Survival (%)	Absent *N* Survival (%)
Surwit et al. 1979[a]	78[b] (47)	39[c] (74)
Bigelow, Vekshtein, and Demopoulos 1983[d]	14 (50)	5 (100)

[a]Altogether 47 patients received preoperative irradiation and 14 were treated by irradiation alone. Effect on findings and survival was not given in paper.
[b]Twenty patients diagnosed on basis of hysterectomy.
[c]Twelve patients diagnosed on basis of hysterectomy.
[d]Hysterectomy specimens only. None of the patients received preoperative radiation therapy.

the corpus. Broadly speaking, recent series have shown patients with stage I disease to have an 85% to 90% and stage II patients to have a 70% to 80% five-year survival rate.

When a patient with endometrial cancer has cervical/isthmic extension, what are the operational risk factors for a good or poor outcome? One is the extent of disease within the cervix. Most investigators (table 23.9) have noted that patients with gross cervical involvement have a worse prognosis than those with only microscopic disease (Kinsella et al. 1980; Homesley et al. 1977; Bruckman et al. 1978; Onsrud et al. 1982). Surwit et al. (1979) also found a difference in survival rate based on the presence (47% three-year survival) or absence (74% three-year survival) of cervical stromal invasion (table 23.10). In addition to the data shown in Table 23.10, Bigelow et al. (1983) reported that stromal invasion in evidence at endocervical curettage (ECC) strongly correlated with the presence of deep myometrial invasion, a well-known adverse prognostic indicator.

Perhaps of greater interest is the relationship of histological grade and myometrial invasion to outcome in stage II endometrial cancer. In the series of Kinsella et al. (1980) five of eight recurrent cancers among the 18 patients with gross disease were grade 3, and all had more than 50% myometrial invasion. Overall, only 1 of 17 grade 1 and 1 of 19 grade 2 cases recurred compared with 8 of 19 grade 3 cases. Surwit et al (1979) also noted a survival relationship to grade for patients with stage

II disease treated by radiation and surgery (grade 1, 89%; grade 2, 66%; and grade 3, 39% of patients were alive at three years). Onsrud et al. (1982) did not find such dramatic differences in the effect of grade on survival of patients with stage II disease (those with grade 1 plus grade 2 had a 19% recurrence rate compared with 25% for those with grade 3), but they observed a large survival differential based on residual myometrial invasion (31.8% recurrence rate with more than 50% invasion vs. 12.9% with less than 50%). Most patients in these series received preoperative radiation. In the predominantly surgical series of Homesley et al. (1977), however, a major relationship of survival to extent of myometrial penetration (68% of patients with one third or less invasion survived compared with 48% in whom invasion was more extensive) was also observed.

The significance of "floaters" in the D&C specimen has only recently been evaluated. In the series of Kadar et al. (1982), all 13 patients with tumor fragments separate from endocervical tissue on ECC survived five years. Bigelow et al. (1983) found, however, that 23% of patients with floaters had cervical extension in the hysterectomy specimen, twice the rate of those with a negative ECC. Onsrud et al. (1982), in a review of curettings from 174 "stage II" cases could find extension into the cervical stroma in only 96 patients. The remaining 78 had a five-year survival identical to their patients with stage I disease (negative ECC).

These data point out the shortcomings of the clinical diagnosis of occult stage II endometrial carcinoma and raise questions about the significance of cervical involvement as a risk factor independent of histological grade and myometrial invasion.

Vascular Space Invasion

A recently appreciated significant prognostic variable in early endometrial cancer is microscopic evidence of vascular space invasion (VSI) within the primary tumor. Although Javert (1952) reported "a very high incidence of spread to the blood vessels of the uterus and paranodal vessels" among 14 patients with endometrial carcinoma and pelvic lymph node metastases and Barber et al. (1962) observed myometrial lymphatic involvement by tumor in 14% of 17 patients with endometrial cancer and lymph node metastasis, little attention was given to VSI in those early years. In 1973, Ng and associates reported VSI in 50% of 68 patients with AS. The frequency of this finding increased with loss of differentiation of the glandular component, ranging from 27% (grade 1) to 67% (grade 3). VSI strongly correlated also with myometrial invasion: among patients with no myometrial invasion, 8.3% had VSI; 43% of those with 50% or less myometrial invasion had VSI; and 88% of those with more than 50% myometrial invasion had vascular invasion.

Aalders in 1982 and Hanson in 1985 correlated the presence of VSI with the recurrence rate in women with stage I endometrial cancer (table 23.11). Altogether, 19.9% of Aalders' patients had VSI, its incidence increasing with the degree of myometrial invasion and tumor dedifferentiation. Hanson et al. found that frequency of VSI increased with age, depth of myometrial invasion (one-third or less, 5%; mid one-third, 24%; outer one-third, 70%), and grade (1, 2%; 2, 25%; 3, 42%). Although the numbers were small, VSI also seemed to occur more frequently

Table 23.11. *Relationship of Vascular Space Invasion to Recurrence in Stage I Endometrial Carcinoma with No Preoperative Irradiation*

Study	Vascular Space Invasion			
	Present *N*	Recurrent (%)	Absent *N*	Recurrent (%)
Aalders 1982	30	(26.7)	121	(9.1)
Hanson et al. 1985	16	(43.7)	95	(2.1)

with AS cancer. In addition, five of seven recurrences among the VSI group were distant metastases, whereas both recurrences in the negative VSI group were local. Common iliac/aortic node metastases were documented in four of eight patients with VSI undergoing selective biopsy. Using discriminant function analysis, Hanson et al. (1985) determined that VSI was a highly significant risk factor ($p < .001$) independent of both histological grade and myometrial invasion.

Residual Disease

The absence of tumor in the uterus after radiation therapy for endometrial carcinoma has long been observed to augur a better outcome for patients than if the tumor had not been eradicated. Furthermore, survival of patients with residual tumor correlated well with depth of residual myometrial penetration. (Of course, absence of residual tumor after D&C without radiation is also a good portent.) What has seldom been investigated, however, is the relationship between preradiation risk factors and the probability of finding carcinoma persistent in the uterus after radiation therapy.

Arnesen et al. observed in 1948 that persistent tumor was found in 26% of patients who had well-differentiated carcinomas compared with 78% who had poorly differentiated tumors (table 23.12). Similar results were reported by Silverberg and DeGiorgi (1974) and most recently by Macasaet et al. (1980). Although DeMuelenaere (1975) did not find that residual endometrial cancer in the uterus after radiation therapy correlated with tumor grade, he observed a correlation with cavity length (among patients with cavities shorter than 10 cm, 30% had residual tumor compared with 43% for those cases with longer cavities) and patient age (among those fewer than ten years postmenopausal, 15% had residual tumor, compared with 57% of patients more than ten years past menopause).

The significance of postradiation residual tumor is twofold. It provides direct evidence first for the radiation sensitivity of endometrial cancer and second for the radiocurability of endometrial cancer without hysterectomy. It does not provide evidence that local radiation therapy contributes to the curability of endometrial cancer when hysterectomy is part of the treatment. Thus, as Silverberg and DeGiorgi (1974) suggested, the major prognostic indicator in these cases is not the presence or absence of residual tumor in the uterus after radiation therapy but the status of the tumor at diagnosis. Whether there is any general difference in radiation sensitivity based on tumor differentiation cannot be concluded from these data. A plausible explanation for these findings is that poorly differentiated cancers tend to be more invasive, bulkier, and more commonly associated with VSI. These are surely more likely explanations for the poorer prognosis of patients with residual tumor than is the residuum per se. Although the time of maximum tumor disappearance is between 5 and 10 weeks postirradiation (Silverberg and DeGiorgi 1974; Wilson et al. 1980), this should be of little concern to the therapist, because waiting until the uterus is tumor-free will not affect prognosis. On the other hand, since the most malignant tumors are least likely to be eradicated, delaying surgical intervention may be harmful.

Tumor Size

Despite the knowledge that tumor size is a prognostic variable in many malignancies, it has received little attention in the literature about endometrial cancer other than descriptions of such indirect indicators as uterine size and length of the uterine cavity. This undoubtedly reflects the long-standing practice of treating endometrial cancer by preoperative radiation.

Schmitz and Schmitz proposed a staging system in 1935 in which stage I incorporated lesions 1 cm or less and stage II, lesions 2 to 3 cm in diameter. In 1956, Lefèvre reported on the relationship of lesion extent within the endometrial cavity, myometrial invasion, and pelvic lymph node metastases. Eleven uteri contained well-defined, plaque-shaped carcinomatous ulcerations up to 3 cm in diameter. Of these, five had deep invasion and one had pelvic node metastases. There were 20 cases with diffuse or cauliflower-shaped lesions with necrosis, occupying most or all of the uterine cavity. Twelve of these had deep invasion and four had nodal involvement.

The most recent data on tumor volume and recurrence came from Anderson et al. in 1980. Using four growth patterns based on bulk (more or less than 3 to 4 mm thick) and area (more or less than 25% involvement of endometrial surface), these investigators found a progressive increase in the frequency of deep myometrial penetration and recurrence. Tumors that were both bulky and diffuse, for example, had deep invasion (more than 30%) in 60% of patients, and there was tumor recurrence in 20% of the group. For lesions neither bulky nor diffuse, these figures were zero in both categories.

Table 23.12. *Relationship between Histological Grade and Frequency of Residual Tumor in the Uterus after Preoperative Radiation*

	Grade 1–2		Grade 3	
Study	*N* Residual	(%)	*N* Residual	(%)
Arneson, Stanbro, and Nolan 1948	23	(26)	9	(78)
Silverberg and DeGiorgi 1971[a]	—	(60)	—	(88)[b]
Macasaet et al. 1980	84	(45)	7	(86)

[a]Study of 76 patients; numbers in grade not specified.
[b]88% for poorly differentiated adenocarcinomas and 82% for adenosquamous carcinomas.

Cytosol Hormone Receptors

The concentration of progesterone and estrogen receptors has been reported to correlate with histological grade (Ehrlich et al. 1981) as well as stage and myometrial invasion (Kauppila et al. 1982b). Two recent papers suggest, furthermore, that survival of endometrial carcinoma is adversely affected by negative estrogen and progesterone status independent of stage, grade, and myometrial invasion (Martin et al. 1983; Creasman et al. 1985).

Clinical Staging

The stage grouping of a malignancy is expected to correlate highly with prognosis because the staging criteria are based on proven prognostic features of the malignancy. The current official FIGO staging system is clinical, that is, stage is assigned without regard to surgical-pathological data. In this system, 75% to 80% of cases are in stage I (malignancy clinically confined to the corpus) and another 5% to 15% are in stage II (malignancy involving the cervix). The stage I cases are subdivided further on the basis of uterine cavity length and histological grade. As has already been pointed out, histological grading based on the curettings contains substantial error. Furthermore, the gradient of survival by cavity length is not a major prognostic factor, and ECC has a substantial false-positive and false-negative rate in the diagnosis of cervical/isthmic extension. Thus, the very risk factors considered to be important in the clinical staging of endometrial carcinoma cannot be optimally assessed or have little prognostic value, whereas such other major prognostic variables as myometrial invasion, VSI, and subclinical extrauterine extension (to nodes and adnexa) are not considered at all. The overall error in underestimating the stage by clinical versus surgical means has been determined in several studies to be 13% to 22% (Kottmeier 1968; Musumeci et al. 1980; Boronow et al. 1984; Cowles et al. 1985). Overstaging occurs also.

Surgical-Pathological Staging

In the United States, the interest in surgical-pathological staging for endometrial cancer generated in the 1950s by Javert and Hofammann (1952), Liu and Meigs (1955), Brunschwig and Murphy (1954), and others was reawakened by the report of Lewis, Stallworthy, and Cowdell from Oxford in 1970. A three-institution pilot study was organized by Boronow in 1973 at the University of Mississippi, Duke University, and the University of Southern California under the auspices of the Gynecologic Oncology Group (GOG). The results of this study confirmed and expanded the Oxford data (Boronow et al. 1984).

Table 23.13 displays the frequency of pelvic node metastasis related to grade of lesion and myometrial invasion in the GOG pilot study, excluding patients with cervical, adnexal, or peritoneal involvement. The pelvic node metastasis rate was 30.7% in patients with more than one-third myometrial invasion who had grade 2 lesions plus grade 3 lesions with any myometrial invasion (12 of 39). The relation-

Table 23.13. *Frequency of Pelvic Node Metastases in Stage I Endometrial Carcinoma*[a] *Relative to Histological Grade and Maximum Depth of Myometrial Penetration*

Histological Grade	Myometrial Invasion			
	None *N* (%)	Inner 1/3 *N* (%)	Mid 1/3 *N* (%)	Outer 1/3 *N* (%)
1	54 (0.0)	24 (0.0)	3 (0.0)	4 (25.0)
2	26 (0.0)	37 (2.7)	6 (33.3)	5 (20.0)
3	7 (0.0)	12 (25.0)	4 (25.0)	12 (41.7)

Source: Boronow et al. 1984.
[a] Surgically corrected: cases with cervical/isthmic, adnexal, and peritoneal involvement excluded.

Table 23.14. *Frequency of Aortic Node Metastases in Stage I Endometrial Carcinoma*[a] *Relative to Histological Grade and Maximum Depth of Myometrial Penetration*

Histological Grade	Myometrial Invasion			
	None *N* (%)	Inner 1/3 *N* (%)	Mid 1/3 *N* (%)	Outer 1/3 *N* (%)
1	54 (0.0)	24 (0.0)	3 (0.0)	4 (0.0)
2	26 (0.0)	37 (0.0)	6 (16.7)	5 (20.0)
3	7 (0.0)	12 (33.3)	4 (0.0)	12 (25.0)

Source: Boronow et al. 1984.
[a] Surgically corrected: cases with cervical/isthmic, adnexal, and peritoneal involvement excluded.

ship of aortic node metastasis to grade and invasion (table 23.14) was similar, but the overall frequency was lower (grade 2 lesions with more than one-third myometrial invasion and all grade 3 lesions with myometrial invasion: 9 of 39, 23.1%). Preliminary data from a subsequent groupwide GOG study indicate that a lower rate of nodal metastases will be detected. Among 528 patients, only 16.1% (46 of 286) had histologically confirmed pelvic node metastases, and 8.4% had aortic node involvement (Morrow et al. 1986). Several other recent reports have been in harmony with these findings in relation to the frequency of pelvic and aortic lymph node metastases in operable endometrial cancer (Masubichi et al. 1979; Musumeci et al. 1980; Piver et al. 1982; Figge et al. 1983).

In 1956, Dahle and Hoeg at the Norwegian Radium Hospital investigated the possibility that the intraperitoneal spread of endometrial carcinoma might result from retrograde passage through the fallopian tubes (Dahle 1956; Hoeg 1956). In a study of 25 patients with adenocarcinoma of the endometrium who had no preoperative radiation therapy, they recovered tumor cells from the fallopian tubes of 15 patients. Of the seven patients with positive cul-de-sac cytological findings, six also had malignant cells in the tubal lumina. Reporting from The University of Texas M. D. Anderson Hospital and Tumor Institute at Houston in 1971, Creasman and Rutledge found that among 100 patients with preoperative radiation therapy and no gross pelvic extrauterine disease at operation, cytological test results were positive in seven. Four of the seven subsequently had recurrences. Other investigators have reported a similar incidence of cancer cells recoverable from the pelvis of patients with endometrial cancer (Morton et al. 1961; Keettel et al. 1974).

In 1981, Creasman et al. reported on the significance of positive peritoneal cytological findings in 167 patients with clinical stage I endometrial AC who underwent surgical staging as part of the GOG pilot study. The overall frequency of positive cytological assay results was 15.5%. Only 13 patients had no evidence of metastasis outside the uterus (no peritoneal implants; no adnexal, pelvic, or aortic metastases) other than the positive cytological findings, and 6 of these 13 died of intraabdominal disease recurrence.

Szpak et al. (1981) reported on 54 patients with stage I endometrial carcinoma, of whom 12 (22%) had positive pelvic washings. Numerous tissue fragments and sheets of AC cells were present in four patients, all of whom died of intraabdominal carcinomatosis within two years. This was compared with two recurrences (site not specified) among the eight patients who had shown a sparse yield of malignant cells. There was no clear relationship to myometrial invasion or tumor grade.

Yazigi et al. (1983), in a study of peritoneal cytology in 93 patients with stage I endometrial cancer, 50 of whom had had preoperative radium treatment, found malignant cells in 11% (10 patients). Again, no obvious correlation was found with grade or invasion. Only one of the ten patients developed recurrence, which was intraabdominal. Preliminary data from the GOG surgical-pathological staging study of early endometrial carcinoma (Morrow et al. 1986), indicated, however, that the frequency of positive pelvic basin cytological findings is influenced by histological grade (grade 1, 6.1%; grade 2 and 3, 13.3%) and myometrial invasion (< mid one-third, 7.6%; > inner one-third, 15.2%). Overall, in 10.5% of the 528 patients, cytological tests were positive. Positive peritoneal cytological specimens were found in 7.8% of 447 patients who had no other evidence of extrauterine spread, compared with 25.9% of 81 patients with metastases to the adnexa, pelvic nodes, or aortic nodes. Only 5 recurrences (14.3%) were reported among the 35 patients who had positive pelvic cytological findings without other evidence of extrauterine spread. These results are summarized in Table 23.15.

Table 23.15. *Frequency of Positive Pelvic Cytology in Endometrial Cancer*

Study	Stage	All Patients	Positive (%)
Dahle 1956		25	(28.0)
Morton, Moore, and Chang 1961		24	(16.7)
Creasman and Rutledge 1971	No gross extra-uterine disease	100	(7.0)
Keettel, Pixley, and Buchsbaum 1974	I	39	(12.0)
GOG pilot study 1981[a]	I	167	(15.5)
Yazigi, Piver, and Blumenson 1983	I	93	(11.0)
GOG groupwide study 1985[b]	I and II (occult)	528	(10.5)
	I (surgical)	447	(7.8)
	Extrauterine spread	81	(25.9)

Note: GOG, Gynecologic Oncology Group.
[a] Reported by Creasman et al. 1981.
[b] Reported by Morrow et al. 1986.

Commentary

It could be argued that the improved survival rate for endometrial carcinoma patients observed over the past 50 years is almost entirely the result of earlier diagnosis, increased operability, and changes in the staging system, rather than improvements in therapy. Although many important risk factors were recognized before 1950 (myometrial invasion, cervix extension, histological grade, uterine size) they were often not taken into account in treatment planning or the reporting of treatment results. Consequently, much of the experience accumulated in treating this disease is unevaluable and uninformative. Much of the clinical research effort in the past, as well as today, has focused on defining the roles of radiation therapy in endometrial cancer management. That hysterectomy is indispensable for optimal results was settled long ago. After more than half a century, however, a life-sparing effect of adjuvant radiation has not been clearly established (although local control is enhanced). This is surely the result of faulty study design relative to risk factors. The widespread preference for preoperative radiation preempted the optimal use of the more accurate and more significant surgical-pathological prognostic variables.

As this review reveals, the risk factors assessable preoperatively are often inaccurate and less predictive than many of the indicators that can be determined by surgical-pathological staging. Uterine enlargement is more often caused by myometrial hyperplasia and fibroids than tumor bulk; in about 20% of patients, the histological grade of the hysterectomy specimen will be higher than that of the curettings; endocervical curettage has a 10% false-negative rate and a false-positive rate as high as 50%, depending on the criteria used. Histological grade in this scheme appears to be the most important risk factor identifiable preoperatively in early endometrial carcinoma.

Surgical-pathological staging, on the other hand, not only assures more accurate determination of tumor type, histological grade, and cervical involvement, it permits the determination of VSI, the degree of myometrial infiltration, the peritoneal cytology status, and whether or not metastases to the peritoneum, adnexa, pelvic and aortic lymph nodes have occurred. The accuracy with which these risk factors can be identified during surgical procedures is diminished by preoperative radiation to a degree that depends on dose of radiation, means of administration, and time interval to hysterectomy. The effect on these risk factors has been quantified only for myometrial invasion. Preoperative radiation reduces the apparent frequency of deep invasion of the uterine wall by two-thirds (Morrow et al. 1976). Thus, surgical-pathological staging is inherently less informative after radiation therapy.

The prognostic value of the surgical-pathological staging data is just beginning to get sorted out, but it is a common observation in oncology that metastases override the significance of most or all local risk factors. Preliminary results of the large, groupwide GOG study (Morrow et al. 1986) show a recurrence risk at two years of 30% for patients with aortic node metastases, 18% for adnexal metastases, 14% for positive pelvic cytological specimens, and 4% for pelvic node metastases as isolated extrauterine risk factors in 536 patients with endometrial carcinoma surgically staged without preoperative radiation (table 23.16). Half of the recurrences in this

Table 23.16. *Gynecologic Oncology Group Surgical Staging Study: Preliminary Data on Recurrence Risk Versus Prognostic Variables*

Positive Prognostic Variable	Patients in Group	Recurrence at Two Years (%)
Single positive variable[a]		
Pelvic nodes	26	(4)
Aortic nodes	10	(30)
Adnexa	11	(18)
Pelvic cytology	35	(14)
Vascular space invasion	23	(22)
Two or more positive variables	42	(43)
All variables negative	412	(5)

Source: Morrow et al. 1986.
[a]Cases in each group negative for all other sites of involvement.

Table 23.17. *Gynecologic Oncology Group Surgical Staging Study: Risk Ratio Calculations for Various Risk Factors in Endometrial Cancer Derived by Multivariate Analysis*

Risk Factor	Risk Ratio
Aortic node metastasis	3.35[a]
Grade 3 histology	2.50
Vascular space invasion	1.87
Outer one-third muscle invasion	1.71
Cervical extension	1.57

Source: Bundy 1985 (personal communication).
[a]Risk ratio for recurrent cancer.

select group of 105 patients occurred among the 31 patients with tumor extension to the isthmus/cervix. With two or more extrauterine risk factors present (42 patients), nearly 50% recurred at two years of follow-up. Among the 412 patients in whom all evaluated extrauterine risk sites were negative for tumor (adnexa, pelvic and aortic nodes, cytological specimens, and peritoneum), only 5.5% had recurrences at two-year follow-up. Table 23.17 shows the risk ratios for recurrences in relation to the various risk factors (B. Bundy, personal communication, 1985).

It has been recognized during the past decade that surgical staging protocols were needed to define the pattern of extrauterine spread accurately and to correlate these findings with pathological risk factors in the hysterectomy specimen. In this manner, patients at high risk for or documented to have extrauterine spread can be identified for adjuvant therapy by conventional or investigational treatment protocols, whereas the low-risk patients can be spared unnecessary treatment. Patients identified as being at high risk for extrauterine spread are also candidates for surgical staging protocols to define the appropriate boundaries of their treatment field. As the data accumulate from studies employing surgical staging, multivariate analysis, and randomization, we can look forward to more precise individualization of treatment based on the most accurate, most reliable, and most predictive prognostic variables.

References

Aalders JG, Abeler V, Kolstad P, Onsrud M. 1980. Post-operative external irradiation and prognostic parameters in stage I endometrial carcinoma. *Obstet Gynecol* 56:419–426.

Aalders JG. 1982. *Prognostic Factors and Treatment of Endometrial Carcinoma: A Clinical and Histopathological Study*. Groningen: Drukkeru Dijkstra Niemeyer BV.

Alberhasky RC, Connelly PJ, Christopherson WM. 1982. Carcinoma of the endometrium. IV. Mixed adenosquamous carcinoma. *Am J Clin Pathol* 77:655–664.

Anderson B, Louis F, Watring WG, Edinger DD. 1980. Growth patterns in endometrial carcinoma. *Gynecol Oncol* 10:134–145.

Arneson AN. 1953. An evaluation of the use of radiation in the treatment of endometrial cancer. *Bulletin of the New York Academy of Sciences* 29:395–410.

Arneson AN, Stanbro WW, Nolan JF. 1948. The use of multiple sources of radium within the uterus in the treatment of endometrial cancer. *Am J Obstet Gynecol* 55:64–78.

Barber KW, Dockerty MB, Pratt JH. 1962. A clinicopathologic study of surgically treated carcinoma of the endometrium with nodal metastasis. *Surg Gynecol Obstet* 115:568–574.

Bigelow B, Vekshtein V, Demopoulos RI. 1983. Endometrial carcinoma stage II: Route and extent of spread to the cervix. *Obstet Gynecol* 62:363–366.

Boronow RC. 1973. A fresh look at corpus cancer management. *Obstet Gynecol* 42:448–451.

Boronow RC, Morrow CP, Creasman WT, DiSaia PJ, Silverberg SG, Miller A, Blessing JA. 1984. Surgical staging in endometrial cancer: Clinicopathologic findings of a prospective study. *Obstet Gynecol* 63:825–832.

Bruckman JF, Goodman RL, Murthy A, Marck A. 1978. Combined irradiation and surgery in the treatment of stage II carcinoma of the endometrium. *Cancer* 42:1146–1151.

Brunschwig A, Murphy AI. 1954. The rationale for radical panhysterectomy and pelvic node excision in carcinoma of the corpus uteri. *Am J Obstet Gynecol* 68:1482–1488.

Burrell MO, Franklin EW, Powell JL. 1982. Endometrial cancer: Evaluation of spread and follow-up in one hundred eighty-nine patients with stage I or stage II disease. *Am J Obstet Gynecol* 144:181–185.

Christopherson WM, Alberhasky RC, Connelly PJ. 1982a. Carcinoma of the endometrium: I. A clinicopathologic study of clear-cell carcinoma and secretory carcinoma. *Cancer* 49:1511–1523.

Christopherson WM, Alberhasky RC, Connelly PJ. 1982b. Carcinoma of the endometrium. II. Papillary adenocarcinoma: A clinical pathological study of 46 cases. *Am J Clin Pathol* 77:534–540.

Christopherson WM, Connelly PJ, Alberhasky RC. 1983. Carcinoma of the endometrium. V. An analysis of prognosticators in patients with favorable subtypes and stage I disease. *Cancer* 51:1705–1709.

Cowles TA, Magrina JF, Masterson BJ, Capen CV. 1985. Comparison of clinical and surgical-staging in patients with endometrial carcinoma. *Obstet Gynecol* 66:413–416.

Creasman WT, DiSaia PJ, Blessing J, Wilkinson RH, Johnston W, Weed JC. 1981. Prognostic significance of peritoneal cytology in patients with endometrial cancer and preliminary data concerning therapy with intraperitoneal radiopharmaceuticals. *Am J Obstet Gynecol* 141:921–929.

Creasman WT, Rutledge F. 1971. The prognostic value of peritoneal cytology in gynecologic malignant disease. *Am J Obstet Gynecol* 110:773–781.

Creasman WT, Soper JT, McCarty KS Jr, McCarty KS Sr, Hinshaw W, Clarke-Pearson DL. 1985. Influence of cytoplasmic steroid receptor content on prognosis of early stage endometrial carcinoma. *Am J Obstet Gynecol* 151:922–932.

Dahle T. 1956. Transtubal spread of tumor cells in carcinoma of the body of the uterus. *Surg Gynecol Obstet* 103:332–336.

DeMuelenaere G. 1975. The radiosensitivity of endometrial carcinoma. *Br J Radiology* 48:652–655.

De Palo G, Kenda R, Andreola S, Luciana L, Musumeci R, Rilke F. 1982. Endometrial carcinoma: Stage I. *Obstet Gynecol* 60:225–231.

Ehrlich CE, Young PCM, Cleary RE. 1981. Cytoplasmic progesterone and estradiol receptors in normal, hyperplastic, and carcinomatous endometria: Therapeutic implications. *Am J Obstet Gynecol* 141:539–545.

Figge DC, Otto PM, Tamimi HK, Greer BE. 1983. Treatment variables in the management of endometrial cancer. *Am J Obstet Gynecol* 146:495–500.

Frick HC, Munnell EW, Richart RM, Berger AP, Lawry MF. 1973. Carcinoma of the endometrium. *Am J Obstet Gynecol* 115:663–676.

Hanson MB, Van Nagell JR, Powell DE, Donaldson ES, Gallion H, Merhige M, Pavlik EJ. 1985. The prognostic significance of lymph-vascular space invasion in stage I endometrial cancer. *Cancer* 55:1753–1757.

Healy WP, Brown RL. 1939. Experience with surgical and radiation therapy in carcinoma of the corpus uteri. *Am J Obstet Gynecol* 38:1–13.

Hendrickson M, Ross J, Eifel PJ, Cox RS, Martinez A, Kempson R. 1982. Adenocarcinoma of the endometrium: Analysis of 256 cases with carcinoma limited to the uterine corpus. *Gynecol Oncol* 13:373–392.

Hoeg K. 1956. Superficial dissemination of cancer of the uterine body. Cytological examination of smears from the tubes and the pouch of Douglas. *Journal of Obstetrics and Gynaecology of the British Empire* 63:899–902.

Homesley HD, Boronow RC, Lewis JL. 1977. Stage II endometrial adenocarcinoma. *Obstet Gynecol* 49:604–608.

Javert CT. 1952. The spread of benign and malignant endometrium in the lymphatic system with a note on coexisting vascular involvement. *Am J Obstet Gynecol* 64:780–806.

Javert CT. 1958. Prognosis of endometrial cancer. *Obstet Gynecol* 12:556–571.

Javert CT, Hofammann K. 1952. Observations on the surgical pathology, selective lymphadenectomy, and classification of endometrial adenocarcinoma. *Cancer* 5:485–498.

Jones HW. 1975. Treatment of adenocarcinoma of the endometrium. *Obstet Gynecol Surv* 30:147–169.

Julian CG, Daikoku NH, Gillespie A. 1977. Adenoepidermoid and adenosquamous carcinoma of the uterus: A clinicopathologic study of 118 cases. *Am J Obstet Gynecol* 128: 106–116.

Kadar NRD, Kohorn EI, LiVolsi VA, Kapp DS. 1982. Histologic variants of cervical involvement by endometrial carcinoma. *Obstet Gynecol* 59:85–92.

Kauppila A, Gronroos M, Nieminen U. 1982a. Clinical outcome in endometrial cancer. *Obstet Gynecol* 60:473–480.

Kauppila A, Kujansuu E, Vihko R. 1982b. Cytosol estrogen and progestin receptors in endometrial carcinoma of patients treated with surgery, radiotherapy, and progestin. *Cancer* 50:2157–2162.

Keettel WC, Pixley EE, Buchsbaum HJ. 1974. Experience with peritoneal cytology in the management of gynecologic malignancies. *Am J Obstet Gynecol* 120:174–182.

Kinsella TJ, Bloomer WD, Lavin PT, Knapp RC. 1980. Stage II endometrial carcinoma: 10-year follow-up of combined radiation and surgical treatment. *Gynecol Oncol* 10: 290–297.

Kottmeier HL. 1968. Individualization of therapy in carcinoma of the corpus. In *Cancer of the Uterus, Tubes and Ovaries*, pp. 102–108. Chicago: Year Book Medical Publishers.

Kurman RJ, Scully RE. 1976. Clear cell carcinoma of the endometrium: An analysis of 21 cases. *Cancer* 37:872–882.

Lauchlan SC. 1981. Tubal (serous) carcinoma of the endometrium. *Arch Pathol* 105:615.

Lefèvre H. 1956. Node dissection in cancer of the endometrium. *Surg Gynecol Obstet* 102:649–656.
Lewis BV, Stallworthy JA, Cowdell R. 1970. Adenocarcinoma of the body of the uterus. *J Obstet Gynecol* 77:343–348.
Liu W, Meigs JV. 1955. Radical hysterectomy and pelvic lymphadenectomy. *Am J Obstet Gynecol* 69:1.
Lotocki RJ, Copeland LJ, DePetrillo AD, Muirhead W. 1983. Stage I endometrial adenocarcinoma: Treatment results in 835 patients. *Am J Obstet Gynecol* 146:141–145.
Macasaet M, Brigati D, Boyce J, Nicastri A, Waxman M, Nelson J, Fruchter R. 1980. The significance of residual disease after radiotherapy in endometrial carcinoma: Clinicopathologic correlation. *Am J Obstet Gynecol* 138:557–563.
Mahle AE. 1923. The morphologic histology of adenocarcinoma of the body of the uterus in relation to longevity. *Surg Gynecol Obstet* 36:385.
Malkasian GD, Annegers JF, Fountain KS. 1980. Carcinoma of the endometrium: Stage I. *Am J Obstet Gynecol* 136:872–888.
Martin JD, Hähnel R, Woodings TL. 1983. The effect of estrogen receptor status on survival in patients with endometrial cancer. *Am J Obstet Gynecol* 147:322–324.
Masubuchi S, Fujimoto I, Masubuchi K. 1979. Lymph node metastasis and prognosis of endometrial carcinoma. *Gynecol Oncol* 7:36–46.
Miller NF. 1940. Carcinoma of the body of the uterus. *Am J Obstet Gynecol* 40:791–803.
Morrow CP, DiSaia PJ, Townsend DE. 1973. Current management of endometrial carcinoma. *Obstet Gynecol* 42:399–406.
Morrow CP, DiSaia PJ, Townsend DE. 1976. The role of postoperative irradiation in the management of stage I adenocarcinoma of the endometrium. *Am J Roentgenol* 127:325–329.
Morrow CP, Creasman WT, Homesley H, Yordan E, Park R, Bundy BN. 1986. Recurrence in endometrial carcinoma as a function of extended surgical staging data. In *Gynecologic Oncology Proceedings of the 2nd International Conference on Gynecologic Cancer, Edinburgh*, eds. CP Morrow, G Smart. New York: Springer Verlag.
Morton DG, Moore JG, Chang N. 1961. The clinical value of peritoneal lavage for cytologic examination. *Am J Obstet Gynecol* 81:1115–1125.
Musumeci R, De Palo G, Conti U, Kenda R, Mangioni C, Belloni C, Marzi M, Bandieramonte G. 1980. Are retroperitoneal lymph node metastases a major problem in endometrial adenocarcinoma? *Cancer* 46:1887–1892.
Ng ABP. 1968. Mixed carcinoma of the endometrium. *Am J Obstet Gynecol* 102:506–515.
Ng ABP, Reagan JW, Storaasli JP, Wentz WB. 1973. Mixed adenosquamous carcinoma of the endometrium. *Am J Clin Pathol* 59:765–781.
Norris CC, Vogt ME. 1924. Carcinoma of the body of the uterus (with the report of 115 cases). *Am J Obstet Gynecol* 7:550–566.
Onsrud M, Aalders J, Abeler V, Taylor P. 1982. Endometrial carcinoma with cervical involvement (stage II): Prognostic factors and value of combined radiological-surgical treatment. *Gynecol Oncol* 13:76–86.
Photopulos GJ, Carney CN, Edelman DA, Hughes RR, Fowler WC, Walton LA. 1979. Clear cell carcinoma of the endometrium. *Cancer* 43:1448–1456.
Piver MS, Lele SB, Barlow JJ, Blumenson L. 1982. Paraaortic lymph node evaluation in stage I endometrial carcinoma. *Obstet Gynecol* 59:97–100.
Salazar OM, DePapp EW, Bonfiglio TA, Feldstein ML, Rubin P, Rudolph JH. 1977. Adenosquamous carcinoma of the endometrium. *Cancer* 40:119–130.
Schmitz H, Schmitz HE. 1935. An improved technique for radium treatment of carcinoma of the uterine body. *Am J Roentgenol* 34:759.
Silverberg SG, Bolin MG, DeGiorgi LS. 1972. Adenocanthoma and mixed adenosquamous carcinoma of the endometrium: A clinicopathologic study. *Cancer* 30:1307–1314.
Silverberg SG, DeGiorgi LS. 1974. Histopathologic analysis of preoperative radiation therapy in endometrial carcinoma. *Am J Obstet Gynecol* 119:698–704.

Surwit EA, Fowler WC, Rogoff EE, Jelovsik F, Parker RT, Creasman WT. 1979. Stage II carcinoma of the endometrium. *Int J Radiat Oncol Biol Phys* 5:323–326.

Szpak CA, Creasman WT, Vollmer RT, Johnston WW. 1981. Prognostic value of cytologic examination of peritoneal washings in patients with endometrial carcinoma. *Acta Cytol* 25:638–640.

Underwood PB, Luta MH, Kreutner A, Miller MC, Johnson RD, 1977. Carcinoma of the endometrium: Radiation followed immediately by operation. *Am J Obstet Gynecol* 128:86–98.

Wilson JF, Cox JD, Chahbazian CM, del Regato JA. 1980. Time dose relationships in endometrial adenocarcinoma: Importance of the interval from external pelvic irradiation to surgery. *Int J Radiat Oncol Biol Phys* 6:597–600.

Yazigi R, Piver MS, Blumenson L. 1983. Malignant peritoneal cytology as prognostic indicator in stage I endometrial cancer. *Obstet Gynecol* 62:359–362.

Annual Clinical Conference on Cancer, Vol. 29
Gynecologic Cancer: Diagnosis and Treatment Strategies
© 1987 by The University of Texas System Cancer Center

24. Current Management of Endometrial Cancer

Samuel C. Ballon

Endometrial adenocarcinoma is unique among malignant tumors of the female genital organs in that approximately three fourths of patients are considered to have clinical stage I disease at the time of diagnosis (Homesley, Boronow, and Lewis 1976). Numerous reports document excellent survival rates of patients with stage I endometrial carcinoma who have been treated with a variety of therapeutic programs. The emphasis on survival statistics in support of a particular treatment has diverted attention from the study of both clinical and pathological features of prognostic importance. An in-depth understanding of these would facilitate the design of appropriate clinical trials by taking into account specific patterns of spread as well as factors that place patients at risk for recurrence. This deficit in our knowledge is of more than theoretical importance. A comprehensive review of survival data suggests that less than 75% of patients with stage I disease are cured (Kottmeier 1979).

This report emphasizes the role of surgical operation in facilitating the appropriate application and integration of available therapeutic modalities. Data are presented to support an initial operation to overcome deficits in clinical staging and to avoid the inappropriate use of adjunctive ionizing radiation, cytotoxic drugs, or hormones in the treatment of this disease. Knowledge of prognostic factors in endometrial carcinoma can identify patients at risk of recurrence but cannot, in itself, define adequate treatment. Surgery represents the rational first step in the treatment of most patients with endometrial cancer.

Deficits in Clinical Staging

The staging of endometrial carcinoma is based on recommendations of the Cancer Committee of the International Federation of Gynecology and Obstetrics (FIGO) (as shown in table 24.1) and includes measurement of uterine depth from the external cervical os to the top of the endometrial cavity. The degree of histological differentiation of the tumor is determined, as is spread to the cervix (stage II disease), which occurs in 10% to 15% of women with endometrial cancer.

Although the size of the uterus has been shown to influence prognosis, many benign conditions also result in uterine enlargement. Reported series have documented a five-year survival rate of 85% with stage IA disease and a 67% five-year survival rate with stage IB disease. Others, however, have not found this to be true and show identical survival for patients with a similar grade of tumor irrespective of uterine size (Malkasian 1978).

Table 24.1. *FIGO Staging of Carcinoma of the Corpus Uteri*

Stage 0	Carcinoma in situ. Histological findings are suspicious of malignancy; cases of stage 0 should not be included in any therapeutic statistics.
Stage I	The carcinoma is confined to the corpus.
Stage IA	The length of the uterine cavity is 8 cm or less.
Stage IB	The length of the uterine cavity is more than 8 cm.
It is desirable that the stage I cases be subgrouped with regard to the histological type of the adenocarcinoma as follows:	
G1	Highly differentiated adenomatous carcinoma.
G2	Differentiated adenomatous carcinoma with partly solid areas.
G3	Predominantly solid or entirely undifferentiated carcinoma.
Stage II	The carcinoma has involved the corpus and the cervix but has not extended outside the uterus.
Stage III	The carcinoma has extended outside the uterus but not outside the true pelvis.
Stage IV	The carcinoma has extended outside the true pelvis or has obviously involved the mucosa of the bladder or rectum. A bullous edema as such does not permit a case to be allotted to stage IV.
Stage IVA	Spread of the growth to adjacent organs.
Stage IVB	Spread to distant organs.

Of those factors that can be assessed reliably preoperatively, histological grade has great prognostic importance because it correlates with the risk of deep myometrial penetration, metastases to the vaginal vault, and spread to pelvic lymph nodes (Cheon 1969). Cervical extension and hematogenous spread also are more frequent with poorly differentiated tumors (De Muelenaere 1976). Thus, although grade can be used to predict the risk of recurrence, it does not define the precise sites of metastases in a given patient. Similarly, cervical involvement by other than anaplastic cancer is unusual and suggests only that both regional and distant sites can harbor metastatic disease. Designating a tumor as stage II cannot, therefore, serve as the basis for a rational treatment plan.

A variety of histological subtypes of endometrial carcinoma and their relative frequency of occurrence have been identified (Berman et al. 1980). They include adenocarcinoma (67.1%), adenoacanthoma (20.3%), adenosquamous carcinoma (12.6%), clear cell carcinoma (including the papillary serous variant [< 1%], and squamous carcinoma [< 1%]). Some of these, such as the papillary serous variant, have demonstrated an unusually high frequency and unique pattern of spread and recurrence. At present, however, histological type is not included in the FIGO staging system.

A large uterus, anaplastic tumor, deep myometrial penetration, cervical spread, and a specific histological subtype of endometrial cancer define the risk of recurrence after hysterectomy. Rational treatment demands, in addition, knowledge of the precise area or areas of involvement. This knowledge can be obtained by an initial operative approach.

Goals of Treatment

The success of a program of therapy can be judged only in the context of its intended goal. In patients with endometrial carcinoma, an initial operation can determine not only the need for adjunctive therapy, but whether available techniques permit adjunctive treatment with curative or palliative intent.

A careful pelvic examination and review of all radiographic studies and information obtained at diagnostic curettage should be completed before laparotomy. A vertical incision extending from the symphysis pubis to within 5 cm of the xyphoid process permits inspection and palpation according to a predetermined, reproducible protocol. The status of the anterior parietal peritoneum, paracolic gutters, peritoneum overlying the kidneys, inferior surfaces of the diaphragm, hepatic capsule, and parenchyma, lesser sac and pancreas, small intestine and mesentery, appendix, large intestine, greater and lesser omentum, peritoneum of the anterior and posterior cul de sac, uterine serosa, fallopian tubes, and ovaries should be determined.

If gross extrauterine disease is identified, as much of this tumor as possible should be removed. A hysterectomy and bilateral salpingo-oophorectomy also are performed. A portion of the primary tumor and of a metastatic focus should be submitted to a pathologist for determination of estrogen and progesterone receptor protein content. Appropriate patients can thus be identified as potential candidates for systemic hormonal therapy or treatment with cytotoxic agents. Irradiation, if indicated, should be expected to improve local control rather than survival.

When no extrauterine spread is readily appreciated, washings are obtained from the pelvis, right and left paracolic gutters, and subdiaphragmatic spaces. These are submitted in separate containers for cytological evaluation (Creasman et al. 1981). After hysterectomy and bilateral salpingo-oophorectomy are accomplished, bilateral pelvic and periaortic lymph nodes are extensively sampled whenever the tumor is moderately or poorly differentiated. Pelvic lymph node metastases have been documented in 11% and 27% of patients with these tumor grades, respectively (Boronow 1984). Inasmuch as only 2% of well-differentiated tumors metastasize to pelvic lymph nodes, their removal in these cases is not routinely indicated. Of critical importance is the finding that over 50% of tumors that have metastasized to pelvic lymph nodes also involve the periaortic lymphatics. In addition, periaortic lymph node involvement in the absence of pelvic lymph node metastases is uncommon.

Operation as a Rational Basis for Therapy

If endometrial cancer is confined to the uterus, hysterectomy should cure the patient. If it is not confined to the uterus, the location and extent of extrauterine involvement can be determined at operation. The need for adjunctive therapy, choice of modality, and realistic goals of treatment can be individualized and are communicated to the patient based on a precise understanding of her disease. In addition, initial hysterectomy and staging laparotomy form the most rational basis for the design of clinical trials that can accurately assess the efficacy of a variety of regional or systemic treatment protocols. Surgery cannot provide all of the answers to the problem of endometrial cancer. It does, however, facilitate asking the most appropriate questions.

References

Berman ML, Ballon SC, Lagasse LD, Watring WG. 1980. Prognosis and treatment of endometrial cancer. *Am J Obstet Gynecol* 136:679–688.

Boronow RC, Morrow CP, Creasman WT, DiSaia PJ, Silverberg SG, Miller A, Blessing JA. 1984. Surgical staging in endometrial cancer: Clinical-pathologic findings of a prospective study. *Obstet Gynecol* 63:825–832.

Cheon H. 1969. Prognosis of endometrial carcinoma. *Obstet Gynecol* 34:680–684.

Creasman WT, DiSaia PJ, Blessing J, Wilkinson RH Jr, Johnson W, Weed JC Jr. 1981. Prognostic significance of peritoneal cytology in patients with endometrial cancer and preliminary data concerning therapy with intraperitoneal radiopharmaceuticals. *Am J Obstet Gynecol* 141:921–929.

De Muelenaere GF. 1976. The distribution of neoplasm in patients dying after treatment of endometrial carcinoma. *Br J Obstet Gynaecol* 83:576–579.

Homesley HD, Boronow RC, Lewis JL Jr. 1976. Treatment of adenocarcinoma of the endometrium at Memorial-James Ewing Hospital 1949–1965. *Obstet Gynecol* 47:100–105.

Kottmeier HL, ed. 1979. *Annual Report On the Results of Treatment in Gynecologic Cancer*, vol. 17. Stockholm: International Federation of Gynecology and Obstetrics.

Malkasian GD. 1978. Carcinoma of the endometrium: Effect of stage and grade on survival. *Cancer* 41:966–971.

Annual Clinical Conference on Cancer, Vol. 29
Gynecologic Cancer: Diagnosis and Treatment Strategies
© 1987 by The University of Texas System Cancer Center

25. Preoperative Irradiation in the Treatment of Adenocarcinoma of the Endometrium, Stage I: The U.T. M. D. Anderson Hospital Experience

Luis Delclos, J. Taylor Wharton, Felix N. Rutledge,
Gilbert H. Fletcher, and Arthur D. Hamberger

In 1948 a program combining preoperative irradiation and simple extrafascial hysterectomy was established at The University of Texas M. D. Anderson Hospital and Tumor Institute at Houston for patients with adenocarcinoma of the endometrium (Rutledge, Tan, and Fletcher 1958). Previous reports (Meigs 1929; Way 1951; Javert 1952; Dobbie 1952; Stander 1956; Javert and Douglas 1956) indicated that the incidence of vaginal metastasis (5.4–17.7%) was sufficiently high to cause concern and to justify prophylactic preoperative irradiation.

Preoperative irradiation at U.T. M. D. Anderson Hospital has been administered mainly by intracavitary radium in two insertions, three weeks apart (Chau 1960). The Heyman packing technique was modified by the addition of an intrauterine tandem and colpostats (Delclos and Fletcher 1969). The modified packing has been used for roomy uterine cavities, whereas an intrauterine tandem alone has been used for small uteri. Through the years the dose to the uterine cavity has progressively increased at U.T. M. D. Anderson Hospital from 1,750 to 2,000 mg-hr as recommended by Heyman (1947) and Kottmeier (1954) to 2,500 mg-hr, delivering with Fletcher colpostats a surface dose to the upper vagina of 7,000 rad in 72 hours or 8,000 rad in two insertions of 48 hours each.

External irradiation preceded intracavitary radium treatment for enlarged uterine cavities, for undifferentiated tumors, and for tumor extending to the cervix (stage II, International Federation of Obstetrics and Gynecology [FIGO]). A pelvic central axis dosage of 4,000 rad in four weeks (20 daily fractions) was delivered with parallel opposed fields from a 22 or 25 MeV photon beam; this was followed by only one intracavitary insertion (originally 2,000 mg-hr, later increased to 2,500 mg-hr in the uterus and 4,000 rad surface dose to the upper vagina, in 48 hours). In all patients suitable for a surgical procedure, a simple extrafascial hysterectomy was performed four to six weeks later (Fletcher, Rutledge, and Delclos 1980).

Starting in 1969, patients with a well-differentiated tumor in a normal-size uterus were given one radium insertion for 72 hours (3,000–3,500 mg-hr to the uterus and 7,000 rad surface dose to the upper vagina) followed by a simple extrafascial hysterectomy during the same admission. Analysis of data from 43 patients treated in this manner was done in 1977, and the results were encouraging (Delclos et al. 1978). If this shorter regimen is as effective in terms of central and regional disease control and survival as two intracavitary insertions, this simplified modality would be a superior method because of expedience and decreased cost.

Randomized Clinical Trial

To determine the optimal technique of preoperative irradiation for stage I adenocarcinoma of the endometrium, a randomized study of 90 patients was conducted between December 1977 and June 1981. Patients with normal-size uteri (stage IA) and well-differentiated tumors (grade 1) were excluded from this study because of evidence that they had been treated effectively by a simple extrafascial hysterectomy.

The 90 patients were divided into two groups (table 25.1). The first group, called the "favorable group," included patients with a normal-size uterus (stage IA) and grade 2 tumors and patients with an enlarged uterus (stage IB) and grade 1 tumors. There were 53 patients in this group. Twenty-five patients were randomized to one intracavitary insertion for 72 hours (3,000–3,500 mg-hr in the uterus and, with Fletcher colpostats, a surface dose to the upper vagina of 6,000–7,000 rad at the lowest point of contact between the colpostat and vaginal surface, i.e., 9 o'clock on the right colpostat and 3 o'clock on the left colpostat, computerizing contributions from the intrauterine tandem and the opposite colpostat to these points). Preoperative irradiation was followed by a simple extrafascial hysterectomy two days later at the same admission. Twenty-eight patients were randomized to two intracavitary insertions, three weeks apart (48–50 hours each; 2,500 mg-hr in the uterus each and a total surface dose of 7,000–8,000 rad as stated above) followed by simple extrafascial hysterectomy five to six weeks later.

The second group of patients, called the "unfavorable group," included patients with normal-size uteri (stage IA) and grade 3 tumors and patients with enlarged uteri (stage IB) and grade 2 or 3 tumors. Thirty-seven patients were in this group. Nineteen patients were randomized to two intracavitary insertions three weeks apart, as outlined in the previous group, and 18 patients were randomized to exter-

Table 25.1. *Adenocarcinoma of the Endometrium, Stage I: Preoperative Randomized Trial December 1977 through June 1981; Analysis October 1985*

Favorable Group 53 Patients Treatment Randomization			Unfavorable Group 37 Patients Treatment Randomization		
	Radium × 1	Radium × 2		Radium × 2	External Irradiation and Radium × 1
Stage IA Grade 2	21	22	Stage IA Grade 3	4	4
Stage IB Grade 1	4	6	Stage IB Grade 2	13	10
			Stage IB Grade 3	2	4
Total	25	28		19	18

nal irradiation (4,000 rad midline pelvis in 20 fractions in four weeks with 18 or 25 MeV photon beam with parallel opposed fields) plus one intracavitary insertion in 48 hours (2,500 mg-hr in the uterus and a surface dose of 3,500 to 4,000 rad as specified above). A simple extrafascial hysterectomy was performed five to six weeks later.

Results

The analysis of survival rates was done in October 1985, so that for all patients, there has been a minimum of four years of follow-up. Figure 25.1 shows that the favorable group of patients had a better prognosis than the unfavorable. There was no significant difference in survival in the favorable group between patients having one intracavitary insertion and those having two (fig. 25.2). In the unfavorable group, a comparison of patients having two intracavitary insertions with patients having external irradiation plus one intracavitary insertion showed no significant difference in survival (fig. 25.3).

Patients with grade 3 tumors had a significantly poorer prognosis when compared with patients having grade 1 and 2 tumors (fig. 25.4). This is in agreement with most literature reports. The difference between grades 1 and 2 was not significant.

In patients with grade 1 or 2 tumors, uterine size (fig. 25.5) did not appear to be a significant factor in survival. In contrast to earlier years, we seldom see patients with very enlarged uteri (>10 cm in the midaxis of the uterus measured by hysterometer). In Gusberg's series (Gusberg and Yannopoulos 1964), patients with very

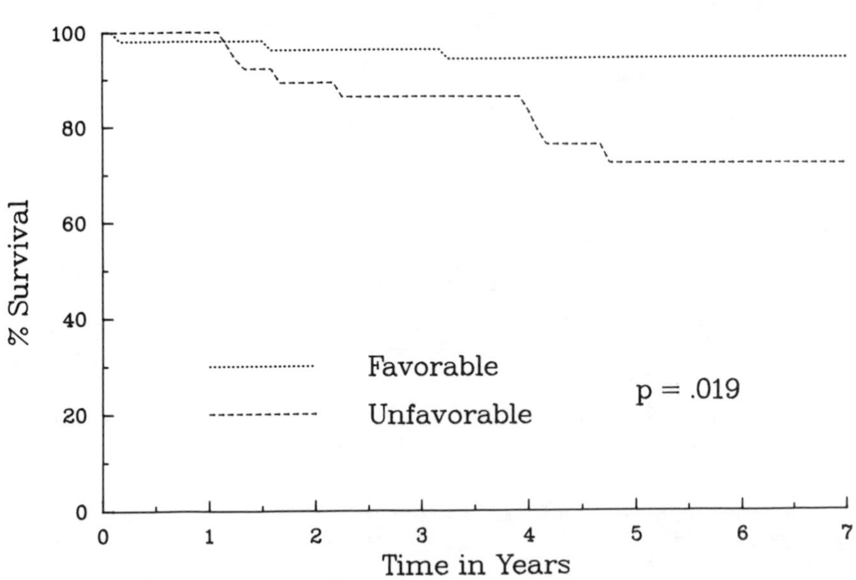

Fig. 25.1. A gradual decline was seen in survival rates for patients in the unfavorable group.

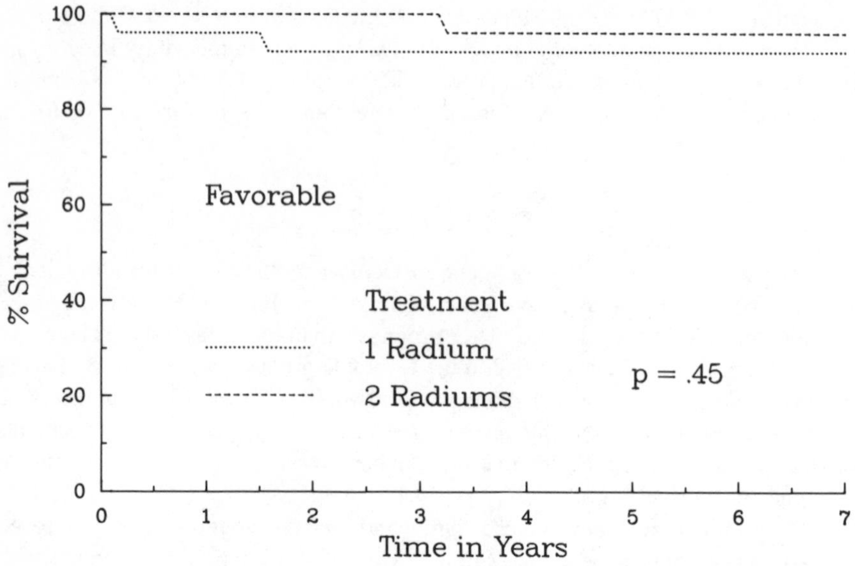

Fig. 25.2. No significant difference in survival rates was observed in the favorable group for the two treatment modalities.

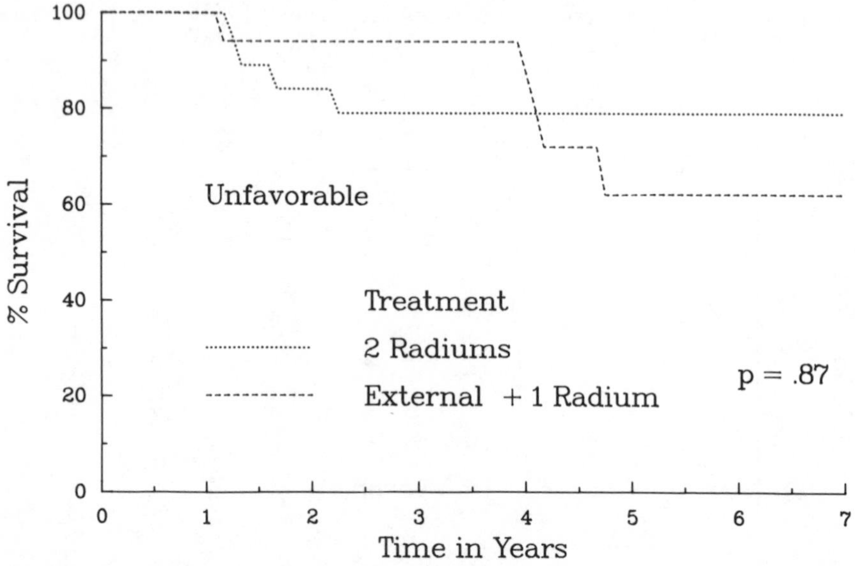

Fig. 25.3. Survival rates in the unfavorable group of patients were not significantly different for patients receiving two intracavitary insertions and those receiving external irradiation and one intracavitary insertion.

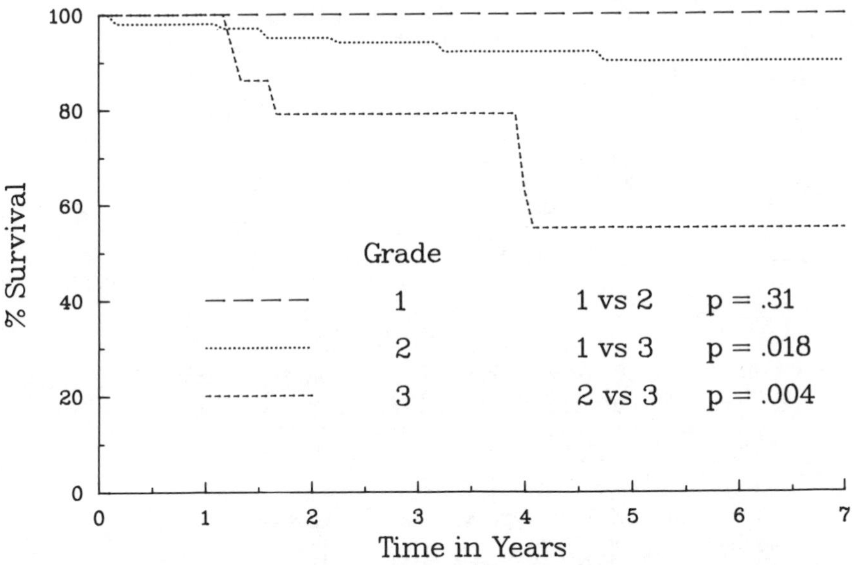

Fig. 25.4 At four years, a marked decline in survival rates was noted in patients with grade 3 tumors.

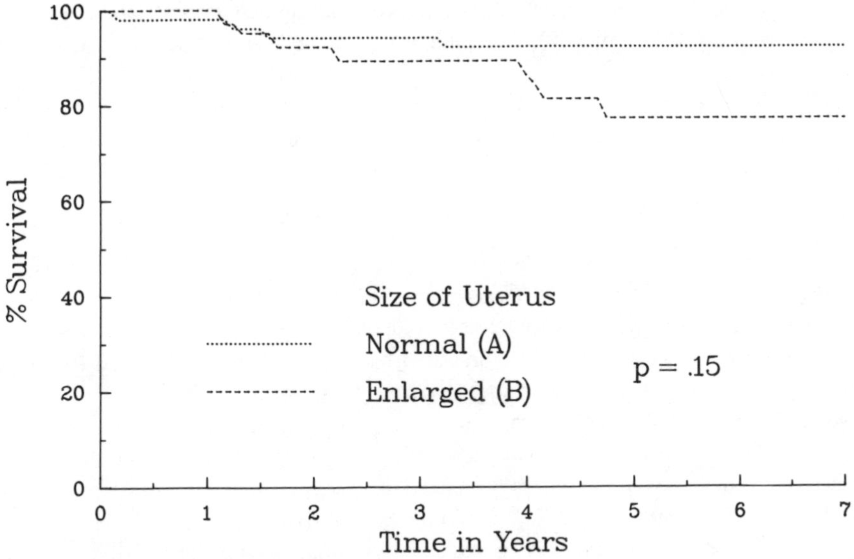

Fig. 25.5 Uterine size did not appear to be an important factor in long-term survival for patients with grade 1 or grade 2 tumors.

Table 25.2. *Correlation of Grade and Uterine Cavity Size with Outcome*

Grade	No. of Patients	Deaths from Tumor
Grade 1 enlarged	10	0
Grade 2 normal	43	3
enlarged	23	1
Grade 3 normal	8	1
enlarged	6	5

large uteri had a poorer prognosis than did patients with uteri smaller than 10 cm. In our series, patients with enlarged uteri and grade 3 tumors also had a poor prognosis (table 25.2).

Correlation of Operative Findings with Outcome

No Disease Outside the Uterus

Three patients died of the disease despite having tumors diagnosed in the early stages as judged by no evidence of disease in the uterus at surgery or by tumor limited to the endometrium. Two had disease recurrence in the abdomen and one had distant metastasis. One patient developed a vault recurrence that was treated with pelvic and vaginal vault irradiation; within one year the patient developed lung metastasis (not proved by biopsy). The patient was treated with hormones and is alive and well six years later.

Of 79 patients with no evidence of disease outside the uterus, 13 were found to have myometrial involvement. None of these 13 patients died of the disease (see table 25.3).

Tumor Outside of the Uterus

Two patients were found to have positive pelvic nodes at surgery (incidence of 2.2%). Both patients had an enlarged uterus (stage IB) and grade 3 tumors. Both patients died at one and one-half years despite chemotherapy. One patient was found to have positive periaortic nodes. She also had pelvic disease unrelated to lymph nodes; the uterus was enlarged (stage IB) and the tumor was grade 3. This patient was also treated with chemotherapy and died of disease at three years.

Nine patients were found to have abdominal tumor spread, and seven died of the disease; of these seven, six had experienced disease recurrence in the abdomen, and only one had distant metastasis. It is of interest that five of nine patients (seven with abdominal spread and two with positive pelvic nodes) who died of their disease were treated postoperatively with hormones or chemotherapy or both, whereas of four patients treated by whole abdominal irradiation with the moving strip technique, only one experienced disease recurrence in the abdomen, one died of distant

Table 25.3. *Operative Findings and Results of Treatment*

Findings	Radium × 1	Radium × 2 or External Irradiation + Radium × 1	Deaths from Tumor
Uterus negative	3	42	2
Endometrium positive	10	11	1
Medial myometrium positive	8	3	0
Lateral myometrium positive	0	2	0
Pelvic nodes	0	2	2
Abdominal spread[a]	4	5	7
Total	25	65	12

[a] One patient also had periaortic nodes.

metastasis, one died of intercurrent disease, and one is alive with no evidence of disease.

Complications

Complications (vaginal necrosis, severe cystitis, severe proctitis, and fistulae) with this combined treatment modality are negligible because doses were kept at conservative levels—below the ones used for the treatment of the uterine cervix. Other factors contributing to a low complication rate were proper selection of applicators and careful techniques of insertion, maintaining the uterus in the axis of the pelvis away from the bladder and rectum, and limiting the vaginal irradiation to the upper third since, in earlier reports, tumor recurrences were predominant in the upper vagina.

Discussion

Earlier reports showed that the incidence of vaginal disease recurrences for patients with cancer of the endometrium treated with surgery alone ranged from 5.4% to 17.7%. With preoperative irradiation, recurrence has been reduced in our series of stage I tumors to 1%.

Landgren et al. (1977) analyzed data on 372 patients treated from 1948 through 1969 and found that with consideration of stage, grade, and specific histology, patients treated preoperatively with intracavitary irradiation alone had fewer disease recurrences in the pelvic region than those treated preoperatively with whole-pelvis irradiation and less intracavitary irradiation. They also found that both regimens led to about the same incidence of distant metastasis. This was in conflict with previous experience, which justified whole-pelvis irradiation because of the reported high incidence of pelvic node metastasis found at surgery in previously untreated patients with endometrial carcinoma (Morrow, DiSaia, and Townsend 1973; Boronow et al. 1984).

After one radium insertion, additional radiation therapy can be administered depending on the operative findings. In this study, none of the patients with positive findings in the myometrium was found to have positive nodes or died of disease. This is in contrast with other reported series (Creasman et al. 1976; Lotocki et al. 1983; Lewis, Stallworthy, and Cowdell 1970).

Among those patients who received two radium insertions *or* external irradiation plus one radium insertion, the number who had no evidence of disease in the uterus at surgery was higher (42 of 65) than that of patients (3 of 25) who received one radium insertion. This may be explained by the higher dose administered and the five- to six-week delay in performing the extrafascial hysterectomy. The presence of tumor cells in the uterus two days after one radium insertion is of no significance, however, because these cells are already devitalized. Thus, the prognosis cannot be based on the evidence of disease in the uterus at that time.

In our series, the low incidence of positive nodes after preoperative irradiation is in agreement with the reported incidence of recurrences in the node-bearing areas of about 1% (Spanos 1979) and also with an earlier lymphadenectomy study at this institution showing that only one of 66 patients was found to have positive nodes at the time of laparotomy (Fletcher, Rutledge, and Delclos 1970). This low incidence is in contrast with reported incidences of 5.6% (Piver et al. 1979; Burrell, Franklin, and Powell 1982) for grade 1 and 26% for grade 3 tumors (Lewis, Stallworthy, and Cowdell 1970) and 4% to 36% depending on histology, grade, and uterine size (Boronow et al. 1984). One may conclude that preoperative irradiation may have been effective in sterilizing disease in the lymph nodes.

Abdominal irradiation may be an effective treatment for widespread abdominal tumor provided that the tumor can be surgically reduced to subclinical levels. This has also been suggested in an analysis of data from 31 patients with intraperitoneal metastasis from adenocarcinoma of the endometrium treated with abdominal irradiation with the moving-strip technique (Greer and Hamberger 1983).

Summary

Preoperative irradiation for stage I adenocarcinoma of the endometrium has been effective and safe, as judged by a reduction of vaginal and pelvic disease recurrences with a minimal incidence of complications.

The techniques of preoperative irradiation can be simplified in the majority of patients by application of only one intracavitary insertion of radium followed by hysterectomy during the same hospital admission.

Whole-abdomen irradiation may be an effective way to control subclinical abdominal tumor spread but needs to be tested, as do new chemotherapy regimens.

Acknowledgment

This investigation was supported in part by Grants CA06294 and CA16672 awarded by the National Cancer Institute, U.S. Department of Health and Human Services.

References

Boronow RC, Morrow CP, Creasman WT, DiSaia PJ, Silverberg SG, Miller A, Blessing JA. 1984. Surgical staging in endometrial cancer: Clinical-pathologic findings of a prospective study. *Obstet Gynecol* 63:825–832.

Burrell MO, Franklin EW, Powell JL. 1982. Endometrial cancer: Evaluation of spread and follow-up in one hundred eighty-nine patients with stage I or stage II disease. *Am J Obstet Gynecol* 144:181–185.

Chau PM. 1960. Technic and evaluation of preoperative radium therapy in adenocarcinoma of the uterine corpus. In *Carcinoma of the Uterine Cervix, Endometrium, and Ovary*, pp. 235–256. Chicago: Year Book Medical.

Creasman WT, Boronow RC, Morrow CP, DiSaia PJ, Blessing J. 1976. Adenocarcinoma of the endometrium: Its metastatic lymph node potential. *Gynecol Oncol* 4:239–243.

Delclos L, Fletcher GH. 1969. Malignant tumors of the endometrium: Evaluation of some aspects of radiotherapy. In *Cancer of the Uterus and Ovary*, pp. 62–72. Chicago: Year Book Medical.

Delclos L, Fletcher GH, Landgren RC, Rodriguez R, Rutledge FN. 1978. The place of radiotherapy in adenocarcinoma of the endometrium. *Revista Interamericana de Radiologia* 3:199–207.

Dobbie MW. 1952. Vaginal recurrences in carcinoma of the body of the uterus and their prevention by radium therapy. *Journal of Obstetrics and Gynaecology of the British Empire* 60:702–705.

Fletcher GH, Rutledge FN, Delclos L. 1970. Adenocarcinoma of the uterus. In *Frontiers of Therapy and Oncology*, ed. JM Vaeth, pp. 262–275. White Plains, New York, Basel, Switzerland: S Karger.

Fletcher GH, Rutledge FN, Delclos L. 1980. Adenocarcinoma of the uterus. In *Textbook of Radiotherapy*, 3rd edition, ed. GH Fletcher, pp. 789–808. Philadelphia: Lea & Febiger.

Greer BE, Hamberger AD. 1983. Treatment of intraperitoneal metastatic adenocarcinoma of the endometrium by the whole-abdomen moving-strip technique and pelvic boost irradiation. *Gynecol Oncol* 16:365–373.

Gusberg SB, Yannopoulos D. 1964. Therapeutic decisions in corpus cancer. *Am J Obstet Gynecol* 88:157–162.

Heyman J. 1947. The radiotherapeutic treatment of cancer corpus uteri. *Br J Radiol* 20: 85–91.

Javert CT. 1952. Spread of benign and malignant endometrium in lymphatic system with note on co-existing vascular involvement. *Am J Obstet Gynecol* 64:780–806.

Javert CT, Douglas RG. 1956. Treatment of endometrial adenocarcinoma: A study of 381 cases at The New York Hospital. A preliminary report. *AJR* 75:508–514.

Kottmeier HL. 1954. Carcinoma of the corpus. Its classification and treatment. *Gynaecologia* 138:287–310.

Landgren RD, Fletcher GH, Gallager HS, Delclos L, Wharton JT. 1977. Treatment failure sites according to irradiation technique and histology in patients with endometrial cancer. *Cancer* 40:131–135.

Lewis BV, Stallworthy JA, Cowdell R. 1970. Adenocarcinoma of the body of the uterus. *Journal of Obstetrics and Gynaecology of the British Commonwealth* 77:343–348.

Lotocki RJ, Copeland LJ, De Petrillo AD, Muirhead W. 1983. Stage I endometrial adenocarcinoma: Treatment results in 835 patients. *Am J Obstet Gynecol* 146:141–145.

Meigs JV. 1929. Adenocarcinoma of fundus of uterus: Report concerning vaginal metastases of this tumor. *N Engl J Med* 201:155–160.

Morrow CP, DiSaia PJ, Townsend DE. 1973. Current management of endometrial carcinoma. *Obstet Gynecol* 42:399–406.

Piver MS, Yazigi R, Blumenson L, Tsukada Y. 1979. A prospective trial comparing hysterectomy, hysterectomy plus vaginal radium, and uterine radium plus hysterectomy in stage I endometrial carcinoma. *Obstet Gynecol* 54:85–89.

Rutledge FN, Tan SK, Fletcher GH. 1958. Vaginal metastases from adenocarcinoma of the corpus uteri. *Am J Obstet Gynecol* 75:167–174.

Spanos WJ, Fletcher GH, Wharton JT, Gallager HS. 1979. Patterns of pelvic recurrence in endometrial carcinoma. *Gynecol Oncol* 6:495–502.

Stander RW. 1956. Vaginal metastases following treatment of endometrial carcinoma. *Am J Obstet Gynecol* 71:776–779.

Way S. 1951. Vaginal metastases of carcinoma of body of uterus. *Journal of Obstetrics and Gynaecology of the British Empire* 58:558–572.

Annual Clinical Conference on Cancer, Vol. 29
Gynecologic Cancer: Diagnosis and Treatment Strategies
© 1987 by The University of Texas System Cancer Center

26. Chemotherapy for Endometrial Cancer

Jan C. Seski, Geri-Lynn Kasper, and Alan J. Kunschner

Endometrial cancer is the most common malignancy of the female genital tract. The overall survival rate for all stages of endometrial cancer is between 60% and 70%. Between 30% and 40% of patients present initially with advanced disease or develop a recurrence after primary therapy (Kottmeier 1979).

Hormonal therapy with progestins has been the most common treatment for metastatic endometrial cancer. Progestin therapy is attractive because it is easy to administer and has few side effects (Ehrlich, Young, and Cleary 1981; Hunter, Longcope, and Jordan 1980; Creasman et al. 1980; Rodriquez et al. 1979). However, overall response to progestins is only 15% to 30%, with well-differentiated tumors most likely to respond and poorly differentiated tumors only responding infrequently (Piver et al. 1980). Since most advanced or recurrent endometrial cancers are moderately or poorly differentiated, the majority of patients with advanced disease will probably not respond to progestins.

There exists, then, a sizable population of patients with endometrial cancer who might better benefit from an alternative form of systemic therapy for the disease.

Our efforts to develop an effective regimen of cytotoxic chemotherapy for endometrial cancer began in 1979 with a study using the combination of doxorubicin HCl and cyclophosphamide (Seski et al. 1981b). These two drugs had previously been shown to have activity as single agents against endometrial cancers (Donovan 1974; Thigpen et al. 1979).

Twenty-six patients with metastatic endometrial cancer received the combination. Doxorubicin HCl was administered every four weeks at a dose of 40 to 50 mg/m^2 together with cyclophosphamide at a dose of 400 to 500 mg/m^2. Of 26 patients, 8 (31%) had a partial response to this combination. The median duration of remission was 4 months, with a range of 2 to 12 months. There were no complete responses. The combination was active against poorly differentiated tumors and was able to reduce the size of large pelvic and abdominal tumor masses in some instances. The toxicity of this regimen was moderate; four patients (15%) developed severe myelosuppression. There was no difference in response to doxorubicin HCl and cyclophosphamide between patients previously treated with progestins and those not previously treated.

The further development of an effective chemotherapeutic regimen for endometrial cancer depended on the discovery of other single agents with activity against these tumors. Hexamethylmelamine was the next drug tested, in 20 patients with metastatic endometrial cancer (Seski et al. 1981a). The drug was administered orally at a dose of 8 mg/kg/day. Six patients (30%) showed a partial response. The median duration of remission was three and a half months, with a range of one to seven months. There were no complete responders. The major toxic effects noted with hexamethylmelamine therapy were nausea, vomiting, and neurotoxicity. In six cases (30%), therapy was discontinued because of side effects. Although the drug had some activity against these tumors, its usefulness was limited because its toxicity precluded prolonged administration.

After the hexamethylmelamine study, we determined that a more active agent was needed. Prior studies on the use of cisplatin had not centered on endometrial cancer and there were few clinical data on its efficacy in such cases beyond the suggestion that the drug was relatively inactive against these tumors (Thigpen 1980). But our preliminary experience suggested that there might be a role for cisplatin in the treatment of endometrial cancers.

For this reason, a phase II clinical trial of cisplatin was started in 1980 (Seski et al. 1982). We treated 26 women who had advanced or recurrent endometrial cancer with cisplatin at a dose of 50, 70, or 100 mg/m^2 every four weeks. An objective response was obtained in 11 of 26 patients (42%), with 10 partial responses and 1 complete response. The median duration of remission was 5 months, with a range of 2 to 11 months. The complete response lasted eight months. Five patients had stable disease, which lasted an average of five months. Differences in response based on the dose of cisplatin were not statistically significant. The major toxicities were gastrointestinal, neurological, and renal, and the drug was discontinued in 8 of 26 cases (31%) because of these side effects.

Cisplatin in this clinical trial demonstrated the most activity of any single agent tested against endometrial cancer. It remained for cisplatin to be combined with other previously tested, active agents to see if improvement in response could be obtained with acceptable toxicity. Therefore, a phase II clinical trial using cisplatin, doxorubicin HCl, and cyclophosphamide for the treatment of endometrial cancer was initiated.

Materials and Methods

In August 1981, 31 women with advanced or recurrent endometrial cancer were entered into our study. So that the activity of the combination of cisplatin, doxorubicin HCl (Adriamycin), and cyclophosphamide—a regimen known as PAC—could be clearly assessed, patients were not started on progestins, tamoxifen, or nonhormonal chemotherapy concomitantly with PAC. Patients with progressive endometrial cancer who had previously received progestins, tamoxifen, or nonhormonal chemotherapy were eligible for PAC.

Each patient received at least two consecutive monthly courses of chemotherapy. Patients were evaluated every four weeks with a complete physical and pelvic examination. When possible, individual tumor masses were carefully measured and the measurements recorded and compared with those of previous examinations. A chest X ray, electrocardiogram, complete blood count, and renal and liver function tests were performed every four weeks prior to the administration of PAC chemotherapy.

Chemotherapy was administered intravenously every four weeks on an inpatient basis. Two dose regimens of PAC were utilized: a low dose of 40 mg/m² doxorubicin HCl, 40 mg/m² cisplatin, and 400 mg/m² cyclophosphamide, and a high dose of 50 mg/m² doxorubicin HCl, 50 mg/m² cisplatin, and 500 mg/m² cyclophosphamide. The dose of PAC was based on a clinical assessment of the patient's performance status and anticipated tolerance for chemotherapy. Debilitated patients or those who had received previous pelvic irradiation usually received the lower dose of PAC.

When a cumulative doxorubicin HCl dose of 450 mg/m² was reached, the drug was stopped and cyclophosphamide was increased to 1,000 mg/m² and cisplatin increased to 70 mg/m². When neurotoxicity or nephrotoxicity (or both) necessitated the discontinuation of cisplatin, cyclophosphamide alone was continued at a dosage of 250 mg/m² orally for five days every four weeks until persistent myelosuppression necessitated its discontinuation.

Renal toxicity was defined as a sustained elevation in the serum creatinine level above 1.6 mg/dl. Neurotoxicity was defined as a peripheral neuropathy manifested by a profound sensory loss in the extremities with absent deep tendon reflexes.

Some patients had disease that was easy to evaluate, either by radiography or clinical examination. Others presented with abdominal disease but had no evaluable disease following cytoreductive surgery. Surgical reexploration ("second look") was performed in these patients after 12 cycles of PAC so that the effect of chemotherapy could be assessed.

A response to chemotherapy was judged to be a complete clinical remission when all existing disease disappeared for at least one month. A complete surgical remission was defined as the absence of visible disease at second-look laparotomy. A complete surgical response was further defined based on a review of biopsies that were either microscopically positive for tumor (S+) or microscopically negative for tumor (S−).

A partial clinical response was defined as a 50% or greater reduction, lasting for a minimum of one month, in the sum of the two greatest diameters of measurable disease. A partial surgical response occurred when a 50% or greater reduction in the sum of the tumor masses was noted at second-look laparotomy. Disease was classified as stable when no change occurred or when less than a partial response was seen.

The technique of second-look laparotomy was similar to that used for ovarian cancer. A generous midline incision was used and the entire abdomen explored thoroughly. Cytological washings were obtained from the pelvis and paracolic gutters. Two peritoneal biopsies were obtained from the right and left pelvic walls, from the cul-de-sac, from over the bladder, and from high in both paracolic gutters. The infundibulopelvic and round ligaments were partially excised. Any adhesion or nodule was sampled, as was the residual omentum. A complete pelvic lymphadenectomy was performed and the paraaortic lymph nodes at the level of the renal vessels removed. In those cases in which the second look was negative for tumor (S−), all therapy was discontinued and patients were followed closely. Patients with persistent disease at second look, either grossly or microscopically positive (S+), were continued on chemotherapy.

The clinical information regarding each patient's age, stage and histological grade

Table 26.1. *Clinical Characteristics and Response of Patients Treated by Cisplatin-Doxorubicin-Cyclophosphamide Chemotherapy for Advanced or Recurrent Endometrial Cancer*

Patient No.	Age (Yr.)	Stage	Grade	Prior Therapy	Dose of Chemo	Duration of Chemo (Mo.)	Disease-Free Interval (Mo.)	Site of Disease	Response	Duration of Response (Mo.)
1	38	IV	III	HSO Cytored	High	12		Abd Pelvis	CR	S−
2	58	II	II	HSO XRT	High	13	10	Lungs	CR	11
3	59	IB	II	HSO XRT Progestin	Low	32	34	Lungs	CR	43
4	78	IA	II	HSO Progestin	High	9		Abd Lungs	CR	9[a]
5	59	IA	I	HSO Cytored	High	12	9	Abd	CR	S−
6	73	II	II	HSO Cytored	High	12		Abd	CR	S−
7	65	IB	III	HSO Cytored	High	25		Abd	CR	23
8	52	IB	II	HSO XRT Cytored	Low	17	9	Abd Pelvis	CR	S+
9	55	IB	III	HSO Cytored	High	12		Abd Pelvis	CR	S+
10	61	III	II	HSO XRT Cytored	Low	22	11	Abd Pelvis	CR	20[a]
11	75	IB	II	HSO Cytored	High	14		Pelvis	CR	14
12	75	IV	II	HSO Cytored	Low	11		Abd Pelvis	PR	11
13	68	IB	III	HSO XRT	Low	7	18	Pelvis Lungs	PR	4
14	63	IA	II	HSO Progestin	High	10		Abd Lungs	PR	10
15	66	IB	II	XRT Cytored Progestin Tamoxifen	Low	8		Abd Lungs	PR	7

16	59	IV	II	HSO XRT	High	7	16	Abd Lungs	PR	4
17	71	III	III	HSO Cytored	High	7		Abd	PR	7
18	76	IB	III	HSO Cytored	High	7		Abd Pelvis	PR	7
19	65	III	III	HSO Cytored	High	10		Abd Pelvis	PR	8
20	58	IV	III	HSO Cytored	High	6		Abd	PR	4
21	65	II	III	HSO XRT	Low	6	26	Abd	PR	6
22	62	IB	III	HSO Cytored	High	12	11	Abd	NR	
23	65	IV	I	HSO	Low	2		Abd Lungs	NR	
24	64	IB	II	HSO XRT Progestin	Low	13	36	Abd Pelvis	NR	
25	64	II	III	HSO XRT	Low	7	17	Abd Lungs	NR	
26	52	IB	II	HSO XRT Progestin	Low	9	34	Abd	NR	
27	66	II	II	HSO	High	2		Abd Pelvis	NR	
28	72	II	II	HSO XRT	Low	3	33	Abd	NR	
29	59	III	II	HSO Cytored	High	4		Abd Pelvis	NR	
30	62	IV	III	None	High	3		Abd Lungs Pelvis	NR	
31	59	IB	II	HSO	High	3		Abd	NR	

Note: Chemo, chemotherapy; HSO, abdominal hysterectomy and bilateral salpingo-oophorectomy; XRT, pelvic irradiation; Cytored, cytoreductive surgery; Abd, abdomen; S−, negative second look; S+, positive second look; CR, complete response; NR, no response; PR, partial response.

[a] Died of unrelated causes.

of tumor, previous therapy, duration and dose of chemotherapy, disease-free interval, site of recurrence, response, and duration of response is summarized in table 26.1.

Results

General Features

The median age of the group of 31 patients was 64 years, with a range of 38 to 78 years. Two patients had grade I tumors, 17 had grade II tumors, and 12 had grade III tumors. Thirteen patients developed recurrent endometrial cancer following hysterectomy and salpingo-oophorectomy (HSO), in 12 of the cases after additional pelvic or vaginal irradiation. The other 18 patients presented with advanced disease. Prior to starting PAC chemotherapy, 17 of these underwent HSO and, in 12 cases, further cytoreductive surgery. Disease was present in the lungs alone in 2 cases; in the abdomen or pelvis in 21 cases; and in the lungs, abdomen, and pelvis in 8 cases. Six patients had prior exposure to progestins and one had also received tamoxifen. No patient had received prior cytotoxic chemotherapy.

Response To Therapy

An objective response to PAC chemotherapy was seen in 21 (68%) of the 31 patients. Eleven patients (35.5%) had a complete response and ten patients (32.3%) had a partial response.

Among the 11 complete responders, there were 4 apparent complete cures. In three cases, the complete disappearance of all disease was confirmed by second-look laparotomy. These three patients have remained free of disease. There was complete regression of pulmonary metastases in the fourth patient after 32 months of chemotherapy; she has remained free of disease for another 11 months. The median duration of remission for the four apparent cures was 28 months, with a range of 18 to 38 months.

Two other patients who were also complete responders died of unrelated causes while continuing to remain free of disease. The five other complete responders initially had complete clinical remission but eventually developed progressive disease. The median duration of remission for these seven patients was 12 months, with a range of 9 to 13 months.

Of 11 patients with complete responses, 5 underwent second-look laparotomy after 12 cycles of chemotherapy. One of these patients had had a pelvic recurrence following HSO and pelvic irradiation, and the other four presented initially with advanced disease. All five patients underwent cytoreductive surgery prior to starting PAC chemotherapy.

Three of five patients who had second-look laparotomy were S− and have continued to remain free of disease at 6, 12, and 16 months after surgery. In two other complete responders, there was microscopic evidence of disease at the time of second-look laparotomy. Both have since developed progressive disease despite further chemotherapy.

Another patient with a complete response following cytoreductive surgery and PAC chemotherapy refused second-look laparotomy and developed progressive disease after 14 cycles of chemotherapy.

There was a partial response to PAC chemotherapy in ten patients. Six had widespread intraabdominal disease and four of these also had pulmonary metastases. The median duration of remission for these patients was 6.5 months, with a range of 3 to 11 months.

There was no relationship between response to PAC chemotherapy and patient age, performance status, tumor grade or site, disease-free interval, dose of PAC, or prior therapy, including progestins.

Clinical Toxicity

All patients receiving PAC chemotherapy experienced alopecia; most suffered from nausea with or without vomiting. Four patients (13%) developed leukopenia (white blood cell count less than 1,000/mm^3) and sepsis requiring hospitalization and parenteral antibiotics. There was no severe neurotoxicity, although there was evidence of mild peripheral neuropathy in all patients who received more than 500 mg/m^2 cisplatin.

In two instances, cisplatin was discontinued because of nephrotoxicity. Both patients had preexisting hypertension and began therapy with a mildly elevated serum creatinine level. One patient developed congestive heart failure after receiving a total of 720 mg doxorubicin HCl. Another patient suffered from hemorrhagic cystitis that abated after cyclophosphamide was discontinued.

Discussion

The combination of cisplatin, doxorubicin HCl, and cyclophosphamide represents the culmination of our efforts to develop an effective chemotherapeutic regimen for endometrial cancer.

Although response rates and toxicity—not treatment comparisons—were involved in this phase II trial, comparisons with other phase II studies are inevitable. The 68% overall response, 35% complete response, and 12% apparent cure rates associated with PAC therapy represent a significant improvement over results reported in our previous chemotherapeutic trials (Seski et al. 1981a, 1981b, 1982).

The addition of cisplatin to doxorubicin HCl and cyclophosphamide substantially enhanced the activity of each of the individual drugs without an increase in toxicity. Among patients treated with doxorubicin HCl and cyclophosphamide alone, 15% suffered myelosuppression. Only 13% of patients receiving PAC developed myelosuppression.

Plans for future investigations into chemotherapy for endometrial cancer should not only center around phase II trials using newer chemotherapeutic agents, but should also include phase III trials, in which differences in treatment efficacy can further be explored.

The integration of hormonal and nonhormonal chemotherapy into the treatment of endometrial cancer has been somewhat imprecise. The random addition of progestins to various chemotherapeutic regimens has made many of these therapeutic trials difficult to evaluate. Cytosol estrogen and progesterone receptors may help serve as indicators for the selection of endocrine or nonhormonal chemotherapy, or combinations of both, in future clinical trials.

Second-look laparotomy has been shown to be an invaluable diagnostic tool for assessing response to therapy in women with cancer of the ovary. Second-look laparotomy proved especially helpful in this phase II trial with PAC in which complete cure was not expected and response was difficult to assess in the irradiated pelvis, the retroperitoneum, and within small peritoneal implants. In the future, second-look laparotomy should be integrated into chemotherapeutic trials for endometrial cancer as an additional method for assessing response.

References

Creasman WT, McCarty KS Sr, Barton TK, McCarty KS Jr. 1980. Clinical correlates of estrogen- and progesterone-binding proteins in human endometrial adenocarcinoma. *Obstet Gynecol* 55:363–370.

Donovan JF. 1974. Nonhormonal chemotherapy of endometrial adenocarcinoma: A review. *Cancer* 34:1587–1592.

Ehrlich CE, Young PC, Cleary RE. 1981. Cytoplasmic progesterone and estradiol receptors in normal, hyperplastic, and carcinomatous endometria: Therapeutic implications. *Am J Obstet Gynecol* 141:539–546.

Hunter RE, Longcope C, Jordan VC. 1980. Steroid hormone receptors in adenocarcinoma of the endometrium. *Gynecol Oncol* 10:152–161.

Kottmeier HL. 1976. Presentation of therapeutic results in carcinoma of the female pelvis: Experience of the annual report on the results of treatment in carcinoma of the uterus, vagina, and ovary. *Gynecol Oncol* 4:13–19.

Piver MS, Barlow JJ, Lurain JR, Blumenson LE. 1980. Medroxyprogesterone acetate (Depo-Provera) vs. hydroxyprogesterone caproate (Delalutin) in women with metastatic endometrial adenocarcinoma. *Cancer* 45:268–272.

Rodriquez J, Sen KK, Seski JC, Menon M, Johnson TR Jr, Menon KM. 1979. Progesterone binding by human endometrial tissue during the proliferative and secretory phases of the menstrual cycle and by hyperplastic and carcinomatous endometrium. *Am J Obstet Gynecol* 133:660–665.

Seski JC, Edwards CL, Copeland LJ, Gershenson DM. 1981a. Hexamethylmelamine chemotherapy for disseminated endometrial cancer. *Obstet Gynecol* 58:361–363.

Seski JC, Edwards CL, Gershenson DM, Copeland LJ. 1981b. Doxorubicin and cyclophosphamide chemotherapy for disseminated endometrial cancer. *Obstet Gynecol* 58:88–91.

Seski JC, Edwards CL, Herson J, Rutledge FN. 1982. Cisplatin chemotherapy for disseminated endometrial cancer. *Obstet Gynecol* 59:225–228.

Thigpen JT. 1980. Cisplatin in the treatment of advanced or recurrent cervical and uterine cancer. In *Cisplatin: Current Status and New Developments*, ed. AW Prestayko, ST Crooke, SK Carter, pp. 420–430. New York: Academic Press.

Thigpen JT, Buchsbaum HJ, Mangan C, Blessing JA. 1979. Phase II trial of Adriamycin in the treatment of advanced or recurrent endometrial carcinoma: A Gynecologic Oncology Group study. *Cancer Treat Rep* 63:21–27.

Annual Clinical Conference on Cancer, Vol. 29
Gynecologic Cancer: Diagnosis and Treatment Strategies
© 1987 by The University of Texas System Cancer Center

27. Current Status of Steroid Hormonal Therapy for Endometrial Cancer

Clarence E. Ehrlich

Treatment of advanced endometrial adenocarcinoma with progesterone was first reported by Kelley (1951). Ten years later Kelley and Baker (1961) published the first report on the efficacy of a synthetic progestin in treating endometrial cancer. Subsequently, over 30 years of clinical experience have shown that about one third of the patients with advanced endometrial carcinoma treated with progestins have objective measurable responses (Kauppila 1984).

The strategy of progestin therapy is only partly established regarding choice of drug, dose, and route of administration; combination with other drugs to enhance its activity; and selection of hormonally responsive cancers. The purpose of this chapter is to review the current status of steroid hormone therapy for endometrial cancer, emphasizing methods for selecting hormonally responsive cancers.

Adjuvant Progestin Therapy

The effectiveness of progestins against advanced endometrial cancer without significant toxicity has logically led to several studies using progestins as adjuvant therapy. Preoperative intracavitary application of progestin has produced complete disappearance of all histopathological evidence of endometrial carcinoma in 24 of 60 patients (40%) (Richardson 1978; Bonte 1979). In another study, after systemic administration of a progestin either intramuscularly or orally in 161 patients, 10% of surgical specimens were completely free of cancer (Bonte 1979). In addition, several studies have suggested a radiation-potentiating effect of progestins for endometrial cancer (Bonte et al. 1978; Mussey and Malkasian 1966). In spite of these data on adjuvant preoperative intrauterine or systemic progestins, they have not found a role in the management of early-stage endometrial cancers.

Several investigators have studied postoperative and postradiotherapy progestin therapy for endometrial cancer. Conflicting results have been produced by these studies (Richardson 1978; Lewis et al. 1974; Malkasian and Decker 1978; Kauppila, Gronroos, and Nieminen 1982). Considering all the available data on adjuvant preoperative or postoperative progestin therapy in endometrial cancer, the value of such treatment remains unproved and awaits a large controlled randomized trial.

Treatment of Advanced Endometrial Cancer

Although an objective response is observed in only one third of patients, progestins are the most commonly used systemic therapy for advanced recurrent endometrial cancer (table 27.1). Kauppila reviewed and calculated response data from 17 studies in which the authors included more than 20 patients and used standardized criteria to define response. The rate of objective response in 1,068 patients treated with medroxyprogesterone, megestrol acetate, or 17α-hydroxyprogesterone was 34%. Despite this response rate, administration of pharmacological doses of a progestin has become the accepted mode of therapy for advanced or recurrent endometrial adenocarcinoma. Unfortunately, this trial-and-error approach means that two thirds of patients are treated ineffectively. In an attempt to address this problem, several means of enhancing the efficacy of progestin therapy have been attempted. These attempts have included changing treatment strategies and identifying progestin-sensitive tumors. Changes in treatment strategies have included use of various types of progestins, modification of dose schedule and dose, route of administration, and combining progestins with other chemotherapeutic agents.

From table 27.1 it is apparent that the type of progestin makes little difference (i.e., objective response rate for medroxyprogesterone is 36%; megestrol acetate, 39%; and 17α-hydroxyprogesterone caproate, 27%). One must view the minimal differences carefully, considering that these were nonrandomized studies conducted over a period of years.

Kohorn (1976) summarized many dosage schedules in his review article. He concluded that no known pharmacological dosage schedule was superior to another schedule. There are some indications that the response may be related to the dose of progestin. Geisler (1973) observed an objective response rate after 40 mg of megestrol acetate per day of 14.3%, while 80 mg per day gave a response rate of 42.8% and 160 mg per day gave 48.3%. In other studies of medroxyprogesterone using a weekly dose of 1,000 mg or more, a 51% objective response rate was observed, and a 31% objective response rate was observed in other studies using lower doses (Kauppila 1984).

Both medroxyprogesterone and megestrol acetate have been used in combination with cytotoxic agents. Cytotoxic agents have included melphalan, cyclophosphamide, 5-fluorouracil, and doxorubicin HCl. Although early studies were promising

Table 27.1. *Response of Endometrial Adenocarcinomas to Progestin Therapy*

Progestin	Patients (*N*)	Response (%)
17α-Hydroxyprogesterone caproate (Delalutin)	404	27
Medroxyprogesterone	510	36
Megestrol acetate (Megace)	154	39
Total	1,068	34

Source: Cumulative series reported in Kauppila 1984.
Note: Average duration of response, 16 to 28 months; average survival time, 18 to 33 months.

(Bruckner and Deppe 1977; Cohen, Deppe, and Bruckner 1977), subsequent studies have not been. In the combined data from seven clinical trials with 349 patients, an objective remission rate of only 35% was observed (Kauppila 1984). The Gynecologic Oncology Group compared oral megestrol acetate, doxorubicin HCl, cyclophosphamide, and 5-fluorouracil to oral megestrol acetate, 5-fluorouracil, and melphalan and observed a 36.8% response rate in each arm of the study. These larger studies found a response rate no better than that for progestin alone (Kauppila 1984).

Antiestrogens such as tamoxifen have been shown to be effective against advanced endometrial cancer, producing a 35% response rate (Bonte et al. 1981; Broens, Mouridsen, and Soerensen 1980; Kauppila and Vihko 1981; Quinn et al. 1981; Swenerton et al. 1979). Acting by a mechanism different from progestins, tamoxifen may produce a response in endometrial cancers resistant to progestins. Study of tamoxifen's effect on endometrial cancer transplanted to nude mice has shown that it augments progesterone receptor concentrations (Satyaswaroop, Zaino, and Mortel 1984). Based on this observation, Satyaswaroop and colleagues (1984) postulated that tamoxifen may increase the degree and duration of response of endometrial carcinoma to progestin therapy. They found in the nude mouse model that treatment with tamoxifen and medroxyprogesterone was superior to medroxyprogesterone alone or estradiol plus medroxyprogesterone for a sex steroid receptor–positive endometrial carcinoma. Schwartz et al. (1983) performed serial cytosol estradiol and progestin receptor measurements during hormonal therapy on an endometrial cancer metastatic to the groin. They observed a substantial increase in progestin receptor levels during treatment with tamoxifen. Thus, on a theoretical basis, tamoxifen might potentiate the effect of progestins. Although responses have been reported using tamoxifen and a progestin, the optimal administration of tamoxifen and a progestin, simultaneous or sequential, remains to be resolved in future studies (Kauppila 1984; Carlson et al. 1984).

Tseng et al. (1984) have shown that malignant endometria synthesize estrogen in a capacity higher than that in normal endometria. They hypothesized that aromatase may play an important role in estrogen production by endometrial carcinomas, resulting in cell growth promotion in estrogen-sensitive tumors. Aromatase inhibitors, such as aminoglutethimide, have induced responses in endometrial cancers (Quinn 1981). Thus, the endocrine treatment of endometrial cancer may involve several modalities. As our knowledge and understanding of the endocrinology of the endometrium and endometrial cancer increases, the optimal hormone therapy will evolve.

Predicting Progestin Sensitivity of Endometrial Cancers

Clinical Factors

As early as 1961, Kelley and Baker observed that response to progestin therapy was more likely in the case of histologically well-differentiated adenocarcinoma or adenoacanthoma. The correlation between response and histological grade of the tumor was later confirmed by Malkasian et al. (1971), Geisler (1973), and Rozier and Underwood (1974). Kohorn (1976) reported a cumulative series from the literature of 58 grade I and 45 grade III endometrial cancers and found a 51.7% and 15.5% response rate, respectively. This further supports the concept that tumor grade affects response of the cancer to progestin therapy.

Kelley and Baker (1961), Varga and Henrikson (1961), and Kennedy (1963) compared a group of patients that responded to 17α-hydroxyprogesterone caproate with a nonresponding group and noted that the cancers of the responders were of long duration and slow growth, whereas those of the nonresponders appeared to grow rapidly. Reifenstein (1974) found that the number of responders was significantly greater in patients with slowly growing tumors, in those who had been treated for 12 or more weeks, and in younger women.

Some authors have observed a better response rate in younger patients (Smith 1969; Wait 1973), but this has by no means been a universal experience. Reifenstein (1974) analyzed 314 patients treated with 17α-hydroxyprogesterone acetate and found no association between age and response. The relationship between age and response is further complicated by the studies of Ng and Reagan (1970) and Wade, Kohorn, and Marris (1967) who reported that anaplastic tumors are more frequent in older patients but well-differentiated tumors occur more frequently in younger women. This would adversely affect the response rate observed in older women if the observations regarding the relationship between response and tumor grade are true.

Kelley and Baker (1970) reporting on 165 patients treated with 17α-hydroxyprogesterone caproate showed a superior response rate for pulmonary and osseous metastasis, but Reifenstein (1974) found that pelvic recurrences responded just as well as pulmonary and osseous metastases. Kohorn (1976) likewise analyzed cases reported in the literature that were treated with medroxyprogesterone, megestrol acetate, and medrogestone and could find no relationship between recurrence site and response.

Reifenstein (1974) found that prior radiation had a negative effect on progestin response in nonpulmonary lesions but that efficacy was increased in the case of metastatic lesions limited to the pulmonary area and in women given radiation and progestin concomitantly. Some investigators have suggested a synergistic effect of radiation and progestin (Gorski et al. 1968; Bonte et al. 1978b), but more data are necessary.

In his analysis of 314 cases of endometrial cancers, Reifenstein (1974) found that neither obesity nor the dosage of 17α-hydroxyprogesterone caproate significantly influenced the response rate. Efficacy of progestins in the treatment of endometrial cancers was decreased in black women. He noted also that cytotoxic chemotherapy given simultaneously had no effect on the efficacy of progestins.

Despite the apparent association of response of recurrent or advanced endometrial adenocarcinomas to progestin therapy with certain clinical parameters such as age and tumor grade, these clinical factors have not proved useful in selecting patients for progestin treatment (Reifenstein 1974; Rozier and Underwood 1974; Malkasian et al. 1971; Smith 1969).

Steroid Receptors

Selection of hormonal or cytotoxic therapy based on the presence or absence of cytoplasmic estradiol receptors (ER) and progesterone receptors (PR) has enhanced the effectiveness of hormonal therapy in advanced breast cancer (Wittliff 1984). Selection of progestin therapy for endometrial adenocarcinomas based on clinical parameters or tumor characteristics has not proved useful since response to progestin does not consistently correlate with any of these factors. Attempts to select progestin-sensitive endometrial adenocarcinomas in vitro have been made with the use of explanted organ cultures (Nordqvist 1964, 1969, 1970b; Kohorn and Tchao 1968), inhibition of DNA and RNA synthesis in short-term endometrial tissue incubations (Nordqvist 1970a; Gerulath and Borth 1977), and induction of 17β-estradiol dehydrogenase by progestin (Tseng, Gusberg, and Gurpide 1977; Tseng and Gurpide 1975; Gurpide, Gusberg, and Tseng 1976; Pollow et al. 1975; Pollow, Schmidt-Gollwitzer, and Nevinney-Stickel 1977). To date, none of these has proved useful for selecting progestin–sensitive endometrial adenocarcinomas.

Assuming that progesterone and estrogen act on human endometrium and mammary gland through similar mechanisms, it might be anticipated that the presence or absence of cytoplasmic PR or ER in endometrial adenocarcinomas could identify the progestin-sensitive cancers. Considerable improvement in the treatment of advanced or recurrent endometrial adenocarcinomas and possibly early-stage endometrial cancer could be achieved if progestin–responsive endometrial adenocarcinomas could be identified in vitro.

ERs and PRs have been documented in the cytoplasm of normal endometrium, endometrial hyperplasia, and carcinomas (Ehrlich, Young, and Cleary 1981; Creasman et al. 1980; Mortel et al. 1981). The physical and biochemical properties of the receptors identified in endometrial hyperplasia and carcinoma are also very similar, if not identical, to those present in normal endometrium (Ehrlich, Young, and Cleary 1981; Mortel et al. 1981; Janne et al. 1980). There have been 127 cases of

Table 27.2. *Response of Recurrent or Advanced Endometrial Adenocarcinoma to Progestin and Progesterone Receptors*

	Responders		Nonresponders	
Study	PR+	PR−	PR+	PR−
McCarty et al. 1979	4	0	1	8
Martin et al. 1979	13	1	0	6
Creasman et al. 1980	3	1	2	7
Benraad et al. 1980	6	2	0	5
Kauppila et al. 1984	2	1	2	16
Quinn, Cauchi, and Fortune 1985	3	0	7	13
Ehrlich, Young, and Cleary 1981	7	1	1	15
Total	38 (86%)	6 (14%)	13 (16%)	70 (84%)

Note: PR+, progestin and progesterone receptor levels high; PR−, progestin and progesterone receptor levels low.

endometrial carcinoma reported in which a correlation has been made between receptor levels and response to progestins (table 27.2). Eighty-six percent of patients responding were PR positive or rich and 14% responding were PR negative or poor. Eighty-four percent of nonresponders were PR negative or poor and 16% PR positive or rich. Thus, data from our laboratory and the literature strongly support the hypothesis that the presence of cytoplasmic PR provides a reliable marker of progestin responsiveness of recurrent or advanced endometrial adenocarcinoma.

Hormone Receptors and Prognosis

Cytoplasmic steroid receptor concentration in breast cancer is an important independent factor in determining prognosis after primary therapy (Knight, Osborne, and Yachmowitz 1980). In endometrial cancers, steroid receptor status has been shown to be strongly associated with several known clinicopathological prognostic factors (Christopherson, Connelly, and Alberhasky 1983), especially histological differentiation. Martin et al. (1983) studied the correlation between estrogen receptors and 87 endometrial cancers. They found women with estrogen receptor–positive adenocarcinomas of the endometrium had survival time significantly increased over that of those with estrogen receptor–negative tumors. This prognostic variable was in addition to and independent of that provided by the histological grade and myometrial penetration of the tumors.

Kauppila, Kujansun, and Vihko (1982) studied a small group of patients with advanced endometrial malignancies and correlated survival duration with receptor status. They observed that in the advanced malignancies (through stage IV) all ten patients with receptor-negative tumors died of carcinoma within 18 months, whereas two of the six patients with PR-positive and ER-positive tumors were alive and disease free 24 months after primary therapy. Creasman et al. (1980) observed that in cases of endometrial carcinoma with deep myometrial invasion, the receptor-negative tumors progressed more often than receptor-positive tumors.

Creasman et al. (1985) studied 105 stage I and II endometrial carcinomas using receptor status as the sole discriminating factor and showed that the disease-free survival rate was dependent on receptor status. Disease-free survival was improved for ER-positive lesions, PR-positive lesions, and lesions positive for both receptors when evaluated separately within each clinicopathological category. They concluded that steroid receptor status should be obtained on all primary endometrial carcinomas with the possible exception of grade I lesions. Evaluating receptor content may predict prognosis better than histological assessment of differentiation and also be helpful in predicting responses to therapy at the time of recurrence.

Conclusions

First, there is no proven role for progestins as preoperative or postoperative adjuvant therapy for endometrial adenocarcinoma. Second, progestins have been shown to be effective against advanced endometrial adenocarcinomas, producing a 30%

objective remission rate. Third, recent studies show that PR levels predict for response of endometrial adenocarcinomas to progestin therapy. Fourth, ER- and PR-rich or positive endometrial carcinomas appear to have a better prognosis than receptor-poor or -negative endometrial carcinomas.

References

Benraad TJ, Friberg LG, Koenders AJM, Kullander S. 1980. Do estrogen and progesterone receptors (E2R and PR) in metastasizing endometrial cancers predict the response to gestagen therapy? *Acta Obstet Gynecol Scand* 59:155–159.

Bonte J. 1979. Developments in endocrine therapy of endometrial and ovarian cancer. *Reviews on Endocrine-Related Cancer* 3:11–17.

Bonte J, Decoster JM, Ide P, Billiet G. 1978. Hormonoprophylaxis and hormonotherapy of endometrial adenocarcinoma by means of medroxyprogesterone acetate. *Gynecol Oncol* 6:60–75.

Bonte J, Ide P, Billiet G, Wynants P. 1981. Tamoxifen as possible chemotherapeutic agent in endometrial adenocarcinoma. *Gynecol Oncol* 11:140–161.

Broens J, Mouridsen HT, Soerensen HM. 1980. Tamoxifen in advanced endometrial carcinoma. *Cancer Chemother Pharmacol* 4:213–217.

Bruckner HW, Deppe G. 1977. Combination chemotherapy of advanced endometrial adenocarcinoma with Adriamycin, cyclophosphamide, 5-fluorouracil and medroxyprogesterone acetate. *Obstet Gynecol* 50:105–125.

Carlson JA, Allegra JC, Day TG, Wittliff JL. 1984. Tamoxifen and endometrial carcinoma: Alterations in estrogen and progesterone receptors in untreated patients and combination hormonal therapy in advanced neoplasia. *Am J Obstet Gynecol Oncol* 149:149–153.

Christopherson WM, Connelly PJ, Alberhasky RC. 1983. Carcinoma of the endometrium: An analysis of prognosticators in patients with favorable subtypes and stage I disease. *Cancer* 51:1705–1709.

Cohen CJ, Deppe G, Bruckner HW. 1977. Treatment of advanced adenocarcinoma of the endometrium with melphalan, 5-fluorouracil and medroxyprogesterone acetate: A preliminary study. *Obstet Gynecol* 50:415–417.

Creasman WT, McCarty KS Sr, Barton TF, McCarty KS Jr. 1980. Clinical correlates of estrogen- and progesterone-binding proteins in human endometrial adenocarcinoma. *Obstet Gynecol* 55:363–370.

Creasman WT, Soper JT, McCarty KS Jr, Hinshaw W, Clarke-Pearson DL. 1985. Influence of cytoplasmic steroid receptor content on prognosis of early stage endometrial carcinoma. *Am J Obstet Gynecol* 151:922–932.

Ehrlich CE, Young PC, Cleary RE. 1981. Cytoplasmic progesterone and estradiol receptors in normal, hyperplastic, and carcinomatous endometria: Therapeutic implications. *Am J Obstet Gynecol* 141:539–546.

Geisler HE. 1973. The use of megestrol acetate in the treatment of advanced malignant lesions of the endometrium. *Gynecol Oncol* 1:340–344.

Gerulath AH, Borth R. 1977. Effect of progesterone and estradiol-17β dehydrogenase in normal and abnormal human endometrium. *Am J Obstet Gynecol* 128:772–776.

Gorski J, Toft DO, Shyamala G, Smith D, Notides A. 1968. Hormone receptors: Studies on the interaction of estrogen with the uterus. *Recent Prog Horm Res* 24:45–80.

Gurpide E, Gusberg SB, Tseng L. 1976. Estradiol binding and metabolism in human endometrial hyperplasia and adenocarcinoma. *J Steroid Biochem* 7:891–896.

Janne O, Kauppila A, Kontula K, Syrjala P, Vierikko P, Vihko R. 1980. Female sex steroid receptors in human endometrial hyperplasia and carcinoma. In *Steroid Receptors and Hormone-Dependent Neoplasia*, ed. J Wittliff, O Dapunt, pp. 37–44. New York: Masson Publishing.

Kauppila A. 1984. Progestin therapy of endometrial, breast, and ovarian carcinoma. *Acta Obstet Gynecol Scand* 63:441–450.

Kauppila A, Gronroos M, Nieminen U. 1982. Clinical outcome in endometrial cancer. *Obstet Gynecol* 60:473–480.

Kauppila A, Kujansuu E, Vihko R. 1982. Cytosol estrogen and progestin receptors in endometrial carcinoma of patients treated with surgery, radiotherapy, and progestin: Clinical correlates. *Cancer* 50:2157–2162.

Kauppila A, Vihko R. 1981. Endometrial carcinoma insensitive to progestin and cytotoxic chemotherapy may respond to tamoxifen. *Acta Obstet Gynecol Scand* 60:589.

Kelley RM. 1951. Discussion. In *Proceedings of the Second Conference of Steroids and Cancer, Council of Pharmacy and Chemistry*, pp. 116–118. Chicago: American Medical Association.

Kelley RM, Baker WH. 1961. Progestational agents in the treatment of carcinoma of the endometrium. *N Engl J Med* 264:216–222.

Kelley RM, Baker WH. 1970. Progestational agents in the treatment of carcinoma of the genitourinary tract. In *Progress in Gynecology*, ed. SH Sturgis, ML Taymor, pp. 362–378. New York: Grune & Stratton.

Kennedy BJ. 1963. A progestagen for treatment of advanced endometrial cancer. *JAMA* 184:758–761.

Knight WA, Osborne CK, Yachmowitz MG. 1980. Steroid hormone receptors in the management of human breast cancer. *Ann Clin Res* 12:202–207.

Kohorn EI. 1976. Gestagens and endometrial cancer. *Gynecol Oncol* 4:398–411.

Kohorn EI, Tchao R. 1968. The effects of hormones on endometrial carcinoma in organ culture. *Br J Obstet Gynaecol* 75:1262–1268.

Lewis GC, Slack NH, Mortel R, Bross DJ. 1974. Adjuvant progestagen therapy in the primary definitive treatment of endometrial cancer. *Gynecol Oncol* 2:368–376.

McCarty KS Jr, Barton TK, Fetter BF, Creasman WT, McCarty KS Sr. 1979. Correlation of estrogen and progesterone receptors with histologic differentiation in endometrial adenocarcinoma. *Am J Pathol* 96:171–183.

Malkasian GD Jr, Decker DG. 1978. Adjuvant progesterone therapy for stage I endometrial carcinoma. *Int J Gynaecol Obstet* 16:48–52.

Malkasian G, Decker D, Mussey E, Johnson C. 1971. Progestogen treatment of recurrent endometrial carcinoma. *Am J Obstet Gynecol* 110:15–19.

Martin JD, Hahnel R, McCartney AJ, Woodings TL. 1983. The effect of estrogen receptor status on survival in patients with endometrial cancer. *Am J Obstet Gynecol* 147: 322–324.

Martin PM, Rolland PH, Gammerre M, Serment H, Toge M. 1979. Estradiol and progesterone receptors in normal and neoplastic endometrium: Correlations between receptors, histopathologic examinations and clinical responses under progestin therapy. *Int J Cancer* 23:321–329.

Mortel R, Levy C, Wolff JP, Nicholas JC, Baulieu EE. 1981. Female sex steroid receptors in postmenopausal endometrial carcinoma and biochemical response to an antiestrogen. *Cancer Res* 41:1140–1147.

Mussey E, Malkasian GD. 1966. Progestagen treatment of recurrent carcinoma of the endometrium. *Am J Obstet Gynecol* 94:78–85.

Ng A, Reagan J. 1970. Incidence and prognosis of endometrial carcinoma by histologic grade and extent. *Obstet Gynecol* 35:437–443.

Nordqvist RSB. 1964. Hormone effects on carcinoma of the human uterine body studied in organ culture. *Acta Obstet Gynecol Scand* 43:296–307.

Nordqvist RSB. 1970a. The synthesis of DNA and RNA in human carcinomatous endometrium in short-term incubation in vitro and its response to oestradiol and progesterone. *J Endocrinol* 48:29–38.

Nordqvist S. 1969. *Hormonal Responsiveness of Human Endometrial Carcinoma Studies In Vitro and In Vivo*. Lund, Sweden: Tornblad Institute.

Nordqvist S. 1970b. Survival and hormonal responsiveness of endometrial carcinoma in organ culture. *Acta Obstet Gynecol Scand* 49:275–283.

Pollow K, Boquoi E, Lubbert H, Pollow B. 1975. Effect of gestagen therapy upon 17β-hydroxysteroid dehydrogenase in human endometrial adenocarcinoma. *J Endocrinol* 67: 131–132.

Pollow K, Schmidt-Gollwitzer M, Nevinney-Stickel J. 1977. Progesterone receptors in normal human endometrium and endometrial carcinoma. In *Progesterone Receptors in Normal and Neoplastic Tissue*, ed. WL McGuire, JP Raynaud, EE Baulieu, pp. 313–338. New York: Raven Press.

Quinn MA, Campbell JJ, Murray R, Pepperell RJ. 1981. Tamoxifen and aminoglutethimide in the management of patients with advanced endometrial carcinoma not responsive to medroxyprogesterone. *Aust NZ J Obstet Gynaecol* 21:226–230.

Quinn MA, Cauchi M, Fortune D. 1985. Endometrial carcinoma: Steroid receptors and response to medroxyprogesterone acetate. *Gynecol Oncol* 21:314–319.

Reifenstein EC. 1974. The treatment of advanced endometrial cancer with hydroxyprogesterone caproate. *Gynecol Oncol* 2:377–414.

Richardson GS, MacLaughlin DT, eds. 1978. The response of hyperplastic, dysplastic, and neoplastic endometrium to progestational therapy. In *Hormonal Biology of Endometrial Cancer*, vol. 42, pp. 155–172. International Union Against Cancer Technical Report Series. Geneva: UICC.

Rozier J, Underwood P. 1974. Use of progestational agents in the treatment of carcinoma of the endometrium. *Obstet Gynecol* 44:60–64.

Satyaswaroop PG, Zaino RJ, Mortel R. 1984. Estrogen-like effects of tamoxifen on human endometrial carcinoma transplanted into nude mice. *Cancer Res* 44:4006–4010.

Schwartz PE, MacLusky N, Naftolin F, Phil D, Eisenfeld A. 1984. Tamoxifen-induced increase in cytosol progestin receptor levels in a case of metastatic endometrial cancer. *Gynecol Oncol* 16:41–48.

Smith J. 1969. Hormone therapy for adenocarcinoma of the endometrium. In *Cancer of the Uterus and Ovary*, ed. SH Sturgis, pp. 73–83. Chicago: Year Book Medical.

Swenerton KD, Shaw D, White GW, Boyes DA. 1979. Treatment of advanced endometrial carcinoma with tamoxifen. *N Engl J Med* 301:105–106.

Tseng L, Gurpide E. 1975. Induction of human endometrial estradiol dehydrogenase by progestins. *Endocrinology* 97:825–833.

Tseng L, Gusberg SB, Gurpide E. 1977. Estradiol receptor and 17β-dehydrogenase in normal and abnormal human endometrium. *Ann NY Acad Sci* 286:190–198.

Tseng L, Mazella J, Funt I, Mann WJ, Stone ML. 1984. Preliminary studies of aromatase in human neoplastic endometrium. *Obstet Gynecol* 63:150–154.

Varga A, Henriksen E. 1961. Clinical and histopathologic evaluation of the effect of 17α-hydroxyprogesterone-17-N-caproate on endometrial carcinoma. *Obstet Gynecol* 18: 658–672.

Wade ME, Kohorn EI, Marris JML. 1967. Adenocarcinoma of the endometrium: Evaluation of preoperative irradiation and factors influencing prognosis. *Am J Obstet Gynecol* 99: 869–876.

Wait RB. 1973. Megestrol acetate in the management of advanced endometrial carcinoma. *Obstet Gynecol* 41:129–136.

Wittliff JL. 1984 Steroid-hormone receptors in breast cancer. *Cancer* 53: 630–643.

Annual Clinical Conference on Cancer, Vol. 29
Gynecologic Cancer: Diagnosis and Treatment Strategies
© 1987 by The University of Texas System Cancer Center

28. Joanne Vandenberge Hill Award and William O. Russell Lecture in Anatomical Pathology: The More Aggressive Subtypes of Endometrial Carcinoma

William M. Christopherson

The increased interest in endometrial carcinoma in recent years has to some extent been engendered by an increase in the incidence of the disease. This increase cannot be entirely accounted for by increased longevity in the general population or more accurate diagnosis. The proportion of cervical to endometrial carcinoma, which has been one of the standard guidelines for judging changes in frequency, is an undependable measurement for obvious reasons, but often is the only data available for institutional monitoring. Through a population-based uterine tumor registry, we have been able to monitor both the incidence and the death rates of the various forms of uterine cancer since 1953. A unique factor about the registry is that it provides access to all the histological material for pathological review and has helped to standardize the diagnoses made over a quarter of a century by a number of pathologists. This brief report will focus on that review and the long-term follow-up of the registry patients.

Histological Subtypes of Endometrial Carcinoma

The majority of endometrial cancers in our review of nearly 1,000 cases were classified as subtypes with low malignant potential. In fact, 82.8% were either adenocarcinomas without specific features or adenoacanthomas. A few such tumors showed secretory activity (secretory carcinoma) or mucin formation (mucinous carcinoma). Because these features had no effect on prognosis, however, secretory and mucinous carcinomas were not considered to be separate subtypes in this review. The end results of treatment were considered to be very good for the patients with low malignant potential subtypes: 9.9% of the treated patients were dead of disease at five-year follow-up, and 14.1% were dead of disease at ten-year follow-up.

The remaining subtypes of endometrial carcinoma, however, all exhibited much more aggressive behavior and are the subject of this report. They include papillary carcinoma of the non–clear cell type, mixed adenosquamous carcinoma (including glassy cell carcinoma), and clear cell carcinoma of the endometrium. The glassy cell carcinomas, which are very uncommon, are believed to be a variant of adenosquamous carcinoma and will be so considered in this presentation.

The relative frequency of the different subtypes and the vital status of patients at five years for all disease stages are shown in table 28.1. Table 28.2 shows the five-

Table 28.1. *Relative Frequency of Endometrial Carcinoma Subtypes and Patient Status after Five Years for All Disease Stages*

	Patients		Five-Year Follow-up	
	N	(%)	Alive (%)	DOD (%)
Adenocarcinoma	604	61.1	75.2	9.7
Adenoacanthoma	215	21.7	87.0	6.0
Papillary adenocarcinoma	46	4.7	51.1	33.3
Mixed adenosquamous carcinoma	68	6.9	47.5	42.4
Clear cell carcinoma	56	5.7	35.2	61.1

Note: DOD, dead of disease.

Table 28.2. *Five-Year Follow-up in Patients with Stage I Disease Treated with Complete Hysterectomy*

	Patients	
	Alive (%)	DOD (%)
Adenoacanthoma	87.5	6.3
Adenocarcinoma	79.8	6.2
Papillary carcinoma	69.7	21.2
Mixed adenosquamous carcinoma	53.1	32.7
Clear cell carcinoma	44.2	51.2

Note: DOD, dead of disease.

year mortality attributed to endometrial cancer and the survival rates for each of the subtypes in patients with stage I disease. The minimum treatment for all patients included in table 28.2 was a complete hysterectomy. Those treated with radiation alone or partial hysterectomy were excluded because of a poor salvage rate.

Age at the time of diagnosis has been shown to be an important prognostic determinant of endometrial carcinoma (Christopherson, Connelly, and Alberhasky 1983). The median age of patients at time of diagnosis was 60 years for the low malignant potential subtypes, 63 for papillary carcinomas, and 67 for both mixed adenosquamous and clear cell carcinomas. At this stage of life, because there are many competing causes of death, death from disease is a much more significant factor than is five-year survival.

Race has also been shown to be an important determinant of treatment outcome—even after disease staging. The survival differential by race is found in all tumor subtypes. Although the relative frequency of endometrial carcinoma is lower in blacks, this frequency differential tends to disappear in the more aggressive subtypes (Christopherson and Nealon 1981).

Papillary Carcinoma

Papillary carcinoma of the endometrium has long been recognized as a distinct morphological variant. Cullen illustrates such a tumor in his publication of 1900. Most reports include only a few cases and emphasize the presence of psammoma bodies rather than the more aggressive behavior (Factor 1974; Hameed and Morgan 1972; Li Volsi 1977; Spjut, Kaufman, and Carrig 1964). Some authors have emphasized the aggressiveness of the tumor (Boutselis 1978; Cefis et al. 1979; Hendrickson and Kempson 1980; Hendrickson et al. 1982; Lauchlan 1981; Christopherson, Alberhasky, and Connelly 1982b).

In our review of 989 cases of invasive endometrial carcinoma, we found 90 tumors with a predominantly papillary pattern. Forty-four of those, however, were examples of papillary clear cell carcinoma, which we chose to classify as clear cell carcinoma (Christopherson, Alberhasky, and Connelly 1982a). Hendrickson et al. (1982), on the other hand, apparently included such tumors in their classification of uterine papillary serous carcinomas. In their series of 26 stage I papillary tumors, those with a clear cell component made up slightly over one-third. Our reason for separating the two types is that patients with the clear cell variant had an even worse prognosis, and there was only a 35.2% survival rate in those patients at five years (Christopherson, Alberhasky, and Connelly 1982a). The papillary pattern and the absence of a major clear cell component provide the basis for the classification as papillary carcinoma. Many endometrial carcinomas have a villus type pattern on the surface and should not be classified as papillary carcinomas because they demonstrate a much less aggressive behavior.

Papillary carcinoma of the endometrium, like papillary carcinoma of other sites, has a tendency towards psammoma-body formation, and this has been the focus of interest in several of the reports. Hendrickson et al. (1982) noted the tendency for deep invasion, serosal involvement, and lymphatic permeation.

As with all endometrial cancers, stage of disease is a very important determinant of treatment outcome. No patient among the 46 with papillary carcinoma of greater than stage I disease survived for five years. The average length of survival of those who died of disease was only 17.2 months.

In general, we found that the nuclear grading is a more sensitive predictor of outcome than is the International Federation of Gynecology and Obstetrics (FIGO) or World Health Organization (WHO) grading system. This is especially true for patients with papillary carcinoma wherein 9.1% with grade 1, 50.0% with grade 2, and 71.4% with grade 3 tumors were dead of disease within five years.

Mixed Adenosquamous Carcinoma

Adenosquamous carcinoma differs from adenoacanthoma in that the squamous component of the former is malignant. The tumors differ clinically in that adenoacanthoma is more apt to be diagnosed at stage I and has an excellent prognosis, whereas adenosquamous carcinoma is less frequently diagnosed at stage I and has one of the worst prognoses of all endometrial carcinomas. It would appear that, in the past, the distinction between these two tumor types was not always made in a critical manner; hence, considerable confusion exists as to the criteria for diagnosis as well as the aggressiveness of these two tumors (Alberhasky, Connelly, and Christopherson 1982).

In the pathological review of endometrial cancers by Alberhasky's group, 68 patients with mixed adenosquamous carcinoma of the endometrium were identified. The predominant component in 35 was adenocarcinoma. Squamous carcinoma predominated in 20, and both elements were found in approximately equal proportion in 13. Neither the proportion of the two elements nor the subtype of the squamous element affected the outcome. It should be noted that only two patients with disease beyond stage I survived for five years.

Five of the tumors in the series had a glandular component with clear cell features. Another five tumors were of the glassy cell type, and four of those exhibited a very aggressive behavior (Christopherson, Alberhasky, and Connelly 1982c). The glassy cell carcinoma has long been recognized to occur in the cervix (Glucksman and Cherry 1956), but only recently was it recognized as primary disease in the endometrium (Alberhasky, Connelly, and Christopherson 1982). Glucksman, as well as several subsequent investigators, noted the aggressive behavior of the cervical cancer and thought the tumor to be a variant of mixed adenosquamous carcinoma, a concept with which most subsequent investigators agree. A detailed description of the histological variations in these tumors can be found in the literature (Christopherson, Alberhasky, and Connelly 1982c; Ng 1968, Ng et al. 1973; Silverberg, Bolin, and DeGiorgi 1972). The squamous elements of adenoacanthoma may have three patterns with considerable overlapping: surface metaplasia of the adenocarcinoma, morular metaplasia, or a diffuse squamous metaplasia. Adenoacanthoma with morular metaplasia as described by Dutra (1959) is readily recognized and is rarely misdiagnosed as mixed adenosquamous carcinoma. Such adenoacanthomas have a predictably favorable outcome. Adenoacanthoma with the surface or diffuse squamous element is much more difficult to distinguish from mixed adenosquamous carcinoma, especially when there is atypia of the squamous element. In our review, we identified 30 such cases with moderate pleomorphism of the squamous epithelium. When we reviewed the treatment results of this small subset, it appeared that they had behaved precisely like adenoacanthomas and not in the more aggressive fashion suggested in previous reports.

On the other side of the scale, mixed adenosquamous carcinoma must be distinguished from poorly differentiated carcinoma of the endometrium. Indeed, the majority of these tumors are grade 3; but if a sufficient sample is available for examination, individual cell keratinization can be found. This is often accentuated in cases of prior irradiation. Finally, the squamous nature of the epithelium has been shown by electron microscopy, and a malignant squamous element may be found in metastases from these tumors.

Adenosquamous carcinoma had many of the other features associated with a poor prognosis. These included deep myometrial invasion, a tendency toward a more advanced stage, lymph vascular or blood vascular invasion, and poor differentiation. The WHO grading system was used to grade the glandular component of these tumors: 60% were grade 3; 39%, grade 2; and a single case, grade 1. The patient with the grade 1 tumor was a long-term survivor. However, there was little difference in the outcome between patients with grade 2 and grade 3 lesions.

As in the other types of endometrial carcinoma, there was a much better survival rate in women who were diagnosed prior to age 50 than in older women.

Several investigators have suggested an increasing frequency in adenosquamous carcinoma (Ng et al. 1973; Silverberg, Bolin, and DeGiorgi 1972). Time trends in our study did not reveal an increase during the years from 1953 to 1976. It should be noted that Ng's observations were based on an institutional experience, whereas ours were population based.

Although it is not the purpose of this study to discuss treatment of endometrial cancer, it is worth noting that combined radiation and surgery appeared superior to hysterectomy alone for these mixed adenosquamous carcinomas (57.3% vs. 33.3% survival at five years).

Clear Cell Carcinoma

Clear cell adenocarcinoma of the vagina and cervix has been the focus of considerable interest since Herbst, Ulfelder, and Poskanzer (1971) described the lesion in the offspring of diethylstilbestrol (DES)-exposed females during the first trimester of pregnancy. Similar DES-related tumors may also occur in the ovary, endometrium and, less commonly, in the parametrium.

The concept of "mesonephroma" was introduced by Schiller in 1939 for a type of ovarian carcinoma. More recently, compelling evidence that the clear cell carcinoma is of müllerian—rather than mesonephric—origin has been thoroughly discussed by Kurman and Scully (1976). One of the best bits of evidence is its demonstrated origin in the endometrium, which is of müllerian derivation. In 1973, Silverberg and DeGiorgi reported 12 cases of clear cell carcinoma of the endometrium, including two that had been previously reported. Among their 12 cases were 4 that generally would be considered secretory carcinoma. In 1976, Kurman and Scully reported 21 cases of clear cell carcinoma of the endometrium. The reports from both these sources indicated that clear cell tumor had a less favorable prognosis than the usual type of endometrial adenocarcinoma, but that more cases with long-term follow-up were needed to prove that the prognosis was significantly different. Other reports also indicated that patients with this tumor type tend to be older and have an overall poorer survival than that generally reported for adenocarcinoma of the endometrium (Photopulos et al. 1979).

Our review of endometrial cancer revealed 56 tumors that met the usual criteria for clear cell carcinoma. These were carefully separated from 15 other tumors with clear cytoplasm that we considered to be secretory carcinoma. The latter type did not demonstrate the aggressive behavior of clear cell carcinoma, and the patients with secretory carcinoma had a mean age of only 58 years compared with 67 years for patients with clear cell carcinoma.

With the exception of only one patient followed for three years, all patients had a follow-up period that lasted at least five years or until death. The average follow-up was 11 years. It is interesting to note that no five-year survivor subsequently died of tumor. The average length of survival for those in whom treatment failed was only 19 months. As in cases of papillary carcinoma, no patient with disease beyond stage I survived for five years.

As with the other subtypes of endometrial carcinoma, depth of myometrial invasion, age at diagnosis, and race were important determinants of treatment outcome. Clear cell carcinoma was equally common in black and white women; however, the five-year survival was only 12.5% in black women compared with 39.1% in white women. Only 3 of the 56 women with clear cell carcinoma developed disease before age 50, and all 3 were five-year survivors.

Those who have questioned whether clear cell carcinoma should be separated from other types of endometrial carcinoma (Eastwood 1978) now have an objective basis on which to make that judgment. There is also overwhelming evidence that secretory carcinoma with its favorable prognosis can—and should—be separately designated.

Many endometrial carcinomas have small foci of differing histology. We included as clear cell carcinoma only tumors that had 50% or more of that component. Thirty-eight tumors were pure clear cell. The remainder had admixtures of ordinary adenocarcinoma. In order of frequency, the patterns were papillary (44 cases), glandular (31 cases), solid (24 cases), and tubulocystic (16 cases). Usually there was an admixture of two, or even three, patterns, and only 15 tumors had a single pattern throughout.

Details of the histology of clear cell carcinoma may be found in reports by Christopherson, Alberhasky, and Connelly (1982a) and Kurman and Scully (1976). The histological diagnosis is usually not difficult and its appearance is indistinguishable from similar tumors occurring in the cervix, vagina, and ovary. Pleomorphism of nuclei is an important characteristic that is not often found in the conventional endometrial carcinoma. Histological grading of clear cell carcinoma of the endometrium utilizing the WHO or FIGO criteria is not applicable to this group of tumors. The four distinctive patterns or combinations thereof, in fact, make such an attempt a worthless exercise. Although, in our review, a higher proportion of patients with papillary components survived for five years (29%) than did those having tubular (25%), glandular (23%), or solid components (18%), the tendency for an admixture of histological patterns and the small number of survivors make the significance of these data questionable. Nuclear grading also proved to be ineffective for this subtype. The majority of tumors were grade 2 or grade 3, but there was no correlation between these tumor grades and survival.

In 64% of the tumors, there were distinctive round hyalin bodies contained within the cytoplasm or lying within a lumen. This material was periodic acid-Schiff (PAS)-positive and resistant to prior diastase digestion. Although the hyalin bodies appeared to be a reliable tumor marker for this tumor subtype, we have thus far been unsuccessful in determining the precise nature of the material.

The suggestion that these lesions have become more prevalent in recent years (Silverberg and DiGiorgi 1973) was not supported by a time-trend analysis of this series, which is the largest series yet examined. In fact, based on the frequency of the tumor from 1953 to 1963, 30 cases would have been expected in the period from 1966 to 1976; however, only 25 occurred.

Summary and Conclusions

Histological subtypes were analyzed in relation to treatment outcome in about 1,000 women with confirmed endometrial carcinoma. The common subtypes, adenoacanthoma and adenocarcinoma, including secretory and mucinous carcinoma, represented almost 83% of the endometrial tumors and were associated with favorable clinical outcomes. Only 9.9% of these patients were dead of disease at four years, and 14.1% were dead of disease at ten years. The more aggressive subtypes were papillary carcinoma, mixed adenosquamous carcinoma (including glassy cell carcinoma), and clear cell carcinoma. The five-year survival rates were 51.1%, 47.5%, and 35.2% for each subtype, respectively. Death rates from disease for each subtype were 33.3%, 42.4%, and 61.1%, respectively. No patient with papillary or clear cell carcinoma that had progressed beyond stage I at diagnosis survived for five years. Only two patients with mixed adenosquamous carcinoma in more advanced stages survived. Nuclear grade, an important determinant of outcome in most endometrial carcinomas, was of no significance in mixed adenosquamous or clear cell carcinoma. Other parameters such as age, race, depth of myometrial invasion, and vascular invasion were important prognostic determinants.

References

Alberhasky RC, Connelly PJ, Christopherson WM. 1982. Carcinoma of the endometrium. IV. Mixed adenosquamous carcinoma. A clinical pathological study of 68 cases with long-term follow-up. *Am J Clin Pathol* 77:655–664.

Boutselis JG. 1978. Endometrial carcinoma: Prognostic factors and treatment. *Surg Clin North Am* 58:109–119.

Cefis F, Carinelli SG, Marzi MM, Serzani F. 1979. Endometrial adenocarcinoma with psammoma bodies. *Tumori* 65:359–362.

Christopherson WM, Alberhasky RC, Connelly PJ. 1982a. Carcinoma of the endometrium. I. A clinicopathological study of clear cell carcinoma and secretory carcinoma. *Cancer* 49:1511–1523.

Christopherson WM, Alberhasky RC, Connelly PJ. 1982b. Carcinoma of the endometrium. II. Papillary adenocarcinoma. A clinical pathological study of 46 cases. *Am J Clin Pathol* 77:534–540.

Christopherson WM, Alberhasky RC, Connelly PJ. 1982c. Glassy cell carcinoma of the endometrium. *Hum Pathol* 13:418–421.

Christopherson WM, Connelly PJ, Alberhasky RC. 1983. Carcinoma of the endometrium. V. An analysis of prognosticators in patients with favorable subtypes and stage I disease. *Cancer* 51:1705–1709.

Christopherson WM, Nealon NA. 1981. Uterine cancer: A comparative study of black and white women. In *Cancer Among Black Populations*, ed. C. Mettlin and GP Murphy, pp. 185–195. New York: Alan R. Liss.

Cullen TS. 1900. *Cancer of the Uterus: Its Pathology, Symptomatology, Diagnosis and Treatment,* p. 374. New York: D. Appleton.

Dutra F. 1959. Intraglandular morules of the endometrium. *Am J Clin Pathol* 31:60–65.

Eastwood J. 1978. Mesonephroid (clear cell) carcinoma of the ovary and endometrium: A comparative prospective clinico-pathological study and review of literature. *Cancer* 41:1911–1928.

Factor SM. 1974. Papillary adenocarcinoma of the endometrium with psammoma bodies. *Arch Pathol* 98:201–205.

Glucksmann A, Cherry C. 1956. Incidence, histology and response to radiation of mixed carcinomas (adenoacanthomas) of the uterine cervix. *Cancer* 9:971–979.

Hameed K, Morgan DA. 1972. Papillary adenocarcinoma of the endometrium with psammoma bodies. Histology and fine structure. *Cancer* 29:1326–1335.

Hendrickson MR, Kempson RL. 1980. *Surgical Pathology of the Uterine Corpus,* pp. 333–388. Philadelphia: W. B. Saunders.

Hendrickson M, Ross J, Eifel P, Martinez A, Kempson R. 1982. Uterine papillary serous carcinoma: A highly malignant form of endometrial adenocarcinoma. *Am J Surg Pathol* 6:93–108.

Herbst AL, Ulfelder H, Poskanzer DC. 1971. Adenocarcinoma of the vagina: Association of maternal stilbesterol therapy with tumor appearance in young women. *N Engl J Med* 284:878–881.

Kurman RJ, Scully RE. 1976. Clear cell carcinoma of the endometrium: An analysis of 21 cases. *Cancer* 37:872–882.

Lauchlan SC. 1981. Tubal (serous) carcinoma of the endometrium. *Arch Pathol Lab Med* 105:615–618.

Li Volsi VA. 1977. Adenocarcinoma of the endometrium with psammoma bodies. *Obstet Gynecol* 50:725–728.

Ng ABP. 1968. Mixed carcinoma of the endometrium. *Am J Obstet Gynecol* 102:506–515.

Ng ABP, Reagan JW, Storaasli JP, Wentz WB. 1973. Mixed adenosquamous carcinoma of the endometrium. *Am J Clin Pathol* 59:765–781.

Photopulos GJ, Carney CN, Edelman DA, Hughes RR, Fowler WC, Walton LA. 1979. Clear cell carcinoma of the endometrium. *Cancer* 43:1448–1456.

Schiller W. 1939. Mesonephroma ovari. *Am J Cancer* 35:1–21.

Silverberg SG, Bolin MG, DeGiorgi LS. 1972. Adenoacanthoma and mixed adenosquamous carcinoma of the endometrium. *Cancer* 30:1307–1314.

Silverberg SG, DeGiorgi LS. 1973. Clear cell carcinoma of the endometrium. Clinical, pathologic, and ultrastructural findings. *Cancer* 31:1127–1140.

Spjut HG, Kaufman RH, Carrig SS. 1964. Psammoma bodies in the cervico-vaginal smear. *Acta Cytol* 8:352–355.

TROPHOBLASTIC DISEASE

Annual Clinical Conference on Cancer, Vol. 29
Gynecologic Cancer: Diagnosis and Treatment Strategies
© 1987 by The University of Texas System Cancer Center

29. Managing High-Risk Gestational Trophoblastic Tumors

Kenneth D. Bagshawe

The chemotherapy of choriocarcinoma has made many advances in the 30 years since the first reports of the use of cytotoxic agents. At the same time, this use has introduced several new problems. In this chapter, I shall review our experience at Charing Cross Hospital in London but not attempt to review the work of other groups. Many of the most difficult cases that my colleagues and I have seen in recent years have been referred to us from Europe and the Middle East, often after prolonged and unsuccessful chemotherapy.

Because most trophoblastic tumors are now eradicable and about 40% of our patients are childless, hysterectomy is undesirable as a means of obtaining a histological diagnosis. As a result, it is neither necessary nor practicable to make a distinction between invasive mole and choriocarcinoma in all cases. After a woman has a hydatidiform mole, persisting trophoblastic activity is detected by the presence of human chorionic gonadotropin (HCG) in serum, and often persisting abnormalities in the uterine pattern are detected by ultrasound examination. In our experience, however, these do not distinguish invasive mole from choriocarcinoma, and curettage rarely provides tissue that allows a decisive histological diagnosis. Statistically, the probability that a trophoblastic proliferation after a hydatidiform mole is choriocarcinoma increases with length of time after evacuation. In any case, the distinction in the early period after mole treatment may be academic, and chemotherapeutic failures have now been virtually eliminated in this group. It is, however, relevant to point out that our criteria for chemotherapeutic intervention are relatively stringent: we treated 7.75% of 5,124 patients who had hydatidiform moles between 1973 and 1983, compared with the 20% to 36% of mole patients in the U.S. series that Lurain, Brewer, and Torok (1983) treated.

There has been no death in the series from invasive mole. Further, all cases following nonmole pregnancies for whom adequate material has been available for histological examination have proved to be choriocarcinoma with the exception of a small group of patients we now recognize as having placental-site tumor.

Placental-Site Tumor

Placental-site tumor is a rare form of gestational trophoblastic neoplasm that has several features distinguishing it from choriocarcinoma (Eckstein, Paradinas, and Bagshawe 1982; Kurman, Scully, and Norris 1976). It appears to arise predominantly from nonmole pregnancy. Histologically, it is distinguished by relatively uniform fields of cytotrophoblastic cells with less syncytium formation than choriocarcinoma. The reduced amount of syncytium probably accounts for the finding that few cells stain for HCG, but many cells stain for human placental lactogen (HPL) and also with a cytotrophoblastic monoclonal antibody (Loke et al. 1984). The serum HCG values tend to be much lower than levels associated with a similar body burden of choriocarcinoma. A further distinctive feature is the occurrence in some patients of nephrotic syndrome—edema, proteinuria, and hypertension, which hysterectomy reversed in the only two cases of this syndrome in our experience. The most important reason for distinguishing this rare tumor from choriocarcinoma is that its response to cytotoxic agents is very limited, and if detected, hysterectomy should be performed at an early stage in the hope of preventing metastases. It is possible that some of the therapeutic failures in our series of "choriocarcinomas" between 1958 and 1980 were unrecognized examples of placental-site tumor.

Retrospective Analysis of Causes of Death

Between 1958 and 1982, 860 patients were treated by chemotherapy for invasive mole or choriocarcinoma, and 109 of these patients died. There were two principal causes of death, which we define as early and late causes.

Causes of Early Death

Twenty-six of the 109 deaths occurred in the first month of treatment and most of these in the first two weeks. These early deaths were attributable to the initial extent of disease or to metastases in specific anatomical sites. The sites of importance are lung, liver, brain, and gastrointestinal tract. The problem arises also from the fact that when tumors are first exposed to intense cytotoxic action, physical changes perhaps of an edematous nature develop and may convert a critical situation into a fatal one.

Although pulmonary metastases tend to be silent, the situation changes when they become extensive and confluent. Dyspnea and cyanosis may then be present at rest or on slight exertion. During the first few days of chemotherapy in such patients, a fall in arterial diatomic oxygen tension may occur followed by a loss of pulmonary compliance and ensuing respiratory failure. This is sometimes referred to as "the tumor lysis syndrome," though it is by no means clear what mechanisms are involved. Patients with liver metastases may suffer intrahepatic or intraabdominal hemorrhage. Brain metastases may undergo edematous change with an increase in intracranial pressure or hemorrhage.

In all these situations it seems important that the first course of chemotherapy and possibly the second course should be given at reduced dosages to minimize these risks. Respiratory assistance is better introduced early rather than after respiratory failure has developed. In the case of brain metastases, it may be appropriate to alert the neurosurgical team as well as to make use of dexamethasone and possibly diuretics to control intracranial pressure.

In the case of metastases in the gastrointestinal tract, it is important to recognize that these may be multiple and very small, so resection should not be attempted. They may also be large and even grow into gut and through the anterior abdominal wall, producing fecal fistulas. All these lesions seem capable of resolution with judicious chemotherapy, transfusions, antibiotics, and careful nursing.

The use of reduced chemotherapeutic dosages is, of course, also necessary in patients with impaired renal or hepatic function. Creatinine clearance measurements are essential before administering high-dose methotrexate. But when reduced dosage levels are used, care has to be taken not to increase the risk of drug resistance at a later stage in therapy. Full dosage should be used as soon as the patient's general condition permits.

Causes of Late Death

Seventy-five of the 109 deaths in the series occurred after chemotherapy had been in progress for many months, and these deaths were attributable to drug resistance. All but two of the six drug-induced "toxic" deaths were related to the intensification of chemotherapy in response to drug resistance.

The avoidance of drug resistance has been a major objective from the start of these studies. It is still not widely known that very few, if any, advanced cases of choriocarcinomas are completely eradicated by methotrexate alone. Our earliest attempt to avoid drug resistance was the use of 6-mercaptopurine with methotrexate, and this combination appeared to be much more effective than methotrexate alone (Bagshawe and McDonald 1960). Although 6-mercaptopurine is only a weak antitrophoblastic agent, good use of it has been made in China (Sung, Wu, and Ho 1963). Combining actinomycin D and methotrexate was found to cause substantial mucositis. In 1963 we found that methotrexate with folinic acid (Leucovorin) was effective and nontoxic in many cases, so this combination became for several years our standard initial therapy (Bagshawe and Wilde 1963). When patients developed drug resistance, other drugs were then introduced. Subsequent analysis showed that although this approach was very satisfactory for many patients, there were also many failures, and in some patients resistance to methotrexate appeared to confer resistance to other drugs. It was clear that there was a broad spectrum of heterogeneity in trophoblastic neoplasms, some of which responded readily and others only after great difficulty.

Three hundred seventeen cases treated between 1958 and 1973 were analyzed for factors that might indicate the propensity of the tumor for drug resistance (Bagshawe 1976). Twelve prognostic factors were identified, and numerical scores were assigned for each of these. A total prognostic score was obtained for each patient by adding the scores for each factor. Low-scoring patients all survived, but those with the highest scores all died. A somewhat simpler scoring system, which eliminates factors that cannot be measured in all patients, has been published subsequently by the World Health Organization (WHO).

This prognostic score indicates the probability that the tumor will become resistant with a sequential introduction of cytotoxic agents. The fact that there were many deaths in the high-scoring group raised the question of whether it would be advantageous to introduce all the known effective agents early in treatment. On this basis, we have stratified our treatment protocols at three levels for low, middle, and high risk.

Low-Risk Patients

Low-risk patients are those scoring up to 5 on the WHO prognostic scale (less than 50 on the earlier scale [Bagshawe 1976]). Although we call this our low-risk group, it includes many patients meeting criteria that put them into the high-risk category of other series, such as the interval of more than three months from the end of antecedent pregnancy. In our series, 405 patients were treated in this risk category between 1958 and 1983. The only death was from pneumonia during an influenza epidemic. Virtually all of these patients were treated with our methotrexate and folinic acid regimen (table 29.1). Approximately 30%, however, have required additional therapy with other drugs either to achieve complete remission or to accelerate attainment of remission. Treatment is given during alternating weeks and continued until HCG is undetectable (i.e., less than 2 IU/L) for six weeks.

Medium-Risk Patients

Medium-risk patients are those who score 6 to 9 on the WHO scale (60–90 on the earlier scale). They have been treated since 1974 with a protocol that provides single drugs or simple drug combinations in quick succession (e.g., A, B, C, D, A, B, etc.) (table 29.1). Retaining this pattern of drug administration has been valuable for identifying new agents effective against choriocarcinoma. This led to identifying etoposide as a powerful drug for choriocarcinoma (Newlands and Bagshawe 1977).

Between 1958 and 1983 there were 232 patients in this category, and 3 of them died from drug resistance despite the use of all effective agents. There have been no deaths in this group since the introduction of etoposide. Treatment in this group is generally continued until HCG is undetectable for eight to ten weeks.

High-Risk Patients

The patients in the high-risk group all have scores of 10 or more (>100 on earlier scale). Following the prognostic analysis in the mid-1970s we introduced a protocol, initially known as *CHAMOMA*, which included cyclophosphamide, hydroxyurea, actinomycin D, methotrexate, vincristine (Oncovin), melphalan, and doxorubicin HCl (Adriamycin), which was later replaced by *CHAMOCA* (cyclophosphamide replaced melphalan). The principle of the regimen was to combine all known effective agents in a protocol that would incur toxicity but would minimize the emergence of drug resistance. Toxicity proved to be variable but was high in some patients, necessitating a recovery period between courses of treatment that was rarely less than 10 days and sometimes as much as 20 days.

Following this we retained many of the features of CHAMOCA in a new protocol EMA-CO (table 29.1). EMA-CO differs from CHAMOCA in two important respects. First, it introduces etoposide. Second, it provides treatment on a weekly basis. Also, the patient requires hospitalization for only one night every two weeks, and though the total drug dosage over a period of time is higher than with CHAMOCA, it is much better tolerated.

Between 1958 and 1983 there were 223 patients in the high-risk category and 105 of them died. With CHAMOCA alone the survival rate of the high-risk group was 75%, and when a five-day course of etoposide was given alternately with CHAMOCA, this rate improved to 83%. EMA-CO has given a similar survival rate (83%) at a much lower cost in toxicity. Treatment in this category is generally continued for 11 to 13 weeks after HCG has been undetectable (i.e., $< 1-2$ IU/L). The extension of therapy well beyond normalization of HCG values is important in successful therapy. HCG at the 1.0 IU/L level in serum corresponded with the estimated presence of some 10^4 to 10^5 trophoblastic tumor cells in earlier studies.

Patients who become resistant to EMA-CO receive an alternative regimen, and the response to cisplatin is assessed in a combination with vincristine and methotrexate (methotrexate and cisplatin on different days) (Newlands and Bagshawe 1979) or with vincristine, methotrexate, and bleomycin. We have avoided using cisplatin as a first agent because we do not yet know its long-term effects on fertility and because it may be useful to hold at least one potentially powerful drug in reserve.

CNS Metastases

Even in the early 1960s there were patients who presented with brain metastases who have survived. But until the late 1970s patients who developed brain metastases during treatment all died. We have made use of the serum: cerebrospinal fluid/HCG ratio as well as computerized tomography scanning to detect central nervous system (CNS) diseases (Bagshawe and Harland 1976; Rushworth, Orr, and Bagshawe 1968).

We have emphasized the importance we attach, first, to the detection of brain metastases at the outset of therapy and, second, to the prevention of brain metastases in the course of chemotherapy. As long as there is viable tumor in the lung, the patient is at risk of developing brain deposits. Established disease in the CNS is treated by increased systemic methotrexate dosage (1 g/m^2 in the EMA-CO protocol). Provided there is no evidence of increased intracranial pressure, methotrexate (10 mg) is given intrathecally at the time of systemic CO (cyclophosphamide and Oncovin [vincristine]). Prophylactic therapy is essentially the same as the CNS therapeutic regimen except that the standard dose of methotrexate in the EMA protocol is used and intrathecal methotrexate is given in the same way with each CO protocol.

CNS metastases occurring late during chemotherapy have been successfully treated in recent years with surgery and chemotherapy (Athanassiou et al. 1983).

Table 29.1. *Treatment Protocols for Low-, Medium-, and High-Risk Patients*

Regimen	Drug	Dose	Administration[a]	Schedule
Low-risk[b]	Methotrexate	50 mg (or 1 mg/kg with maximum 70 mg)	IM	Every 48 hours for 4 injections
	Folinic acid (Leucovorin, calcium folinate)	6 mg	IM or PO	30 hours after each methotrexate injection
Medium-risk[c]				
Course A	Etoposide	100 mg/m^2	IV in 200 ml saline	30-minute infusion daily for 5 consecutive days
Course B	Hydroxyurea	0.5 g	PO	Day 1; repeated after 12 hours
	Low-risk regimen			Days 2–8
	6-mercaptopurine	75 mg		Days 2–8, but only on days folinic acid given
Course C	Dactinomycin	0.5 mg (or 10–12 μg/kg)	IV	Daily for 5 days

Course D	Vincristine	1 mg/m^2	IV	Days 1 and 3
	Cyclophosphamide	400 mg/m^2	IV	Days 1 and 3
High-risk[d]				
Course A (EMA)	Etoposide	100 mg/m^2	IV in 200 ml saline	30-minute infusion, day 1 and day 2
	Dactinomycin	0.5 mg	IV	Day 1 and day 2
	Methotrexate	100 mg/m^2	IV	Day 1
	Methotrexate	200 mg/m^2	IV in 1000 ml saline	Day 1, 12-hour infusion
	Folinic acid (Leucovorin, calcium folinate)	15 mg	IM or PO	Every 12 hours for 4 doses beginning 24 hours after starting methotrexate
Course B (CO)	Vincristine	1.0 mg/m^2	IV	Day 8
	Cyclophosphamide	600 mg/m^2	IV in saline	Day 8

[a] IM, intramuscularly; PO, *per os* (by mouth); IV, intravenously.
[b] Courses start day 1, 14, 28, etc.
[c] The sequence of courses is A, B, C, D, A, B, etc., or regimen D may be held in reserve in case one or another proves toxic or ineffective. The sequence then would be A, B, C, A, B, etc. The interval between the end of a course and the start of the next should not be more than seven days unless there is persisting toxicity but should not be greater than ten days unless toxicity is severe.
[d] These courses should be given on days 1 and 2, 8, 15, and 16, etc. The intervals should not be extended without cause.

Despite these measures a small number of patients still develop drug-resistant disease, though as already mentioned it is important to determine whether the tumor is of the placental-site type. Patients with minimal persistent HCG elevation are examined for residual disease with a view to surgery. If conventional radiology, computerized tomography scanning, and magnetic resonance imaging produce no abnormal findings, immunoscintigraphy is used to locate residual tumor using anti-HCG labeled with ^{131}I (Begent et al. 1980). In about half of these drug-resistant patients, disease sites have been identified and surgical resections have achieved sustained remission. Hysterectomy is not usually undertaken unless there is evidence of resistant disease in the uterus.

Follow-up has been maintained for more than 95% of the resident (United Kingdom) patients. Recent analyses indicate no significant increase in infertility, nor in congenital abnormalities in subsequent children (Rustin et al. 1984), and no excess of second malignancies (Rustin et al. 1983).

References

Athanassiou A, Begent RHJ, Newlands ES, Parker D, Rustin GJ, Bagshawe KD. 1983. Central nervous system metastases of choriocarcinoma. *Cancer* 52:1728–1735.

Bagshawe KD. 1976. Risk and prognostic factors in trophoblastic neoplasia. *Cancer* 38: 1373–1385.

Bagshawe KD, Harland S. 1976. Immunodiagnosis and monitoring of gonadotrophin-producing metastases in the central nervous system. *Cancer* 38:112–118.

Bagshawe KD, McDonald J. 1960. Treatment of choriocarcinoma with a combination of cytotoxic drugs. *Br Med J* 11:426–431.

Bagshawe KD, Wilde CE. 1963. Infusion therapy in pelvic trophoblastic tumors. *Journal of Obstetrics and Gynaecology of the British Commonwealth* 72:59–64.

Begent RHJ, Stanway G, Searle F, Jewkes RF, Jones BE, Vernon P, Bagshawe KD. 1980. Radioimmunolocalization of tumours by external scintigraphy after administration of ^{131}I antibody to human chorionic gonadotrophin. *Journal of the Royal Society of Medicine* 73: 624–630.

Eckstein RP, Paradinas FJ, Bagshawe KD. 1982. Placental site trophoblastic tumour. *Histopathology* 6:211–226.

Kurman RJ, Scully RE, Norris HJ. 1976. Trophoblastic pseudotumor of the uterus. *Cancer* 38:1214–1226.

Loke YW, Day S, Butterworth B, Potter B. 1984. Monoclonal antibody to human cytotrophoblast cross reacts with basal layers of some fetal epithelial surfaces. *Placenta* 5:199–204.

Lurain JR, Brewer JI, Torok EE. 1983. Natural history of hydatidiform mole after primary evacuation. *Am J Obstet Gynecol* 145:591.

Newlands ES, Bagshawe KD. 1977. Epipodophyllin derivative (VP16–213) in malignant teratomas and choriocarcinomas. *Lancet* 2:87.

Newlands ES, Bagshawe KD. 1979. Activity of high dose cis-platinum in combination with vincristine and methotrexate in drug resistant choriocarcinoma. *Br J Cancer* 40:943–945.

Rushworth AGJ, Orr AH, Bagshawe KD. 1968. The concentration of HCG in the plasma and spinal fluid of patients with trophoblastic tumours in the central nervous system. *Br J Cancer* 22:253–257.

Rustin GJS, Booth M, Dent J, Salt S, Rustin F, Bagshawe KD. 1984. Pregnancy after cytotoxic chemotherapy for gestational trophoblastic tumours. *Br Med J Clin Res* 288: 103–106.

Rustin GJS, Rustin F, Dent J, Booth M, Salt S, Bagshawe KD. 1983. No increase in second

tumors after cytotoxic chemotherapy for gestational trophoblastic tumors. *N Engl J Med* 308:473–476.
Sung HC, Wu PC, Ho TH. 1963. Treatment of choriocarcinoma and chorioadenoma destruens with 6-mercaptopurine and surgery: A clinical report of 93 cases. *Chin Med J [Engl]* 82:24–38.
World Health Organization Scientific Group. 1983. Gestational trophoblastic diseases. Vol. 692 in the Technical Report Series. Geneva: World Health Organization.

Annual Clinical Conference on Cancer, Vol. 29
Gynecologic Cancer: Diagnosis and Treatment Strategies
© 1987 by The University of Texas System Cancer Center

30. Immunology of Gestational Trophoblastic Neoplasms

Roland A. Pattillo and A. C. F. Ruckert

The detection of choriocarcinoma in the placenta of a patient with gestational choriocarcinoma has been reported, to our knowledge, only nine times in the world literature (Ariel and Pack 1960; Brewer and Gerbie 1966; Buckell and Owen 1954; Daamen, Bloem, and Westerbeck 1961; Driscoll 1963; Emery 1952; Kay and Reed 1953; Mercer et al. 1958; Novak 1954). This may be largely because the placenta is no longer available for study when the diagnosis of choriocarcinoma is made in the mother. The time of transformation from normal trophoblast to choriocarcinoma cannot be determined with certainty, but the fact that several cases have been reported in which the malignancy existed within the placenta indicates that this malignant transformation may take place during the gestational period. Malignant transformation in trophoblast cells retained after expulsion of the placenta cannot be excluded.

Rarely, gestational choriocarcinoma is transmitted transplacentally to the fetus, resulting in the birth of a child with choriocarcinoma or one who manifests the malignancy later. Characteristically, the child of a mother who has gestational choriocarcinoma is normal and does not give evidence of disease. This report concerns a study of 18 mothers with choriocarcinoma and the manifestation of immunologic sensitivity to that malignancy by the mother and the child born of that pregnancy. The mothers and children were studied postnatally with a cytotoxicity assay (modified Hellström assay), which identifies immunologic recognition of choriocarcinoma cells by lymphocytes sensitized to this malignancy in the mother and child. Lymphocytes from all children studied showed immunologic recognition of choriocarcinoma target cells in vitro and displayed no blocking of cytotoxicity. Lymphocytes from all mothers showed immunologic recognition, cytotoxicity, and blocking of cytotoxicity only when choriocarcinoma was present as evidenced by positive human chorionic gonadotropin (HCG) levels. One infant in the study died of metastatic choriocarcinoma.

Children of these mothers with choriocarcinoma have been studied at various times corresponding to key points in maturation of immunologic competence as it relates to the immune system's postnatal development. The data represent only a preliminary report because there are few opportunities to obtain adequate blood samples from infants and children of mothers who have this disease. An attempt to suggest a structural framework for the development of immunologic reactivity to neoplastic trophoblast antigens will, understandably, have limited potential. Nonetheless, the availability of the trophoblastic model in vitro provides the first opportunity to elucidate previously unknown dimensions.

Materials and Methods

At the Medical College of Wisconsin, blocking factor assays recently have been added to HCG monitoring of patients with trophoblastic disease because of about a 10% incidence of recurrent disease after chemotherapy. The blocking factor assay is a new test for agents in the patient's serum that prevent the host from reacting against the tumor; these may be tumor antigen, tumor antibody, or antigen-antibody complex.

The blocking factor assay consists of incubating choriocarcinoma target cells without lymphocytes; with normal control lymphocytes (that do not antigenically recognize the tumor cells and therefore do not adhere to them); and with the patient's lymphocytes, which are specifically sensitized to the tumor, recognize it, and cytotoxically destroy it unless the patient's serum containing the blocking factor is added—it prevents the lymphocytes from adhering to and destroying the tumor. The end point of the assay is terminal tritiated thymidine uptake by target tumor cells not destroyed by the cytotoxic lymphocytes. The blocking index is the difference between cytotoxicity in the presence and cytotoxicity in the absence of the patient's serum containing the blocking factor. The choriocarcinoma cells were derived from five different patients and provided five different assays.

The blocking factor calculation was performed as previously described (Pattillo and Gey 1968; Pattillo, Story, and Ruckert 1979; Pattillo et al. 1979). The choriocarcinoma cells were grown in tissue culture flasks, were transferred (10^3 cells/well) to eight-well Lab-Tek chambers and incubated for 24 hours at 37° C in an atmosphere of 5% CO_2 in air (slide incubation compartments) (Lab-Tek Products, Naperville, Illinois). After incubation, the 3520 medium was removed and replaced with fresh 3520 medium. (This medium is made of 30% Gey's balanced salt solution [BSS], 50% Waymouth medium MB 752-1, and 20% fetal calf serum. [All tissue culture media were obtained from Grand Island Biological Company of Grand Island, New York.]) The fresh medium contained 10^5 of the patient's lymphocytes and was added to the target cells in triplicate culture with 20% patient serum substituted for the 20% fetal calf serum and to target cells in another without the substitution. After a 24-hour incubation, the chambers were washed four times with BSS to remove the lymphocytes, and the remaining undestroyed tumor cells were pulse treated in a two-hour incubation in 3520 medium with tritiated thymidine (10 μCi/ml, 5–30 Ci/mmol).

After the pulse medium was removed, the cells were washed twice with BSS containing excess unlabeled thymidine and frozen. Then the cells were thawed, and the amount of radioactivity incorporated into acid-precipitable material was determined in triplicate. Values were expressed as percentages of radioactivity incorporated by the target cells incubated in the absence of lymphocytes.

The cytotoxicity of the patient's lymphocytes was assessed by comparing values obtained from incubating target cells with patient lymphocytes and those obtained by incubating target cells with normal donor lymphocytes. Blocking of cytotoxicity was assessed by comparing values obtained from incubating target cells with patient lymphocytes in medium containing fetal calf serum and those obtained from incubating target cells with patient lymphocytes in medium containing patient serum. Significance was assessed by Student's *t* test with $p \leq .05$ considered significant.

Results

As described in Materials and Methods, the modified Hellström assay has been used as a cytotoxicity and blocking factor assay and has been shown to correlate with the sensitive tumor marker HCG. Table 30.1, a representative record of assays in one patient studied closely for more than two years, contains data demonstrating positive cytotoxicity results in about three quarters of the tests. Conditions that may produce cytotoxicity blocking include poor growth of target cells, poor dispersion of sensitized lymphocytes, mechanical factors, and others.

Table 30.2 shows a series of mothers with trophoblastic disease, all of whom displayed cytotoxicity in the assay system. Patient 1 (table 30.2) is an example of a

Table 30.1. *Blocking Factor Assay in One Patient*

JAr Cells[a]	Control Lymphocytes	Patient Lymphocytes	Patient Lymphocytes with Autologous Serum	Recognition[b]	Blocking
Feb. 1981	112.1[c] ± 7.6[d]	20.0 ± 6.5	100.4 ± 15.7	+[e]	+[f]
Feb. 1981	123.1 ± 24.5	43.9 ± 5.0	93.7 ± 23.8	+	+
Mar. 1981	132.0 ± 9.5	18.9 ± 12.9	79.2 ± 2.2	+	+
Dec. 1981	85.6 ± 18.1	47.1 ± 7.5	71.2 ± 18.4	+	−
Jan. 1982	102.1 ± 8.6	34.0 ± 3.2	64.9 ± 20.7	+	+
Feb. 1982	93.0 ± 12.5	90.2 ± 27.6	160.4 ± 23.1	−[g]	ND[h]
Feb. 1982	111.4 ± 10.1	49.3 ± 13.0	114.7 ± 29.9	+	+
Apr. 1982	87.1 ± 20.5	88.2 ± 11.7	132.3 ± 73.5	−	ND
Apr. 1982	87.0 ± 12.9	77.7 ± 5.5	142.5 ± 16.6	−	ND
Apr. 1982	88.9 ± 13.7	41.2 ± 9.7	125.8 ± 11.5	+	+
Apr. 1982	134.0 ± 17.7	19.7 ± 4.5	130.0 ± 29.7	+	+
May 1982	105.9 ± 11.7	64.4 ± 0.03	102.1 ± 23.8	+	−
May 1982	105.4 ± 21.9	30.6 ± 24.7	59.8 ± 3.5	+	−
May 1982	106.5 ± 34.4	81.9 ± 14.1	107.6 ± 13.4	−	ND
Jun. 1982	135.8 ± 10.7	72.8 ± 8.7	106.6 ± 15.8	+	+
Jun. 1982	126.0 ± 20.7	64.4 ± 6.1	138.0 ± 34.2	+	+
Apr. 1983	104.9 ± 14.6	40.0 ± 18.1	97.0 ± 15.0	+	+
May 1983	110.3 ± 10.5	38.6 ± 19.8	103.9 ± 23.6	+	+

[a] JAr Cells: established choriocarcinoma cell line.
[b] Recognition: lymphocytes recognize and attach to tumor antigens on the target cell surface.
[c] Percentage of lymphocytes.
[d] Mean ± standard error.
[e] Differs significantly ($p \leq 0.05$) from target cells incubated with control lymphocytes.
[f] Differs significantly ($p \leq 0.05$) from target cells incubated with patient lymphocytes.
[g] Not significantly different.
[h] Not determined.

Table 30.2. *Blocking Factor Assays*

Patient	Target Cell Type[a] and Test Date	Control Lymphocytes	Patient Lymphocytes	Patient Lymphocytes with Autologous Serum	Recognition Cytotoxicity[b]	Blockin
1	*Omega-Z cells*					
	Jan. 1981	109.8[c] ± 22.3[d]	13.1 ± 7.8	115.1 ± 17.5	+[e]	+[f]
	Feb. 1981	105.9 ± 6.6	11.1 ± 7.9	18.8 ± 11.5	+	−
2	*JAr cells*					
	Jan. 1981	108.2[c] ± 9.6[d]	54.1 ± 3.7	128.8 ± 17.9	+[e]	+[f]
	Feb. 1981	82.4 ± 9.1	23.4 ± 4.1	78.6 ± 20.1	+	+
	Feb. 1981	123.1 ± 24.5	18.9 ± 13.9	18.9 ± 3.4	+	−
	Mar. 1981	133.3 ± 5.5	11.3 ± 1.7	28.5 ± 4.1	+	+
	Feb. 1983	141.7 ± 12.1	34.3 ± 6.7	39.1 ± 13.0	+	−
2	*BeWo cells*					
	Mar. 1981	139.8 ± 17.1	4.4 ± 0.8	5.5 ± 1.1	+	−
	Apr. 1981	96.9 ± 18.9	9.4 ± 1.0	13.7 ± 4.0	+	−
2	*ElFa cells*					
	Mar. 1981	148.0 ± 14.2	15.7 ± 2.6	20.1 ± 4.3	+	−
	Apr. 1981	105.1 ± 17.2	0.3 ± 6.5	72.1 ± 4.9	+	+
2	*Omega-Z cells*					
	Jan. 1981	109.8 ± 22.3	28.5 ± 27.7	94.3 ± 35.6	+	−
	Mar. 1981	147.2 ± 12.8	15.6 ± 5.2	16.6 ± 13.8	+	−
3	*JAr cells*					
	Feb. 1983	113.4[c] ± 15.2[d]	43.4 ± 5.4	96.0 ± 23.2	+[e]	+[f]
4	*JAr cells*					
	Jun. 1982	126.0[c] ± 20.7[d]	63.9 ± 11.4	134.2 ± 18.7	+[e]	+[f]
	Jun. 1982	93.4 ± 10.9	56.7 ± 4.2	102.8 ± 14.0	+	+

[a] Target cell types are designated according to source.
[b] Recognition cytotoxicity means patient's sensitized lymphocytes react to choriocarcinoma cells.
[c] Percentage of lymphocytes.
[d] Mean ± standard error.
[e] Differs significantly ($p \leq 0.05$) from target cells incubated with control lymphocytes.
[f] Differs significantly ($p \leq 0.05$) from target cells incubated with patient lymphocytes.

patient who demonstrated recognition, cytotoxicity, and blocking while progressive choriocarcinoma growth was present. After surgical and chemotherapeutic resolution of tumor, her tests continued to show recognition and cytoxocity, but blocking-factor activity had disappeared.

Patient 2 (table 30.2) was studied with four target cell choriocarcinoma systems, all of which showed recognition of choriocarcinoma target cells by the patient's sensitized lymphocytes. These assays confirmed the Hellström phenomenon, which means that lymphocytes from patients bearing histologically similar types of tumor are sensitized to this tumor-associated antigen and cross-react with other tumors of the same histological type. Control assays with other malignant target cells, including cervical, breast, and ovarian cancer target cells, were uniformly negative for cross-reactivity.

Patients 3 and 4 (table 30.2) showed recognition and cytoxicity, but these were persistently blocked with positive HCG titers. These patients were known to have metastatic choriocarcinoma.

Table 30.3 shows data from studies of a mother with choriocarcinoma and her child, beginning soon after the child was born. This woman has been in continuous remission from her gestational choriocarcinoma and, as indicated in the table, continues to show recognition and cytotoxicity against her own choriocarcinoma cells and absence of blocking factor activity. The child's record (table 30.3) similarly shows recognition and cytotoxicity against the placental choriocarcinoma of that gestation and no blocking activity.

In contrast to this case of a healthy child free of choriocarcinoma but demonstrating immunologic memory of the event during pregnancy, the record of the first mother-child pair in table 30.4 shows that the child died at five months of age from metastatic choriocarcinoma. Although the mother remained healthy without clinical evidence of choriocarcinoma, her lymphocytes showed recognition and cytotoxicity without blocking factor activity, which indicated sensitization by this choriocarcinoma tumor-associated antigen.

The next data in table 30.4 record assays of mothers and children conducted at periodic points in the postnatal development of the children of these pregnancies. The second mother-child pair's test results show that, at three years of age, the child showed recognition and cytotoxicity of JAr choriocarcinoma cells in the same fashion as her mother, who was in complete remission. For the third pair, studies done when the child was four years old show recognition and cytotoxicity for both mother and child, without blocking in the mother after resolution of her choriocarcinoma in February 1981. The next pair, studied when the child was five years of age, likewise showed recognition and cytotoxicity (table 30.4).

To determine whether male or female offspring would produce differences in

Table 30.3. *Blocking Factor Assay of One Mother and Child*

JAr Choriocarcinoma Cells[a]	Control Lymphocytes	Patient Lymphocytes	Patient Lymphocytes with Autologous Serum	Recognition Cytotoxicity[b]	Blocking
Mother					
Jun. 1980	100.5 ± 4.6	41.8 ± 15.9	35.4 ± 17.0	+	−
Dec. 1981	130.0 ± 0.1	67.3 ± 1.9	75.0 ± 9.6	+	−
Jun. 1982	93.4 ± 10.9	49.7 ± 8.0	79.1 ± 18.7	+	−
Dec. 1983	113.7 ± 15.2	16.1 ± 5.3	8.5 ± 4.3	+	−
Child					
Jun. 1980	100.5 ± 4.6	53.9 ± 21.6	44.9 ± 19.0	+	−
Dec. 1981	130.0 ± 0.1	44.2 ± 13.4	73.0 ± 11.5	+	−
Dec. 1983	113.7 ± 15.2	7.3 ± 0.4	11.9 ± 2.4	+	−

[a] JAr choriocarcinoma cells designated according to donor.
[b] Recognition cytotoxicity means patient's sensitized lymphocytes react to choriocarcinoma cells.

Table 30.4. *Blocking Factor Assays in Patients and Their Children*

Patient (Choriocarcinoma Cell Type[a]) and Child	Control Lymphocytes	Patient Lymphocytes	Patient Lymphocytes with Autologous Serum	Recognition Cytotoxicity[b]	Blocking
Mother (JAr)					
Dec. 1983	92.1 ± 9.7	51.3 ± 4.5	65.3 ± 21.4	+	–
Child					
boy, 5 months					
Died of metastatic choriocarcinoma					
Mother (JAr)					
Dec. 1983	113.7[c] ± 15.2[d]	19.9 ± 3.2	16.2 ± 2.4	+[e]	–[f]
Child					
girl, 3 years					
Dec. 1983				+	–
Mother (JAr)					
Oct. 1980	154.7 ± 26.5	7.3 ± 3.6	50.7 ± 10.3	+	+
Feb. 1981	82.4 ± 9.1	45.7 ± 14.8	57.1 ± 29.3	+	–
Child					
girl, 4 years					
Dec. 1983	113.7 ± 15.2	10.4 ± 0.4	ND ND	+	ND
Mother (JAr)					
Jan. 1984	94.4 ± 11.1	38.6 ± 15.9	64.7 ± 18.4	+	–
Child					
girl, 5 years					
Jan. 1984	94.4 ± 11.1	40.3 ± 12.6	50.1 ± 5.5	+	–
Mother (type 2)					
Died of metastatic choriocarcinoma					
Child					
girl, 10 years					
Mar. 1982	93.6 ± 15.0	57.6 ± 9.9	26.6 ± 12.8	+	–
Mother (BeWo)					
Died of metastatic choriocarcinoma					
Child					
boy, 10 years					
Jun. 1980	129.8 ± 29.8	31.5 ± 5.2	17.4 ± 2.3	+	–
Mother (BeWo)					
Dec. 1983	76.6 ± 4.6	13.0 ± 4.1	17.4 ± 2.3	+	–
Child					
boy, 10 years					
Dec. 1983	76.6 ± 4.6	12.1 ± 3.1	28.3 ± 8.9	+	–

[a] Choriocarcinoma cells named according to donor.
[b] Recognition cytotoxicity means lymphocytes recognize and attach to tumor antigens on the target cell surface.
[c] Percentage of lymphocytes.
[d] Mean ± significant error.
[e] Differs significantly ($p \leq 0.05$) from target cells incubated with control lymphocytes.
[f] Differs significantly ($p \leq 0.05$) from target cells incubated with patient lymphocytes.

cytotoxicity, we studied the girl and boy, both 10 years old, whose mothers had succumbed to metastatic disease (next two cases, table 30.4). Both daughter and son are living free of disease and show recognition and cytotoxicity to the choriocarcinoma antigens of the mother.

Previous reports have suggested a higher frequency of choriocarcinoma in mothers with blood type A married to fathers with blood type O, and we were interested in determining whether the child of such a pregnancy was different in any way from infants born to other mothers with postgestational choriocarcinoma (Bagshawe et al. 1971). The last mother-child pair shown in table 30.4 showed no difference in assay results of the mother who has JAr choriocarcinoma and blood type A and her offspring, who also has blood type A. The mother, who remains in complete remission, showed cytotoxicity and recognition without blocking, as did the child.

Discussion

Immune reactivity undergoes a chronologic evolution during intrauterine and postnatal gestational life. Although this is best known with regard to immunoglobulin or B cell development, the regulatory role of T and B cell interaction is well recognized. The major immunoglobulin in utero is IgG obtained from the mother through placental transfer. This globulin is detectable early during the first trimester; it peaks at about the twentieth week and remains steady through delivery. The production of antibody in the fetus, as distinguished from IgG transferred from the mother, is mainly in the form of IgM. IgM is detectable in fetal serum at about the twentieth week. If one cultures fetal cells in vitro and measures their capacity to produce immunoglobulins, fetal IgM appears as early as after 10.5 weeks of gestation, and IgG is noted at 12 weeks. The preponderance of the initial reaction in the fetus of IgM as primary immunologic response contrasts with that of the mother, in whom IgM is the major primary response; within a week or so, this is, however, superseded by a predominant IgG response in the mother. In the fetus, IgM response may persist through delivery and well into the postnatal period.

Since malignancy in the placenta may exist during gestation, it is reasonable to conclude that initial fetal sensitization to choriocarcinoma tumor-associated antigens begins at that time. Maturation of immune competence in the placenta and fetus may be a determinant in the outcome of sensitization and be strong enough to protect the fetus from invasion by malignant choriocarcinoma cells.

It might be speculated that the earlier malignant transformation occurs, the less capacity will the placenta and fetus have for mounting an effective immune response. Such an event might lead to unopposed transplacental invasion of malignant choriocarcinoma cells into the fetus. The difference in immunologic response between the infant who succumbed to metastatic choriocarcinoma and all other infants who were free of disease (table 30.4) may be related to the time at which the malignant transformation occurred.

Since transplantation antigens that are present in the fetus generally localize on the plasma membrane, and host cells are programmed to reject foreign tissue, cells similar to transplant rejection phenomena may be expressed through the cytotoxic T cells identified in this study. Neither the mechanism of malignant transformation nor the time of cytotoxic T-cell generation during the intrauterine or postnatal period is known. But the general principle of generation of diverse antigen-binding cells in the bone marrow and thymus and their seeding in specific microenvironments in lymph nodes and spleen sets the stage for necessary antigen processing by macrophages. This processing may bring about sufficient antigen preparation suited for T-cell and B-cell interaction and ultimate generation of active progenitors with killer-cell and immunocytotoxic properties.

Careful dissection of the process of development of immune resistance of cells to neoplastic antigens will require complex models for which the trophoblastic cell system may be well suited. Mechanisms of response to infectious agents, including bacteria and viruses, may also be investigated in such systems. At this time, our initial data point to the exciting potential for new information on placental and fetal immunologic mechanisms.

Summary

Children of mothers who had choriocarcinoma after gestation were examined for their susceptibility or resistance to this malignant disease by in vitro examination of their placental cells. The questions were: Did their lymphocytes become sensitized to the malignancy during intrauterine gestation? Did their lymphocytes retain the memory of this event? And have their lymphocytes retained cytotoxicity to the choriocarcinoma, thus affording them resistance to this disease? All results were affirmative. When possible, the mother's choriocarcinoma cells were grown in vitro. Lymphocytes from mother and child were incubated to determine their recognition and cytotoxic capacity to kill these malignant cells from their own placenta as well as from those of other patients with malignant trophoblastic disease. Two mothers died of resistant widespread disease; one child died at five months of metastatic choriocarcinoma; of the original 18 high-risk mothers, 15 are in remission. The children's lymphocytes were cytotoxic at 2, 3, 4, 5, and 10 years of age. This is the first report of resistance to a tumor antigen developed during gestation.

References

Ariel IM, Pack GT. 1960. *Cancer and Allied Diseases of Infancy and Childhood*. Boston: Little, Brown.

Bagshawe KD, Rawlins G, Pike MC, Lowler SD. 1971. ABO blood groups in trophoblastic neoplasms. *Lancet* 1:553–556.

Brewer JI, Gerbie AB. 1966. Early development of choriocarcinoma. *Am J Obstet Gynecol* 94:692–710.

Buckell EWC, Owen TK. 1954. Chorionepithelioma in mother and infant. *Journal of Obstetrics and Gynaecology of the British Empire* 61:329–330.

Daamen DBF, Bloem GWD, Westerbeck AJ. 1961. Chorionepithelioma in mother and child. *Journal of Obstetrics and Gynaecology of the British Commonwealth* 68:144–149.

Driscoll SG. 1963. Choriocarcinoma. An "incidental finding" within a term placenta. *Obstet Gynecol* 21:96–101.

Emery JL. 1952. Chorionepithelioma in a newborn male child with hyperplasia of the interstitial cells of the testes. *Journal of Pathology and Bacteriology* 64:735–739.
Kay S, Reed WG. 1953. Chorioepithelioma of the lung in a female infant seven months old. *Am J Pathol* 29:555–567.
Mercer RD, Lammert AC, Anderson R, Hazard JB. 1958. Choriocarcinoma in mother and infant. *JAMA* 166:482–483.
Novak E, Seah C. 1954. Choriocarcinoma of uterus: Study of 74 cases from Mathieu Memorial Chorioepithelioma Registry. *Am J Obstet Gynecol* 67:933–961.
Pattillo RA, Gey G. 1968. Establishment of a cell line of human hormone-synthesizing trophoblastic cells in vitro. *Cancer Res* 28:1231–1236.
Pattillo RA, Ruckert ACF, Story MT, Mattingly RF. 1979. Immunodiagnosis in ovarian cancer: Blocking factor activity. *Am J Obstet Gynecol* 133:791–802.
Pattillo RA, Story MT, Ruckert ACF. 1979. Expression of cell-mediated immunity and blocking factor using a new line of ovarian cancer cells in vitro. *Cancer Res* 39:1185–1191.

DIAGNOSTIC PROCEDURES

Annual Clinical Conference on Cancer, Vol. 29
Gynecologic Cancer: Diagnosis and Treatment Strategies
© 1987 by The University of Texas System Cancer Center

31. DNA Flow Cytometry in the Diagnosis of Gynecologic Malignancies

Martin N. Raber, Bart Barlogie, and Tod S. Johnson

The concept that abnormalities of cellular DNA content reflect the biologic behavior of a tumor originated more than 25 years ago. Using the Feulgen method for staining DNA, Atkin and colleagues in England (1964) and Caspersson in Sweden (1979) showed that relatively crude measurements of DNA could be correlated with classic cytogenetic analysis to reflect the ploidy of the tumor cell population. Further studies by Atkin suggested that, with few exceptions, patients with DNA content in the "near diploid" range survived longer than patients having tumors that contained significantly increased cellular DNA contents (aneuploid) (Atkin and Kay 1979). Continued work based on Feulgen methodology has confirmed the results of these early investigations.

At the same time, advances in techniques of cell counting and sizing were adapted to allow relatively high-speed measurements of several parameters on a single-cell basis (Horan and Wheeless 1977). Using fluorescent stains, which bind DNA in a quantitative and specific fashion, flow cytometry (FCM) provides an accurate reflection of each cell's DNA content and has given us new insight into both the ploidy and proliferative activity of human tumors.

Principles of Flow Cytometry

A single-cell suspension of tumor cells is prepared by using mechanical and enzymatic methods of cell separation. The cells are stained with a fluorescent stain and entrained at high speed across a focused light. The light source is provided by either a laser or mercury arc lamp; the fluorescent stain is excited and emits fluorescence, which is measured and displayed on a histogram.

In principle, any cellular component that can be bound in a quantitative fashion by a fluorescent stain can be measured using flow methodology. In practice, numerous phenotypic markers, both membranous and cytoplasmic, have been quantitated and have become routine adjuncts in the diagnosis and classification of hematologic malignancies. In cases involving solid tumors, however, most investigations have focused on staining nucleic acids—particularly DNA. Whereas a number of other probes are currently being evaluated, none has had the worldwide impact of cellular DNA measurements, which provide information on both the ploidy and proliferative activity of a tumor.

With the description of the mammalian cell cycle by Quastler and Sherman

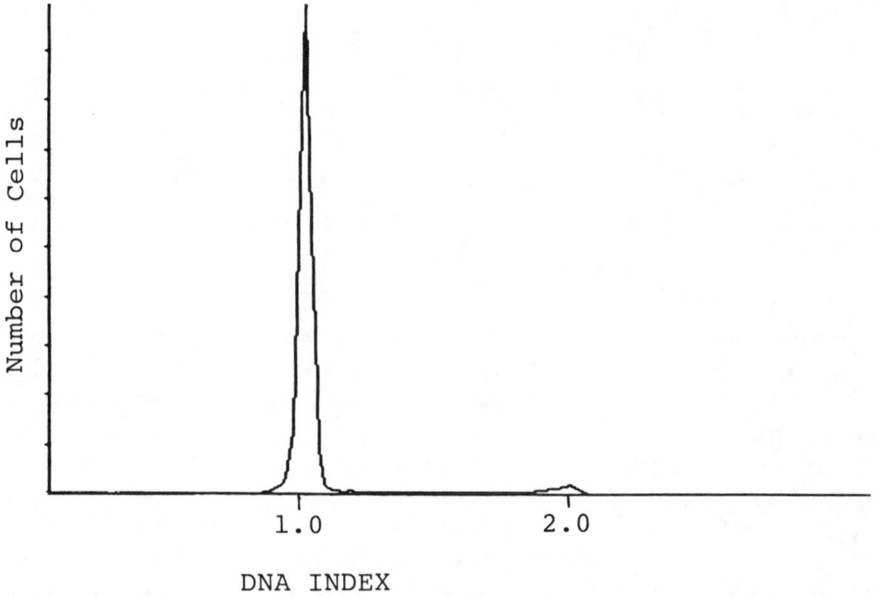

Fig. 31.1. A DNA histogram from a tumor with a diploid DNA content. The DNA content is expressed as DNA index. A DNA index of 1 is considered diploid. The peak with a DNA index of 2 represents cells in the G_2 and mitotic phases of the cell cycle.

(1959), it became apparent that interphase could be divided into three compartments: (1) a period of DNA synthesis during which the chromatin material is copied, referred to as S phase, which is preceded and followed by two GAPS, (2) G_1 and (3) G_2. Thus, if one were to measure the DNA content of a single population of normal cells (fig. 31.1), the cells in the G_1 phase would have the "diploid" quantity of DNA. This population would be the majority. A second, smaller population would have completed DNA synthesis and would be in the G_2 phase. It would contain twice the DNA content of the G_1 population. Between these two extremes would be the S phase, containing a population of cells with intermediate DNA content.

Most tumors contain a mixture of normal stromal and tumor cells. Thus, they provide for comparisons of the DNA contents of G_1 cells in the two populations. Figure 31.2 shows a histogram of a tumor in which the DNA content of the tumor population is markedly different from that of the normal cell population. This population with abnormal DNA content (aneuploid) may have more (hyperdiploid) or less (hypodiploid) DNA than the normal cells. To differentiate between the two populations, the sample can be measured both as it is after staining and with a control population of normal human granulocytes to confirm the diploid position. Thus, with a single parameter one can measure both the ploidy and the proliferative activity of a tumor.

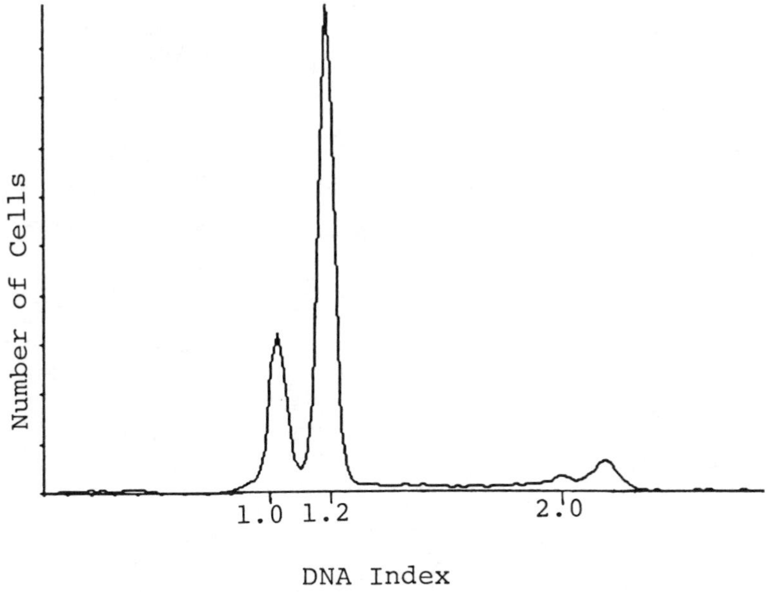

Fig. 31.2. A DNA histogram from a tumor with an aneuploid DNA content. The normal cells in the sample have a DNA index of 1. The tumor cells have a higher DNA content. Their DNA index is 1.2.

Results of DNA Content Analysis

A review of the literature (table 31.1) shows that the results of DNA content analysis of over 4000 tumors have been reported (Barlogie et al. 1983; Raber and Barlogie in press). What conclusions can be drawn from such analyses, and how can these conclusions be applied in the diagnosis of gynecologic malignancies?

The majority of tumors studied have been shown to be aneuploid, and aneuploidy is an excellent marker of the malignant process. In both leukemias (Dosik et al. 1980) and solid tumors (Jakobsen 1985), DNA content appears to accurately reflect karyotypic abnormalities. The abnormality of DNA content appears to be present and stable throughout the course of the disease and is not related to the presence or absence of metastasis. In most tumor types in which sufficient follow-up is available, highly abnormal DNA content is associated with a poorer prognosis than near normal values, a conclusion that supports earlier work based on Feulgen methodology (Atkin and Kay 1979).

Although there is a tendency for aneuploidy to be more common in poorly differentiated tumors, it appears that DNA content is a prognostic variable independent of other known parameters. Ploidy measured by FCM is an easily measured marker of the malignant process; its prognostic importance is currently being further elucidated. The same cannot be said, however, for cell cycle analysis. Although many

Table 31.1. *DNA-Aneuploidy in Solid Tumors*

Tumor Type	*N*	Aneuploid (%) Mean	Range
Bladder	474	88	70–95
Brain	109	43	11–90
Breast	746	73	44–92
Cervix	235	78	68–80
Colon	258	65	39–74
Head and neck	73	86	—
Lung	517	83	79–86
Ovarian	86	58	45–93
Prostate	371	66	36–71
Bone			
sarcoma	236	70	61–98
Skin	220	82	—
squamous cell			
melanoma	715	76	76–78
Testicular	86	58	—
Miscellaneous	315	56	—
Total	4,429	70	11–98

investigators have developed methods for analyzing complex histograms (those with more than a one-cell population), their analyses have been fraught with difficulty. When the tumor and normal cell populations have similar modal DNA contents, analysis cannot be carried out unless one assumes that there are no cycling cells in the normal populations. This is not always a valid assumption. Although highly aneuploid populations are easier to analyze, FCM-derived estimations of the S-phase compartment in solid tumors are consistently higher than those derived from classic labeling studies. The most likely explanation for this discrepancy is that there are noncycling cells present, with S-phase DNA content. Thus, for both theoretical and methodologic reasons, FCM-based cell cycle analysis still cannot be considered a valid prognostic indicator of tumor behavior in patients with solid tumors.

In our own laboratory, simultaneous two-parameter analyses of DNA and RNA are routinely performed on solid tumors. In many instances, the tumor cell population can be distinguished from normal cells on the basis of an increased RNA content (fig. 31.3), thus eliminating the problem of overlapping cell populations. Some investigators are currently using a monoclonal antibody to bromodeoxyuridine, after incubations with the substance, in an attempt to better define the S-phase compartment (Gratzner 1982). Nevertheless, the value of currently reported FCM-derived measurements of S phase remains controversial.

Applications of Flow Cytometry in Patients with Gynecologic Tumors

The major direction of research in gynecologic malignancies has been twofold: an attempt to apply FCM to the problems of diagnosis and an assessment of the impact of ploidy abnormalities on the natural history of these tumors. Almost from the be-

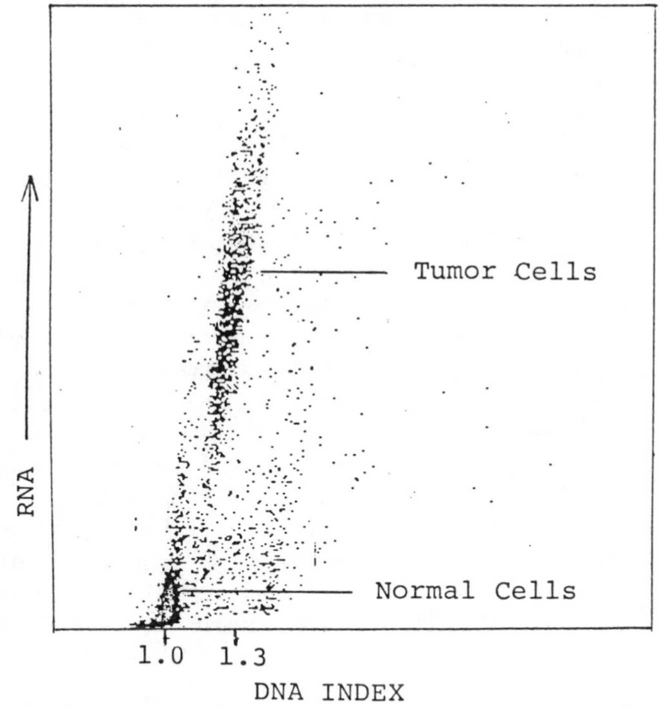

Fig. 31.3. A DNA/RNA histogram from a tumor with an aneuploid DNA content (DNA index 1.3). With the addition of the second parameter (RNA) and an elevated RNA content, the tumor cell population can be clearly distinguished from the normal cells, and overlap has been eliminated.

ginning of solid-tumor FCM research, investigators have been trying to develop a flow-based system for screening cervical preparations. Early observations based on one parameter (DNA) analysis revealed false-negative results at a rate of approximately 10% and false-positive results varying between 10% and 60% (Linden et al. 1980). Using two parameters (DNA and protein) in a relatively small series, Linden et al. reported extremely low false-negative and false-positive rates. They and other workers have indicated that with increasing cytologic atypia, false-negative results are rare, whereas in cases of mild-to-moderate dysplasia, the correlation between FCM and classic cytology is probably not sufficient to rely on a fully automated system (Raber and Barlogie in press).

An innovative approach to this problem has been described by Wheeless and associates (1984) at the University of Rochester. They have developed a multidimensional, slit scan flow system based on measurements of DNA, RNA, nuclear size, cell size, and other morphologic information. Using such a system, they studied 740 specimens in a blinded fashion. On cytologic review, the false-positive rate was 17.6% and the false-negative rate was 2.6%. All false-negative results were related to mild dysplasia. Considering their stated goal of a false-positive rate of less than 20% and a false-negative rate of less than 1%, this technique appears valid. The slit scan flow system, which demands sophisticated instrumentation, is currently being evaluated in a "double-blind" study.

Although the data from a number of FCM centers worldwide are consistent in terms of prognostic information, the importance of aneuploidy remains unclear. In his original observations based on Feulgen staining, Atkin found significant aneuploidy to be a poor prognostic feature in all diseases except cervical carcinoma (Atkin and Kay 1979). Nevertheless, a number of investigators have performed similar studies based on FCM analysis of DNA content. In the largest reported series (Jakobsen 1984) of 171 cases, highly aneuploid DNA content is significantly associated with a poor prognosis. Studies from our own laboratory and others have indicated that DNA content is not significantly correlated with malignancy grade or clinical stage of disease. It thus appears to be an independent prognostic parameter (Raber and Barlogie in press).

Both ovarian (Friedlander et al. 1984) and endometrial (Mosberger et al. 1984) tumors have been analyzed in a similar fashion; in both cases, ploidy appeared to be an independent prognostic variable in which aneuploidy was associated with shorter survival, regardless of therapy. It is important to realize, however, that in an era of successful chemotherapy for some tumors, patients with aggressive tumors that traditionally have denoted a brief life expectancy may actually be more responsive to treatment. Such cases are changing our interpretation of classically poor prognostic signs.

Summary

Flow cytometry provides an easy technique for the measurement of cellular DNA content, permitting an estimation of both the ploidy and proliferative activity of a tumor. It has been applied as a tumor marker, in which aneuploidy appears to be a stable marker of the malignant process. As a means of screening gynecologic samples, single-parameter DNA content analysis is probably unacceptable; however, multiparameter techniques appear promising. In terms of prognostic information, FCM-measured aneuploidy has been associated with shortened survival in cervical, endometrial, and ovarian cancer. It appears to be unrelated to classic prognostic determinants (histology and extent of disease). The importance of FCM-based cell cycle analysis of solid tumors remains unclear, primarily because of the difficulty of interpreting complex histograms. New techniques, including dual-parameter analysis, may help to resolve these difficulties.

References

Atkin NB. 1964. Nuclear size in carcinoma of the cervix: Its relationship to DNA content and prognosis. *Cancer* 17:1391–1399.

Atkin NB, Kay R. 1979. Prognostic significance of modal DNA value and other factors in malignant tumors based on 1465 cases. *Br J Cancer* 40:210–221.

Barlogie B, Raber M, Schumann J, Johnson TS, Drewinko B, Schwartzendruber D, Göhde W, Andreeff M, Freireich EJ. 1983. Flow cytometry in clinical cancer research. *Cancer Res* 43:3982–3997.

Caspersson T. 1979. Quantitative tumor cytochemistry. GHA Clones Memorial Lecture. *Cancer Res* 39:2341–2355.

Dosik G, Barlogie B, Göhde W, Johnston D, Tekell J, Drewinko B. 1980. Flow cytometry of DNA content on human bone marrows: A critical reappraisal. *Blood* 55:734–740.

Friedlander ML, Hedley DW, Taylor IW, Russell P, Coates AS, Tattersall MH. 1984. Influence of cellular DNA content on survival in advanced ovarian cancer. *Cancer Res* 44: 397–400.

Gratzner H. 1982. Monoclonal antibody to 5 bromo and 5 iodo deoxyuridine: A new agent for detection of DNA replication. *Science* 218:474–475.

Horan P, Wheeless L. 1977. Quantitative single cell analysis and sorting. *Science* 198: 149–157.

Jakobsen A. 1984. Prognostic impact of ploidy level in carcinoma of the cervix. *Am J Clin Oncol* 7:475–480.

Jakobsen A. 1985. Flow cytometric analysis of human cervical carcinoma. Doctoral thesis. Arhus Universitet, Arhus, Denmark.

Linden WA, Beck HP, Baisch H, Gebbers JO, Heinenbrok W, Junghanns P, Roters M, Scholz K, Stegner H, Winkler R, Wollner W. 1980. Flow cytometric analyses of cervical smears and solid tumors. In *Flow Cytometry IV*, ed. OD Laerum, T Lundmo, E Thorud, pp. 443–447. Oslo: Universitetsforlaget.

Mosberger B, Auer G, Forsslund G, Mosberger G. 1984. The prognostic significance of DNA measurements in endometrial carcinoma. *Cytometry* 5:430–436.

Quastler H, Sherman F. 1959. Cell population studies in the intestinal epithelium of the mouse. *Exp Cell Res* 17:420–438.

Raber M, Barlogie B. In press. DNA flow cytometry in human solid tumors. In: *Flow Cytometry and Sorting*, ed. M Melamed, ML Mendelson, Y Lindmo. New York: Alan R. Liss.

Wheeless L, Pallen S, Berkan T, Brooks C, Gorman K, Lesh S, Lopez P, Wood J. 1984. Multidimensional slit scan prescreening system: Preliminary results of a single blind clinical study. *Cytometry* 5:1–8.

Annual Clinical Conference on Cancer, Vol. 29
Gynecologic Cancer: Diagnosis and Treatment Strategies
© 1987 by The University of Texas System Cancer Center

32. Tumor Markers for Gynecologic Cancers

Herbert A. Fritsche, Ralph S. Freedman, Frank J. Liu, and Catherine J. Cox

Tumor markers can be defined as biochemical substances that are selectively but not specifically produced by cancer cells. They may be oncofetal proteins that are normally present in embryonic tissues and are later reexpressed by adult tissues when they are involved in the neoplastic process. Tumor markers may also be normal constituents or products of cells that are overexpressed in cancer. Recently, monoclonal antibody technology has permitted the identification of tumor-associated molecular or conformational epitopes contained in presumably normal glycoproteins and glycolipids, and these epitopes may also serve as tumor markers. No tumor marker substance or molecular epitope yet defined has been shown to be specifically related to cancer, however, because these substances can be expressed by benign tumor tissues and normal cells in proliferation. When tumor-associated substances are secreted into the circulation, they can be useful in the clinical management of the cancer patient. Rising or falling levels of the marker in the circulation can reflect changes in tumor burden and permit early assessment of the patient's response to therapy. When used to monitor patients in remission, increasing levels of the tumor marker in the circulation can permit the early detection of disease recurrence.

The clinical usefulness of tumor markers in gynecology has been well documented with the experience of human chorionic gonadotropin (HCG) and alpha fetoprotein (AFP) in germ cell tumors. Recently, a variety of new tumor markers has become available for germ cell tumors, as well as for other neoplastic diseases of the female genital tract. In this report, we will review the current status of these tumor markers in the diagnosis and clinical management of patients with gynecologic cancers.

Alpha Fetoprotein

Alpha fetoprotein is an oncofetal protein, which, in the fetus, is produced by the yolk sac, liver, and gastrointestinal tract (Gitlin and Gitlin 1975). AFP consists of a single polypeptide chain with a molecular weight of 69,000 and contains 4.5% carbohydrate (Ruoslahti and Hirai 1978). The physiological role of AFP remains undefined, although some reports have suggested a role in estrogen metabolism and immunosuppression (Ruoslahti and Hirai 1978). The normal level of circulating AFP in the adult, as determined by immunoassay methods, is 2 to 10 ng/ml (Ruoslahti and Seppala 1971). Abnormal levels of AFP are observed in maternal sera and in the sera of some patients with nonmalignant diseases, including viral hepatitis, cirrhosis, and obstructive jaundice (Seppala and Ruoslahti 1973; Akiyama, Kayama, and Kamada 1972; Abelev 1981). The role of AFP as a tumor marker for hepatocellular carcinoma, adenocarcinoma of the upper gastrointestinal tract, and germ cell tumors of the ovary and testis is well established (Lehman 1975; Waldman and McIntire 1979; Talerman, Haije, and Beggerman 1978b). In gynecologic cancer, the clinical utility of AFP is limited to endodermal sinus tumors (EST) and mixed germ cell tumors that contain elements of EST (Talerman, Haije, and Beggerman 1978a). In EST, serial monitoring with serum AFP has been shown to reflect complete resection of tumor, response of the patient to chemotherapy, and early detection of disease recurrence (Talerman, Haije, and Beggerman 1978b; Sell, Dogaard, and Pederson 1976; Maeyama, Tayama, and Inoue 1984).

It has recently been observed that glycosylation differences exist in AFP derived from yolk sac and liver and that these differences result in the differential binding of AFP to concanavalin A (Tsuchida, Yamashita, and Kobata 1984). Affinity chromatography with concanavalin A can be used in patients with greatly elevated serum AFP to differentiate germ cell tumor from hepatocellular carcinoma. However, the method does not possess the test sensitivity to permit the characterization of AFP at borderline elevations. Thus, the method cannot be used to discriminate between recurrent tumor and liver cell damage that might result from nonmalignant liver disease or hepatotoxic chemotherapy (Buamah, Cornell, and Skillen 1984; Vessella et al. 1984). Attempts are being made to produce monoclonal antibodies that might be able to identify the source of borderline AFP elevations in patients with germ cell tumors, but these efforts have not yet been successful (Brock, Barron, and Heyningen 1984).

Chorionic Gonadotropin

Chorionic gonadotropin is a glycoprotein hormone that is synthesized by the placenta. It has a molecular weight of 46,000 and is composed of two polypeptide chains (Hussa 1981). The beta chain is unique to HCG, whereas the alpha chain is similar to the alpha chains of luteinizing hormone (LH), follicle-stimulating hormone, and thyroid-stimulating hormone (Hussa 1982). The development of the beta chain-specific antiserum has permitted the accurate measurement of HCG in the presence of the pituitary gonadotropins when these are present in the circulation at normal physiological concentrations. However, false elevations of HCG may result from the cross-reaction of LH with the beta-specific HCG antiserum at high levels of LH, which can be observed in the sera of premenopausal women at midcycle and in men with hypogonadal function (Hussa 1981).

The clinical utility of HCG in the diagnosis and clinical management of patients with trophoblastic tumors has been well established (Hussa 1981; Begent and Bagshawe 1983; Schlaerth et al. 1981; Schwartz 1984). The levels of HCG in the circulation of patients with choriocarcinoma correlate with tumor burden. It has been estimated that abnormal serum HCG levels occur when 10^4 to 10^5 tumor cells are present (Bagshawe 1975). In patients with advanced disease, serum values ranging from 10^5 to 10^7 IU/L suggest a tumor burden of 10^{10} to 10^{12} cells. Serial monitoring of HCG levels in patients with trophoblastic disease and germ cell tumors has been shown to reflect accurately the response of the patient to therapy and permit early detection of disease recurrence (Begent and Bagshawe 1983; Schwartz 1984).

It has been recognized that immunoreactive HCG can exist in serum as the whole molecule and as free alpha and beta chains. Radioimmunoassay methods that employ polyclonal beta-HCG antiserum may measure all three entities as HCG (Arends 1978). Double monoclonal immunometric assays are available that can specifically measure whole molecule HCG, whereas other assays may measure both the whole molecule and the free beta chains (Shapiro et al. 1985). Recently, Schwarz and coworkers have developed an immunoassay system that provides simultaneous assessment of alpha and beta chains and the whole molecule form of HCG (Schwarz, Berger, and Georg 1985). The clinical significance of the free alpha and beta chains as tumor markers remains undefined. Some reports have suggested that alpha subunit measurements may provide an earlier assessment of the patient's response to therapy and an earlier signal of disease recurrence than does HCG (Nishimura, Ashitaka, and Togo 1979; Quigley, Tyrey, and Hammond 1980). The presence of free beta chains in the circulation, as well as hyper- and hypoglycosylated forms of HCG, may be one of the reasons why various HCG methods produce discrepant HCG results (Shapiro et al. 1985; Hussa, Rinke, and Schneitzer 1985). Both the whole molecule HCG and the beta chain may exist in a form that lacks a terminal sialic acid or contains varying amounts of carbohydrates (Hussa, Rinke, and Schneitzer 1985). It is clear that additional clinical studies will be required to define the role of the alpha and beta chains and these various glycosylated forms of HCG as tumor markers.

Carcinoembryonic Antigen

Carcinoembryonic antigen (CEA) is by far the most widely used tumor marker, but it has had little application in gynecologic cancers. CEA consists of a family of glycoproteins that differ in their carbohydrate content (Pritchard and Todd 1979). The molecular weight of the predominant form of CEA is 200,000, although species of both higher and lower molecular weight have been described. Approximately 30% to 40% of patients with epithelial ovarian tumors may have elevated serum levels of CEA ($>$ 5.0 ng/ml). In the majority of these cases, however, the CEA level does not exceed 20 ng/ml, which is the level of CEA observed in patients with benign tumors of the ovary (Stall and Martin 1981). Significant elevations of serum CEA are more frequently observed in patients with mucinous tumors than in those with the serous cell type, and in these cases the poorly differentiated tumors are most often associated with CEA production (Khoo and Mackay 1976). Thus, the role of CEA in adenocarcinoma of the ovary appears to be limited to those patients with poorly differentiated mucinous tumors who also have stage III or stage IV disease.

CEA also appears to be of limited value in squamous cell carcinoma of the cervix. Only 20% to 30% of patients with this disease have abnormal serum CEA values. Of these, only about one-fifth have significant elevations of CEA, and most of these CEA elevations are generally observed in patients in stage III or stage IV disease (Fritsche et al. 1982). Kjorstad and Orjaseter (1978) observed that in patients with advanced disease, pretreatment CEA values did not have prognostic significance, but elevated CEA values in stage I patients were suggestive of lymph node involvement. Several reports suggest only a limited role for CEA in monitoring patients for recurrence of disease (Ito, Kurihara, and Nishimura 1977; Kjorstad and Orjaseter 1982).

CEA might play a more prominent role in adenocarcinoma of the cervix. A recent report suggests that pretreatment CEA values have prognostic value in this disease (Kjorstad and Orjaseter 1984). No patients with CEA values greater than 15 ng/ml survived the disease, whereas patients with CEA values of less than 5 ng/ml had an estimated five-year survival rate of 90%. Approximately two thirds of the patients who had CEA values in the range of 5 to 15 ng/ml and were treated with surgery and radiotherapy experienced disease recurrence. The authors suggested that this group of high-risk patients be considered candidates for chemotherapy.

Tumor-Associated Antigen

Tumor-associated antigen (TA-4) is a glycoprotein with a molecular weight of 48,000 that was isolated from squamous cell carcinoma of the uterine cervix (Kato et al. 1979a). It is heat stable at 57°C for at least one hour but is inactivated by neuraminidase treatment. The half-life of TA-4 in the circulation has been estimated to be 24 hours (Kato et al. 1979b). In initial clinical studies of TA-4, serum levels were elevated in 25% to 50% of squamous cell carcinoma patients who had early stage disease (in situ, stage I or II), and from 80% to 100% of patients who had stage III or stage IV disease or recurrence (Kato et al. 1979a, 1979b). However, more extensive studies have shown that significant elevations of serum TA-4 rarely occur in the early stages of the disease and that serum TA-4 may be elevated in approximately 50% of patients with this disease (Kato et al. 1982). Initial tissue localization studies demonstrated that TA-4 was present in normal squamous epithelium of the uterine cervix but not in adenocarcinoma of the uterine cervix, endometrium, and ovary (Morioka 1980). In addition, there was no correlation observed between the tumor content of TA-4 and the circulating level of TA-4 in patients with squamous cell carcinoma of the uterine cervix (Morioka 1980). Serum levels of TA-4 are reported to have prognostic significance and to be of value in monitoring the course of the disease. Kato and coworkers have reported that patients who have significantly elevated serum levels of TA-4 (> 15 U/ml) have a poorer survival rate than those patients with normal values (< 5 U/ml) (Kato et al. 1983).

Recently, Ueda and coworkers (1984) evaluated a commercially available antiserum for TA-4. Their immunoperoxidase studies showed that TA-4 was a component of normal differentiated squamous cells and differentiated cells of squamous cell carcinoma of the cervix. It was also present in some adenocarcinomas of the cervix, endometrium, and ovary (all histological cell types). A commercially available radioimmunoassay for TA-4 that employs the same antiserum demonstrated serum TA-4 elevations to occur in approximately 50% of patients with squamous cell carcinoma (Maruo et al. 1985). Both the serum value of TA-4 and the incidence of elevation increased with the stage of the disease.

TA-4 has now been fractionated by isoelectric focusing into acidic and neutral components (Kato, Nagaya, and Torigoe 1984). The acidic component with a low isoelectric point appears to be associated with cervical squamous cell carcinoma, whereas the neutral component is related to benign squamous cells of the cervix. If this is the case, monoclonal antibodies might be able to discriminate between these forms and improve the clinical specificity of the TA-4 test by reducing the false-positive rate.

Cancer Antigen 125

Cancer antigen 125 (CA 125) is a tumor-associated protein that contains an epitope recognized by the murine monoclonal antibody OC 125 (Bast et al. 1981). This IgG_1 monoclonal antibody was raised against the epithelial cell line OVCA 433. The antigenic site recognized by OC 125 appears to be expressed by cell surface proteins of serous, endometrioid, and clear cell tumors of the ovary, but not by mucinous tumors or normal ovarian cells (Kabawat et al. 1983a). OC 125 also reacts with some adenocarcinoma tissues of the endometrium and fallopian tube, as well as fetal coelomic epithelium (Kato, Nagaya, and Torigoe 1984). Preliminary characterization studies suggest that CA 125, the circulating protein that contains the epitope recognized by OC 125, is a mucin-like glycoprotein that has a molecular weight greater than 500,000. The half-life of CA 125 in the circulation has been estimated to be 4.8 days (Canney et al. 1984). Several types of immunoradiometric assays employing OC 125 have been used to quantitate serum CA 125 levels (Bast et al. 1983; Klug et al. 1984). Using a cutoff value of 35 U/ml, both assays demonstrated elevated serum CA 125 in approximately 80% of patients with ovarian cancer and in 15% to 20% of patients with pancreatic and colorectal cancer. The false-positive rate of the assay was 6% in patients with nonmalignant diseases. Women in the first trimester of pregnancy may have CA 125 levels greater than 35 U/ml, and as many as 20% of these individuals may have CA 125 levels greater than 65 U/ml (Niloff et al. 1984a). No nonmalignant gynecologic diseases have yet been associated with CA 125 levels greater than 65 U/ml (Niloff et al. 1984b). In nonmalignant diseases of other tissues, serum CA 125 levels greater than 65 U/ml were observed in 75% of patients with peritonitis, 38% of patients with acute pancreatitis, and 40% to 80% of patients with cirrhosis of the liver, metastatic disease to the liver, and hepatoma (Ruibal et al. 1984). These data would suggest caution in the interpretation of CA 125 levels in ovarian cancer patients who may also have cirrhosis of the liver (Ricolleau et al. 1984).

Canney and coworkers have also demonstrated CA 125 elevations to occur in 83% of patients with ovarian cancers, but in contrast to prior reports, they found six of six patients with mucinous ovarian cancer to have elevated serum CA 125 values (Canney et al. 1984). At least one report suggests that serum levels of CA 125 may also be elevated in a significant number of patients with adenocarcinomas of the cervix, endometrium, and fallopian tube (Niloff et al. 1984a). In that study, elevated CA 125 levels in endometrial cancer were observed only in patients who had stage IV or recurrent disease.

There appears to be a consensus on the usefulness of CA 125 for monitoring the response to therapy and disease progression in patients with adenocarcinoma of the ovary. Rising or falling CA 125 values in the circulation have been correlated with the clinical status of the disease in 85% to 93% of the cases (Canney et al. 1984; Bast et al. 1983; Brioschi et al. 1985; Ricolleau et al. 1984; Niloff et al. 1985). In one study, second-look procedures helped to identify tumor recurrences in 22 of 36 patients with normal levels of CA 125 (Niloff et al. 1985). However, in all of these cases, the tumor mass did not exceed a diameter of 1 cm. In the same study, 19 of 20 patients with elevated serum CA 125 were confirmed to have recurrence of disease at second-look operations. No studies have been reported on the number of patients who demonstrate CA 125 elevations prior to other clinical signs of recurrence and the amount of lead time that can be obtained with CA 125 serial monitoring of patients. When CA 125 is used to monitor the response of patients to complete surgical resection, the serum CA 125 level might be expected to fall by 50% at the end of every half-life of 4.8 days (Canney et al. 1984). However, this approach should be used cautiously until the clearance mechanisms for CA 125 have been well defined. Transient rises of CA 125 may also occur in patients who are responding to chemotherapy (Canney et al. 1984). Such paradoxical rises of CA 125 and other tumor markers are attributed to tumor lysis in situ.

Cancer Antigen 19-9

Cancer antigen 19-9 (CA 19-9) is a tumor-associated protein that contains an epitope recognized by the IgG_1 murine monoclonal antibody 19-9 (Magnani et al. 1983). The epitope is a Lewis A active pentasaccharide that is present in a monosialoganglioside in tissues and is also expressed by a high-molecular-weight mucin in the circulation of patients with gastrointestinal and pancreatic cancer (Magnani et al. 1983). Tissue localization studies have also revealed the presence of CA 19-9 in epithelial tumors of the ovary. It is estimated to be found in 76% of mucinous, 40% of endometrioid, 27% of serous, and 25% of mesodermal mixed tumors; in 57% of clear cell carcinomas; and in 45% of Brenner tumors (Charpin et al. 1982). However, preliminary studies of serum CA 19-9 in epithelial ovarian cancer patients suggest that elevations of this marker may occur in only 17% to 25% of the patients (Ricolleau et al. 1984; Bast et al. 1984). In most of these cases, the CA 19-9 elevations occurred in patients who also demonstrated serum elevations of CA 125. Thus, the utility of CA 19-9 as a marker for mucinous adenocarcinoma of the ovary remains to be determined.

Ovarian Cancer-Associated Antigens

Bhattacharya and coworkers have described six glycoproteins that contain antigenic determinants expressed by ovarian cystadenocarcinomas (OCAA) (Barlow and

Bhattacharya 1983). OCAA is a high-molecular-weight glycoprotein containing 30% to 40% carbohydrate. OCAA-1 has a molecular weight of 50,000 and is immunologically distinct from OCAA. OCAAs 2 to 4 are high-molecular-weight proteins that are present in the circulation of ovarian cancer patients and in normal and malignant tissues of the lung and the gastrointestinal tract. OCAA-5 is a CEA-like antigen that appears to be present only in mucinous ovarian tumors.

NB/70K, another ovarian cancer antigen, is a glycoprotein with a molecular weight of 70,000. It is a component of the tumor-associated fraction previously called OCA (Knauf and Urbach 1981). NB/70K appears to be an antigen common to serous, mucinous, and endometrioid histological cell types of ovarian cancer (Bizzari, Mackillop, and Buick 1983). Elevated levels of NB/70K have been observed in the circulation of ovarian cancer patients and those with benign gynecologic tumors (Dembo, Chang, and Urbach 1985). Nonmalignant gynecologic disease and liver failure may be associated with borderline elevations of NB/70K. Recently, a monoclonal antibody has become available for NB/70K, and this may improve the clinical specificity of the test (Knauf et al. 1985). NB/7OK has been shown to be immunologically distinct from both CA 125 and CEA (Bizzari, Mackillop, and Buick 1983; Knauf et al. 1985).

Another new tumor marker that may have application in ovarian cancer is detected by the monoclonal antibody 29-1 (Brockhaus et al. 1983). This antibody is directed against the carbohydrate moiety, lacto-N-fucopentaose III (LNF III), which is expressed by gastrointestinal and ovarian tumors (Ordonez, Freedman, and Herlyn in press). It has previously been described as both the LeX and stage-specific mouse embryonic antigen (SSEA-1). A circulating protein containing the LNF III determinant has been reported in the serum of patients with ovarian cancer (Cox, Freedman, and Fritsche 1986). In that preliminary report, elevated levels of LNF III expression were observed in 12 of 18 patients with serous cell carcinoma of the ovary. Serial patterns of LNF III correlated well with CA 125 serial patterns, and both markers accurately reflected the clinical course of the disease.

Initial clinical studies have demonstrated that the ovarian cancer antigens OCAAs 1 to 5, NB/70K, and LNF III all may have potential for use as tumor markers for adenocarcinoma of the ovary. It is clear, though, that before their usefulness can be established, each of these putative tumor markers will require more extensive characterization studies and validation of their clinical utility.

Pregnancy-Related Proteins

HCG and AFP are, of course, the most well researched tumor markers of pregnancy-related proteins. However, a number of other placental and pregnancy-related proteins have been identified, several of which may have application as markers for trophoblastic tumors (Horne, Rankin, and Bremner 1984). The pregnancy-specific glycoprotein SP-1 is a product of the syncytiotrophoblast (Bohn and Kraus 1977). A glycoprotein, it contains 29% carbohydrate and has a molecular weight of 90,000. It has been previously identified as the pregnancy-associated plasma protein C (PAPP-C) and trophoblast-specific B-1 glycoprotein (TSG). Serum SP-1 is elevated in a high percentage of patients with gestational trophoblastic tumors, and it correlates well with HCG in following the course of the disease (Than et al. 1982; Lee et al. 1981). The serum SP-1/HCG ratio may reflect the degree of differentiation of trophoblasts and may be useful for differentiating between choriocarcinoma and invasive mole. In six cases of choriocarcinoma, the ratio ranged from 0.68 to 0.7; in four cases of invasive mole, the ratio ranged from 1.1 to 1.8 (Sakuragi 1982).

Placental protein 5 (PP-5) and pregnancy-associated plasma protein A (PAPP-A) are also produced by the trophoblast and may have potential as tumor markers (Bohn and Kraus 1977). In one study, PP-5 was reported to be able to discriminate between hydatidiform mole and choriocarcinoma (Lee et al. 1981). Levels of PP-5 in nine cases of choriocarcinoma were below 4 μg/L, whereas PP-5 levels in 14 cases of hydatidiform mole were greater than 4 μg/L. Recently, a monoclonal antibody to placental alkaline phosphatase (PLAP) has been used to study the expression of this marker in epithelial tumors of the ovary (Nouwen et al. 1985). Serum levels of PLAP were elevated in 46% of the patients with adenocarcinoma of the ovary. Thus, the use of monoclonal antibodies may significantly improve the role of PLAP as a tumor marker.

Summary

Considerable progress has been made in the application of tumor markers to the neoplastic diseases of the female genital tract. CA 125 appears to be a valuable new marker for epithelial tumors of the ovary. CA 19-9, NB/70K, LNF-III, and placental alkaline phosphatase all have potential application to this neoplastic disease and may complement the CA 125 test. Similarly, the placental proteins SP-1, PP-5, and PAPP-A may complement HCG as serum markers for trophoblastic tumors. Finally, TA-4 may have application as a tumor marker for squamous cell carcinoma of the uterine cervix, a disease for which no tumor marker now exists. It is highly likely that monoclonal antibody technology will continue to identify other new tumor-associated substances that may have use in the diagnosis and clinical management of cancer.

References

Abelev G. 1981. Alpha fetoprotein in oncogenesis and its association with malignant tumors. *Adv Cancer Res* 14:295–358.

Akiyama T, Kayama T, Kamada T. 1972. Alpha fetoprotein in acute viral hepatitis. *N Engl J Med* 287:989–992.

Arends J. 1978. Limitations in the specificity of the assay of human chorionic gonadrotrophin using beta subunit antiserum. *Scand J Immunol* 8 [Suppl 8]:583–585.

Bagshawe KD. 1975. Medical aspects of malignant disease. In *Medical Oncology*, ed. KD Bagshawe, pp. 453–467. London: Blackwell.

Barlow J, Bhattacharya M. 1983. Tumor associated antigens for cystadenocarcinoma of the ovary. *Clin Obstet Gynecol* 10:187–196.

Bast R, Feeney M, Lazarus H, Nadler L, Colvin R, Knapp R. 1981. Reactivity of a monoclonal antibody with human ovarian carcinoma. *J Clin Invest* 68:1331–1337.

Bast R, Klug T, St. John E, Jenison E, Niloff J, Lazarus H, Berkowitz R, Leavitt T, Griffiths CT, Parker L, Zurawski V, Knapp R. 1983. A radioimmunoassay using monoclonal antibody to monitor the course of epithelial ovarian cancer. *N Engl J Med* 309:883–887.

Bast R, Klug T, Schaetzl E, Lovin P, Niloff J, Greber T, Zurawski V, Knapp R. 1984. Monitoring human ovarian carcinoma with a combination of CA 125, CA 19-9 and carcinoembryonic antigen. *Am J Obstet Gynecol* 149:553–559.

Begent R, Bagshawe K. 1983. Treatment of advanced trophoblastic disease. In *Gynecologic Oncology*, ed. CT Griffiths, AF Fuller, pp. 155–186. Boston: Martinus Nijhoff.

Bizzari J, Mackillop W, Buick R. 1983. Cellular specificity of NB/70K, a putative human ovarian tumor antigen. *Cancer Res* 43: 864–867.

Bohn H, Kraus W. 1977. Isolation and characterization of the pregnancy specific B-1 glycoprotein in the urine of pregnant women. *Arch Gynecol* 223:33–39.

Brioschi P, Bischof P, Ropin C, DeToten M, Irion O, Krauer F. 1985. Longitudinal study of CEA and CA 125 in ovarian cancer. *Gynecol Oncol* 21:1–6.

Brock D, Barron L, Heyningen V. 1984. Approaches to the production of monoclonal antibodies specific for concanavalin A binding and non-binding forms of alpha fetoprotein. *Tumor Biology* 5:171–178.

Brockhaus M, Magnani J, Herlyn M, Blaszczyk M, Steplewski Z, Koprowski H, Ginsburg V. 1983. Monoclonal antibodies directed against the sugar sequence of lacto-N-fucopentaose III are obtained from mice immunized with human tumors. *Arch Biochem Biophys* 217: 647–651.

Buamah P, Cornell C, Skillen A. 1984. Affinity chromatography used in distinguishing alpha fetoprotein in serum from patients with tumors of hepatic parenchyma and of germ cells. *Clin Chem* 30:1257–1258.

Canney P, Moore M, Wilkinson P, James R. 1984. Ovarian cancer antigen CA 125: A prospective clinical assessment of its role as a tumour marker. *Br J Cancer* 50:765–769.

Charpin C, Bhan A, Zurawski V, Scully R. 1982. Carcinoembryonic antigen (CEA) and carbohydrate determinant 19-9 (CA 19-9) localization in 121 primary and metastatic ovarian tumors: An immunohistochemical study with the use of monoclonal antibodies. *Int J Gynecol Pathol* 1:231–245.

Cox C, Freedman R, Fritsche H. 1986. Lacto-N-fucopentaose III activity in the serum of patients with ovarian carcinoma. *Gynecol Obstet Invest* 21:164–168.

Dembo A, Chang P, Urbach G. 1985. Clinical correlations of ovarian cancer antigen NB/70K: A preliminary report. *Obstet Gynecol* 65:710–714.

Fritsche H, Freedman R, Liu F, Acomb LD, Collinsworth W. 1982. A survey of tumor markers in patients with squamous cell carcinoma of the uterine cervix. *Gynecol Oncol* 14: 230–235.

Gitlin D, Gitlin J. 1975. Fetal and neonatal development of human plasma proteins. In *The Plasma Proteins II*, ed. FN Putnam, pp. 264–320. New York: Academic Press.

Horne C, Rankin R, Bremner R. 1984. Pregnancy specific proteins as markers for gestational trophoblastic disease. *Int J Gynecol Pathol* 3:27–40.

Hussa R. 1981. Clinical utility of human chorionic gonadotrophin and alpha subunit measurements. *J Obstet Gynecol* 60:1–12.

Hussa R. 1982. Human choronic gonadotrophin—A clinical marker. *Ligand Review* 3 [Suppl 2]:6–43.

Hussa R, Rinke M, Schneitzer P. 1985. Discordant human chorionic gonadotropin results: Causes and solutions. *Obstet Gynecol* 65:211–219.

Ito H, Kurihara S, Nishimura C. 1977. Serum carcinoembryonic antigens in patients with carcinoma of the cervix. *Obstet Gynecol* 57:468–471.

Kabawat S, Bast R, Bhan A, Welch R, Knapp R, Colvin R. 1983a. Tissue distribution of a coelomic-epithelium-related antigen recognized by the monoclonal antibody OC 125. *Int J Gynecol Pathol* 2:275–285.

Kabawat S, Bast R, Welch W, Knapp R, Colvin R. 1983b. Immunopathologic characterization of a monoclonal antibody that recognizes common surface antigens of human ovarian tumors of serous, endometrioid, and clear cell types. *Am J Clin Pathol* 79:98–104.

Kato H, Miyauchi F, Morioka H, Fugino T, Torigoe T. 1979a. Tumor antigen of human cervical squamous cell carcinoma: Correlation of circulating levels with disease progress. *Cancer* 43:585–590.

Kato H, Morioka H, Aramaki S, Tamai K, Torigoe T. 1983. Prognostic significance of the tumor antigen TA-4 in squamous cell carcinoma of the uterine cervix. *Am J Obstet Gynecol* 145:350–354.

Kato H, Morioka H, Aramaki S, Torigoe T. 1979b. Radioimmunoassay for tumor antigen of human cervical squamous cell carcinoma. *Cell Mol Biol* 25:51–56.

Kato H, Morioka H, Tsutsui H, Aramaki S, Torigoe T. 1982. Value of tumor-antigen (TA-4) of squamous cell carcinoma in predicting the extent of cervical cancer. *Cancer* 50:1294–1296.

Kato H, Nagaya T, Torigoe T. 1984. Heterogeneity of a tumor antigen TA-4 of squamous cell carcinoma in relation to its appearance in the circulation. *Gann* 75:433–435.

Kato H, Torigoe T. 1977. Radioimmunoassay for tumor antigen of human cervical squamous cell carcinoma. *Cancer* 40:1621–1628.

Khoo S, Mackay J. 1976. Carcinoembryonic antigen in ovarian cancer. *Br J Obstet Gynaecol* 83:753–761.

Kjorstad K, Orjaseter H. 1978. Carcinoembryonic antigen levels in patients with squamous cell carcinoma of the cervix. *Obstet Gynecol* 51:536–539.

Kjorstad K, Orjaseter H. 1982. The prognostic value of CEA determinations in the plasma of patients with squamous cell cancer of the cervix. *Cancer* 50:283–287.

Kjorstad K, Orjaseter H. 1984. The prognostic significance of carcinoembryonic antigen determinations in patients with adenocarcinoma of the cervix. *Gynecol Oncol* 19:284–289.

Klug T, Bast R, Niloff J, Knapp R, Zurawski V. 1984. Monoclonal antibody immunoradiometric assay for an antigenic determinant (CA 125) associated with human epithelial ovarian carcinomas. *Cancer Res* 44:1048–1053.

Knauf S, Anderson D, Knapp R, Bast R. 1985. A study of the NB/70K and CA-125 monoclonal antibody radioimmunoassays for measuring serum antigen levels in ovarian cancer patients. *Am J Obstet Gynecol* 152:911–913.

Knauf S, Urbach G. 1981. Identification, purification and radioimmunoassay of NB/70K, a human ovarian tumor associated antigen. *Cancer Res* 41:1351–1357.

Lee J, Salem H, Al-Ani A, Chard T. 1981. Circulating concentrations of specific placental proteins (human choronic gonadotrophin, pregnancy specific beta-1 glycoprotein, and placental protein 5) in untreated gestational trophoblastic tumors. *Am J Obstet Gynecol* 139:702–704.

Lehman F. 1975. Early detection of hepatoma. *Ann NY Acad Sci* 259:196–210.

Maeyama M, Tayama C, Inoue S. 1984. Serial serum determination of alpha fetoprotein as a marker of the effect of postoperative chemotherapy in ovarian endodermal sinus tumor. *Gynecol Oncol* 17:104–116.

Magnani J, Steplewski Z, Koprowski H, Ginsburg V. 1983. Identification of the gastrointestinal and pancreatic cancer-associated antigen detected by monoclonal antibody 19-9 in the sera of patients as a mucin. *Cancer Res* 43:5489–5492.

Maruo T, Shibata K, Kimura A, Hoshina M, Mochizuki M. 1985. Tumor associated antigen, TA-4, in the monitoring of the effects of therapy for squamous cell carcinoma of the uterine cervix. *Cancer* 56:302–308.

Morioka H. 1980. Tumor antigen of squamous cell carcinoma—Its tissue distribution and its relationship to serum TA-4 concentrations. *Asia Oceania J Obstet Gynaecol* 6:91–97.

Niloff J, Bast R, Schaetzl E, Knapp R. 1985. Predictive value of CA 125 antigen levels in second-look procedures for ovarian cancer. *Am J Obstet Gynecol* 151:981–986.

Niloff J, Klug T, Schaetzl E, Zurawski V, Knapp R, Bast R. 1984a. Evaluation of serum CA 125 in carcinomas of the fallopian tube, endometrium, and endocervix. *Am J Obstet Gynecol* 148:1057–1058.

Niloff A, Knapp R, Schaetzl E, Reynolds C, Bast R. 1984b. CA 125 antigen levels in obstetric and gynecologic patients. *Obstet Gynecol* 64:703–707.
Nishimura R, Ashitaka Y, Togo S. 1979. The clinical evaluation of the simultaneous measurements of human chorionic gonadotrophin and its alpha subunit in sera of patients with trophoblastic diseases. *Endocrinol Jpn* 26:575–583.
Nouwen E, Pollet D, Schelstraete J, Erdekens M, Hansch C, Van de Voorde A, DeBroe M. 1985. Human placental alkaline phosphatase in benign and malignant ovarian neoplasia. *Cancer Res* 45:892–902.
Ordonez N, Freedman R, Herlyn M. In press. Lewis and related tumor-associated determinants on ovarian carcinoma. *Gynecol Oncol.*
Pritchard D, Todd CW. 1979. The chemistry of carcinoembryonic antigen. In *Immunodiagnosis of Cancer Part I*, ed. R Herberman, K McIntire, pp. 165–181. New York: Dekker.
Quigley M, Tyrey L, Hammond C. 1980. Alpha subunit in sera of choriocarcinoma patients in remission. *J Clin Endocrinol Metab* 50:98–103.
Ricolleau G, Chatal J, Fumoleau P, Kremer M, Douillard J, Curtet C. 1984. Radioimmunoassay of the CA 125 antigen in ovarian carcinomas: Advantages compared with CA 19-9 and CEA. *Tumor Biol* 5:151–159.
Ruibal A, Encabo G, Miralles E, Muralles E, Murcia C, Capderila J, Salgado A, Martinez-Vasquez J. 1984. CA 125 seric levels in nonmalignant pathologies. *Bull Cancer (Paris)* 71:145–148.
Ruoslahti E, Hirai H. 1978. Alpha fetoprotein. *Scand J Immunol* 8 [Suppl 8]:3–26.
Ruoslahti E, Seppala M. 1971. Studies of carcino-fetal proteins III. Development of radioimmunoassay for alpha fetoprotein in serum of healthy human adults. *Int J Cancer* 8:374–384.
Sakuragi N. 1982. Serum SP-1 and HCG levels in choriocarcinoma, invasive mole, and hydatidiform mole—clinical significance of SP-1/HCG ratio. *Gynecol Oncol* 13:393–398.
Schlaerth J, Morrow P, Kletyky O, Nalick R, D'Ablaing G. 1981. Prognostic characteristics of serum human chorionic gonadotrophin titer regression following molar pregnancy. *Obstet Gynecol* 58:478–482.
Schwartz P. 1984. Combination chemotherapy in the management of ovarian germ cell malignancies. *Obstet Gynecol* 64:564–572.
Schwarz S, Berger P, Georg W. 1985. Epitope-selective, monoclonal antibody based immunoradiometric assays of predictable specificity for differential measurement of choriogonadotrophin and its subunits. *Clin Chem* 31 (8):1322–1328.
Sell A, Dogaard H, Pederson B. 1976. Serum alpha fetoprotein as a marker for the effect of postoperative radiation therapy and chemotherapy in eight cases of ovarian endodermal sinus tumor. *Int J Cancer* 18:574–580.
Seppala M, Ruoslahti E. 1973. Alpha fetoprotein: Physiology and pathology during pregnancy and application to antenatal diagnosis. *J Perinat Med* 1:104–113.
Shapiro A, Wu T, Ballon S, Lamb E. 1985. Use of an immunoradiometric assay and radioimmunoassay for the detection of free B-human chorionic gonadotrophin. *Obstet Gynecol* 65:546–549.
Stall K, Martin E. 1981. Plasma carcinoembryonic antigen levels in ovarian cancer patients. *J Reprod Med* 26:73–79.
Talerman A, Haije W, Beggerman L. 1978a. Histological patterns in germ cell tumors associated with raised serum alpha fetoprotein. *Scand J Immunol* 8 (Suppl 9):97–102.
Talerman A, Haije W, Beggerman L. 1978b. Serum alpha fetoprotein in diagnosis and management of endodermal sinus tumor and mixed germ cell tumors of the ovary. *Cancer* 41:272–278.
Than G, Csaba I, Bohn H, Szabo D, Szalmasy M, Menczer G. 1982. Monitoring therapy in trophoblastic diseases by radioimmunoassay of pregnancy specific B-1 glycoprotein and the B unit of human chorionic gonadotrophin. *Oncodev Biol Med* 3:315–323.
Tsuchida Y, Yamashita K, Kobata A. 1984. Structure of the sugar chain of alpha fetoprotein

purified from a human yolk sac and its reactivity with concanavalin A. *Tumor Biology* 5:33–40.

Ueda G, Inoue Y, Yamasaki M, Inoue M, Tanaka Y, Hiramatsu K, Saito J, Nishino T, Abe Y. 1984. Immunohistochemical demonstration of tumor antigen TA-4 in gynecologic tumors. *Int J Gynecol Pathol* 3:291–298.

Vessella R, Santrach M, Bronson D, Smith C, Klicka M, Lange CP. 1984. Evaluation of AFP glycosylation heterogeneity in cancer patients with AFP-producing tumors. *Int J Cancer* 34:309–314.

Waldman T, McIntire K. 1979. Use of sensitive assays for alpha fetoprotein in monitoring the treatment of malignancy. In *Immunodiagnosis of Cancer: Part I*, ed. RB Herberman, KR McIntire, pp. 130–147. New York: Dekker.

Annual Clinical Conference on Cancer, Vol. 29
Gynecologic Cancer: Diagnosis and Treatment Strategies
© 1987 by The University of Texas System Cancer Center

33. Imaging Techniques in Gynecologic Cancer

Errol Lewis

A variety of invasive and noninvasive procedures are used in the radiological detection and staging of pelvic malignancies. The available modalities include conventional radiography, tomography, intravenous urography, gastrointestinal barium studies, radionuclide scintigraphy, ultrasonography, computerized tomography (CT), lymphangiography, angiography, and percutaneous biopsy. Today, pelvic pneumography and hysterosalpingography are rarely used. The roles of digital subtraction angiography (DSA) and magnetic resonance imaging (MRI) are still to be determined.

Ten years ago, less invasive techniques such as plain films, intravenous pyelography, and barium enema studies could be used to detect gross soft tissue masses and bony metastases. However, these techniques were not consistent when used to determine the extent of disease to the contiguous soft tissues and the pelvic and retroperitoneal lymph nodes. In recent years—particularly with the advent of the cross-sectional imaging techniques such as ultrasonography, CT, and MRI—less invasive techniques have become more important than the older diagnostic modalities in the diagnosis and staging of pelvic malignancies. In addition to the advantage of being noninvasive, these modalities can aid physicians in determining the entire degree and extent of a patient's pathological process. Radiologists have also become more involved in the management of patients with gynecologic malignancies by performing transcatheter intraarterial infusion and occlusion, percutaneous biopsies, aspiration and injection of cystic or necrotic neoplasms, and nephrostomy.

In this chapter, I will discuss the applications of all available imaging modalities used in the diagnosis of gynecologic cancer. The primary emphasis will be on the diagnosis of ovarian and cervical cancer.

Diagnosis of Ovarian Cancer

Ovarian cancer is the leading cause of deaths from gynecologic cancer and the fourth most frequent cause of cancer death in women, after breast, colon, and lung cancer. The five-year survival rate ranges from 29% to 32% (American Cancer Society 1980; Cutler, Myers, and Green 1975). Unless there is ovarian torsion or rupture, early ovarian cancer is usually silent. Pelvic discomfort or pain (57%), abdominal distension (51%), and bleeding (25%) are usually manifestations of advanced disease. In one series of patients with ovarian cancer (Piver, Barlow, and Lele 1978), subclinical metastases in stage I ovarian carcinoma was noted with the following rates of incidence: diaphragmatic metastases, 11.3%; aortic lymph node metastases, 13.3%; pelvic lymph node metastases, 8.1%; omental metastases, 3.2%; and evidence of malignancy in peritoneal washings, 32.9%. Because ovarian carcinoma is often diagnosed in the late stages, the diagnostic effort of the radiologist is primarily directed toward determining the extent of the disease.

Conventional Radiology

Plain Radiography

The radiograph of the abdomen may reveal soft tissue masses that displace gas-filled loops of bowels (fig. 33.1). Calcification, dental-like structures, or fat within a mass may indicate the presence of a dermoid. Approximately 12% of patients with serous cystadenoma or cystadenocarcinoma develop psammomatous calcification in the

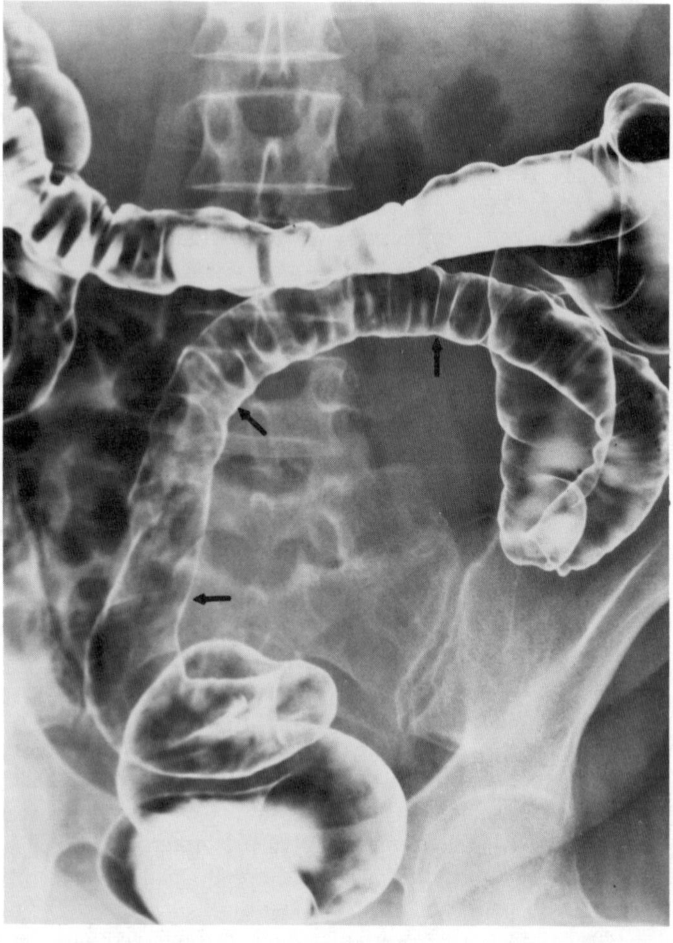

Fig. 33.1. Mucinous cystadenocarcinoma. The radiograph from the barium enema demonstrates a large soft tissue mass displacing and elevating the sigmoid colon (*arrows*).

primary tumor or the metastases. In these types of tumors, malignancy may be suggested by the presence of distorted bowels, ascites, and rarely, skeletal metastases (Stevens 1971).

Chest radiographs are useful for detecting pulmonary metastases and pleural effusions and, subsequently, for monitoring responses to chemotherapy. In patients with ovarian carcinoma, pleural effusions occur frequently on the right side. Routine chest tomography is not necessary in cases involving lung metastases, which represent advanced disease that is usually preceded by other findings such as peritoneal carcinomatosis and ascites.

Because of an extremely low incidence of skeletal metastasis, a regular radiographic bone scan is not necessary in the staging of ovarian carcinoma. In a study by Metler et al. (1982), less than 3% of 104 patients with ovarian carcinoma had osseous metastases at initial staging. All the patients with skeletal metastases had stage III, grade III adenocarcinoma and all had experienced bone pain. None of the patients with skeletal metastases had elevated alkaline phosphatase levels.

Excretory Urography

Urography, which is frequently performed in a patient with a pelvic mass, may reveal the vague outlines of distortion of the bladder or obstruction of the ureters by the mass. However, the efficacy of routine excretory urography in the staging of gynecologic malignancies has been questioned. Hillman, Clark, and Babbitt (1984) demonstrated that the urogram is extremely inaccurate in evaluating the extent of gynecologic malignancies. In their study, the true positive rate ranged from 7% to 33%. The excretory urogram is useful for locating the position of the ureters and for demonstrating the presence of obstruction or unsuspected urinary tract abnormalities, all of which can be obtained by sonography and, more specifically, by CT. CT is also more accurate for assessing the primary mass and the degree and extent of malignancy. The continued use of excretory urography in the preoperative staging of gynecologic malignancies is, therefore, related to traditional application and the physician's skill in interpreting urograms. When considering the cost, the low sensitivity and specificity of urography in preoperative staging, and the redundancy of information obtainable by more efficacious methods, it appears unnecessary to perform routine excretory urograms.

Barium Studies

Metastases to the small and large bowel may occur by hematogenous spread, direct extension, or serosal seeding (Levitt et al. 1982). Because ovarian cancer is primarily a disease of the peritoneum, intraperitoneal seeding with serosal spread is the most common metastatic pattern. Malignant neoplasms that arise in the ovaries eventually break through the organ's capsule and spread along the visceral peritoneum to invade the wall of the adjacent bowel. The findings from barium enema studies, therefore, reflect the degree of desmoplastic response elicited by the tumor as well as the extent of the involvement of the bowel wall. The findings within the bowel may include fixation or angulation of the bowel loops, traction changes, and mass effect. These changes—individually or in any combination—suggest that there is no specific pattern or degree of growth in tumor involvement of the bowel (Gedgaudas et al. 1983). A more subtle manifestation of serosal implants, "the striped colon," has also been described (Ginaldi et al. 1980).

The spread of abdominal malignancy as it relates to the dynamics and distribution of ascites has been examined (Meyers 1973; Meyers and McSweeney 1972). Four sites of ovarian metastases are common: the pouch of Douglas, right lower quadrant, sigmoid colon, and right paracolic gutter. In Meyers' series of 35 cases with ascites and abdominal carcinomatosis, 15 were of ovarian origin (Meyers 1973; Meyers and McSweeney 1972; Meyers 1975; Khilnani et al. 1966).

Generally, the small bowel is affected by metastases far more frequently than the large bowel. In a recent study by Yuhasz et al. (1985) of patients with ovarian carcinoma, all of the abnormalities of the small bowel were due to metastatic disease. Presently, radiation therapy is not the primary mode of treatment in ovarian patients; therefore, radiation damage to the bowel is uncommon in these patients. This contrasts sharply with cases of cervical cancer wherein obstruction may be due to metastases, radiation, or adhesions. Furthermore, it is possible that the site of obstruction may be used as a differential point for diagnosis. In the study by Yuhasz et al., all proximal obstructions (duodenum or jejunum) were caused by metastastic growth and all distal obstructions (ileum) were caused by radiation.

It is also possible for metastatic growth to invade the transverse colon by contiguous spread from the greater omentum. In barium studies, this is demonstrated by involvement of the superior border of the transverse colon with a mass effect, nodularity, and tethered mucosal folds; focal or diffuse areas of circumferential narrowing may also be identified. Conventional barium studies provide only indirect evidence of omental disease (Rubesin and Levine 1985), whereas CT scan usually detects omental masses larger than 2 cm and sometimes as small as 1 cm.

Radionuclide Scanning

Since the emergence of cross-sectional imaging modalities such as ultrasonography and CT, the vast majority of radionuclide scans performed in staging ovarian malignancies have become redundant. This includes screening for liver metastasis by hepatic scintigraphy, which has shown both low specificity and high false-positive rates. In patients with ovarian carcinoma, a high percentage of extrahepatic disease can be detected by ultrasonography and by CT examinations but not by scintigraphy (Doiron and Bernardino 1981; Sonnendecker and De Souza 1984; Harbert 1984).

Metler et al. (1982) found that less than 3% of their patients with ovarian carcinoma had osseous metastases at initial staging. Radionuclide bone scanning need not be performed routinely but should be reserved specifically for patients with symptoms. Studies such as lymphscintigraphy and contrast peritoneography have been superseded by lymphography, ultrasonography, and CT (Bloomer 1983; Yoonessi, Abdel-Dayem, and Shalaby 1982).

In the future, radionuclide monoclonal antibodies may prove to be reliable for defining the primary, recurrent, metastatic, and even occult carcinoma. The research is in its infancy (Epenetos et al. 1984; DeLand and Goldenberg 1985).

Lymphangiography

Drainage in the ovarian lymphatic system is from the aortic bifurcation to the paraaortic lymph nodes, the renal hilar nodes, and, occasionally, to the nodes of the external and common iliac lymph groups. Once there is neoplastic involvement of the ovarian capsule and fallopian tubes, foci of metastases are more likely to appear in the iliac and inguinal lymphatics and nodes. Because anastomoses exist between the ovarian lymph vessels and those of the uterus and fallopian tubes, however, other variations may occur.

In a study of 289 patients, Fuks (1975) had positive results on lymphangiograms in 21% of the patients with stage I or stage II epithelial carcinoma of the ovary. In the same study, aortic node dissection confirmed lymph node involvement in all patients whose lymphangiogram results had been positive, but there was a 17% false-negative rate. In a study that included 72 lymphangiograms performed on 66 patients, Athey et al. (1975) found metastatic involvement in the paraaortic nodes in 70%, the iliac nodes in 58%, and the inguinal nodes in 27%. In germ cell tumors, paraaortic nodes were involved with a 90% incidence and iliac nodes with a 30% incidence.

Ultrasonography

Two types of ultrasonographic imaging devices are available for evaluation of a patient with a pelvic mass: articulated arm or static B-mode scanners and real-time equipment. The static imaging device affords serial tomographic evaluation of the pelvis and surrounding structures and a global picture of the entire pelvis and surrounding structures. The development of the wide-angle, high-resolution, real-time scanners permits a more flexible approach for the diagnostic evaluation of the patient with a pelvic mass. The real-time scanner allows far more flexibility in scanning techniques in any plane—transverse, sagittal, or oblique. In addition, with real-time scanning, a quick survey of the abdomen can be performed. The kidneys can be examined for the presence of obstructive uropathy; the liver for hepatic metastases, texture abnormalities, and dilated bile ducts; the paracolic recesses, hepatorenal space, and cul-de-sac for the presence of ascites; and the peritoneal surfaces for tumor implants.

A requirement for ultrasonography of the pelvis is a full urinary bladder to create a sonic fluid-filled window for visualization of the pelvic structures. The distended bladder displaces gas-containing bowel out of the pelvis and, most important, displaces the antiflexed uterus to a more horizontal position. It is well known that bowel loops may create "pseudolesions"; however, with the aid of real-time sonography, peristalsis may be observed. If not, the water enema technique is extremely useful in determining whether pelvic masses represent bowel loops (Kurtz et al. 1979). The main advantages of ultrasonography are a low cost (compared with that of CT) and the absence of radiation. It can therefore be safely used in pediatric patients, pregnant women with suspected pelvic masses, women of child-bearing age, and other patients with suspected nonneoplastic masses.

The accuracy of ultrasonography is extremely dependent on the expertise of the operator and the resolution of the scanning device used. CT scanning is far less operator dependent. One disadvantage of ultrasonography is that it cannot detect neoplastic involvement of the bowel and bladder. Extension of tumor to involve the bony pelvis is difficult to evaluate by sonography. Overlying intraluminal bowel gas may hamper sonographic imaging, especially in the retroperitoneum. Peritoneal and omental metastases of less than 2 cm cannot be detected by ultrasonography (Yeh 1979) nor can a predominately cystic mass be detected when there are ascites and fluid-filled bowel within the pelvis. An ovarian mass that is predominately cystic could eventually merge with the ascites and fluid-filled bowel.

Normal-size adult ovaries can be routinely identified by ultrasonography; however, with age and cessation of ovulation and menstruation, the ovaries shrink. In postmenopausal women, the ovaries are rarely palpable by physical examination and are rarely visualized with ultrasonography (Sample 1980; Sample, Lippe, and Gyepes 1977; Athey 1981). Therefore, an ovarian neoplasm should be suspected when postmenopausal ovaries are palpable or well visualized and appear to contain cystic activity on ultrasonography (Barber and Grober 1971). In addition to the initial diagnosis and staging of tumor, ultrasonography may be used to identify postoperative complications such as abscesses, hematomas, lymphoceles, and tumor recurrence with a high degree of accuracy.

The accuracy of ultrasonography in detecting a pelvic mass and in determining its size, location, and consistency has been reported to be as high as 91% (Lawson and Albarelli 1977). A technically adequate study may disclose a cystic mass smaller than 2 cm in diameter if the mass is echo free and has sharply defined margins; however, a solid mass of less than 2 cm to 3 cm may escape recognition. It should be noted that the appearance of these tumors is nonspecific except for a few features that may suggest the histological diagnosis. These include a functioning simple ovarian cyst, cystadenoma with fine septation, and cystadenocarcinoma with solid nodules (Lawson and Albarelli 1977; Fleischer et al. 1978; Berland et al. 1980; Walsh et al. 1979; Requard, Mettler, and Wicks 1981; Paling and Shawker 1981). The sonographic appearance of an ovarian tumor correlates well with the tumor's gross morphology but very poorly with the histology. However, the ultrasonographer's role is primarily to indicate whether a suspected adnexal mass is of a benign or malignant nature (fig. 33.2).

Although pathognomonic patterns are not present in ultrasonography, certain sonographic criteria may help considerably in narrowing the differential diagnosis. A recent study by Moyle et al. (1983) demonstrated that anechoic lesions have a greater likelihood of being benign tumors—usually mucinous cystadenoma or serous cystadenoma. As the percentage of echogenic material (solid tissue) increases in the mass, the likelihood of malignancy also increases (fig. 33.2). The exceptions are benign teratomas that contain very echogenic foci and tumors that are completely or almost completely echogenic. Ultrasonic features that suggest a malignancy include the following: a multiloculated cystic mass with a diameter greater than 5 cm in a perimenopausal or postmenopausal woman; thick septation, especially with coexistent solid nodules; a complex mass inseparable from the

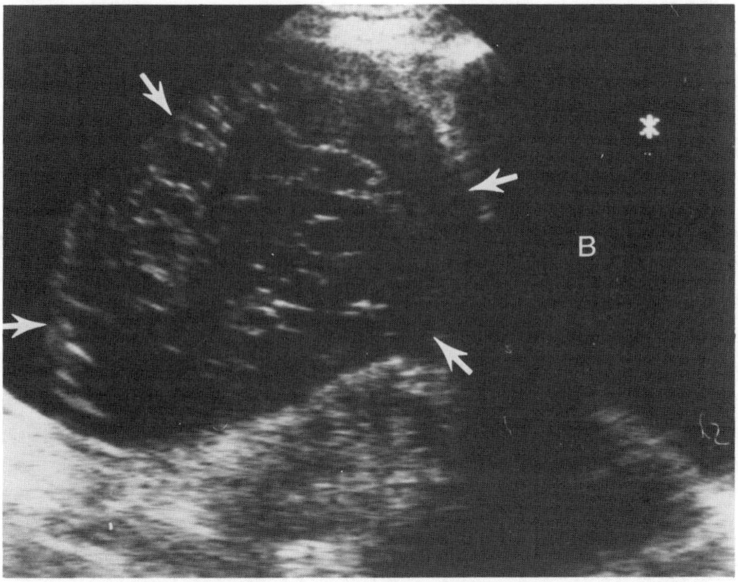

Fig. 33.2. Mucinous cystadenocarcinoma. A sagittal sonogram through the pelvis demonstrates a large, multiseptated, predominantly cystic mass (*arrows*) superior to the bladder (*B*). This corresponds with the soft tissue mass seen in figure 1.

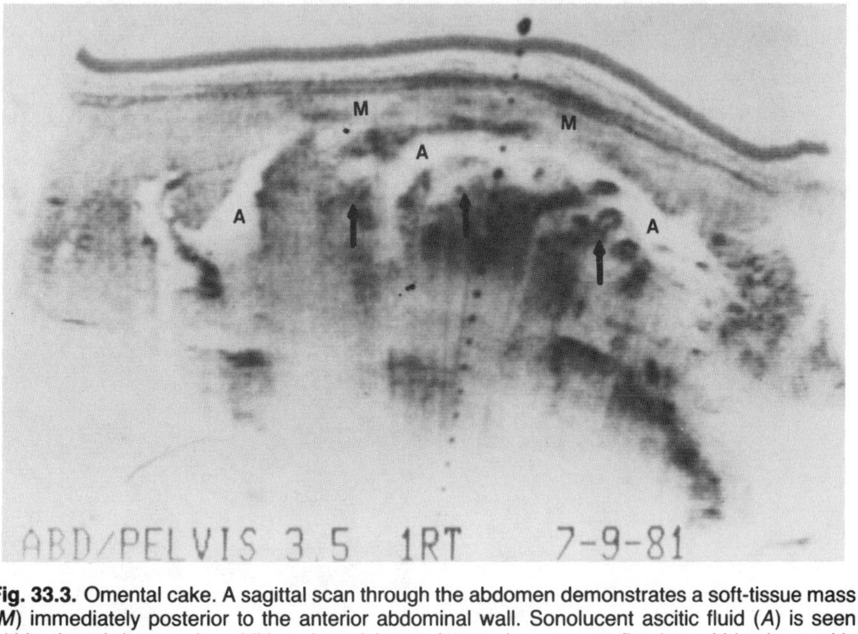

Fig. 33.3. Omental cake. A sagittal scan through the abdomen demonstrates a soft-tissue mass (*M*) immediately posterior to the anterior abdominal wall. Sonolucent ascitic fluid (*A*) is seen within the abdomen. In addition, bowel loops (*arrows*) are seen floating within the ascitic fluid (*A*).

uterus (fig. 33.2); ascites; "omental cake" (mesenteric metastases) (fig. 33.3); para-aortic lymph node enlargement; and hepatic metastases. Two ultrasonography studies of ovarian carcinoma (Requard, Mettler, and Wicks 1981; Paling and Shawker 1981) disclosed ascites in 37% to 41% of patients, extrapelvic disease in 40%, and hydronephrosis in 14%. In 20% of patients, there was omental or peritoneal involvement with a high false-negative rate probably related to the presence of small metastatic implants that were impossible to differentiate from omental fat and bowel gas.

Ascites also may hinder the recognition of omental and mesenteric metastases. In addition, in 2% to 5% of mucinous tumors, peritoneal spread of mucin-secreting cells with gelatinous material results in "pseudomyxoma peritonei."

Ultrasonography may predict uterine involvement by revealing a tumor mass that is inseparable from the uterus, but it is insensitive in defining tumor invasion into the bladder or bowel (Bowie 1977). When a mass is detected, full abdominal ultrasonography should be performed to determine the presence of ascites, hydronephrosis, retroperitoneal disease, and liver metastases. Because of the absence of ionizing radiation, ultrasonography is useful in identifying an ovarian mass in the pregnant patient (Czernobilsky 1982; Novak and Woodruff 1979).

Of all tumors of the ovary, 10% are attributed to metastatic disease of genital or extragenital origin (Blaustein 1982). Adenocarcinoma of the endometrium is the most common tumor to metastasize to the ovary. The most common extragenital

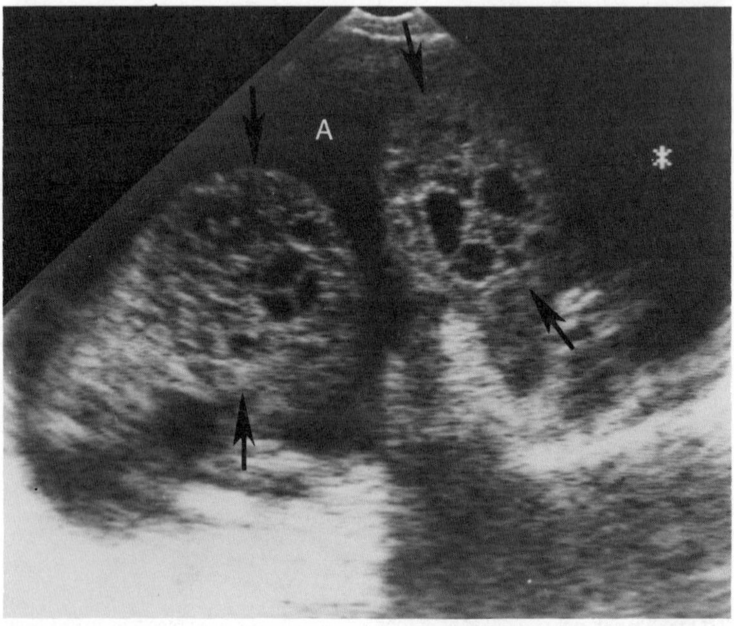

Fig. 33.4. Krukenberg tumors. Transverse scan through the pelvis demonstrates bilateral complex masses with cystic components (*arrows*). These masses are noted to be floating within a sea of ascites (*A*). The patient was a young woman with primary gastric carcinoma.

sites of origin are the gastrointestinal tract and the breast. Ovarian metastases from breast carcinomas are revealed at autopsy in about 20% of breast cancer patients and are bilateral in 60% to 80% of cases. Tumors arising in the gastrointestinal tract may metastasize to the ovary, producing extremely large masses. The stomach is the primary source in over 90% of cases. The classification of Krukenberg tumor should be restricted to tumors that contain the typical mucin-secreting "signet-ring" cells. On ultrasonography, the Krukenberg tumor is a complex-appearing mass with solid components, which may be impossible to distinguish from a primary carcinoma of the ovary (Novak and Woodruff 1979; Blaustein 1982; Rochester et al. 1977) (fig. 33.4). Other tumors that commonly metastasize to the ovaries stem from lymphoma and leukemia and appear ultrasonographically as solid masses (Bickers et al. 1981).

Differential diagnoses for ovarian malignancies include multicystic ovary from ovarian hyperstimulation syndrome, which may closely simulate ovarian malignancy; inflammatory processes of the adnexa; matted loops of bowel originating from appendicitis, diverticulitis, or inflammatory bowel disease; and other tumors that may arise in the pelvis, including pelvic sarcomas, bowel tumors, and sacropelvic girdle masses (Fleischer et al. 1978; McArdle and Sacks 1980; Rankin and Hutton 1981).

Computerized Tomography

In the last decade, CT has probably been more advantageous in the staging of tumors than any other diagnostic imaging modality. This is primarily because of an increased resolution and the ability to demonstrate subtle differences in the radiographic densities of bone, air, soft tissue, and fat in a cross-sectional dimension. Therefore, primary tumors such as those containing fat (dermoid) or calcification (psammomatous or dental calcification) (fig. 33.5), as well as cystic or solid masses and masses containing septations can be determined (Amendola et al. 1981). The advantages of CT include the ease of performance, predictable accuracy with bulk disease, and assessment of areas—largely in the upper retroperitoneum, mesentery, and abdominal viscera—not visualized by lymphangiography. However, it should be noted that the limitations of CT include an inability to detect an abnormality in normal-size lymph nodes and a proper anatomic resolution only in very thin patients who have a paucity of retroperitoneal fat (Lee et al. 1978; Walsh et al. 1980). Besides detecting soft tissue masses and determining the extent of tumor pathology, CT has become an extremely valuable tool for performing percutaneous interventional procedures such as abdominal fluid aspiration, abscess drainage, or tumor biopsy. Although simpler radiographic techniques can guide percutaneous invasive procedures of more accessible lesions, in small or deeply situated abnormalities, extreme precision is required, such as that offered by CT (van Sonnenberg et al. 1982; Martin et al. 1982; Haaga 1979; Ferruci et al. 1980; Isler et al. 1981).

In a randomized study of 53 patients with palpable abdominal masses, Dixon et al. (1981) compared the utility of CT with that of conventional imaging. The time to diagnosis was significantly shorter in the patients undergoing CT. Although the cost of imaging investigations was greater in the CT group, the cost for hospitalization

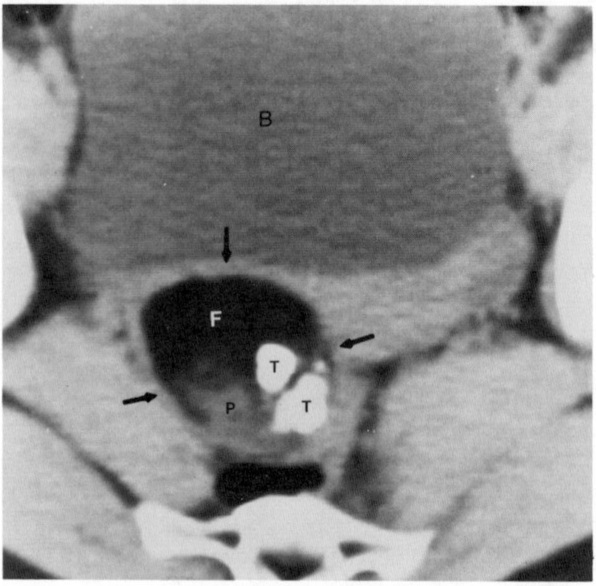

Fig. 33.5. Dermoid. A CT scan through the pelvis demonstrates a mass (*arrows*) containing teeth (*T*). In addition, the low-density component within the mass corresponds to fat (*F*), and the higher density in the lower aspect of the mass is the dermoid plug (*P*; *B*, bladder).

was significantly less in the CT group than in the group not undergoing CT. Others have observed a decrease in the use of invasive tests such as abdominal angiography, lymphangiography, and endoscopic retrograde pancreatography, along with a concomitant increase in the use of CT. In a study by Fineberg et al. (1983), it was noted that the referring physicians also advocated the use of CT for noninvasive imaging.

Recently, Sanders et al. (1983) compared the utility of CT and ultrasonography in 74 patients who appeared to have pelvic masses on clinical examination and in 110 patients who were suspected of having recurrent pelvic tumors. There was no statistical difference in the ability of the two modalities to identify masses in order to predict the extent of disease. The sensitivities of the two techniques were virtually identical with 96% accuracy for CT and 91% accuracy for ultrasonography. Both modalities had an accuracy of 81% in the detection of recurrent disease; however, in the staging of newly diagnosed tumors, CT was slightly more accurate (68%) than ultrasonography (56%) when their results were compared with pathological staging following surgery.

Because of the nature of ovarian carcinoma, the majority of patients are classified at stage III or stage IV disease at the time of initial clinical presentation. CT scanning cannot replace surgery as a staging technique because of the need for obtaining histological samples. Often the only evidence of metastasis is the presence of small peritoneal seedlings that cannot be identified, especially in the presence of ascites (fig. 33.6). CT will not supplant ultrasonography as the initial modality for examining the pelvis (Gross et al. 1983); however, the greatest advantage of CT over other imaging techniques is its ability to reveal disease both within and outside the pelvic area (i.e., in the liver, retroperitoneum, and omentum). In cases of ovarian carcinoma, CT is a preferred imaging technique for demonstrating tumor invasion of the bowel, pelvic sidewall, and ureter and for revealing retroperitoneal and pelvic lymph node metastases (Amendola et al. 1981; Kerr-Wilson et al. 1984; Johnson et al. 1983; Whitley et al. 1981).

Some of the diverse features depicted on CT scan of ovarian tumors are thick, irregular cyst walls; solid areas of soft tissue components; internal septations; and soft tissue or wall calcifications (fig. 33.7). CT is superior to surgical exploration in the detection of intrahepatic metastases and in the assessment of intrauterine disease (Kerr-Wilson et al. 1984; Johnson et al. 1983; Whitley et al. 1981). Although intrahepatic metastases are thought to be uncommon, in a study by Paling and Shawker (1981) 39% of patients presented with intrahepatic metastases.

Computerized tomography may be far better and more accurate than ultrasonography in determining the degree and extent of metastases to the small bowel serosa and omentum; however, with CT, small peritoneal metastases less than 1 cm cannot be detected. Dunnick et al. (1979) detected small peritoneal implants by CT after the intraperitoneal instillation of water-soluble contrast. The newest CT scanners have both increased spatial resolution and faster scan times, which may obviate the need for instillation of contrast solution in the future.

Therefore, CT is most useful in ovarian carcinomas when used as a noninvasive imaging technique to delineate the entire extent of known areas of tumor and to reveal unsuspected sites of disease in both the abdomen and pelvis. It is also extremely useful in following the response of the tumor to therapy and in detecting the

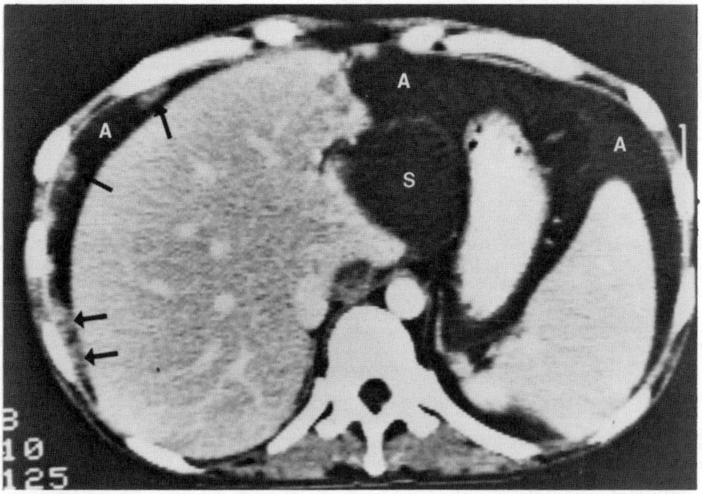

Fig. 33.6. Peritoneal metastases. A CT scan of a patient with ovarian carcinoma demonstrates several small, soft-tissue masses (*arrows*) adherent to the peritoneum. These are due to peritoneal metastases. In addition, ascites (*A*) is noted lateral to the liver and anterior to the stomach and spleen. Ascites is also present within the lesser sac (*S*).

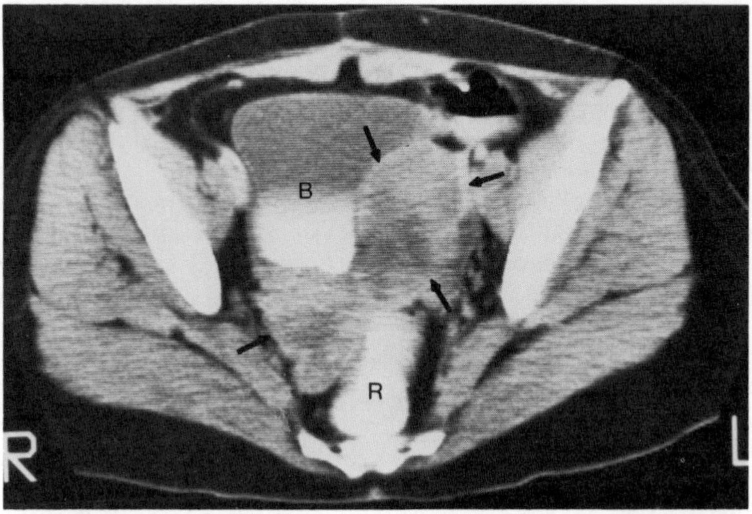

Fig. 33.7. Bilateral ovarian carcinomas. A CT scan of the pelvis demonstrates bilateral solid masses (*arrows*) within the pelvis. Central areas of low density suggest either necrosis or fluid density (*B*, bladder; *R*, rectum).

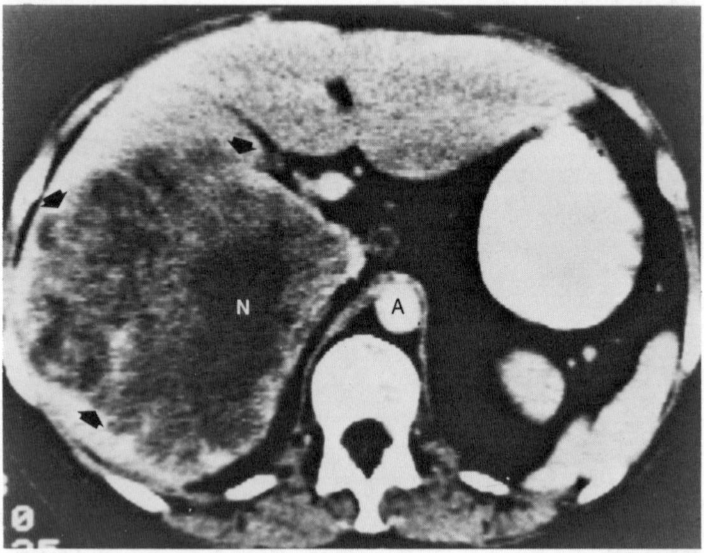

Fig. 33.8. Hepatic metastases. This CT scan of the liver demonstrates a large mass of mixed attenuation occupying virtually the entire right lobe of the liver (*arrows*). There are central areas of decreased attenuation due to necrosis (*N*; *A*, aorta).

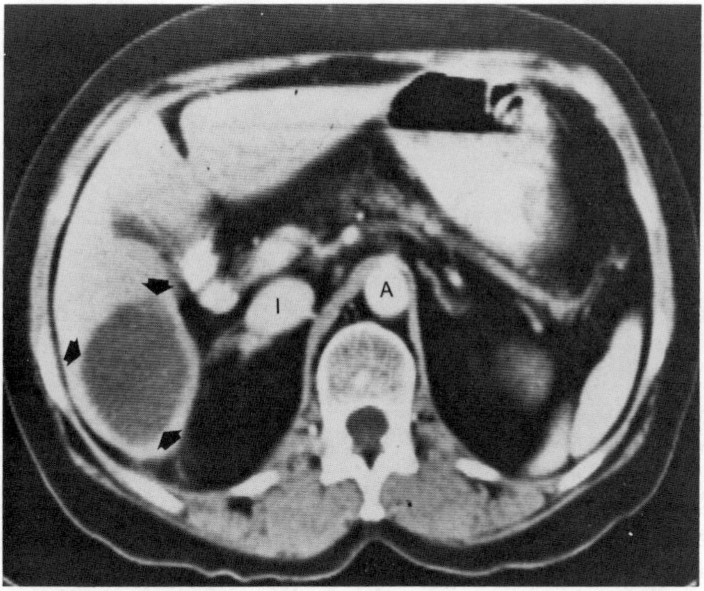

Fig. 33.9. Regression of the hepatic metastases. This CT scan was obtained following several courses of intraarterial chemotherapy. The low-density metastases (*arrows*) are noted to have decreased markedly in size since the previous scan (fig. 33.8) (*A*, aorta; *I*, inferior vena cava).

presence of residual tumor after cytoreductive surgery (Whitley et al. 1981) (figs. 33.8 and 33.9). Serial CT scans at three- to four-month intervals may also provide important prognostic information. In many instances, CT is preferred to ultrasonography for diagnostic imaging, particularly ultrasound, especially in assessing response to treatments because it allows recognition of more disease sites without interference from overlying gas artifact and also provides superior anatomic display between the edges of normal and abnormal structures.

Recently, Brenner et al. (1985), in a study of 52 patients with ovarian carcinoma undergoing second-look laparotomy to confirm tumor status, compared the results of preoperative abdominopelvic CT scan with postoperative findings. In 42% of cases, negative results on CT scans were associated with positive findings at laparotomy. A large percentage of these cases represented microscopic residual tumor, which was defined as positive peritoneal washings with grossly negative exploration. In view of the low sensitivity in this group of patients as well as the large number of false-negative examinations, it appears that the findings of a negative CT scan prior to second-look laparotomy are not significant. Positive findings confirmed by needle aspiration under CT guidance would therefore eliminate the need for laparotomy in about 25% of such patients, thus decreasing morbidity and costs (figs. 33.10 and 33.11).

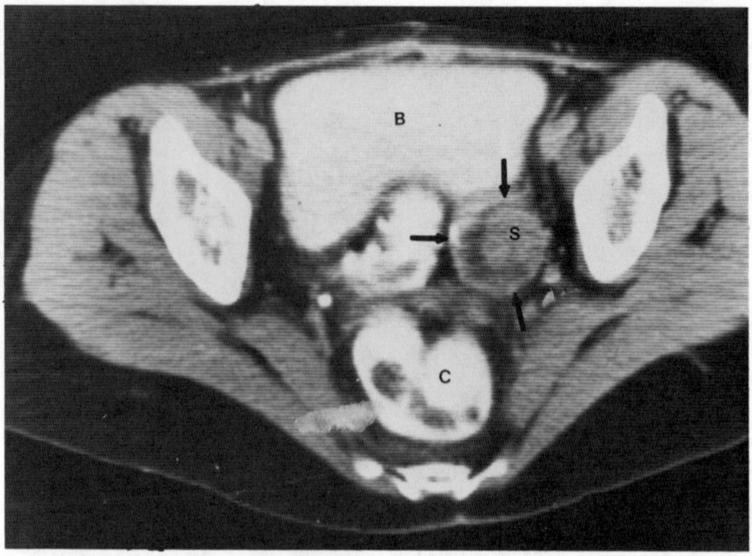

Fig. 33.10. Recurrent ovarian carcinoma. The CT scan of the pelvis demonstrates a mass in the left adnexa (*arrows*). An extrinsic solid component (*S*) is present. This is consistent with recurrent carcinoma (*B*, bladder; *C*, sigmoid colon).

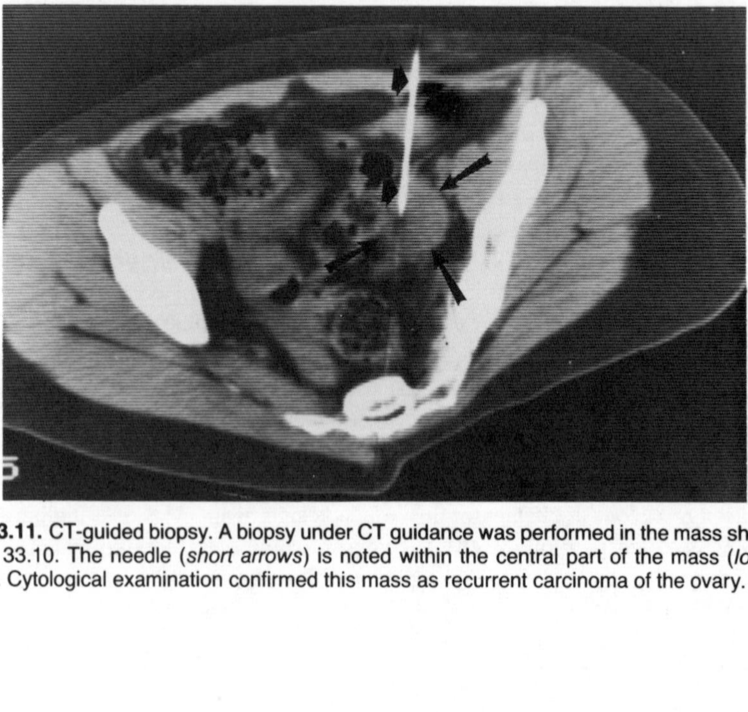

Fig. 33.11. CT-guided biopsy. A biopsy under CT guidance was performed in the mass shown in figure 33.10. The needle (*short arrows*) is noted within the central part of the mass (*long arrows*). Cytological examination confirmed this mass as recurrent carcinoma of the ovary.

Magnetic Resonance Imaging

MRI is a relatively new technique, involving the use of radiofrequency waves in varying magnetic fields to produce cross-sectional images of the body. The image depends on the number of hydrogen nuclei in the body tissues and the extent to which hydrogen is bound within each organ molecule. MRI is noninvasive, avoids ionizing radiation, and involves no observable side effects. The imaging plane can be electronically selected for direct coronal, sagittal, or routine transverse plane imaging. The pelvis is particularly well suited to MRI scanning because of the high degree of natural contrasts provided by pelvic fat, urine in the bladder, and gas within the bowel. In addition, there is less motion blurring in the pelvic area than in the upper abdomen and chest. Therefore, MRI is potentially a very promising modality for characterizing pelvic masses and for the staging of pelvic malignancies. At present, the primary disadvantages of MRI include a long scanning time and the high cost of purchasing the equipment and performing the examinations.

Although the utilization of MRI scanning in the pelvis is still in its infancy, there have been several reports of MRI examinations of both the normal and abnormal female pelvis (Bryan et al. 1983; Hricak et al. 1983; Johnson et al. 1984; Butler et al. 1984). Because of the limited experience with pelvic examination by MRI, no definite conclusions can be drawn regarding the future role of this technique. Thus far, MRI has been primarily used for examining ovarian cysts and dermoids, which have diverse appearances on the MRI scans. The major tissue in a dermoid is fat, along with small amounts of hair, bone, and other matter. Therefore, the fat content accounts for the high signal level in most dermoids examined by MRI. In a dermoid containing a negligible amount of fat, a mass with low signal intensity will be imaged. The different degrees of intensities obtained in an MRI image of a dermoid are related to the various solid and fluid components of the mass (Johnson et al. 1984; Butler et al. 1984). MRI should be assessed in terms of its capability to determine tumor extent to the sidewall of the pelvis and to detect metastases in lymph nodes that are not enlarged. It remains to be determined whether the increased contrast resolution of MRI will be adequate to show tumor in normal-size nodes. At present, lymphadenopathy can be detected on MRI by signal-producing masses by their contrast to adjacent vessels such as the iliac vessels, which produce no signal. Thereby, MRI imaging is superior to CT scanning in the pelvic area in that small nodes can be differentiated from the adjoining vessels (fig. 33.12).

The advantages and disadvantages of MRI versus other types of noninvasive diagnostic imaging techniques can be summarized as follows: (1) MRI does not assign unique values to disease processes (i.e., a malignant process cannot be differentiated from a benign process); (2) the definition of normal structures on present, early-generation MRI scans approaches that of CT and sonography, though the ability of MRI to define edges of bowel is an advantage over sonography; (3) the similar appearance of pathological processes such as cystadenomas on CT and sonography does not guarantee a similar appearance on MRI; (4) the ability of MRI to scan in several planes can be used to significant advantage in some cases; and (5) the lack of

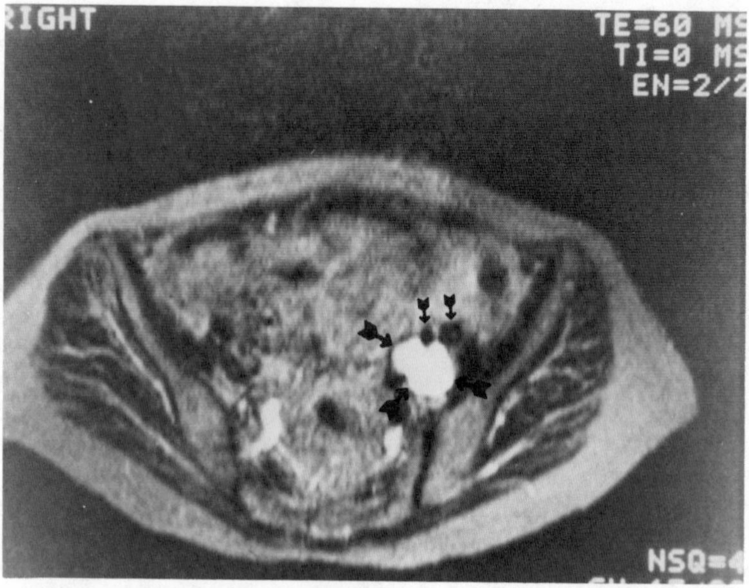

Fig. 33.12. Pelvic lymphadenopathy. An MRI scan demonstrates a mass of high-intensity (*large arrows*) adjacent to the external iliac vessels (*small arrows*) of low intensity. The appearance of the low-intensity blood vessels is due to rapidly flowing blood within the vessels.

radiation exposure is a clear advantage over CT, especially in children and in patients requiring repeated examinations.

It is premature to predict the clinical value MRI will have in the field of noninvasive imaging. It is clear, however, that several years of experience with MRI are required before meaningful clinical data will become available for evaluation.

Interventional Radiology

Angiography

Because of ultrasonography and CT, angiography is only used in selected cases of ovarian tumors. The arterial supply to the ovary originates from two sources: the ovarian arteries usually arise from the aorta, and the adnexal branches of the uterine arteries arise from the internal iliac arteries. Fernstrom (1955) described the use of arteriography in the diagnosis of gynecologic neoplasms. Arteriography is still of considerable value in delineating hepatic metastases. Hepatic angiography, particularly with selective catheterization techniques, is now reserved for tumor staging and in preparation for interventional management such as hepatic arterial infusion with chemotherapy or embolization of the liver.

Most ovarian malignancies and ovarian metastases are relatively hypovascular (Fernstrom 1955). The angiographic evaluation of the left lobe of the liver remains difficult, but selective catheterization of the left hepatic artery adds immeasurably to the diagnostic capabilities (Wallace and Chuang 1982). Together, angiography and CT are very effective for specific diagnostic situations (Prando et al. 1979) where the different imaging modalities supply conflicting information with regard to the extent of the tumor.

Metastatic ovarian carcinoma in the liver is relatively uncommon and difficult to treat. Hepatic arterial infusion or embolization has been successful. Sensitivity of the neoplasm to the chemotherapeutic agent is usually apparent after a single course. The treatment is repeated at monthly intervals as long as the response continues. With stable or progressive disease, sequential embolization of the hepatic arteries with Ivalon (polyvinyl alcohol foam) is undertaken. One lobe is embolized each month, and the entire liver is then reembolized with Ivalon. A combination of infusion and embolization may also be effective (i.e., chemotherapy with cisplatin and Ivalon).

Percutaneous Needle Biopsies

In recent years, diagnostic radiologists have employed percutaneous needle biopsy to establish the diagnosis of lesions throughout the body. With the aid of fluoroscopy, ultrasonography, and CT, percutaneous needle biopsy has been used to detect pelvic masses, tumor recurrences in the pelvis, hepatic metastases, and retroperitoneal adenopathy. In many cases, the use of percutaneous biopsies obviates the need for surgical exploration, thus decreasing patient morbidity and costs. In ovarian neoplasms, percutaneous biopsy of abnormal areas or areas suggestive of tumor detected by radiological means may also obviate the need for a second-look operation.

At The University of Texas M. D. Anderson Hospital and Tumor Institute at Houston, the decision to perform biopsies under fluoroscopy, ultrasonography, or CT is determined by the depth, location, and size of the abnormality. In short, if the lesion is of reasonable size and is fairly accessible, the biopsy will be performed under ultrasonic guidance. Conversely, if the lesion is small and deep-seated, the high precision accuracy afforded by CT is required. Biopsies can be performed in virtually every body site—chest wall, lung, abdomen, pelvis, liver, bone, and heart (Haaga 1979; Ferruci et al. 1980; Isler et al. 1981).

Combining Techniques for Diagnosis

A combination of diagnostic modalities is used to determine ovarian carcinoma. The evaluation should begin with a routine chest radiograph and a sonogram of the pelvis. If the findings suggest carcinoma of the ovary, the examination should be extended to exclude abnormalities in the liver, peritoneal cavity, retroperitoneum, and kidneys. In cases of widespread disease, a CT examination encompassing the entire abdomen and pelvis should be performed to assess the extent of the disease process. CT scanning is also the optimal modality in the follow-up of an ovarian cancer patient to determine the response to therapy and disease status.

Because the urinary tract is rarely involved in cases of ovarian carcinoma, routine excretory urography prior to surgery is no longer necessary. The assessment of the upper urinary tract as well as the patency and anatomical placement of the ureters can be adequately assessed with ultrasonography and, more specifically, with CT examination. The inadequacy of both ultrasonography and CT for detecting minimal serosal implantations of the bowel is well known. Therefore, when these imaging modalities do not detect mesenteric or serosal metastases to the bowel, then regular upper and lower barium studies should also be performed. This is important because of ovarian carcinoma's marked propensity to metastasize to the bowel.

When retroperitoneal lymphadenopathy is revealed by ultrasonography or CT, a biopsy may be performed for confirmation. However, if both cross-sectional modalities produce negative results (i.e., no other metastatic disease is demonstrated), a lymphangiogram should then be performed. When necessary, invasive procedures such as arteriography, CT, sonographically guided percutaneous biopsy, nephrostomy, and percutaneous biliary drainage procedures can be performed.

Diagnosis of Cervical Cancer

Cancer of the cervix is the second most common malignancy found in females who are 15 to 34 years old. The squamous type of carcinoma is most prevalent, occurring in 95% of cases; adenocarcinoma is found in 5%. Although most women with cervical cancer are asymptomatic, about one-third present with vaginal bleeding and leukorrhea. Since the introduction of the Papanicolaou test (pap smear) in 1945, the mortality of cervical carcinoma has decreased; however, 20% of women delay seeking medical attention for at least six months following the onset of symptoms.

Conventional Radiology

In a recent series by Griffin, Parker, and Taylor (1976), the incidence of metastases from cervical carcinoma detected by routine radiographic modalities was extremely low (i.e, 7.3% on intravenous pyelography, 3.4% on barium enema, and 1% on chest radiography).

Pulmonary and skeletal metastases seldom appear until the local disease is advanced. Excretory urography demonstrates deviation of ureters or hydronephrosis in 20% of the cases. Barium studies occasionally detect metastatic invasion of the bowel.

Complications of radiation therapy are a small, elevated bladder with a thickened wall, a narrow rigid rectum, increased pelvic fat, and a widened presacral space (Green and Libshitz 1979). Rectovaginal and vesicovaginal fistulas occur only in approximately 1.2% of patients. Fistulas are noted more frequently, however, in cases in which hysterectomy is combined with radiation therapy (Strockbine, Hancock, and Fletcher 1970). In cases of fistulas, barium studies and retrograde cystography are helpful for diagnosis. The development of ureteral obstruction after treatment is almost invariably (95% of cases) due to recurrent tumor rather than radiation fibrosis (5%) and is frequently associated with lower extremity edema secondary to compression of the iliac vein. Radionecrosis of the bony pelvis and aseptic necrosis of the femoral heads may complicate therapy (Cunningham, Fuks, and Castellino 1974).

Lymphangiography

Lymphangiography is the only direct radiological approach to the visualization of the lymph vessels and lymph nodes. Metastatic disease in the lymph nodes is characterized by a change in fluid dynamics of the lymphatics or an alteration in the internal architecture of the lymph nodes. Lymphangiography is the only radiological method that evaluates the internal architecture of the nodes. A nodal defect that has not been traversed by the lymphatic channels is the most reliable criterion for the diagnosis of metastatic disease in a patient with a known primary neoplasm (fig. 33.13). A nodal defect in such a case is caused by tumor emboli that grow and destroy nodal tissue. The defect is usually peripheral, and the remaining functioning portion of the node is frequently crescent shaped ("rim sign"). A defect as small as 5 mm can be defined by lymphangiography when it replaces only a portion of the

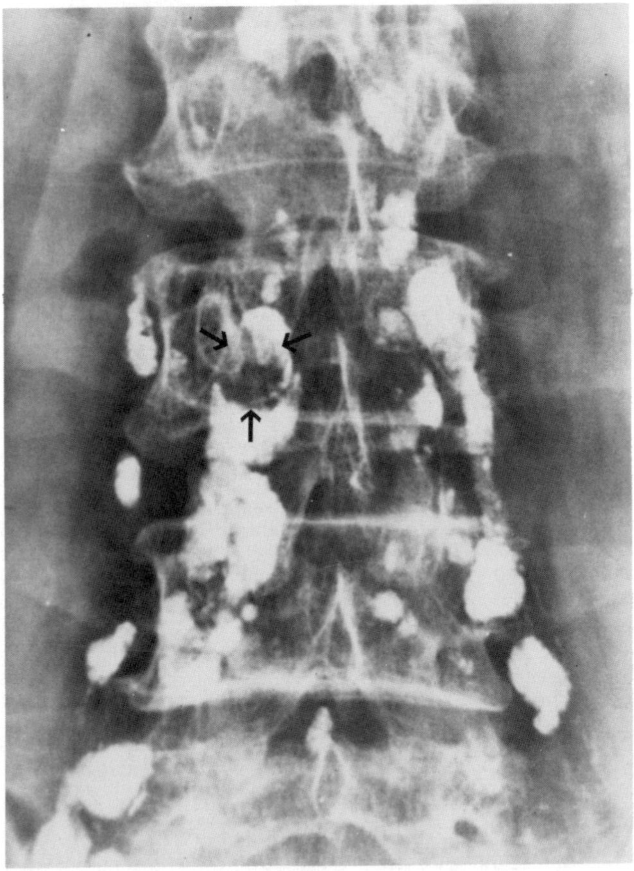

Fig. 33.13. Metastatic nodal cervical carcinoma. The nodal phase of the lymphangiogram demonstrates a typical filling defect (*arrows*) within this small retroperitoneal node. This was confirmed to be due to metastatic cervical carcinoma. (See fig. 33.17.)

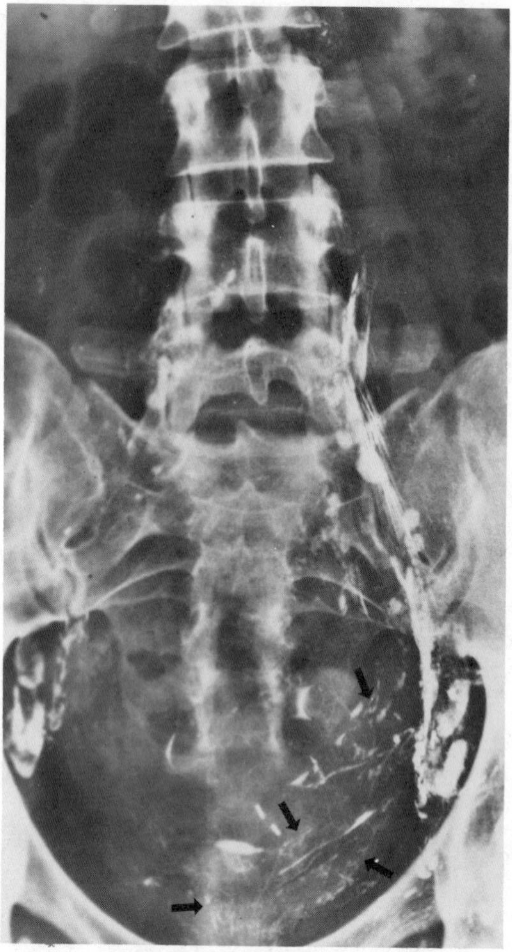

Fig. 33.14. Inadequate filling of the retroperitoneal nodes. The lymphangiogram demonstrates inadequate filling of the retroperitoneal nodes. In addition, there is evidence of lymphatic venous collateral circulation (*arrows*) within the pelvis. A subsequent CT scan (see fig. 33.18) confirmed the presence of adenopathy at the level of the renal vessels. This was due to metastatic cervical carcinoma.

node. However, if the node is totally replaced by a neoplasm, it will not be opacified (fig. 33.14), rendering a false-negative lymphangiogram. Other false-negative examinations are due to metastases that are too small to detect and failure of opacification of the involved nodes (Wallace and Jing 1977).

Bipedal lymphangiography usually opacifies most of the lymph nodes in the inguinal, external, and common iliac areas in addition to the paracaval, paraaortic, and interaortacaval nodes. But the hypogastric and presacral lymph nodes are only occasionally visualized. Another pitfall of lymphangiography is its failure to opacify such abdominal lymph nodes as mesenteric, portohepatic, splenic, and renal hilar nodes, and those above the cisterna chyli, including retrocaval nodes.

The modes of lymphatic metastases depend upon the normal distribution of lymphatic drainage; the variations of normal drainage; and the collateral pathways, which, in the event of extensive obstruction of normal channels, include lymphatic to lymphatic, lymphatic to paralymphatic, and lymphatic to venous. Utilizing the diagnostic criteria mentioned previously, the positive diagnosis of nodal metastases by lymphangiography in conjunction with other modalities—specifically CT—can yield a very high positive pathological correlation of 90% to 95%.

The lymphatics in the uterine cervix form a rich plexus. The collecting trunks drain to the lymph nodes of the external iliac and hypogastric chains as well as to the presacral area.

The results of lymphangiography in cervical carcinoma show a wide range of sensitivity (28%–83%) and specificity (47%–100%) (Brown et al. 1979; de Muylder et al. 1984). In part, these ranges reflect the difference in prevalence of nodal involvement in various stages of the disease. The sensitivity and specificity of CT average 71% and 92%, respectively (Brenner et al. 1982; Whitley et al. 1982). The accuracy of lymphangiography in detecting metastases in patients with stage I carcinoma of the cervix is low. The metastases in this group are usually in the pelvis and are most likely included within the usual radiation portals.

At U.T. M. D. Anderson Hospital, in one series of 103 patients with advanced cancer of the cervix, including bulky stage I lesions and postirradiation recurrence, metastases were diagnosed by lymphangiography in 42 (Piver, Wallace, and Castro 1971). Exploratory laparotomy confirmed the presence of metastases in 41 of 53 of these patients (sensitivity, 77%). Of the cases determined to be negative by lymphangiography, 49 of 50 were true negatives (specificity, 98%) and 12 were found to have lymph node metastases. The overall accuracy was 87%. The high percentage of false negatives (12%) supports the contention that only a definite diagnosis of positive disease is clinically useful (Wallace and Jing 1977; Wallace et al. 1979). Microscopic neoplastic foci are not detected by lymphangiography, nor are all the pelvic and paraaortic lymph nodes opacified.

At U.T. M. D. Anderson Hospital in 1981, 36 patients with carcinoma of the uterine cervix were examined by lymphangiography and followed within a month by CT to assess the findings of both modalities and their impact on management. Lymphangiography results were negative for lymph node metastases in 24 patients and positive in the remaining 12. CT findings were negative in 23 patients and positive in 13. Pathological correlation by biopsy or surgery was obtained in 15 patients. Lymphangiography showed evidence of nodal metastases in six and an overall accuracy of 93%. Five patients had nodal metastases by CT and the overall accuracy was 73%. There were two false negatives (13%) with CT. Two cases (13%) showed false-positive findings on CT resulting from lymphoid hyperplasia and postirradiation fibrosis.

In cases of advanced lesions or follow-up after irradiation or surgery when lymphangiography showed lymphatic obstruction in the pelvic region with non-opacification of the nodes above the interruption, CT showed either normal nodes with no evidence of metastases or nonopacified nodal metastases in the paraaortic area. In addition, CT revealed local extension of the lesion of the cervix and extranodal metastases, such as to the urinary tract, liver, and skeleton.

In a recent series (Legasse et al. 1980), 6% of clinical stage IB and 18% of clinical stage IIA cervical carcinoma patients had paraaortic nodes found to be positive at the time of surgery. In this group of patients, detection of positive nodes prior to surgery would have obviated the need for surgical intervention, and the patients could have undergone radiotherapy with extended fields. Therefore, even if lymphangiogram and CT readings are normal, there is still a possibility of metastases. Positive results on CT or lymphangiogram are only of clinical significance; therefore, when possible, histological material should be obtained with fine-needle aspiration.

Ultrasonography

In the early stages of cervical carcinoma, ultrasonography offers little in diagnostic capability except in patients in whom clinical examination is extremely difficult. Ultrasonography is useful in identifying large, exophytic fungating masses or masses involving the cervix and parametrium with enlargement of the pelvic lymph nodes in stage III or IV carcinoma. Involvement of the pelvic wall, bladder, and rectum may be difficult to define by ultrasonography. The kidneys can be examined routinely for hydronephrosis, which indicates stage III disease (Sanders and James 1980; Requard, Wicks, and Metter 1981).

Computerized Tomography

The main role of CT in patients with cervical carcinoma is to determine the extent of disease (i.e., the tumor size, uterine size, endometrium invasion, parametrial and pelvic side wall extension, and pelvic adenopathy). Extrapelvic metastases to the liver, skeleton, and paraaortic lymph nodes, as well as hydronephrosis, are readily detected. In a recent series by Walsh and Goplerud (1981) examination of 75 patients with cervical carcinoma determined that CT was inaccurate in differentiating stage IB from stage IIB lesions but was extremely accurate in the diagnosis and staging of advanced lesions (i.e., those greater than stage IIIB).

A primary neoplasm of the cervix is frequently of water density or less and is best seen at the level of the femoral heads. Parametrial extension is determined by extension to the obturator internis or piriformis muscle. Bladder and rectal invasion are difficult to assess but may be manifested by irregular thickening of the adjacent walls with obliteration of the posterior perivesical and anterior rectal fat planes (fig. 33.15).

A further difficulty in diagnosis is the differentiation between tumor recurrence and radiation fibrosis. Both entities may be seen as irregular, soft tissue densities within the pelvis (fig. 33.16). Differentiation between the two would have to be determined by CT-guided fine-needle aspiration. Positive findings on needle aspiration would obviate the need for further laparotomy.

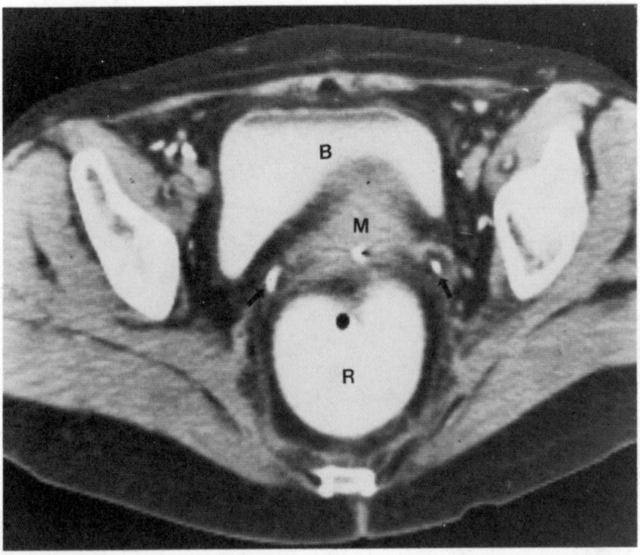

Fig. 33.15. Mass (*M*) with irregular margins in the cervical region. Periureteral extension of the tumor mass is seen (*arrows*). This is due to stage IIB cervical carcinoma (*B*, bladder; *R*, rectum).

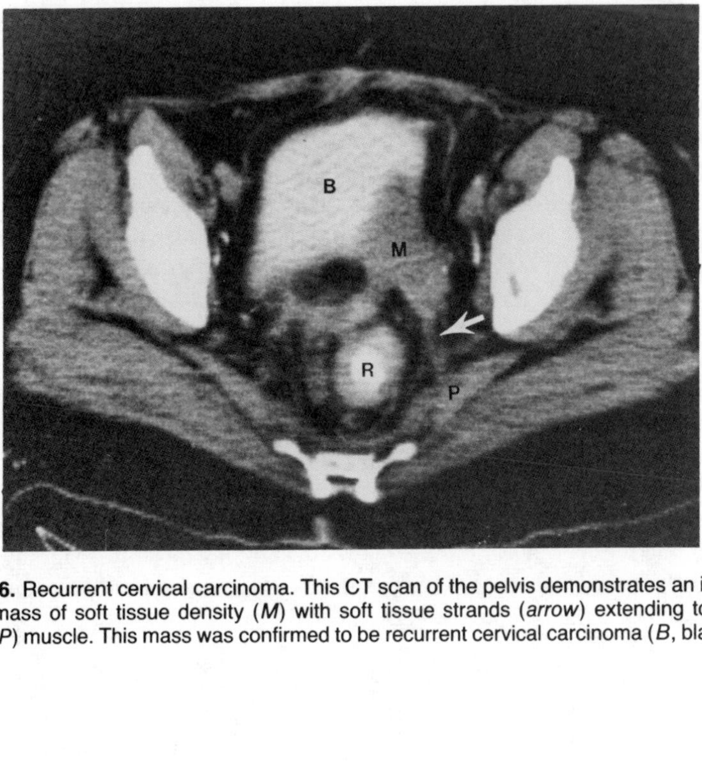

Fig. 33.16. Recurrent cervical carcinoma. This CT scan of the pelvis demonstrates an irregular-shaped mass of soft tissue density (*M*) with soft tissue strands (*arrow*) extending to the left piriform (*P*) muscle. This mass was confirmed to be recurrent cervical carcinoma (*B*, bladder; *R*, rectum).

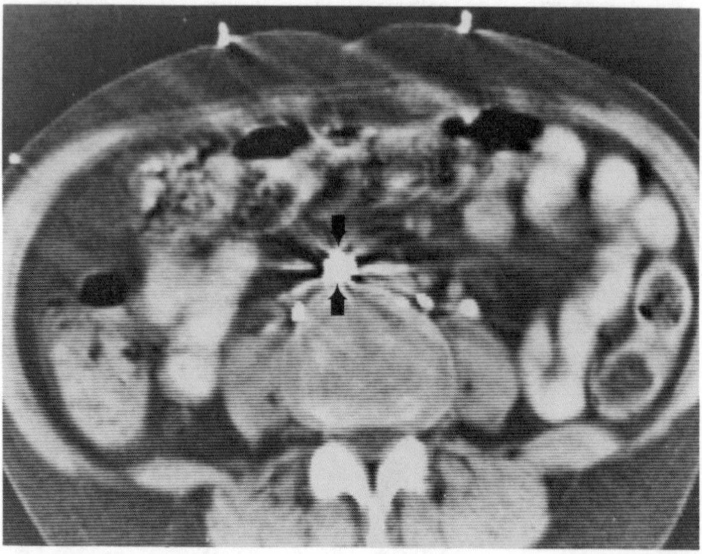

Fig. 33.17. Metastases within normal-size nodes. Corresponding to the lymphangiogram shown in figure 33.13, this CT scan shows an opacified retroperitoneal node (*arrows*) of normal size. This illustrates the greatest disadvantage of CT—its inability to detect metastases within normal-size metastatic nodes.

The obturator, hypogastric, external, and common iliac lymph nodes are the most frequent sites of metastases and are considered abnormal when they are 1.5 cm or greater in diameter. Because of the incidence of secondary infection with carcinoma of the cervix, the presence of metastases producing isolated enlargement of the lymph nodes must be established histologically by biopsy (percutaneous or surgical) or by lymphangiography. Metastases to nodes of normal size and microscopic spread will therefore escape detection (Whitley et al. 1982; Kilcheski et al. 1981; Walsh and Goplerud 1981; Ginaldi et al. 1981; Walsh et al. 1981) (fig. 33.17). There have been several reports concerning the CT diagnosis of lymph node metastases from carcinoma of the cervix. Whitley et al. (1982) used CT to diagnose metastases in 17 patients and reported a sensitivity of 80%, specificity of 83%, and overall accuracy of 83%. The false-positive results (11.7%) were caused by lymphoid hyperplasia, while the false-negative results (5.8%) were caused by microscopic metastases in nodes less than 1.5 cm in diameter. In a series of 75 patients studied by Walsh and Goplerud (1981), the overall accuracy was 74%.

CT has also been used for mapping radiotherapy portals. The detection of pelvic side wall and retroperitoneal disease allows the radiotherapist to adapt the therapy portals to the tumor bulk and to alter the portals according to changes in tumor size. The postradiation changes are well documented by CT.

Magnetic Resonance Imaging

On MRI images, carcinoma of the cervix may be viewed as a mass with increased intensity. Extension into the parametrial tissues may also be demonstrated as areas of high intensity. With further improvement in techniques and resolution, MRI may play a role in distinguishing stage IIA from stage IIB lesions, which is of obvious clinical importance. Radiotherapy is indicated for stage IIB lesions, whereas surgery is recommended for stage IIA lesions. A further advantage of MRI may be its ability to scan the sagittal plane to determine uterine and vaginal extension. It has also been suggested that the differentiation between uterine invasion and an obstructed uterus with hematometria is far better visualized on MRI than with CT (Bryan et al. 1983; Hricak et al. 1983; Butler et al. 1984).

In the future, MRI may be more useful than CT in revealing the presence of both pelvic and retroperitoneal nodes. The presence of nodes would be demonstrated by soft tissue of medium intensity adjacent to the blood vessels of low intensity (because of rapid blood flow). It should be noted, however, that the differentiation between benign and malignant nodes currently cannot be determined by MRI examination.

Interventional Radiology

The rationale for arterial infusion is to expose the neoplasm to a high local concentration (compared with intravenous administration) of a chemotherapeutic agent without increasing toxicity. Utilizing bilateral, internal iliac artery infusion of bleomycin alone or in combination with mitomycin C and vincristine for the treatment of recurrent cervical carcinoma, Morrow et al. (1977) observed 2 of 16 objective remissions and Swenerton et al. (1979) reported 3 of 20. Ohta (1978), Oku, Iwaski, and Tojo (1979), and other Japanese investigators suggested the application of arterial infusion prior to definitive radiotherapy.

At U.T. M. D. Anderson Hospital, nine patients with squamous cell carcinoma of the uterine cervix were treated by bilateral internal iliac artery infusion of cisplatin. Of these, six had had unresectable pelvic recurrence following radiation therapy and three had had large, previously untreated primary tumors. Three patients (33%) experienced a partial response. Recently, cisplatin was combined with bleomycin intraarterially while vincristine and mitomycin C were delivered intravenously in seven patients. All showed a partial response (50% or more reduction in size of the pelvic mass); two have possibly been cured with the addition of local radiation therapy.

The control of hemorrhage in patients with carcinoma of the cervix may be lifesaving and may allow more specific therapy by surgery, irradiation, or chemotherapy. It is our preference to use Ivalon particles (250–500 μm) and Gelfoam cubes (3 mm) for peripheral embolization and Gelfoam segments and stainless steel coils for central vascular occlusion. Embolization of the anterior branches of both internal iliac arteries has been helpful in controlling vaginal hemorrhage from carcinoma of the cervix. Bleeding from the cervix, bladder, and rectum after radiation therapy has been successfully treated in approximately 50% of patients by embolization of the internal iliac or inferior mesenteric arteries.

In a case of gynecologic malignancy, the most common reason for performing a nephrostomy is ureteral obstruction secondary to pelvic or retroperitoneal disease. Urinary tract diversion by percutaneous nephrostomy has been used for postoperative and postradiotherapy fistulas. Prior to arterial chemotherapy with cisplatin, a renal toxic agent, nephrostomy to relieve urethral obstructions becomes a necessity. This is performed under fluoroscopic or ultrasonic guidance. After a percutaneous nephrostomy has been performed, it may be percutaneously converted to an internal ureteral stent (Pfister, Yoder, and Newhouse 1981).

Fine-needle aspiration biopsy under CT guidance has been found to be accurate in the pretreatment staging of carcinoma of the cervix (Edeiken-Monroe and Zornoza 1982). By demonstrating dissemination of tumor to the pelvic and paraaortic lymph nodes, it reduces the need for exploratory laparotomy or lymphadenectomy. Percutaneous, retroperitoneal lymph node biopsies revealed that 129 patients had carcinoma of the cervix. In those patients, lymphangiogram results had been positive or showed possible metastatic disease. Of the 159 biopsies performed, 114 were done on external iliac lymph nodes and 45 were done on paraaortic lymph nodes. An overall accuracy of 68% was obtained without significant complications. The sensitivity of the test was 58%, and specificity was 100%. Percutaneous biopsy did not reveal metastases in 32% of patients with questionable disease. The predictive value of a negative test was 42%, whereas the predictive value of a positive test was 100%. This reiterates the view that only a biopsy with positive results is significant.

Combining Techniques for Diagnosis

Clinical examination is of utmost importance in the diagnosis of cervical carcinoma. The imaging modalities are important in staging the patient's disease. With the exception of a chest radiograph, diagnostic techniques such as barium studies, bone radiographs, and excretory urography are believed to be no longer necessary unless specific clinical indications are present.

In cases of cervical carcinoma, the initial imaging modality should be a CT scan of the abdomen and pelvis to assess pelvic disease, including possible extension to the side wall or extrapelvic disease. In patients with cervical carcinoma, the lymphangiogram and CT are effective combined modalities. If abnormal adenopathy is not shown by CT, then a lymphangiogram should be performed to determine whether metastatic nodal disease is present within normal-size nodes. When an abnormality is detected by CT or lymphangiography, it should be confirmed with a fine-needle aspiration biopsy performed with CT guidance or fluoroscopy (fig. 33.18).

The role of MRI is still to be determined. It is hoped that in the future MRI will aid in determining metastatic invasion into the parametrium or the uterus and also in determining whether nodes are malignant or benign. Interventional techniques such as intraarterial infusion, percutaneous nephrostomies, and ureteral stenting will continue to play major roles in disease management. In addition, percutaneous drainage of postoperative fluid collections such as abscesses, urinomas, and lymphoceles can be performed.

In an era of cost-effective medicine, the work-up of patients should be quick, thorough, and as practical as possible to arrive at the correct diagnosis. However, the diagnostic sequence utilized should be individualized depending on the clinical presentation and circumstances of each patient and should be designed to avoid superfluous studies that may result in unnecessary radiation exposure, morbidity, and

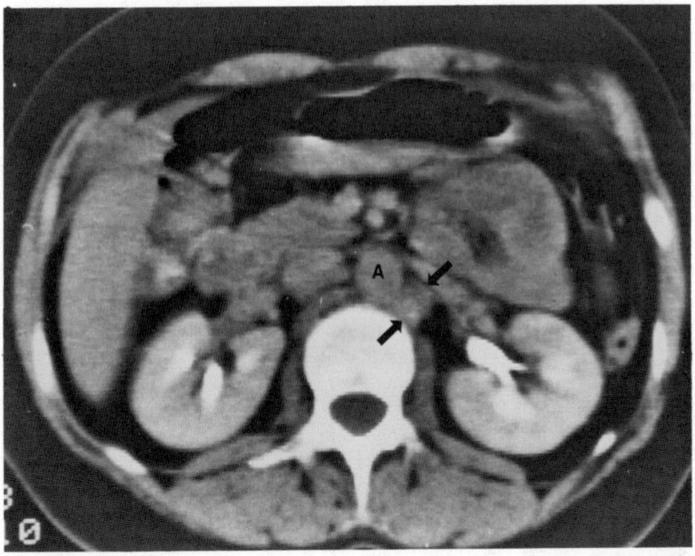

Fig. 33.18 Metastatic retroperitoneal adenopathy. The CT scan of the midabdomen demonstrates a lymph node (*arrows*) just to the left of the aorta (*A*). This adenopathy corresponds to that in the lymphangiogram (fig. 33.14) showing obstructed lymphatic vessels. Spread to this lymph node was due to metastatic cervical carcinoma that was confirmed by percutaneous biopsy.

mortality, as well as financial burden and inconvenience. The availability of the equipment and personnel, as well as expertise for performing and interpreting the various procedures, must be considered.

References

Amendola MA, Walsh JW, Amendola BE, Tisnado J, Hall DJ, Goplerud DR. 1981. Computed tomography in the evaluation of carcinoma of the ovary. *J Comput Assist Tomogr* 5:179–186.

American Cancer Society. 1980. *1980 Cancer Facts and Figures*. New York: ACS.

Athey PA. 1981. Sonographic appearance of the female pelvis. In *Ultrasound in Obstetrics and Gynecology*, ed. PA Athey, FP Hadlock, pp. 104–123. St. Louis: CV Mosby.

Athey PA, Wallace S, Jing B-S, Gallager HS, Smith SP. 1975. Lymphangiography in ovarian cancer. *AJR* 123:106–113.

Barber HRK, Grober EA. 1971. The PMPO syndrome (postmenopausal palpable ovary syndrome). *Obstet Gynecol* 38:921–923.

Berland LM, Lawson TL, Albarelli JN. 1980. Ultrasonic diagnosis of ovarian and adnexal disease. *Seminars in Ultrasound* 1:17–29.

Bickers GH, Seibert JJ, Anderson JC, Golladay S, Berry DL. 1981. Sonography of ovarian involvement in childhood acute lymphocytic leukemia. *AJR* 137:399–401.

Blaustein A. 1982. Metastatic carcinoma in the ovary. In *Pathology of the Female Genital Tract*, ed. A Blaustein, pp. 705–715. New York: Springer-Verlag.

Bloomer WD. 1983. Lymphoscintigraphy in gynecologic malignancies. *Semin Nucl Med* 13:54–59.

Bowie JD. 1977. Ultrasound of gynecologic pelvic masses: The indefinite uterus and other patterns associated with diagnostic error. *Journal of Clinical Ultrasound* 5:323–328.

Brenner DE, Shaff MI, Jones HW, Grosh WW, Greco FA, Burnett LS. 1985. Abdomino-pelvic computed tomography: Evaluation in patients undergoing second-look laparotomy for ovarian carcinoma. *Obstet Gynecol* 65:715–719.

Brenner DE, Whitley NO, Prempee T, Villa Santa U. 1982. An evaluation of the computed tomographic scanner for the staging of carcinoma of the cervix. *Cancer* 50:2323–2328.

Brown RC, Buchsbaum HJ, Tewfik HH, Platz CE. 1979. Accuracy of lymphangiography in the diagnosis of paraaortic lymph node metastases from carcinoma of the cervix. *Obstet Gynecol* 54:571–575.

Bryan P, Butler HE, LiPuma JP, Haaga JR, El Yousef S, Resnick MI, Cohen AM, Maluija VK, Nelson AD, Clampitt M, Alfidi RJ, Cohen J, Morrison CS. 1983. NMR scanning of the pelvis: Initial experience with a 0.3 T system. *AJR* 141:1111–1118.

Butler H, Bryan PJ, LiPuma JP, Cohen AM, El Yousef S, Andriole JG, Lieberman J. 1984. Magnetic resonance imaging of the abdominal female pelvis. *AJR* 143:1259–1266.

Cunningham JJ, Fuks ZY, Castellino RA. 1974. Radiographic manifestations of carcinoma of the cervix and complications of its treatment. *Radiol Clin North Am* 12:93–108.

Cutler SJ, Myers MH, Green SB. 1975. Trends in survival rates of patients with cancer. *N Engl J Med* 293:122–124.

Czernobilsky B. 1982. Primary epithelial tumors of the ovary. In *Pathology of the Female Genital Tract*, ed. A Blaustein, pp. 511–560. New York: Springer-Verlag.

DeLand FH, Goldenberg DM. 1985. Diagnosis and treatment of neoplasms with radio-nuclide-labeled antibodies. *Semin Nucl Med* 15:2–11.

de Muylder X, Bélanger R, Vauclair R, Audet-Lapointe P, Cormier A, Methot Y. 1984. Value of lymphography in stage IB cancer of the uterine cervix. *Am J Obstet Gynecol* 148: 610–613.

Dixon AK, Fry IK, Kingham JGC, McLean AM, White FE. 1981. Computed tomography in patients with an abdominal mass: Effective and efficient? A controlled trial. *Lancet* 1: 1199–1201.

Doiron MJ, Bernardino ME. 1981. A comparison of noninvasive imaging modalities in the melanoma patient. *Cancer* 47:2581–2584.

Dunnick NR, Jones RB, Doppman JL, Speyer J, Myers CE. 1979. Intraperitoneal contrast infusion for assessment of intraperitoneal fluid dynamics. *AJR* 133:221–223.

Edeiken-Monroe BS, Zornoza J. 1982. Carcinoma of the cervix: Percutaneous lymph node aspiration biopsy. *AJR* 138:655–657.

Epenetos AA, Shepherd J, Britton KE, Hawkins L, Nimmon CC, Taylor-Papadimitriou J, Durbin H, Malpas JS, Mather S, Granowska M, Duke D, Bodmer WF. 1984. Radioimmu-nodiagnosis of ovarian cancer using ^{123}I-labelled, tumor-associated monoclonal antibodies. *Cancer Detect Prev* 7:45–49.

Fernstrom I. 1955. Arteriography of the uterine artery. *Acta Radiol [Suppl] Stockh* No. 122.

Ferruci JT Jr, Wittenberg J, Mueller PR, Simeone JF, Harbin WP, Kirkpatrick RH, Taft PD. 1980. Diagnosis of abdominal malignancy by radiologic fine-needle aspiration biopsy. *AJR* 134:323–330.

Fineberg HV, Wittenberg J, Ferruci JT Jr, Mueller PR, Simeone JF, Goldman J. 1983. Clinical value of body computed tomography over time and technologic change. *AJR* 141:1067–1072.

Fleischer AC, James AE Jr, Millis JB, Julian C. 1978. Differential diagnosis of pelvic masses by gray scale sonography. *AJR* 131:469–476.

Fuks Z. 1975. External radiotherapy of ovarian cancer: Standard approaches and new frontiers. *Semin Oncol* 2:253–256.

Gedgaudas RK, Kelvin FM, Thompson WM, Rice RP. 1983. The value of the preoperative barium-enema examination in the assessment of pelvic masses. *Radiology* 146:609–613.

Ginaldi S, Lindell MM Jr, Zornoza J. 1980. The striped colon: A new radiographic observation in metastatic serosal implants. *AJR* 134:453–455.

Ginaldi S, Wallace S, Jing B-S, Bernardino ME. 1981. Carcinoma of the cervix: Lymphangiography and computed tomography. *AJR* 136:1087–1091.

Green B, Libshitz HI. 1979. Bladder and ureter. In *Diagnostic Roentgenology of Radiotherapy Change*, ed. HI Libshitz, pp. 123–136. Baltimore: Williams & Wilkins.

Griffin WG, Parker RG, Taylor WJ. 1976. An evaluation of procedures used in staging carcinoma of the cervix. *Am J Roentgenol* 127:825–827.

Gross BH, Moss AA, Mihara K, Goldberg HI, Glazer GM. 1983. Computed tomography of gynecologic diseases. *AJR* 141:765–773.

Haaga JR. 1979. New techniques for CT-guided biopsies. *AJR* 133:633.

Harbert JC. 1984. Efficacy of liver scanning in malignant disease. *Semin Nucl Med* 14: 287–295.

Hillman BJ, Clark RL, Babbitt G. 1984. Efficacy of the excretory urogram in the staging of gynecologic malignancies. *AJR* 143:997–999.

Hricak H, Alpers C, Crooks LE, Sheldon PE. 1983. Magnetic resonance imaging of the female pelvis: Initial experience. *AJR* 141:1119–1128.

Isler RJ, Ferruci JT Jr, Wittenberg J, Mueller PR, Simeone JF, Van Sonnenberg E, Hall DA. 1981. Tissue care biopsy of abdominal tumors with a 22-gauge cutting needle. *AJR* 136:725–728.

Johnson IR, Symonds EM, Worthington DM, Johnson J, Gyngell M, Hawkes RC. 1984. Imaging ovarian tumours by nuclear magnetic resonance. *Br J Obstet Gynaecol* 91:260–264.

Johnson RJ, Blackledge G, Eddleston B, Crowther D. 1983. Abdomino-pelvic computed tomography in the management of ovarian carcinoma. *Radiology* 146:447–452.

Kerr-Wilson RHJ, Shingleton HM, Orr JW Jr, Hatch KD. 1984. The use of ultrasound and computed tomography scanning in the management of gynecologic cancer patients. *Gynecol Oncol* 18:54–61.

Khilnani MT, Marshak RH, Eliasoph J, Wolf BS. 1966. Roentgen features of metastases to the colon. *AJR* 96:302–310.

Kilcheski TS, Arger PH, Mulhern CB, Coleman BG, Kressel HY, Mikuta JI. 1981. Role of computed tomography in the presurgical evaluation of carcinoma of the cervix. *J Comput Assist Tomogr* 5:378–383.

Kurtz AB, Rubin CS, Kramer FL, Goldberg BB. 1979. Ultrasound evaluation of the posterior compartment. *Radiology* 132:677–682.

Lawson TL, Albarelli JN. 1977. Diagnosis of gynecologic pelvic masses by gray scale ultrasonology: Analysis of specificity and accuracy. *AJR* 128:1003–1006

Lee JKT, Stanley RJ, Sagel SS, McClennan BL. 1978. Accuracy of CT in detecting intraabdominal and pelvic lymph node metastases from pelvic cancers. *AJR* 131:675–679.

Legasse LD, Creasman WT, Shingleton HM, Ford JH, Blessing JA. 1980. Results and complications of operative staging in cervical cancer: Experience of the gynecologic oncology group. *Gynecol Oncol* 9:90–98.

Levitt GR, Koehler RE, Sagel SS, Lee JKT. 1982. Metastatic disease of the mesentery and omentum. *Radiol Clin North Am* 20:501–510.

Martin EC, Karlson KD, Frankuchen EJ, Cooperman A, Casarella WJ. 1982. Percutaneous drainage of postoperative intraabdominal abscess. *AJR* 138:13–15.

McArdle CR, Sacks BA. 1980. Ovarian hyperstimulation syndrome. *AJR* 135:835–836.

Metler FA Jr, Christie JH, Crow NE Jr, Garcia JF, Wicks JD, Bartow SA. 1982. Radionuclide bone scan, radiographic bone survey, and alkaline phosphatase. *Cancer* 50:1483–1485.

Meyers MA, McSweeney J. 1972. Secondary neoplasms of the bowel. *Radiology* 105:1–11.

Meyers MA. 1973. Distribution of intra-abdominal malignant seeding: Dependency on dynamics of flow of ascitic fluid. *AJR* 119:198–206.

Meyers MA. 1975. Metastatic seeding along the small bowel mesentery. *AJR* 123:67–73.

Morrow CP, DiSaia PJ, Mangan CF, Lagasse LD. 1977. Continuous pelvic arterial infusion with bleomycin for squamous carcinoma of the cervix recurrent after irradiation therapy. *Cancer Treat Rep* 61:1403–1405.

Moyle JW, Rochester D, Sider L, Shrock K, Krause P. 1983. Sonography of ovarian tumors: Predictability of tumor type. *AJR* 141:985–991.

Novak ER, Woodruff JD. 1979. *Novak's Gynecologic and Obstetrical Pathology*. Philadelphia: W.B. Saunders.

Ohta A. 1978. Basic and clinical studies on the simultaneous combination treatment of cervical cancer with a carcinostatic agent and radiation. *Journal of Tokyo Medical College* 36:529.

Oku T, Iwasaki M, Tojo S. 1979. Study on surgical chemotherapy for advanced carcinoma of the uterine cervix—particularly on the problem of clinical effect and drug concentration. *Acta Obstet Gynecol Jpn* 31:1833.

Paling MR, Shawker TH. 1981. Abdominal ultrasound in advanced ovarian carcinoma. *Journal of Clinical Ultrasound* 9:435–441.

Pfister RC, Yoder IC, Newhouse JH. 1981. Percutaneous uroradiologic procedures. *Semin Roentgenol* 16:135–151.

Piver MS, Barlow JJ, Lele SB. 1978. Incidence of subclinical metastases in stage I and II ovarian carcinoma. *Obstet Gynecol* 52:100–104.

Piver S, Wallace S, Castro J. 1971. The accuracy of lymphangiography in carcinoma of the uterine cervix. *AJR* 111:278–283.

Prando A, Wallace S, Bernardino ME, Lindell MM. 1979. Computed tomographic arteriography of the liver. *Radiology* 130:697–701.

Rankin RN, Hutton LC. 1981. Ultrasound in the ovarian hyperstimulation system. *Journal of Clinical Ultrasound* 9:473–476.

Requard CK, Mettler FA Jr, Wicks JD. 1981. Preoperative sonography of malignant ovarian neoplasms. *AJR* 137:79–82.

Requard CK, Wicks JD, Metler FA. 1981. Ultrasonography in the staging of endometrial adenocarcinoma. *Radiology* 140:781–785.

Rochester D, Levin B, Bowie JD, Kunzman A. 1977. Ultrasonic appearance of the Krukenberg tumor. *AJR* 129:919–920.

Rubesin SE, Levine MS. 1985. Omental cakes: Colonic involvement by omental metastases. *Radiology* 154:593–596.

Sample WF. 1980. Gray-scale ultrasonography of the normal female pelvis. In *The Principles and Practice of Ultrasonography in Obstetrics and Gynecology* (ed 2), ed. RE Sanders, AE James, pp. 75–89. New York: Appleton-Century-Crofts.

Sample WF, Lippe BM, Gyepes MT. 1977. Gray-scale ultrasonography of the normal female pelvis. *Radiology* 125:477–483.

Sanders RC, James AE, eds. 1980. *The Principles and Practice of Ultrasonography in Obstetrics and Gynecology* (ed 2). New York: Appleton-Century-Crofts.

Sanders RC, McNeil BJ, Finberg HJ, Hessel SJ, Siegelman SS, Adams DF, Alderson PO, Abrams HL. 1983. A prospective study of computed tomography and ultrasound in the detection and staging of pelvic masses. *Radiology* 146:439–442.

Sonnendecker EWW, De Souza JJL. 1984. Screening of liver metastases from ovarian cancer with serum carcinomaembryonic antigen and radionuclide hepatic scintiphotography. *Br J Obstet Gynaecol* 91:187–192.

Stevens GM. 1971. *The Female Reproductive System: An Atlas of Tumor Radiology*. Chicago: Year Book Medical.

Strockbine MF, Hancock JE, Fletcher GH. 1970. Complications in 831 patients with squamous cell carcinoma of the intact uterine cervix treated with 3,000 rads or more whole pelvis irradiation. *AJR* 108:293–304.

Swenerton KD, Evers JA, White GW, Boyes DA. 1979. Intermittent pelvic infusion with vincristine, bleomycin, and mitomycin C for advanced recurrent carcinoma of the cervix. *Cancer Treat Rep* 63:1379–1381.

van Sonnenberg E, Ferruci JT Jr, Mueller PR, Wittenberg J, Simeone JF. 1982. Percutaneous drainage of abscesses and fluid collections: Techniques, results, and applications. *Radiology* 142:1–10.

Wallace S, Chuang VP. 1982. The radiologic diagnosis and management of hepatic metastases. *Der Radiologe* 22:56–64.

Wallace S, Jing B-S. 1977. Carcinoma lymphangiography in carcinoma. In *Clinical Lymphography (sect 7)*, ed. ME Clouse, pp. 185–273. Baltimore: Williams & Wilkins.

Wallace S, Jing B-S, Zornoza J, Hammond JA, Hamberger A, Herson J, Freedman R, Wharton T. 1979. Is lymphangiography worthwhile? Current concepts in cancer: Updated cervix cancer II. Stages IB and II. *Int J Radiat Oncol Biol Phys* 5:1873–1876.

Walsh JW, Amendola MA, Hall DJ, Tisnado J, Goplerud DR. 1981. Recurrent carcinoma of the cervix: CT diagnosis. *AJR* 136:117–122.

Walsh JW, Amendola MA, Konerding KF, Tisnado J, Hazra TA. 1980. Computed tomographic detection of pelvic and inguinal lymph-node metastases from primary and recurrent pelvic malignant disease. *Radiology* 137:157–166.

Walsh JW, Goplerud DR. 1981. Prospective comparison between clinical and CT staging in primary cervical carcinoma. *AJR* 137:997–1003.

Walsh JW, Taylor KJ, Wasson JF, Schwartz PE, Rosenfield AT. 1979. Gray-scale ultrasound in 204 proved gynecologic masses: Accuracy and specific diagnostic criteria. *Radiology* 130:391–397.

Whitley N, Brenner D, Francis A, Kwon T, Villa Santa U, Aisner J, Wiernik P, Whitley J. 1981. Use of the computed tomographic whole body scanner to stage and follow patients with advanced ovarian carcinoma. *Invest Radiol* 16:479–486.

Whitley NO, Brenner DE, Francis A, Villa Santa U, Aisner J, Wiernik PH, Whitley J. 1982. Computed tomographic evaluation of carcinoma of the cervix. *Radiology* 142:439–446.

Yeh H. 1979. Ultrasonography of peritoneal tumors. *Radiology* 133:419–424.

Yoonessi M, Abdel-Dayem HM, Shalaby OFO. 1982. The use of scintigraphic and contrast peritoneography in gynecologic malignancies. *Diagn Gynecol Obstet* 4:75–78.

Yuhasz M, Laufer I, Sutton G, Herlinger H, Caroline DF. 1985. Radiology of the small bowel in patients with gynecologic malignancies. *AJR* 144:303–307.

Annual Clinical Conference on Cancer, Vol. 29
Gynecologic Cancer: Diagnosis and Treatment Strategies
© 1987 by The University of Texas System Cancer Center

34. Nuclear Medicine in Gynecologic Oncology: Recent Practice

Lamk M. Lamki

Nuclear medicine tests tell more about the physiological function of an organ than about its anatomy. This is in contrast to several other modalities in current use in the field of diagnostic imaging. Some of these newer modalities, such as computerized tomography (CT), offer a better resolution of the anatomy of the organ being examined. This has caused physicians to drift away from certain nuclear medicine tests, specifically those that focus primarily on the anatomy. When CT scanning is available, for instance, it is no longer advisable to perform a scintigraphic brain scan in search of metastasis; CT scanning is more accurate overall and more likely than a nuclear study to result in a specific diagnosis. In certain cases of diffuse cortical infections like herpes encephalitis, however, a scintiscan is still superior to a CT scan.

The tendency has been to replace the nuclear liver scan with CT or ultrasonography. Routine screening of the liver for metastasis with the isotope liver scan is not justified in gynecologic cancer (Harbert 1984). But it is appropriate for follow-up of a patient who has a known lesion, and it is certainly cost-effective (Silberstein, Gilbert, and Pu 1985). The advantage of CT, magnetic resonance imaging (MRI), and ultrasonography over nuclear medicine is that other organs are examined simultaneously; retroperitoneal masses, for example, may be detected during examination of the liver.

Today's practice of nuclear medicine in gynecologic oncology may be divided into the three categories—(1) time-tested function-oriented scintiscans, (2) innovations of established nuclear tests, and (3) newer pathophysiological scintistudies. I shall discuss here, briefly, each of these categories, giving three examples of each.

Time-Tested Function-Oriented Scintiscans

Among the three best examples of scintiscans that have withstood the test of time are the bone scan, nuclear venogram, and ventilation perfusion lung scan. These tests have not been easy to replace for several reasons, including the ease of the procedures, their noninvasiveness, the relatively low radiation exposure, and the low cost.

Bone Scan

The bone scan is performed using methyl diphosphonate (MDP) labeled with technetium 99m. Two hours after intravenous injection of 20 mCi of ^{99m}Tc MDP, when maximum uptake has taken place in the bones and background activity has been cleared by the kidneys, total body images are taken from anterior and posterior views. Occasionally, blood flow or blood pool images are taken immediately after the injection to rule out other pathological conditions, but these extra images are rarely necessary under normal circumstances for diagnosing metastatic lesions from gynecologic cancer. The focal areas of increased activity in the bone scan reflect the increased metabolic state of the osteoblasts stimulated by the metastatic lesions. This may occur long before blastic or lytic lesions are obvious in the radiograph. The radiographic evidence of bone metastasis may remain long after the metastatic lesion has healed. Thus the bone scan not only can detect metastasis earlier, but it can also reflect healing and response to therapy more accurately than a radiograph. The other advantage of the bone scan is that all the bones in the body can be examined simultaneously without exposing the patient to additional radiation. The specific utility of the bone scan in gynecologic oncology was reviewed by McNeil (1984). Its diagnostic yield in early stages (I and II) of endometrial carcinoma, cervical cancer, and ovarian cancer is poor, but it is substantial in stages III and IV. In follow-up examinations for recurrence of disease, abnormalities can be seen in 8% to 15% of bone scans of patients with ovarian and endometrial carcinoma, and additional renal abnormalities may be detected in the bone scans of patients who have cervical cancer.

Radionuclide Venogram

The bilateral nuclear venogram of the lower limbs is of special interest to the gynecologic oncologist. It tests the patency of lower inferior vena cava (IVC) and bilateral common iliac and external iliac veins as well as the deep venous system of the thighs down to the popliteal vessels. Simple and noninvasive, the test consists of the intravenous injection of macroaggregates of albumin (MAA) labeled with ^{99m}Tc into the veins of the feet—a total of 3 mCi (1.5 mCi for each foot) in three divided doses—one for the pelvis, followed by injection for the thigh veins, and last for the calves, while the tourniquets are applied just tightly enough to stop flow into the superficial veins and thus force the ^{99m}Tc MAA into the deep venous system. This method is more sensitive than contrast radiographic venography for the thigh and pelvic deep veins but not the calf veins, which is why contrast studies for the calf veins are recommended. In young women, a nuclear venogram of the pelvic veins has the added advantage of examining the iliac veins with minimal radiation exposure of the gonads. In addition, collateral vessels may be recorded in the abdominal wall and liver without additional radiation exposure. A few minutes after the tourniquets are released, there should be no residual radioactivity in the lower limbs or pelvic veins. The presence of residual activity may suggest acute thrombosis because ^{99m}Tc MAA adheres electrostatically to a thrombus.

Other agents that may be used to study the deep venous patency include red blood cells tagged with ^{99m}Tc. Although it is rarely needed in gynecologic practice, a bilateral upper limb venous flow study is an excellent indicator of patency of the axillary vein, subclavian vein, and superior vena cava (SVC). This may be needed in mediastinal metastasis or in parenteral feeding (central venous line). At The University of Texas M. D. Anderson Hospital and Tumor Institute at Houston, we prefer to use ^{99m}Tc diethylene triamine pentacetic acid (DTPA) instead of the labeled MAA for upper limb venograms because with the latter compound, lung activity obscures the field of view. Partial or complete obstruction of the central veins or SVC can be diagnosed accurately by this test, and it is a good follow-up method of checking treatment of SVC or subclavian vein thrombosis noninvasively and with minimum radiation exposure. All these venous flow studies can be performed by taking a mobile gamma camera to the patient's bedside.

Ventilation-Perfusion Lung Scan

Ventilation-perfusion lung scan is still the best overall test for diagnosing pulmonary embolism. After the venogram described above (using 3 mCi of ^{99m}Tc MAA), six views of the chest will provide a complete perfusion lung scan. Wedge-shaped areas of absent radioactivity, especially if pleura-based, indicate perfusion defects. When such areas are large enough to represent two bronchopulmonary segments and the ventilation study shows normal ventilation of the same areas, the probability of pulmonary embolus (PE) is high. Moreover, if the chest X ray taken on the same day shows no local abnormality to explain the perfusion defects, the probability of PE is higher than 85% (Neumann 1980). When the perfusion defect is only subsegmental, or not in the pleura, or when the perfusion defect is only diminished rather than absent, the probability of PE is low, which means it is lower than 27%. This is also the case when the perfusion defect is large but there is a matching ventilation defect or when an abnormality seen on a radiograph explains the perfusion defect.

A finding of only one bronchopulmonary perfusion defect suggests a moderate probability of PE even if results of the ventilation study and chest X ray are normal. Such a probability indicates that the patient should have a pulmonary angiogram unless the physician can clearly explain why it is not needed. Indeterminate probability means that technical or other findings make it impossible to establish a probability rating for PE (e.g., presence of significant chronic obstructive lung disease). Normal findings on a perfusion lung scan effectively rule out PE (Biello, Matter, and McKnight 1979).

For the ventilation study, commonly performed using ^{133}Xe gas, a recording is made of the patient's first breath of the gas and again after two minutes of xenon inhalation to show the lung volume at equilibrium; then "washout" images are recorded every two minutes to check for gas trapping that may occur as in obstructive lung disease. A combination of chest X ray, perfusion lung scan, and ventilation study are needed to determine the probability of PE. A ventilation study may also be performed with the use of krypton 81m, which has a short half-life and so allows the administration of more gas to obtain additional views without significant increase in the patient's radiation exposure. A mobile ventilation study may be done even for patients on artificial ventilators in intensive care by using ^{99m}Tc-labeled aerosols, for example, ^{99m}Tc DTPA or ^{99m}Tc sulfur colloid rather than xenon gas. Aerosol studies cannot, however, be performed for some patients—those who have high amounts of secretion in the bronchial tree, for example, or those patients whose clinical conditions (such as excessive coughing) prevent the aerosols from reaching the lung periphery.

Once a diagnosis of PE is established, only a perfusion lung scan is needed for follow-up during treatment with heparin or streptokinase. The scan may be repeated in three days if needed, and certainly at least one follow-up scan is recommended before the patient is discharged from the hospital. A return of the scan's results to normal will be an important reference point if a comparison is needed in the future.

Innovative Uses of Established Nuclear Tests

The three tests that have been improved and are used most frequently in gynecologic oncology are gated cardiac blood pool studies, renal perfusion and diuretic renographic tests, and the gallium 67 lung scan.

Gated Cardiac Blood Pool Studies

Gated cardiac blood pool scintigraphy is recognized as a reliable test in the management of ischemic heart disease. It is also an important tool in the follow-up examinations of cancer patients who are receiving such cardiotoxic chemotherapeutic agents as doxorubicin HCl (Adriamycin) and related bisanthrene drugs. Gated cardiac scintigraphy is performed by labeling the patient's own red cells with ^{99m}Tc and reinjecting them intravenously. A gamma camera with an on-line computer can acquire rapid-sequence images, for example, 20 images for each cardiac cycle starting with each R wave as the gated trigger. After this is done continuously for about five minutes, all the data are combined and reduced to 20 images of a "representative" cardiac cycle. When these images are looped to give a cinematic representation of the cardiac cycle, we can study the wall motion of the ventricles during systole and diastole. Doxorubicin toxicity is manifested by generalized reduction in contraction (global hypokinesia) of the left ventricle during the wall motion study, but it may start as apical hypokinesia. A pure focal hypokinesia, typical of ischemic heart disease, is seen after blocking of one or part of one coronary artery and is not found in doxorubicin toxicity.

The data in the 20 frames may be used also to calculate the ejection fraction of the left ventricle. The counts in the first or second frame immediately after the R wave represent the radioactivity (volume) in end-diastole, and one of the midcycle frames, typically the seventh or eighth, represents the end-systolic volume. These may be selected automatically by the computer or manually by the operator. An appropriate background area is chosen just lateral to the left ventricle blood pool for background counts, and the ejection fraction is calculated as follows:

$$EF = \frac{(ED - BK) - (ES - BK)}{ED - BK},$$

where *EF* is the ejection fraction, *ED* is end-diastolic volume, *BK* is the background activity, and *ES* is the end-systolic volume. A normal ejection fraction varies with different laboratory standards, but it is somewhere between 50% and 60%. A heart that cannot eject 50% of its end-diastolic volume will usually be shown to have at least some degree of hypokinesia in the wall motion part of the study. Both ejection fraction and wall motion studies should be repeated at regular intervals for patients receiving more than 300 mg in cumulative doses of doxorubicin HCl. Ideally, these studies are done just before the patient's next dose.

The above study may be performed while the patient is exercising, for example, using a bicycle ergometer. Data collection takes place first at rest and then is repeated during each level of exercise and again at exercise completion. Such ejection fraction measurements are a test of cardiac reserve. If, for example, the baseline ejection fraction is borderline low, a substantial rise of ejection fraction with exercise indicates good reserve. Before doxorubicin therapy is begun, it may be used also to detect preexisting coronary ischemia in which the ejection fraction drops with exercise, unlike the normal response of a rise in ejection fraction.

Renal Perfusion and Diuretic Renography

A gynecologic oncologist often becomes very concerned when, after an operative procedure, the patient develops anuria or oliguria or even nonoliguric uremia. In most cases, a renal perfusion study and, if necessary, a diuretic study will be diagnostic. Renal perfusion may be done even at bedside using a mobile camera with an on-board computer. The patient is injected intravenously with 10 mCi of ^{99m}Tc DTPA. A good bolus is essential in showing the perfusion of the two kidneys clearly. With the patient supine, the study is performed from the posterior view unless the intensive care beds are not radiolucent. A two-minute rapid sequence recording will identify the kidneys clearly if they are perfused normally, but usually the study is continued for several minutes (up to 30 minutes) to show function and rule out obstruction. Surgical damage to the renal arteries or the ureter may thus be ruled out within a few minutes by a noninvasive technique at the patient's bedside, with minimum radiation exposure and maximum cost-effectiveness.

Reasonably good perfusion or only a moderate reduction in perfusion but extremely poor function is a classic sign of vasomotor nephropathy or acute tubular necrosis (ATN). Occasionally, however, a drug-induced interstitial nephritis may look very much like vasomotor nephropathy or ATN, although ^{67}Ga can differentiate between the two because it is not taken up in ATN but is taken up intensely in the case of drug-induced interstitial nephritis (Linton et al. 1985). On the other hand, perfusion that is reasonably good and a collecting system that is active but not reaching the bladder suggests an obstruction. Therefore, at 20 minutes into the test, the patient is injected intravenously with furosemide (0.5 mg/kg body weight), and the study is continued for another 20 minutes. The test results will then differentiate a dilated baggy collecting system from an actively obstructed collecting system. An unobstructed dilated system will reduce the radioactivity level by 50% in 20 minutes. This study may also show whether extravasation is present in cases of ureteral damage.

Technetium 99m DTPA renography, with or without a diuretic, has an advantage over other methods because the radiopharmaceutical used in this type of renography is not toxic to the patient, unlike the contrast media used in contrast urography to study renal failure. Furthermore, nuclear renography can be done at the patient's bedside, and it can detect small amounts of extravasation that may be missed by contrast intravenous urography.

Gallium 67 Lung Scan

Gallium 67 citrate given intravenously will localize normally in the liver, spleen, and bone marrow, and some will be excreted by the colon. It will also localize, however, in infected areas and in several types of malignant neoplasms. These are the established uses of this test. The innovative use of the gallium scan is in diagnosing the presence or absence of an inflammatory process in the lung when a patient is taking chemotherapeutic agents that have pulmonary toxicity. The best studied agent is bleomycin. Its pulmonary toxicity is common, and unfortunately, the abnormalities do not show up early enough in a plain chest radiograph. With the use of ^{67}Ga citrate, however, the lung abnormalities may be picked up long before they are obvious in x-ray film or clinically. Typically, both lung fields show increased diffuse uptake of ^{67}Ga, which is graded from 0 to 4+ in intensity. Zero is normal, 1+ is barely above background activity, 2+ marks bone activity, 3+ means more than bone activity, and 4+ represents an uptake intensity that is higher than that of the liver and higher than any other in the body. A 1+ uptake is regarded as a warning sign, but it is not a contraindication to further treatment. A grade of 2+ is, however, regarded as a sign of bleomycin toxicity if the patient had a previous baseline study that showed normal or zero gallium uptake. The best use of a gallium scan is to perform it before each dose of bleomycin, which applies also to other chemotherapeutic agents that may produce pulmonary toxicity. A dose of 7 mCi ^{67}Ga intravenously is typical, and views of the rest of the body may be simultaneously recorded to check for metastasis or infection.

Newer Pathophysiological Scintistudies

Several newer pathophysiological scintistudies have augmented the nuclear physician's ability to help the gynecologic oncologist. The three best examples, and the most representative of this group, are catheter placement studies, ^{111}In-labeled leukocyte studies, and labeled monoclonal antibody studies.

Catheter Placement Studies

Injection of ^{99m}Tc MAA into an arterial catheter in place has been used for a long time, particularly in liver studies, to measure relative blood supply. Only recently has this technique become a commonly used clinical tool for studying distribution patterns of the catheterized hepatic artery (or its branches) during intraarterial infusion of chemotherapeutic agents in the hope of avoiding extrahepatic distribution of the high concentrations of the chemotherapeutic agents. In gynecologic oncology, the catheter placement study of greater relevance is that of the pelvic arteries. Specifically, when the catheter is placed in the internal iliac artery or the bilateral internal iliac arteries for pelvic tumor infusion of a chemotherapeutic agent, one would like to know the distribution pattern from the tip of the catheter. The catheters are usually inserted from femoral arteries to either the ipsilateral or contralateral internal iliac artery. Depending on the site of the tumor, the desired distribution may be in the true pelvis only, or it may need to be more extensive, thus requiring the use of both the anterior and posterior branches of the internal iliac artery (catheter tip in the main trunk). The latter will, of course, result in the distribution of a high concentration of the chemotherapeutic agent to the gluteal areas and to the genitalia. Thus, undesirable "burning" of normal tissue may result. The highly selective anterior branch catheterization may result in highly focal drug distribution to benefit the cervix and upper vagina. Occasionally, the catheter tip is erroneously placed in the common iliac artery, which means that the chemotherapeutic agent is likely to travel up the abdominal wall by the inferior epigastric branch and down the thigh through the external iliac artery. Nuclear medicine specialists at U.T. M. D. Anderson Hospital use computer analysis to study regions of interest, at least in difficult cases, in order to reach the relative percentage of distribution between true pelvis, buttock, and genitalia of each injection, right and left. This information then helps clinicians to judge the clinical utility of the catheter in place and to choose the relative amounts of chemotherapeutic agents to be injected into the left and right catheters. Typically, this varies from 25/75 to 50/50 (right/left), depending on which catheter distributes more drug to the tumor and which one sends more to undesirable areas. Occasionally, the catheter is so misplaced that it is totally unacceptable for therapeutic purposes.

The major advantage of the nuclear medicine study over contrast arteriography for understanding the distribution of the catheterized artery is that the nuclear medicine study is performed under normal pressure injection, at least at the same pressure as will be used to infuse the chemotherapeutic agent whether by pump or direct injection. Contrast arteriography, because it is done with high-pressure injection, does not truly reflect what will happen during therapeutic infusion. Also it does not readily provide oblique and lateral views.

Regular and pulsatile pumps are used at U.T. M. D. Anderson Hospital for therapeutic infusions, and the radionuclide catheter placement study is performed with the pump that will eventually be used for the patient's drug perfusion. Sometimes, in order to determine whether to use a regular or a pulsatile pump, both flow studies must be performed and a computer subtraction study used to compare the relative distribution achieved with each pump. Occasionally the two are significantly different.

Indium 111 Leukocyte Studies

Mixed leukocytes labeled with ^{111}In have been used in clinical medicine for the last six or seven years, mainly to detect the site of infection (Marcus 1984). This is, of course, particularly useful in the abdomen and pelvis because the alternative nuclear medicine study is with ^{67}Ga, which is normally secreted into the bowel lumen and therefore will obscure a small site of activity like that of a small abscess. Another advantage of radiolabeled leukocytes over ^{67}Ga is that ^{67}Ga will localize not only in infected tissue but also in tumor, whereas labeled leukocytes will concentrate only in infected or inflamed areas and not at sites of malignancy (McAfee and Samin 1985). This may be of special importance for patients with ovarian carcinoma in whom pelvic inflammation is suspected. Gallium 67 will be taken up by both types of tissue, but leukocytes will localize only at the inflamed sites and not in ovarian carcinoma.

We have also been using leukocytes labeled with ^{111}In in an experimental protocol to monitor the use of biologic response modifiers (BRM), specifically, a study of the use of viral oncolysate immunotherapy directed by Dr. Ralph S. Freedman. After intraperitoneal injection of a viral oncolysate for metastatic ovarian carcinoma, labeled leukocytes are injected intravenously and can be shown to localize in the peritoneal cavity with foci of increased activity around the tumor masses. This suggests stimulation of immune response by the BRM. The results are still preliminary, however, and we are continuing the study, using both mixed leukocytes and also lymphocytes.

Other uses of leukocytes labeled with ^{111}In in gynecologic oncology include localization of intraabdominal abscesses after surgery. Using subtraction technique (^{99m}Tc sulfur colloid scan of the liver from the ^{111}In leukocyte scan), subphrenic or subhepatic abcesses can be detected. In addition, such general inflammatory conditions as acute respiratory distress syndrome of the adult, from a variety of causes, may be diagnosed with the use of ^{111}In leukocytes.

Labeled Monoclonal Antibodies

In oncology, the use of monoclonal antibodies labeled with radioactive isotopes has escalated in the last few years, and their use is fairly advanced in treatment of patients with melanoma (Larson and Carrasquillo 1984) and colon cancer. At U.T. M. D. Anderson Hospital, nuclear medicine specialists and clinical immunologists are using the 96.5 antimelanoma murine monoclonal antibody labeled with ^{111}In directed to the P-97 melanoma surface antigen (Murray et al. 1985), as well as the ZME-018 antibody directed against the GP240 high molecular-weight melanoma antigen. We are also studying an anti-carcinoembryonic antigen monoclonal antibody labeled with ^{111}In for colon cancer. Researchers in Great Britain are already engaged in clinical trials of iodine-labeled antibodies for ovarian carcinoma (Jackson et al. 1985) and for breast cancer (Rainsbury 1984), but the results are too preliminary to predict their clinical uses. Part of the problem is the lack of highly specific antiovarian antibody (Epenetos 1982).

Emission Computerized Tomography

Emission computerized tomography can be single photon (SPECT) or positron (PET). SPECT, which is a mode of collecting the data, can be done for any of the studies described above. The image is then reconstructed into transaxial, coronal, or sagittal slices. This can be done for low-energy studies performed with ^{99m}Tc or medium-energy studies like those using ^{67}Ga and ^{111}In. Although SPECT generally improves sensitivity and specificity, like radiographic transmission CT, it is time-consuming. PET scanning requires special cameras and positron-emitting radioisotopes (e.g. carbon 11, nitrogen 13, oxygen 15). These radioisotopes are short-lived and therefore have to be produced on site, requiring expensive medical cyclotrons. Most of the positron-emitting radioisotopes have the great advantage of being elements found naturally in biological constituents, e.g. carbon, oxygen, nitrogen. Carbon 11 may be incorporated in glucose to study brain metabolism during neuronal activities, e.g., with eyes open and eyes closed. Metastasis will likely manifest a different metabolic pattern of oxygen 15- and nitrogen 13-ammonia compounds. A new vista in the study of metabolic behavior of malignancy is thus opened to the gynecologic oncologist.

References

Biello DR, Matter AG, McKnight RC. 1979. Ventilation-perfusion studies in suspected pulmonary embolism. *American Journal of Radiology* 133:1033–1037.

Epenetos AA, Mather S, Granovska M, Nimmon CC, Hawkins LR, Britton KE, Shepherd J, Taylor-Papadimitriou J, Durbin H, Malpas JS. 1982. Targeting of iodine-123 labeled tumor-associated monoclonal antibodies to ovarian, breast and gastrointestinal tumors. *Lancet* ii:999–1004.

Harbert JC. 1984. Efficacy of liver scanning in malignant disease. *Semin Nucl Med* 14: 287–295.

Jackson PC, Pitcher EM, Davies JO, Davies ER, Sadowski CS, Staddon GE, Stirrat GM, Surderland CA. 1985. Radionuclide imaging of ovarian tumours with a radiolabelled (^{123}I) monoclonal antibody ($NDOG_2$). *Eur J Nucl Med* 11:22–28.

Larson SM, Carrasquillo JA. 1984. Nuclear oncology. 1984. *Semin Nucl Med* 14(4): 268–276.

Linton AL, Richmond JM, Clark WF, Lindsay RM, Driedger AA, Lamki LM. 1985. Gallium^{67} scintigraphy in the diagnosis of acute renal disease. *Clin Nephrol* 24:84–87.

Marcus CS. 1984. The status of indium-111 oxine leukocyte imaging studies. *Noninvasive Medical Imaging* 1(3):213–226.

McAfee JD, Samin A. 1985. In-111 labeled leukocytes: A review of problems in image interpretation. *Radiology* 155:221–229.

McNeil BJ. 1984. Value of bone scanning in neoplastic disease. *Semin Nucl Med* 14:277–286.

Murray JL, Rosenblum MG, Sobol RE, Bartholomew RM, Plager CE, Haynie TP, Jahns MF, Glenn HJ, Lamki L, Benjamin RS, Papadopoulos N, Boddie AW, Frincke JM, David GS, Carlo DJ, Hersh EM. 1985. Radioimmunoimaging in malignant melanoma with ^{111}In-labeled monoclonal antibody 96.5. *Cancer Res* 45:2376–2381.

Neumann RD, Sostman HD, Gottschalk A. 1980. Current status of ventilation-perfusion imaging. *Semin Nucl Med* 10:198–217.

Rainsbury RM. 1984. The localization of human breast carcinomas by radiolabelled monoclonal antibodies. *Br J Surg* 71:805–812.

Silberstein EB, Gilbert LA, Pu MY. 1985. Comparative efficacy of radionuclide, ultrasound, and computed tomographic liver imaging for hepatic metastases. *Current Concepts in Diagnostic Nuclear Medicine* 2(3):3–9.

NEW TREATMENT MODALITIES

Annual Clinical Conference on Cancer, Vol. 29
Gynecologic Cancer: Diagnosis and Treatment Strategies
© 1987 by The University of Texas System Cancer Center

35. Use of Murine Monoclonal Antibodies as Immunotherapeutic Agents for Gastrointestinal Adenocarcinoma

Henry F. Sears

Immunotherapy of human adenocarcinoma of the gastrointestinal tract using murine monoclonal antibodies is conceptually an attractive treatment strategy. Numerous animal in vivo studies and early clinical trials have demonstrated some tumoricidal activity (Sears et al. 1983, 1985; Miller et al. 1982; Houghton et al. 1985; Oldham et al. 1984; Foon et al. 1984; Dillman et al. 1984). Localization and binding studies have shown selective uptake of both intact antibody and antibody fragment conjugates (Chatal et al. 1982; Moldofsky et al. 1983, 1984; Mach et al. 1983). Case reports describing improved clinical courses after exposure to murine monoclonal antibodies have been encouraging (Sears et al. 1983, 1985; Miller et al. 1982). Nonetheless, a variety of problems related to serotherapy with murine immunoglobulin has been identified in early trials. Among these, a predominant problem has been the marked heterogeneity of antigen expression on human tumors and the modulation of these antigens after antibody binding. This variability of antigen expression from cell to cell within a particular tumor (Ernst et al. in press) becomes more pronounced as the tumor becomes more clinically detectable or metastatic. Undifferentiated tumors do not express many of the antigens found on more differentiated tumor types.

A second major problem associated with the use of murine immunoglobulin in patients is immunization to the foreign protein (Sears et al. 1983, 1985; Miller et al. 1982; Houghton et al. 1985; Oldham et al. 1984; Foon et al. 1984; Dillman et al. 1984). In many patients whose own immune systems have not been altered by their tumor therapy, murine immunoglobulin is recognized as a foreign protein, and an immune response is mounted against it. Though a single administration of murine immunoglobulin has proved safe in a number of studies, an antimouse immunoglobulin antibody response can be expected in a majority of patients (Sears et al. 1983, 1985). Potentially severe allergic reactions have occurred after multiple injections of murine monoclonal antibody (Sears et al. 1983). Thus, strategies to reduce the amount of circulating human antimouse immunoglobulin produced after an initial injection of monoclonal antibody have been explored. Using therapeutic reagents that contain a number of monoclonal antibodies, the problem of tumor cell heterogeneity may be addressed by directing the antibodies against differing epitopes of multiple tumor-associated antigens.

In this presentation, I will review the outcome of three clinical trials using a single murine immunoglobulin, 1083-17-1A, a gamma 2A isotypical antibody, which is cytotoxic for human colorectal adenocarcinoma cells (Herlyn et al. 1979, 1980; Herlyn and Kaprowski 1982). The tumor cytolysis seen in in vitro antibody-dependent cellular cytotoxicity assays is mediated by activation of human mononuclear effector cells. The dramatic tumor destruction produced by this reagent in the xenotransplant nude mouse model can be completely abrogated by interference with the monocyte-macrophage function (Herlyn and Koprowski 1982). The administration of monoclonal antibody leads to cure in the animal model only when the tumor burden is small. Only infrequently have my colleagues and I had the opportunity to treat patients who have small tumor burdens.

Phase I Trial of Monoclonal Antibody 1083-17-1A

Twenty patients with advanced adenocarcinomas of the gastrointestinal tract were entered in the initial phase I evaluation of murine immunoglobulin 17-1A, which is capable of binding to and killing human adenocarcinoma cells. This study was designed to evaluate toxicity, immunopharmacology, and binding specificity. Selected patients were those with tumors that had not been controlled by previous therapeutic intervention and for whom no alternate treatment strategies existed. The protocol also required that each patient have a complication of adenocarcinoma necessitating surgery so that normal and tumor tissues could be simultaneously obtained to assess monoclonal antibody binding after an intravenous administration. Intravenous dosages of murine monoclonal antibody varied from 15 mg to 1,000 mg. Clinical data from the phase I trial, which ran from December 1980 to January 1983, are presented in table 35.1.

In this group of patients there was minimal or no toxicity demonstrated, and there were no symptomatic allergic reactions to the initial administration of murine immunoglobulin. Antibody binding to tumor was documented (Shen et al. 1984). Serological evidence of an immune response to the monoclonal antibody was detected in one half of the patients. The only patient to receive multiple injections of monoclonal antibody in this initial trial experienced a vascular bronchospastic response during his fifth injection, which was easily reversed, however, with intravenous epinephrine. Immune responses were noted in eight of nine patients who had small initial injections of monoclonal antibody compared with an immune response in only one of nine patients who received initial large doses of antibody.

Tumor responses in the phase I group have been difficult to assess. It should be emphasized that in ten patients, major operative manipulations of the most clinically evident tumors were done during biopsy of the metastasis to provide tissue for detection of antibody binding. Therefore, indicator lesions were sometimes markedly altered. There were two patients, however, in whom a tumor response could be documented. These patients received no other treatment at the time that the monoclonal antibody was administered. Two other patients also had tumor responses, but other chemotherapeutic modalities were being used at the time of the antibody admin-

Table 35.1. *Results of Phase I MAb Immunotherapy*

Patient No.	Sex	Primary Site	Amount of MAb Received (mg)	Survival After Antibody (Mo.)	Current Status	Human Antimouse Antibody
1	M	R	15	43	Dead	+
2	F	C	150	2	Dead	−
3	M	C	150	13	Dead	+
4	M	G	200	3	Dead[a]	+
5	F	C	100	5	Dead	+
6	M	G	72	1	Dead	NT
7	F	R	128	49+	AWD	+
8	M	R	92	30	Dead	+
9	M	C	133	45+	NED	+
10	M	C	135	3	Dead	?
11	M	C	137	3	Dead	+
12	M	C	366	25	Dead	−
13	F	C	440	16	Dead	−
14	M	P	433	40+	NED	−
15	M	C	400	8	Dead	−
16	M	R	380	8	Dead	−
17	M	C	675	5	Dead	+
18	F	C	391	10	Dead	−
19	M	C	1,000	6	Dead	−
20	M	C	611	11	Dead	−

Note: MAb, monoclonal antibody; R, rectum; C, colon; G, gastric; P, pancreas; AWD, alive with disease; NED, no evidence of disease; NT, not tested.
[a] Received multiple doses of MAb.

istration. All four of those patients are living—two with disease recurrence and two with no evidence of recurrence. The duration of tumor-free survival has been 44 months for one of the patients who had retroperitoneal colorectal adenocarcinoma metastasis and 38 months for another patient who had liver metastasis from a pancreatic carcinoma. These results prompted a phase II trial to more accurately assess tumor response.

Phase II Trial of Monoclonal Antibody 1083-17-1A

The phase II trial was designed to assess tumor response to a single injection of murine monoclonal antibody 17-1A. Each patient selected for the study had a measurable metastatic lesion, and in accordance with eligibility requirements, each had undergone a trial of chemotherapy that failed. Of the 20 patients evaluated, there were no complete responders and only two partial responders to the single injection of antibody 17-1A. Partial response in one of the patients lasted for 18 months. The clinical data are listed in table 35.2.

There was an interesting alteration of the tumor in one patient after monoclonal antibody administration. The patient had previously been part of an immunolocalization imaging trial that utilized F(Ab)½ fragments of the 17-1A antibody conju-

Table 35.2. *Phase II Assessment of Response to Single MAb Injections*

Patient No.	Sex	Age (yr.)	Site of Primary Tumor	Site of Metastasis	MAb Dose (mg)	CEA at Time of Antibody Administration	Antimouse Antibody	Duration of Response (Mo.)	Status
21	M	60	Colon	Liver	765	2,540	–	0	Dead
22	F	40	Colon	Lung	255	246	–	0	Dead
23	M	65	Colon	Liver	850	51	+	0	Dead[a]
24	M	58	Colon	Liver	800	260	+	0	Dead
25	M	41	Rectum	Lung	112	293	+	0	Dead
26	M	51	Colon	Ret	200	76	+	0	Dead
27	F	49	Rectum	Ret	770	9.4	+	0	Dead
28	M	65	Rectum	Pelvis	192	81	–	0	Dead
29	F	48	Colon	Lung	207	<2.5	+	0	Dead
30	F	65	Colon	Liver	215	96	–	0	Dead
31	M	55	Colon	Liver	220	1,080	–	0	Dead
32	F	36	Colon	Pelvis	220	<2.5	–	18	AWD[b]
34	F	70	Rectum	Pelvis	220	<2.5	–	12	Dead[b]
35	F	44	Colon	Pelvis	220	<2.5	+	0	Dead
36	M	62	Colon	Liver	220	48.2	–	0	Dead
37	M	47	Colon	Pelvis	207	<2.5	+	0	Dead
39	M	53	Colon	Lung	200	12.6	–	0	AWD
41	M	57	Colon	Lung	200	<2.5	+	0	Dead
42	M	60	Colon	Lung	200	4.4	+	0	Dead
43	F	65	Colon	Ret	200	33.8	–	0	Dead

Note: MAb, monoclonal antibody; CEA, carcinoembryonic antigen; Ret, retroperitoneum; AWD, alive with disease.
[a] Response in liver metastasis but not in abdominal wall metastasis.
[b] Responders.

gated to iodine 131. The patient's large hepatic metastasis imaged easily; however, a comparably sized metastatic lesion of the abdominal wall did not accumulate isotope. When the patient was infused with monoclonal antibody, there was marked response in the hepatic tumor, but there was no response in the abdominal wall metastasis. In fact, the abdominal wall metastasis continued to grow unabated. This case exemplifies the potential problem related to heterogeneous expression of antigen on metastatic tumors.

Review of our phase II trial data indicated that response to serotherapy using a single injection of monoclonal antibody is limited. This is especially true for patients with a large, clinically measurable tumor burden.

Strategies To Allow Multiple Injections

A trial was designed to compare the different immune responses to murine monoclonal antibodies in patients receiving a large initial dose of murine immunoglobulin instead of a smaller more potentially immunogenic dose. Twenty patients with advanced adenocarcinoma of the gastrointestinal tract were in this study (table 35.3), which was randomized so that patients received an initial injection of either 100 mg or 700 mg of antibody. After the first injection, each patient received 100 mg of antibody every other week for four months. Administration of antibody was discontinued if circulating human antimouse immunoglobulin antibody was detected. Patients with poor Eastern Cooperative Oncology Group performance criteria were excluded, as were those who were nutritionally or immunologically compromised by their tumors or by the tumor treatments.

Each of the patients who received the smaller (100 mg) initial injection of monoclonal antibody developed a human antimouse immunoglobulin response, which was detected by serum antibody against mouse protein within two weeks. Six patients who received 700 mg of monoclonal antibody as the initial injection had no detectable circulating antimouse immunoglobulin responses and no toxic or immunologic reactions to subsequent administrations. The duration of this induced tolerance was limited by the length of time in which subsequent injections of 100 mg of antibody were given. When antibody administration was discontinued in three patients who had documented tumor progression, each patient developed a human antimouse immunoglobulin response. In all patients, detection of human antimouse immunoglobulin occurred after antibody administration had been discontinued for at least two weeks. Two patients completed the study protocol while receiving 100 mg of antibody every two weeks and afterwards received only 5 mg of antibody biweekly. Within four weeks of starting the low-dose maintenance schedule, tests of these patients showed very low titers of human antimouse immunoglobulin. One patient who received 700 mg of antibody developed a prompt human antimouse response despite the large initial injection. He had an anaphylactic response to a subsequent injection of antibody, but the symptoms were easily treated. The allergic response actually occurred when there was a steep upward curve in the titers of the patient's human antimouse response. These studies demonstrate that strategies to

Table 35.3. *Comparison of Immune Responses from Initial MAb Injections*

Patient No.	Sex	Site Primary/Metastasis	Antibody Initial Dose (mg)/No. of Doses	Human Antimouse (Days)	Current Status (Mo.)
44	F	Colon/omentum	100/1	5	Dead
45	M	Rectum/liver	700/5	None	Dead
46	F	Rectum/liver	100/2	21	AWD (27)
47	F	Colon/liver	700/2	14	Dead
48	F	Colon/lung	100/1	10	Dead
49	F	Rectum/lung	700/8	None	AWD (26)
50	F	Rectum/lung	100/2	14	Dead
51	M	Colon/liver	700/3	None	Dead
52	M	Colon/lung	100/2	14	AWD (22)
53	M	Rectum/lung	700/6	70	AWD (20)
54	M	Rectum/lung	700/8	94	Dead
55	M	Colon/liver	700/3[a]	14	AWD (18)
56	M	Rectum/lung	700/3	56	AWD (17)
57	F	Colon/pelvis	700/8	97	AWD (16)
58	M	Pancreas/ret	700/2	14	Dead
59	M	Rectum/lung	100/2	14	AWD (15)
60	F	Colon/omentum	100/2	13	AWD (15)
61	F	Pancreas/liver	100/2	14	Dead
62	M	Pancreas/mesentery	100/2	14	AWD (14)
63	M	Pancreas/liver	100/2	14	AWD (14)

Note: AWD, alive with disease; ret, retroperitoneum.
[a] Patient experienced anaphylactic response.

limit human antimouse antibody response can be successfully designed and that levels of human antimurine antibody must be monitored in future trials.

Discussion

These three trials of passive serotherapy using murine monoclonal antibody that has cytotoxic activity against human colorectal adenocarcinoma cells have provided important results. First, murine immunoglobulin may be administered to patients without untoward toxicity if the antigen bound is not circulating in the blood and the antibody does not bind to other blood elements, bone marrow, or stem cells. There is a strong correlation between a patient's development of a human antimouse immunoglobulin response and the quantity in which the antibody is administered. This can lead to symptomatic allergic responses. Strategies to influence, but not completely abrogate, this response are potentially available. Monoclonal antibody with tumor cytotoxic activity (mediated by activation of human effector cells) has the ability to bind to and alter tumor growth. In some patients with a low tumor burden, dramatic responses have been documented, and life expectancy has exceeded even the most liberal estimates of expected survival.

The majority of patients with clinically identifiable metastatic lesions do not have significant responses to a single injection of monoclonal antibody. The data from our preliminary trials have helped to identify several variables that may limit response. First, and probably most significant, is the heterogeneity of expression of antigens on human tumors (Shen et al. 1984). Second is the modulation of antigens in response to binding with an antibody, which clearly affects further binding and tumor response. Third is the dependence on a human effector cell, which may cause these treatment strategies to be compromised by other cytotoxic antitumor therapy. All of these variables will have to be studied in greater detail. Nonetheless, the murine monoclonal antibody represents an exciting new modality for development of treatment strategies for patients with malignant disease. The protocols for using these reagents will be refined by future clinical trials. The unique characteristics of each tumor-associated antigen that binds monoclonal antibody will demand different approaches to effective tumor-altering strategies. After the problems of antigen heterogeneity and host immunization are addressed, the potential of these reagents for effective tumor targeting remains very attractive.

References

Chatal JF, Saccavini JC, Fumoleau P, Curtet C, Le Mevel B. 1982. Photoscanning localization of human tumors using radioiodinated monoclonal antibodies to colorectal carcinoma: Proceedings of the 29th Annual Meeting of the Society of Nuclear Medicine (abstract). *J Nucl Med* 23:28.

Dillman RO, Shawler DL, Dillman JB, Royston I. 1984. Therapy of chronic lymphocytic leukemia and cutaneous T-cell lymphoma with T101 monoclonal antibody. *J Clin Oncol* 2:881–891.

Ernst CS, Shen JW, Sears HF, Atkinson B, Litwin S, Herlyn M, Koprowski H. In press. Multiparameter evaluation of the expression in situ of normal and tumor-associated antigens in human colorectal carcinoma. *JNCI*.

Foon KA, Schroff RW, Bunn PA, Mayer D, Abrams PG, Fer M, Ochs J, Bottino GC, Sherwin SA, Carlo DJ, Herberman RB, Oldham RK. 1984. Effects of monoclonal antibody therapy in patients with chronic lymphocytic leukemia. *Blood* 64:1085–1093.

Herlyn DM, Koprowski H. 1982. IgG2a monoclonal antibodies inhibit human tumor growth through interaction with effector cells. *Proc Natl Acad Sci USA* 79:4761–4765.

Herlyn DM, Steplewski Z, Herlyn MF, Koprowski H. 1980. Inhibition of growth of colorectal carcinoma in nude mice by monoclonal antibody. *Cancer Res* 40:717–721.

Herlyn M, Steplewski Z, Herlyn D, Koprowski H. 1979. Colorectal carcinoma-specific antigen: Detection by means of monoclonal antibodies. *Proc Natl Acad Sci USA* 76: 1438–1442.

Houghton AN, Mintzer D, Cordon-Cardo C, Welt S, Fliegel B, Vadhan S, Carswell E, Melamed MR, Oettgen HF, Old LJ. 1985. Mouse monoclonal IgG3 antibody detecting GD3 ganglioside: A phase I trial in patients with malignant melanoma. *Proc Natl Acad Sci USA* 82:1242–1246.

Mach JP, Chatal JF, Lumbroso JD, Foroni M, Douillard JY, Carrel S, Herlyn DM, Steplewski Z, Koprowski H. 1983. Tumor localization in patients by radiolabeled monoclonal antibodies against colon carcinoma. *Cancer Res* 43:5593–5600.

Miller RA, Maloney DC, Warnke R, Levy R. 1982. Treatment of B cell lymphoma with monoclonal anti-ideotype antibody. *N Engl J Med* 306:517–522.

Moldofsky PJ, Powe J, Mulhern CB, Sears HF, Hammond ND, Gatenby RA, Steplewski Z, Koprowski H. 1983. Metastatic colon carcinoma detected with radiolabeled $F(ab)_2$ monoclonal antibody fragments. *Radiology* 149:549–555.

Moldofsky PJ, Sears HF, Mulhern CB, Hammond ND, Powe J, Gatenby RA, Steplewski Z,

Koprowski H. 1984. Detection of metastatic tumor in normal sized retroperitoneal lymph nodes using radiolabeled monoclonal antibody imaging. *N Engl J Med* 311:106–107.

Oldham RK, Foon KA, Morgan AC, Woodhouse CS, Schroff RW, Abrams PG, Fer M, Schoenberger CS, Farrell M, Kimball E, Sherwin SA. 1984. Monoclonal antibody therapy of malignant melanoma: In vivo localization in cutaneous metastasis after intravenous administration. *J Clin Oncol* 2:1235–1244.

Sears HF, Herlyn D, Steplewski Z, Koprowski H. 1985. Phase II clinical trial of a murine monoclonal antibody cytotoxic for gastrointestinal adenocarcinoma. *Cancer Res* 45: 5910–5913.

Sears HF, Steplewski Z, Herlyn D, Koprowski H. 1983. Effects of monoclonal antibody immunotherapy on patients with gastrointestinal adenocarcinoma. *J Biol Response Mod* 3:2.

Shen JW, Atkinson B, Koprowski H, Sears HF. 1984. Binding of murine immunoglobulin to human tissues after immunotherapy with anticolorectal carcinoma monoclonal antibody. *Int J Cancer* 33:465–468.

Annual Clinical Conference on Cancer, Vol. 29
Gynecologic Cancer: Diagnosis and Treatment Strategies
© 1987 by The University of Texas System Cancer Center

36. Hyperthermia in the Treatment of Gynecologic Cancers

Joseph S. Kong, Peter M. Corry, and Patton B. Saul

Hyperthermia is the elevation of body or tissue temperature above that of the normal physiologic temperature. The possible use of hyperthermia in the treatment of malignant tumors was first suggested in 1866 in a report by Busch, who noticed the spontaneous disappearance of a soft tissue sarcoma in a patient after the patient developed a high fever from erysipelas (Busch 1866). In 1893, Coley attempted to treat his patients with malignant tumors by using pyrogens to induce fever (Coley 1893). Regional hyperthermia was first employed as a local treatment for tumors by Westermark (1898).

Hyperthermia as a cancer treatment modality has gained considerable interest in the last 15 years. From recent research, a large body of knowledge has been gathered that provides a sound biologic basis for the clinical use of hyperthermia. A brief summary of the important biologic aspects of hyperthermia related to the treatment of malignant tumors is presented here.

Biologic Aspects of Hyperthermia

Hyperthermia kills cells in a predictable and reproducible manner. When mammalian cells such as Chinese hamster ovary (CHO) cells are exposed to hyperthermia at different temperatures, the cell survival curves generated are similar to those generated by radiation (fig. 36.1), depicting an exponential cell kill with an initial "shoulder." The degree of cell kill increases with the duration of exposure to hyperthermia. In addition, the slopes of the cell survival curves become steeper with increasing temperatures, indicating a more efficient cell kill.

Hyperthermia enhances the cytotoxic effect of radiation in a complex way. Some demonstrated mechanisms of this enhancement are the inhibition or reduction of repair of sublethal damage and potentially lethal damage that are produced by radiation (Gerweck, Gillette, and Dewey 1975).

In addition, hyperthermia and radiation complement each other in several ways. Cells in the S phase of the cell cycle have been shown to be more sensitive to the damaging effects of hyperthermia than those in the G_1 phase, whereas the reverse is true with radiation (fig. 36.2).

It has been shown that radiosensitivity is reduced in cells that are in a hypoxic condition. In fact, hypoxia in solid tumor centers is often purported to be the cause of radiation failure. However, nutrient deprivation and low pH, which also prevail

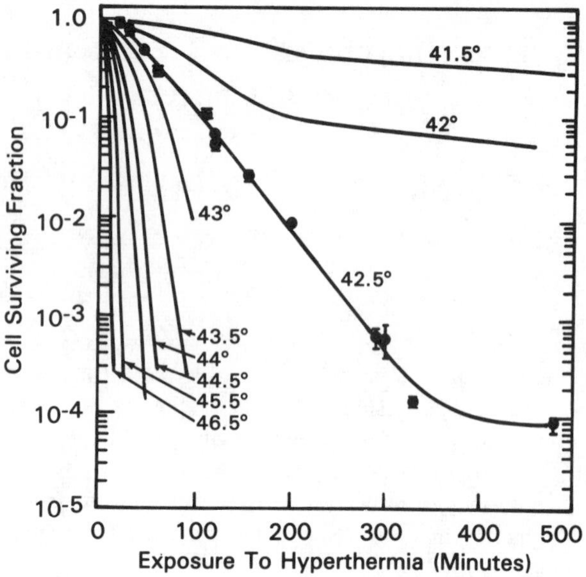

Fig. 36.1. Survival curves of CHO cells after hyperthermia treatments at different temperatures and durations. Reprinted with permission from Dewey et al., Cellular response to combinations of hyperthermia and radiation, *Radiology* (1977; 123:464–477).

at these same tumor centers, appear to enhance the cytotoxicity of hyperthermia (fig. 36.3).

The microvasculature of tumors also renders them more susceptible to heat. In normal tissues, vasodilation occurs when the tissue is heated. The increased perfusion helps to maintain a normal temperature. In contrast, the neovasculature in tumor tissues is known to be tortuous and contain many sinusoids, causing sluggish blood flow or stasis. Hyperthermia above 42°C causes no change or decrease in tumor blood perfusion (Bicher et al. 1980). Clinically, it is not unusual to find that tumor tissues heat up much more easily than surrounding normal tissues.

In addition to the interaction with radiation, hyperthermia has also been shown to potentiate the cytotoxic effect of a number of drugs (table 36.1).

Given these known biologic effects of hyperthermia, it is logical to explore the clinical use of hyperthermia in conjunction with radiation or with chemotherapy. Indeed, clinical trials are proceeding in many centers to study the combined treatment for superficial tumors of various kinds. However, clinical data for deep tumors such as gynecologic cancers are rare. This is due to the lack of current technology to provide well-controlled heating of deep-seated tumors and the lack of noninvasive methods for monitoring temperatures in deep tissues. In the following section, the commonly employed heating methods and thermometry pertaining to their use in pelvic tumors are briefly discussed.

Current Heating Methods and Thermometry

Ultrasound

Ultrasound waves are generated by the excitation of a piezoelectric element in a transducer using an external power source. The ultrasound pressure waves travel down the water column of the transducer into the tissue. Heating is produced by mechanical friction in the tissue caused by the pressure waves. The main advantages of ultrasound are its ease of use, its good depth of penetration in soft tissues, and its potential to be focused to produce more precise heating at depth. A disadvantage of ultrasound is its high absorption in bones, which causes overheating. A more serious problem is its lack of penetration through air-soft tissue interfaces due to reflection. This makes it unsuitable for use in heating pelvic tumors in the presence of bowel gas.

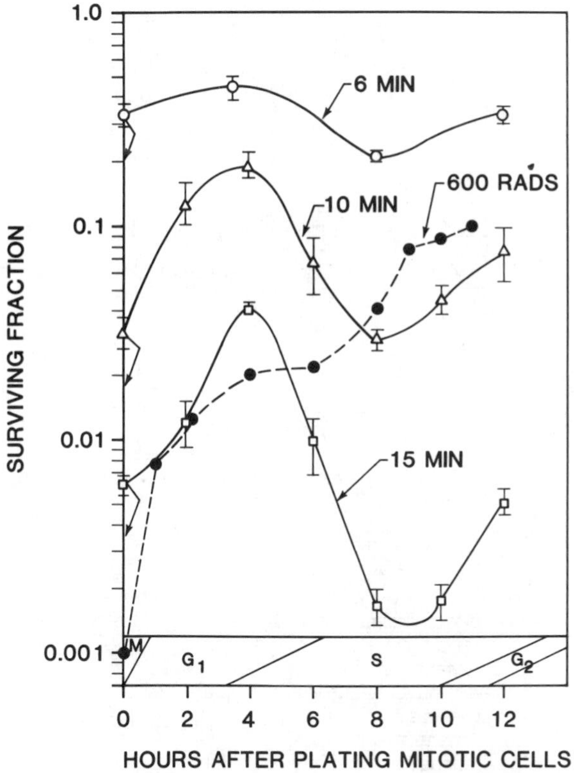

Fig. 36.2. CHO cell survivals by cell age after exposure to radiation or 45.5°C hyperthermia at 6, 10, or 15 minutes. Reprinted with permission from *Int J Radiat Oncol Biol Phys* (1971; 19:467–477). Westra A, Dewey WC, Variation in sensitivity to heat shock during the cell cycle of Chinese hamster cell in vitro. Copyright 1971, Pergamon Press.

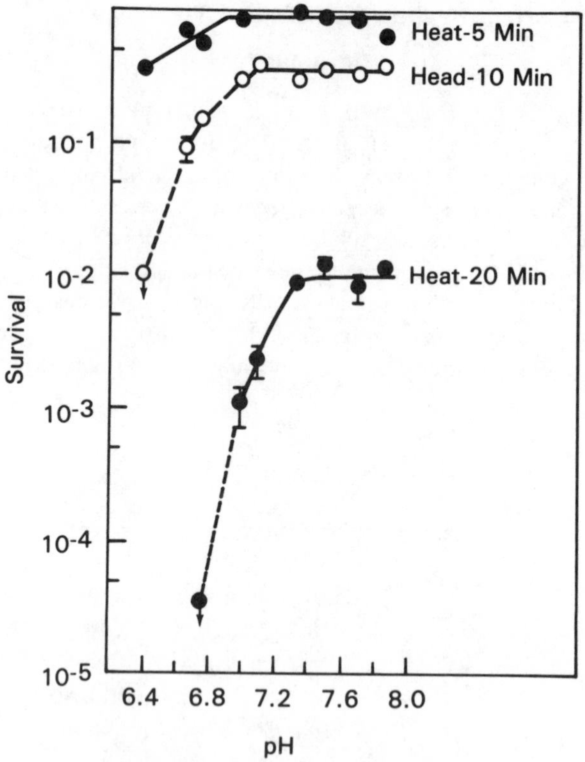

Fig. 36.3. Effects of pH on the survivals of CHO cells after 45.5°C hyperthermia for 5, 10, and 20 minutes. Reprinted from *JNCI* (1977; 58:1837–1839).

Table 36.1. *Drug Cytotoxicity Enhancement by Hyperthermia*

Cytotoxicity increases with temperature
Thiotepa
Nitrosoureas
Mitomycin C
Cis-platinum
Synergistic interaction above threshold temperature
Doxorubicin HCl
Bleomycin
Actinomycin D
Conversion to cytotoxicity by hyperthermia
Cysteamine
Amphotericin B
Lidocaine

Microwaves

Microwaves produce heating by causing rapid dipole movement, primarily in water molecules in the tissue. Microwaves can be applied to superficial tissues using external applicators; however, at commonly used frequencies the penetration into tissues is limited. Therefore, deep tumors cannot be heated by external microwave application. This can be overcome if a microwave antennae array can be implanted directly into the tumor.

Capacitive Heating

Capacitive heating uses an alternating electric field to excite tissue molecules to produce heat. An arrangement of a single pair or multiple pairs of capacitors can be utilized. This method can potentially heat up a large volume of tissue and achieve deep heating. The major disadvantage of a capacitive heating is the preferential deposition of power in fat tissue over that of muscle when the electric field is perpendicular to the fat-muscle interface. Because of this propensity for overheating the subcutaneous and intraperitoneal fat, capacitive heating is undesirable for pelvic tumor treatment.

Magnetic Induction

Magnetic induction utilizes a coil or a set of coils to impose a magnetic field that, in turn, induces eddy currents in the tissue to be heated. Depending on the arrangement of the induction coils, a large volume of tissue can be heated and deep heating is possible. The major drawback of magnetic induction is the limited control of energy deposition, making the heating pattern unpredictable.

Interstitial Heating

Interstitial heating can be performed by implanting microwave antennae or metallic electrodes, usually in arrays, into the tissue to be heated. A properly spaced array can eliminate the problem of limited penetration of the microwaves. Deposition of power by each antenna can be individually controlled. With implanted electrodes, a high-frequency electric current is passed into the tissue through the electrodes. The heat generated is mainly a result of resistive heating in the tissues. Interstitial radiotherapy can be delivered simultaneously with a suitable isotope such as ^{192}Ir or ^{198}Au. The main disadvantage of interstitial heating is its invasive nature. For implantation in pelvic tumors, general anesthesia is required. But the well-controlled power deposition makes interstitial hyperthermia a good heating method for pelvic tumors.

Thermometry

The commonly used thermometers are thermisters, thermocouples, and optical thermometers. They all have the drawback of being invasive thermometers. Another problem with these thermometers is that only a finite number of points in the tissue can be measured at any given time.

Clinical Data

Reports of phase I/II studies using combined hyperthermia and radiotherapy have shown efficacy against various superficial metastases, including those from primary gynecologic cancers. The responses of these metastatic tumors ranged from 30% to 80%, mostly achieved with a low radiation dose (2000–4000 rad) (Arcangeli et al. 1980; Hornback et al. 1977; Kim and Hahn 1979; Marmor et al. 1979; Perez et al. 1981).

The clinical hyperthermia program at The University of Texas M.D. Anderson Hospital and Tumor Institute at Houston was established in 1979. Thus far, more than 400 patients have been treated with hyperthermia alone, or in combination with chemotherapy or radiotherapy. Among these 400 patients, six received combined hyperthermia and radiotherapy for metastatic gynecologic cancers. Radiotherapy treatments were given in 200 rad per daily fraction, five days each week, or 400 rad per fraction thrice weekly to a total tumor dose of up to 5000 rad. Hyperthermia at tumor temperatures of 43° to 46°C is given immediately prior to each radiation fraction using ultrasound or magnetic induction (table 36.2). Five patients completed the planned course of treatment, and of those, four achieved a complete response lasting from 10 to 52 weeks. One patient was lost to follow-up after completing her treatment. The acute toxic reactions in these six patients included pain, erythema, and tissue swelling, but no skin burns or ulceration.

For deep pelvic tumors, we have recently initiated a protocol employing interstitial hyperthermia and radiotherapy. To date, four patients with large, unresectable, recurrent pelvic tumors have been treated for palliation of severe pain that required chronic narcotics administration (table 36.3). All four patients received full-dose radiotherapy as the initial treatment for primary carcinoma of the cervix. In the combined treatment, a laparotomy was performed to expose the tumor and to facilitate the insertion of thermocouples to monitor the temperatures in the tumor and the surrounding normal tissues. Electrodes for heating and radioactive gold (^{198}Au) grains were intraabdominally implanted into the tumor in the first two patients. In the other two patients, instead of gold grains, hollow electrodes were implanted transcutaneously through the perineum into the tumor; they were afterloaded with radioactive iridium (^{192}Ir) to deliver the radiation. The total radiation dosage given by the implants in these four patients ranged from 4,000 rad to 8,700 rad. Hyperthermia at a target tumor temperature of 43°C was administered with high-frequency current once daily for one hour over four to ten days. As a result of the combined treatment, two patients had stable disease for two and six months, respectively, with complete relief of pain. The remaining two patients had progressive disease.

A more extensive pilot study using a similar technique of transcutaneous perineal implant was reported by the University of Arizona (Surwit et al. 1983). Of a total of 21 patients who had recurrent carcinoma of the cervix treated by radioactive implant and hyperthermia, seven patients achieved a complete response with a median duration of 11 months. Ten patients achieved a partial response with a median dura-

Table 36.2. *Combined Hyperthermia/Radiotherapy for Metastatic Gynecologic Cancers*

Patient No.	Primary Cancer	Metastatic Site Treated	Heating Method	XRT Dose Fractionation	Response/Duration
1	Squamous carcinoma of cervix	Supraclavicular	US	4000 rad / 20 fractions	CR/52 weeks
2	Uterine sarcoma	Supraclavicular	US/MI		Intolerance to hyperthermia
3	Ovarian carcinoma	Inguinal	US	2400 rad / 6 fractions	CR/36 weeks
4	Endometrial carcinoma	Abdominal	MI		Lost to follow-up
5	Adenocarcinoma of cervix	Supraclavicular	US	2800 rad / 7 fractions	CR/15 weeks
6	Endometrial carcinoma	Supraclavicular	US	4400 rad / 11 fractions	CR/10 weeks

Note: US, ultrasound; MI, magnetic induction; CR, complete response; XRT, radiotherapy.

Table 36.3. *Combined Treatment for Palliation of Cancer: Recurrent Pelvic Tumors*

Patient No.	Primary Cancer	Isotope Implant	Implant Dose	Number of Hyperthermia Treatments	Response/Palliation	Duration
1	Squamous carcinoma of cervix	^{198}Au	8400 rad	10	SD/complete pain relief	6 months
2	Squamous carcinoma of cervix	^{198}Au	8700 rad	5	PD	
3	Squamous carcinoma of cervix	^{192}Ir	4000 rad	6	SD/complete pain relief	2 months
4	Squamous carcinoma of cervix	^{192}Ir	4000 rad	4	PD	

Note: SD, stable disease; PD, progressive disease.

tion of three months. Major complications occurred in four patients in the form of enterovaginal or vesicovaginal fistulization.

Future Directions

Although the results of the combined treatment for metastatic and recurrent tumors are encouraging, further clinical investigations, including randomized trials, are necessary to determine whether hyperthermia has a role as one of the primary modalities of treatment for gynecologic cancers. A prerequisite for these further trials is the development of better deep-heating equipment and noninvasive thermometry.

The current research efforts in the development of deep-heating equipment center around the design of applicator arrays whereby energy is deposited in deep tissues through multiple portals. Examples of such arrays are the ultrasound systems that are being tested at Stanford University (Fessenden et al. 1984) and the University of Arizona, and the annular dielectric heating array (ADAS) developed by the BSD Corporation (Sapozink et al. 1984). Another system that shows promise for focused deep heating is the hybrid radiofrequency applicator, which is being developed at U.T. M. D. Anderson Hospital by Boddie et al. (1984). It is a complex antenna system using multiple paired inductors situated between capacitor plates. By manipulating the spatial arrangement and the energization of the inductors, specific energy deposition patterns by radiowaves can be created in deep tissues.

Noninvasive thermometry methods currently under study include the use of nuclear magnetic resonance, computerized tomography number, and various radiometric methods (Cetas 1984). However, practical application of these methods is not expected to be realized in the near future.

Acknowledgment

This work was supported in part by Grants CA06294, CA16672, CM17524, and CA17891 from the National Cancer Institute, Department of Health and Human Services.

References

Arcangeli G, Barni E, Cividalli A, Mauro F, Morelli D, Nervi C, Spano M, Tabocchini A. 1980. Effectiveness of microwave hyperthermia combined with ionizing radiation: Clinical results on neck node metastases. *Int J Radiat Oncol Biol Phys* 6:143–148.

Bicher HI, Hetzel FW, Sandhu TS, Frinka S, Vaupel P, O'Hara MD, O'Brien T. 1980. Effects of hyperthermia on normal and tumor microenvironment. *Radiology* 137:523–530.

Boddie AW, Yamanashi WS, Frazer J, McBride CM, Martin R. 1984. Superficial and deep focused hyperthermia in animals with a hybrid radiofrequency applicator. In *Proceedings of the 4th International Symposium on Hyperthermic Oncology*. ed. Jens Overgaard, pp. 629–632. Aarhus, Denmark: Taylor and Francis.

Busch W. 1866. Uber den Einfluss welchen heftigere Erysipelen zuweilen auf Organiserke Neubildungen ausuben. *Yerhandlungen des Naturh: Preuss Rheinl* 23:28–30.

Cetas TC. 1984. Will thermometric tomography become practical for hyperthermia treatment monitoring? *Cancer Research* [Suppl] 44:4805S–4808S.

Coley WB. 1893. The treatment of malignant tumors by repeated inoculations of erysipelas with a report of 10 original cases. *Am J Med Sci* 105:487–511.

Dewey WC, Hopwood LE, Sapareto SA, Gerweck LE. 1977. Cellular response to combinations of hyperthermia and radiation. *Radiology* 123:464–477.

Fessenden P, Lee ER, Anderson TL, Strohbehn JW, Meyer JL, Samulski TV, Marmor JB. 1984. Experience with a multitransducer ultrasound system for localized hyperthermia of deep tissues. *IEEE Trans Biomed Eng* BME-31:126–135.

Freeman ML, Dewey WC, Hopwood LE. 1977. Effect of pH on hyperthermic cell survival. *JNCI* 58:1837–1839.

Gerweck LE, Gillette EL, Dewey WC. 1975. Effect of heat and radiation on synchronous Chinese hamster cells: Killing and repair. *Radiat Res* 64:611–623.

Hornback NB, Shupe RE, Shidnia H, Joe BT, Sayoc E, Marshall C. 1977. Preliminary clinical results of combined 433 megahertz microwave therapy and on patients with advanced cancer. *Cancer* 40:2854–2863.

Kim JH, Hahn EW. 1979. Clinical and biological studies of localized hyperthermia. *Cancer Res* 39:2258–2261.

Marmor JB, Pounds D, Postic TB, Hahn GM. 1979. Treatment of superficial human neoplasms by local hyperthermia induced by ultrasound. *Cancer* 43:188–197.

Perez CA, Kopecky W, Rao DV, Baglan R, Mann J. 1981. Local microwave hyperthermia and irradiation in cancer therapy: Preliminary observations and directions for future clinical trials. *Int J Radiat Oncol Biol Phys* 7:765–772.

Sapozink MD, Gibbs FA Jr, Gates KS, Stewart JR. 1984. Regional hyperthermia in the treatment of clinically advanced, deep seated malignancy: Results of a pilot study employing an annular array applicator. *Int J Radiat Oncol Biol Phys* 10(6):775–786.

Surwit EA, Manning MR, Aristizabal SA, Oleson JR, Cetas TC. 1983. Interstitial thermoradiotherapy in recurrent gynecologic malignancies. *Gynecol Oncol* 15:95–102.

Westermark F. 1898. Uber die Behandlung des Ulerirended Cerixacarcinoms. Mittle Konstanter Warme. *Abl Gynak* 1335–1339.

Westra A, Dewey WC. 1971. Variation in sensitivity to heat shock during the cell cycle of Chinese hamster cell in vitro. *Int J Radiat Oncol Biol Phys* 19:467–477.

REHABILITATION

Annual Clinical Conference on Cancer, Vol. 29
Gynecologic Cancer: Diagnosis and Treatment Strategies
© 1987 by The University of Texas System Cancer Center

37. Sexual Rehabilitation of the Patient with Gynecologic Cancer

Leslie R. Schover

Gynecologic cancers strike women in their most vulnerable areas—not only physically, but emotionally. In our society, women have until quite recently based their self-esteem on traditional female qualities such as physical attractiveness, sexual responsiveness, fertility, and ability to provide nurturance. Women treated for gynecologic cancer often must endure changes in their physical appearance, impairment of sexual function, loss of reproductive capacity, and even a reduction in the energy needed for mothering the rest of the family. Now that most women work outside of the home and many are single parents, they must also shoulder the burden of the family's continued financial and daily-life functioning during their periods of illness.

The Section of Sexual Rehabilitation at The University of Texas M. D. Anderson Hospital and Tumor Institute at Houston provides clinical services and carries out research not just to prevent and treat sexual dysfunction, but to help gynecologic cancer patients cope with changes in body image, infertility, and relationship issues related to the illness. My colleagues and I in the Section of Sexual Rehabilitation include a woman's husband or sexual partner in education and counseling whenever possible. Sexual problems are couple issues and are treated most effectively within the context of a relationship.

The Integrated Model of Sexual Problems in Cancer Patients

We believe that sexual problems in gynecologic cancer patients have multiple causes and often require interdisciplinary treatment plans. Figure 37.1 illustrates the integrative model that guides our work. Assessment of a sexual problem should include attention to a woman's individual psychological and sexual history, her current marital and family relationships, and the medical impact of her cancer and its treatment on sexual function.

Sexual problems are often complex. Occasionally a woman has just one sexual complaint, such as difficulty reaching orgasm during intercourse after a radical hysterectomy. Most patients have multiple problems, however. For example, a woman who has undergone total pelvic exenteration may experience a loss of desire for sex because of her negative feelings about her body. If she tries, nevertheless, to have sexual activity with her husband, she does not feel excitement or pleasure. Her neovagina also cannot produce its own lubrication, and if she is not motivated to use an

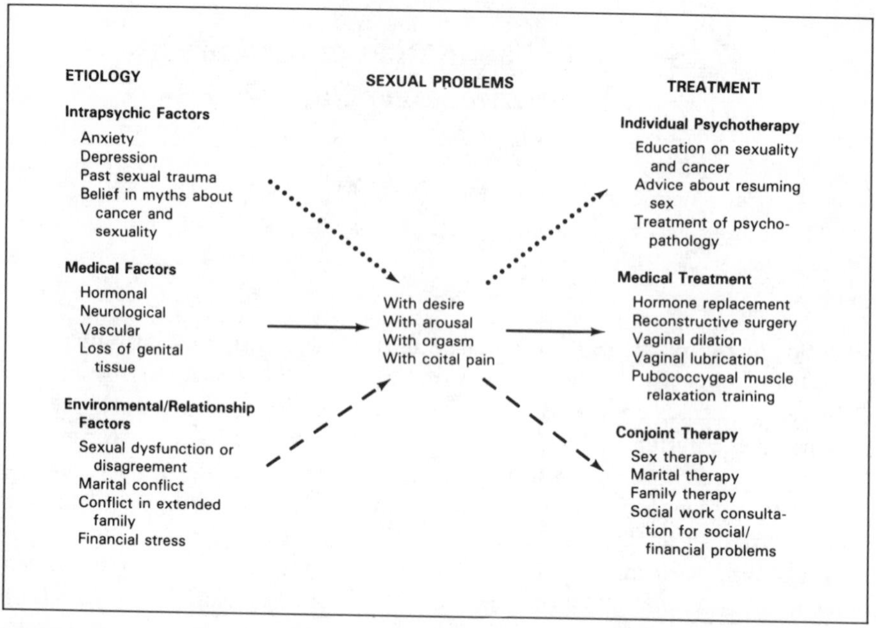

Fig. 37.1. An integrative model of etiology and treatment of sexual problems in gynecologic cancer patients.

extra lubricant, intercourse may be painful for her. Because she is not in the mood for sex, even caressing of her clitoris does not help her to reach orgasm. A clinician should be aware of the multiaxial nature of sexual dysfunction (Schover et al. 1982) and not overlook the effects of cancer treatment on the several phases of the sexual response cycle.

Figure 37.1 also suggests the range of treatment components that may be combined to create a comprehensive rehabilitation plan for a woman's sexual problem after gynecologic cancer therapy. The choice of treatment modalities should be dictated by the causes of the sexual problem. If a woman was sexually molested as a child and presents with a sudden sexual phobia or aversion after radiotherapy and hysterectomy for uterine cancer, individual psychotherapy may help her deal with her reactivated fears of violation and loss of control over her sexuality. Couple sessions could also be useful in helping the husband understand his wife's feelings and as a vehicle for prescribing sex therapy homework exercises to guide the couple in resuming nonpressured touching. The touching could gradually become more sexual as the wife overcomes her fears. A gynecologist might collaborate with the mental health clinician, reassuring the patient that sexual activity was healthy and advising her on use of a water-based vaginal lubricant or, if necessary, teaching her to use a set of graduated vaginal dilators to become comfortable again with vaginal penetration.

Techniques of Brief Sexual Counseling

Every woman treated for a gynecologic cancer should be offered education about the effects of her proposed cancer treatment on sexual function. The optimal scheduling for such a brief session of counseling is at the start of the cancer therapy. We suggest that the educator be a physician, social worker, oncology nurse, or a psychologist or sex therapist. For effective communication, simple, dignified language should be used, and we recommend that models or pictures of genitals be incorporated into the counseling. Whenever possible, the partner should be included in sessions. The counselor should emphasize the ability to return to normal sexual function, and follow-up visits to check for problems should be scheduled. Topics to be covered should include the sexual response cycle, genital anatomy, sexual side effects of cancer treatment, myths about sex and cancer, when and how to resume sex, the use of water-based lubricants, the use of vaginal dilators, the pros and cons of hormone therapy, and techniques of coping with ostomy appliances during sex.

We try to include the male partner because women are often too embarrassed or unassertive to pass on what they have learned to the mate. Men often fear that sexual activity after cancer treatment will harm the woman or might even transmit cancer to the partner.

We begin all education sessions by showing the couple a lifelike model of the external genitals and internal pelvic organs, explaining the function of each anatomic area (vulva, inner and outer labia, clitoris, urethra, vagina, bladder, rectum, cervix, uterus, ovaries, and fallopian tubes). We summarize the physiological changes that occur with arousal and orgasm as well as during the menstrual cycle. We make sure that each partner understands the information; the use of simple words is important here. Rather than just lecturing, we ask questions to engage the couple. For example, we might say: "The only job of the clitoris is to send messages of pleasure to the brain when it is touched. For many women, caressing of the clitoris is the easiest way to reach an orgasm or climax. How important is the clitoris in your lovemaking together?"

This dialogue lays the groundwork for an explanation of the effects of cancer therapy on sexuality. Topics for discussion may include changes in vaginal size, effects of radiotherapy on vaginal expansion and lubrication, vaginal irritation (stomatitis) during chemotherapy, symptoms of sudden menopause, loss of genital tissue as in vulvectomy or vaginectomy, and remaining sexually active while wearing an ostomy appliance. We focus on women's success in overcoming initial dyspareunia or dryness, and in learning to reach orgasm through stimulation of remaining erotic zones even after such major operations as total pelvic exenteration (Andersen and Hacker 1983a).

Both men and women usually have only a sketchy knowledge of pelvic and genital anatomy. Many still do not know the location or function of the clitoris, and some women still believe they urinate through their vaginas. Most of our patients have never looked at their own vulvas in a mirror and have no idea that their vaginas deepen and widen with sexual arousal. They are astounded to hear that vaginal lubrication is produced by the cells lining the vagina and not by a gland or by the cervix. Few even know where the cervix is or how it is shaped.

Women also have many misconceptions about hormones and menopause. They fear that cancer treatments that cause hormone deficiencies will make them lose desire for sex, become depressed, gain weight, or grow a mustache. Unfortunately, they are often ignorant of the real side effects of sudden menopause, such as hot flushes and vaginal dryness. Young women who are eligible for replacement hormones sometimes refuse to take them because of fear that estrogens cause cancer. Such patients need a clear explanation of the risks and benefits of hormone therapy, including a discussion of osteoporosis and hormonal protection from cardiovascular disease.

We find that women are not very compliant about using vaginal dilators. Many of our patients disclose that they have never felt comfortable using a tampon and certainly have not explored the inside of their vaginas with their own fingers. They feel that a dilator is really just like a dildo, and that vaginal dilation is a form of masturbation. Such women need desensitization by a health care professional who can take the time to help the patient look at her genitals in a mirror, identify the various parts, watch while a dilator is gently inserted into her vagina, and then practice inserting the dilator herself. We often suggest that women use the dilator in the bathtub or while watching TV or reading during private time, taking the dilator out of a sexual context. Support from the partner is very important, too. Some men feel threatened by the dilator, worrying that their wives will prefer masturbation to partner sex or will become overly sexual.

Women who have radical pelvic surgery such as vulvectomy or exenteration need special care. They must adjust to the changes in their appearance and to new sensations in their genitals (Andersen and Hacker 1983b; Schover and Fife 1986). They can benefit from advice on avoiding pain during sexual activity and on relearning how to achieve sexual pleasure. Books such as *For Yourself* (Barbach 1974), *For Each Other* (Barbach 1982), and *Becoming Orgasmic* (Heiman, LoPiccolo, and LoPiccolo 1976) can be helpful. They are written for healthy women who wish to be more easily orgasmic, but the techniques they suggest can also aid women in becoming more aroused and reaching orgasm after cancer surgery.

Some basic sex therapy exercises can also help couples stay sexually active during and after cancer treatment. A clinician does not have to be a sex therapist to suggest these, but he or she ought to read a basic textbook such as *The New Sex Therapy* (Kaplan 1974). The sensate focus exercises, which emphasize gentle, nonpressured erotic touching with gradual progression toward sexual stimulation and arousal, provide a helpful structure for couples in resuming sexual activity. Instructions are contained in many self-help books, including *For Each Other* (Barbach 1982), *Becoming Orgasmic* (Heiman, LoPiccolo, and LoPiccolo 1976), and *Prime Time: Sexual Health for Men Over Fifty* (Schover 1984). These books also discuss sexual communication, often a crucial skill in restoring satisfying lovemaking. Couples may need to be more experimental than usual in trying new types of caressing or positions for intercourse.

One area often ignored in counseling cancer patients is advice on contraception. Gynecologic oncology patients are often rendered infertile by treatment, but the gynecologist should not ignore the women of childbearing age who must cope with uncertain fertility during chemotherapy or who may remain fertile after operations to remove one malignant ovary or excise vulvar cancer. Oncologists treating young women for nonpelvic cancer may need to consult gynecologic oncologists. We have seen several tragic pregnancies that occurred during chemotherapy or hormonal therapy because a woman believed herself to be infertile and failed to use contraception. The consequences have ranged from miscarriage, to elective abortion of an abnormal fetus, to carrying the pregnancy to term and giving the baby up for adoption. In all cases, however, the woman had to cope with the emotional pain of an unwanted pregnancy over and above the stress of her cancer treatment. All of these pregnancies could have been prevented by proper education before the start of cancer therapy.

Referral for Intensive Therapy

The great majority of patients need only brief sexual counseling, but a small group, perhaps 10% to 20%, could have a better quality of life with more intensive therapy. Intensive therapy, as noted in figure 37.1, may consist of one or several modalities such as individual psychotherapy, hormone replacement therapy, reconstructive surgery, or formal sex therapy that includes both partners.

A patient's need for referral is often apparent early in the cancer treatment process. High-risk groups include women who are highly anxious about sexual issues, who are in new relationships, who are childless and face infertility, or who have histories of emotional distress or marital and family conflict. Women undergoing major operations such as radical vulvectomy or total pelvic exenteration should routinely receive intensive evaluation.

Other women do not seem distressed until a follow-up visit, when a sensitive physician may elicit a story of sexual dysfunction or marital disruption. Often the sexual problem is just one aspect of generalized emotional troubles. It may be the only complaint, however, that a woman feels justified in voicing, because she sees her cancer treatment as having physically damaged her sexual function. The referral process may involve reframing the problem as a response to the stress of cancer, stating explicitly that even normal, well-adjusted people need help in coping with illness. Otherwise, a woman may believe that her gynecologist is fobbing her off on a "psychiatrist" because the problem is "all in her head."

Sexuality and Cervical Cancer: An Interim Report on Successful Counseling

The principles of sexual rehabilitation set forth above have guided a research project on sexual function in women with early-stage invasive cervical cancer. The study was designed to compare the impact of radical hysterectomy with that of definitive radiotherapy on sexual and marital relationships. The data also support our approach to sexual rehabilitation, however. Although the project is still a year from completion, I will highlight our findings from the first two years (coinvestigators are myself, Michael Fife, M.S.W., and David M. Gershenson, M.D., all on the staff of U.T. M. D. Anderson Hospital).

Background

Previous researchers studying women treated for early-stage cervical cancer observed high rates of sexual dysfunction and marital dissolution (Abitbol and Davenport 1974; Adelusi 1980; Decker and Schwartzman 1962; Hansen 1981; Siebel, Freeman, and Graves 1982). Radiotherapy was seen as even more destructive than radical hysterectomy. The one study that was really well designed, however, including a prospective assessment of sexual function and age-matched women randomly assigned to a treatment group, found similar rates of sexual impairment after treatment, whether it was surgery or radiotherapy (Vincent et al. 1975). None of the studies included a really detailed assessment of sexual function across the response cycle or of the quality of a couple's marital relationship.

Subjects and Methods

At U.T. M. D. Anderson Hospital, women with stage I through stage IIA cervical cancer are evaluated and assigned to treatment by joint consultation between the gynecologist and radiotherapist. From August 1983 through August 1985, we invited all English-speaking women treated with radical hysterectomy or with a combination of external-beam and intracavitary radiotherapy to participate in a study on sexuality. Partners were also asked to participate.

Each woman or couple was interviewed at the beginning of treatment about their relationship, sexual function in the past year, and reactions to the cancer diagnosis. The interviewer was a clinical psychologist with specialized training in sex therapy. Each partner filled out a multiple-choice questionnaire on relationship happiness, anxieties about sexuality and cancer, and sexual function. Another questionnaire, the Brief Symptom Inventory, was administered to measure psychological distress. Sexual counseling, as described earlier in this chapter, was provided to the couple or at least to the woman. The interview and questionnaires were repeated six months and one year after treatment. Many women were also interviewed at their three- and nine-month follow-up visits. Although a few received extra sessions of sexual counseling, none required formal, intensive sex therapy.

At the time of interim data analysis, 51 women had been evaluated initially and were at least six months posttreatment. Follow-up data were available on 41 women with an average follow-up date of seven months. The group was young, with a mean age of 38 years (range, 25–60). Only seven women were postmenopausal at the time of cancer diagnosis. Eighteen of the women (35%) underwent radical hysterectomy for cancer; four of these also had bilateral salpingo-oophorectomy. Seven (14%) were treated with radical hysterectomy and postoperative radiotherapy, 21 (41%) with radiotherapy alone (external beam and intracavitary), and 5 (10%) with cut-through hysterectomy and radiotherapy.

Cancer Risk Factors and Life History

Although we did not design the study to gather epidemiological data, the women's life histories were compatible with the theory that cervical cancer is caused or promoted by a sexually transmitted virus (Hulka 1982; Rapp and Jenkins 1981). Forty-three percent had been married more than once and 18% had six or more children. We soon realized that our typical patient had a life of turmoil, and often victimization. At least a third of the women had lived with an alcoholic partner, and a third had been physically abused by a spouse. The incidence of rape, incest, and sexual molestation of the women's own children appeared high, but unfortunately we did not assess these events in all women when the study first began.

Marital Relationships

The women's relationship status at the time of cancer diagnosis is listed in table 37.1. Seventy-four percent of relationships remained stable at the time of follow-up. The quarter of women who would change relationship status was strikingly easy to identify. After the initial interview, the psychologist rated the woman's relationship as having no, mild, or moderate-to-severe conflict. All relationships that changed fell into the category of "moderate to severe." Women also rated their own marital happiness on a seven-point scale from "extremely unhappy" to "perfect." Eighty-six percent of women whose relationship status changed had initially rated themselves in the lowest two categories of the scale. Thus, cancer did not destroy good relationships. It was merely a catalyst for separation in those that already had conflict. For the group as a whole, relationship happiness averaged in the range of "very happy" both before and after cancer treatment.

Sexual Frequency

This group of women did not decrease their frequency of expression of affection, sexual desire, sexual activity with a partner, or masturbation after cancer treatment (table 37.2). The types of sexual caressing that made up their sexual routine also did not change over time in any obvious way (table 37.3). There was no evidence that couples' lovemaking became more perfunctory or restricted.

Sexual Satisfaction

Corroborating evidence for continued good sexual function comes from questionnaire items on the quality of the sexual interaction (table 37.4). Women spent as

Table 37.1. *Relationship Status at Cancer Diagnosis*

Status	*N*	%	Years (mean)
Married	36	70	12
Separated/divorced	11	22	5
Widowed	1	2	1
Single	1	2	—
Living with partner	2	4	2

Table 37.2. *Sexual Frequency over Time*

	At Diagnosis			At Follow-up		
Variable	*N*	Mean	Label	*N*	Mean	Label
Frequency of affection	47	1.43	1/day	38	1.13	1/day
Frequency of sex	49	3.39	2/week	38	3.34	2/week
Frequency of desire	48	2.94	2/week	38	3.21	2/week
Frequency of masturbation	47	6.98	<1/month	37	6.84	<1/month

Note: There are no significant differences.

Table 37.3. *Percentage of Women Engaging in Sexual Activities*

Activity	At Diagnosis	At Follow-up
Penile-vaginal intercourse	96	92
Breast caressing	92	84
Caressing of female genitals	90	87
Caressing of male genitals	84	82
Cunnilingus	52	43
Fellatio	47	43
Anal intercourse	16	5

Note: The mean number of activities was 4.70 at diagnosis (SD = 1.78) and 4.35 at follow-up (SD = 1.90). Three women were sexually inactive at diagnosis, and two were inactive at follow-up.

Table 37.4. *Sexual Satisfaction over Time*

	At Diagnosis			At Follow-up		
Variable	*N*	Mean	Label	*N*	Mean	Label
Duration of foreplay	44	4.20	7–10 minutes	32	4.38	7–10 minutes
Female achieves arousal	51	1.51	75% of time	36	1.86	75% of time
Orgasm with masturbation	23	1.78	75% of time	17	1.82	75% of time
Noncoital orgasm	38	2.10	75% of time	28	2.39	75% of time
Coital orgasm	50	2.06	75% of time	37	2.43	75% of time
Dyspareunia	49	2.59	25% of time	35	3.03	25% of time
Sexual satisfaction	47	5.15	Moderately satisfied	35	4.94	Moderately satisfied

much time in foreplay as they had before the cancer. They were still able to feel subjectively aroused, lubricate vaginally, and reach orgasm on most occasions. Dyspareunia occurred about a quarter of the time before and after cancer treatment, and sexual satisfaction remained moderate.

A number of women did have minor complaints about vaginal dryness or types of genital pain (table 37.5). Only four women (11%), however, reported that dyspareunia was severe enough to interfere with sexual frequency and pleasure. The others characteristically said that the discomfort was mild and disappeared as sexual arousal increased. Perhaps if we had only asked for complaints instead of assessing sexual function more broadly, our picture of sexuality would have resembled results from past research.

Anxieties about Sexuality and Cancer

At the initial assessment, each woman rated how often she had worried about seven areas of anxiety about sexuality and cancer since her cancer diagnosis (table 37.6). An average anxiety score was computed for each subject. Women higher in sexual anxiety also initially presented with more psychological distress (Brief Symptom Inventory scores), more symptoms of vaginismus, and more frequent dyspareunia. By the time of follow-up, the women having high anxiety were still more emotionally distressed and were more unhappy in their relationships. The anxiety score was thus a good indicator of women at high risk for sexual and marital problems and could be used in the future to identify patients in need of early, intensive treatment.

Table 37.5. *Sexual Complaints at Follow-up*

Complaint	*N*	%
Vaginal dryness	19	37
Pain with deep thrusting	14	37
Postcoital vaginal soreness	13	35
Increased latency to reach orgasm	10	27
Usually need extra lubrication	9	24
Postcoital spotting of blood	12	24
Vagina feels too short	9	23
Pain on penetration	8	21
Dyspareunia interferes with pleasure	4	11
Need to change intercourse position	4	11
Vagina feels too narrow	4	10
Decreased orgasmic intensity	1	3

Table 37.6. *Anxieties at Diagnosis about Sexuality and Cancer*

Anxiety	Mean Level	Often or Constantly Worried (%)
Fear that sex caused cancer	Once or twice	4
Fear that sex exacerbates cancer	Once or twice	11
Fear of venereal contagion of cancer	Never	2
Fear of losing attractiveness	Once or twice	23
Fear that cancer will interfere with sex	Once or twice	19
Fear of inability to have orgasm after cancer treatment	Once or twice	8
Fear of infertility	Once or twice	14

Note: The average level of anxiety for the sample group was "once or twice." On the average, only 2% worried "often or constantly."

Resumption of Daily Life Activities

Most women not only stayed sexually active and maintained their close relationships, but they also resumed other daily life activities, including jobs outside of the home, household chores and care of the family, hobbies, and social activities (table 37.7). A significant correlation existed between age and returning to jobs outside of the home. Older women were more likely to take early retirement after cancer treatment.

Surgery Compared with Radiotherapy

Strikingly few differences could be found between women treated with hysterectomy alone, radiotherapy alone, or a combination of the two treatments. The few significant findings we observed are listed in table 37.8. Women primarily treated with radiotherapy were slightly older, which probably accounts for the fact that they experienced less frequent sexual desire and were less likely to return to jobs after cancer treatment. The one difference that looks important is in psychological distress (Brief Symptom Inventory score). Both treatment groups began by being mildly distressed. Across all women, scores on depression, anxiety, and interpersonal sensitivity decreased significantly over time. It appears, however, that this decrease took place mainly in the hysterectomy group. Perhaps the finality of surgery was easier to endure than two months of radiotherapy. More long-term data on a

Table 37.7. *Women Resuming Daily Life Activities*

Activity	Same as Before Cancer (%)	Somewhat Less (%)	No Resumption (%)	*N*
Job outside home	67	15	18	34
Household chores	73	25	2	40
Care of family	74	26	0	40
Active hobbies	74	17	9	35
Quiet hobbies	87	10	3	39
Social life	85	15	0	40

Note: Not all subjects participated in all activities before diagnosis ($N = 41$).

Table 37.8. *Differences Between Treatment Groups*

Variable	Radical Hysterectomy		Radiotherapy		*p*
	N	Mean or %	*N*	Mean or %	
Age	25	35 years	26	41 years	.05
Frequency of desire at follow-up	18	2.33	20	4.00	.01
Global Symptom Index at follow-up	16	33.06	17	82.94	.05
Resumption of job at follow-up	13	100%	10	70%	.05

larger sample of women will be available next year; we await these data to see if the present findings are confirmed. At that time, we will also be able to provide information about the effects on sexuality of hormone replacement therapy, vaginal dilation, and the male partner's involvement in sexual rehabilitation.

Conclusion

Although these women with cervical cancer often had histories of relationship turmoil, over three-quarters were able to maintain stable relationships up to seven months after cancer treatment. Changes in relationship status were accurately predicted by the amount of conflict that existed at the time of cancer diagnosis. Measures of sexual frequency, types of stimulation used, function, and satisfaction remained stable for women, whether the women received surgical or radiotherapeutic treatment. Some women complained of minor vaginal dryness or pain, but the discomfort rarely interfered with sexual desire or the ability to reach orgasm. Most women also resumed normal daily life activities, including jobs, household chores, hobbies, and social life. Psychological distress decreased from diagnosis to follow-up, especially for women who had radical hysterectomies. Women initially high in sexual anxiety continued to be more emotionally distressed and unhappy in their relationships at follow-up.

Finally, we believe that the brief sexual education and counseling we provided to women and their partners may account for the positive outcomes in our data compared with outcomes reported in previous research. We did not think that it was ethical to withhold counseling from half the subjects, allowing a comparison with an untreated control group. Thus, we cannot prove that the counseling was crucial. Our patient group included relatively young women who received all the supportive services and care provided by a major cancer center. We hope, however, that other clinicians will take note of these preliminary findings and adapt our techniques to their own settings. Sexual rehabilitation should be an integral part of the care of gynecologic oncology patients.

References

Abitbol MM, Davenport JH. 1974. Sexual dysfunction after therapy for cervical carcinoma. *Am J Obstet Gynecol* 119:181–189.

Adelusi B. 1980. Coital function after radiotherapy for carcinoma of the cervix uteri. *Br J Obstet Gynaecol* 87:821–823.

Andersen BL, Hacker NF. 1983a. Psychosexual adjustment following pelvic exenteration. *Obstet Gynecol* 61:331–338.

Andersen BL, Hacker NF. 1983b. Treatment for gynecologic cancer: A review of the effects on female sexuality. *Health Psychology* 2:203–221.

Barbach L. 1974. *For Yourself.* New York: Anchor Press/Doubleday.

Barbach L. 1982. *For Each Other.* New York: Anchor Press/Doubleday.

Decker WH, Schwartzman E. 1962. Sexual function following treatment for carcinoma of the cervix. *Am J Obstet Gynecol* 83:401–405.

Hansen JK. 1981. Surgical and combination therapy of the cervix uteri stages IB and IIA. *Gynecol Oncol* 12:S7–S24.

Heiman JR, LoPiccolo L, LoPiccolo J. 1976. *Becoming Orgasmic*. Englewood Cliffs, N.J.: Prentice-Hall.

Hulka BS. 1982. Risk factors for cervical cancer. *J Chronic Dis* 35:3–11.

Kaplan HS. 1974. *The New Sex Therapy*. New York: Brunner/Mazel.

Rapp F, Jenkins FJ. 1981. Genital cancer and viruses. *Gynecol Oncol* 12:S25–S41.

Schover LR. 1984. *Prime Time: Sexual Health for Men Over Fifty*. New York: Holt, Rinehart & Winston.

Schover LR, Fife M. 1986. Sexual counseling of patients undergoing radical surgery for pelvic or genital cancer. *Journal of Psychosocial Oncology* 3:21–41.

Schover LR, Friedman J, Heiman JR, Weiler SJ, LoPiccolo J. 1982. Multiaxial problem-oriented system for sexual dysfunctions: An alternative to DSM III. *Arch Gen Psychiatry* 39:614–619.

Siebel M, Freeman MG, Graves WL. 1982. Sexual function after surgical and radiation therapy for cervical carcinoma. *South Med J* 75:1195–1197.

Vincent CE, Vincent B, Griess FC, Linton EB. 1975. Some marital-sexual concomitants of carcinoma of the cervix. *South Med J* 68:552–558.

JEFFREY A. GOTTLIEB MEMORIAL LECTURE

Annual Clinical Conference on Cancer, Vol. 29
Gynecologic Cancer: Diagnosis and Treatment Strategies
© 1987 by The University of Texas System Cancer Center

38. Clinical Cancer Research—Sunrise or Sunset?

C. Gordon Zubrod

Clinical research was at one time a much-to-be-desired career for young physicians—a career that today has few applicants. One has only to read some of the many papers documenting this phenomenon (Booth 1979, 1980; Feinstein, Koss, and Austin 1967; Fredrickson 1981; Gill 1984; Legato 1981; Oliver 1977; Wyngaarden 1979). Alvan Feinstein and coworkers in 1967 in a scholarly analysis of the content of papers submitted for the Atlantic City meetings called attention to the turning away from clinical research (Feinstein, Koss, and Austin 1967). Jim Wyngaarden, now the director of the National Institutes of Health (NIH), spoke several years at the Atlantic City meetings of the disappearance of the clinical traineeships and in 1979 published his study (Wyngaarden 1979). At the same time, fundamental research has exploded in productivity, so almost every day there are new exciting discoveries about the nature of cancer and the potential for its cure or prevention. Where are the clinical investigators who will be able to make use of this new knowledge to control cancer? As we gaze at this reddened sky, do we watch the sun rising or setting on clinical research? I thought I would examine this question today, using some personal observations of clinical investigation I've made since I first stepped onto the wards. Let me summarize by saying that in my various opportunities to observe clinical research, it prospered most when there was long-term stability for the academic physician.

Let me go back to my beginnings. When I was a medical student and later a house officer at Columbia and Presbyterian in New York, the Department of Medicine was filled with superb physicians, each of whom was an active clinical investigator. A list of some of these would include Walter Palmer, Robert Loeb, Dana Atchley, Alphonse Dochez, Randolph West, Franklin Hanger, Martin Dawson, Michael Heidelberger, Alvin Coburn, and Alexander and Ethel Gutman. They, with the exception of Dana Atchley, saw few private patients and did a good deal of teaching but spent most of their time on research. There were no research grants and only three to four full-time faculty positions, yet there was little turnover of staff. The reason for this happy situation came to me a few years later when Bob Berliner, the real star of our house staff, asked one of them about the possibility of a career in clinical investigation. He was told that unless he had a large family fortune, he should enter private practice. So the reason for this extraordinary stability of the clinical investigators in the 1930s was presumably personal financial independence.

As I was finishing my residency, World War II engulfed our country and everyone's career plans. While I awaited my commission, Drs. Palmer and Loeb called me in and asked me to go see a certain Dr. James A. Shannon who was starting a malaria research team and needed clinical helpers. Malaria was the primary health problem for the armed forces, because the Allies faced a long war in the mosquito-rich areas of the South Pacific, China, India, Burma, and North Africa. Quinine was grown only in the Dutch East Indies, then in Japan's possession. Atabrine (quinacrine) was a little-studied drug, and its secrets were held tightly by the I. G. Farben cartel in Germany. Dr. Shannon assembled a team in the New York University division of Goldwater Hospital in New York. The early members (1942–1946), in addition to Shannon, included David Earle, Robert Berliner, John Taggart, Bernard Brodie, Sidney Udenfriend, Thomas Kennedy, Irving London, Eugéne Knox, and Roger Greif. This team was the clinical and pharmacology component of a large national drug development program. In a relatively short time Atabrine was synthesized, studied for toxicity and pharmacological disposition, and shown to be much better than quinine. A prophylactic regimen was developed that kept the Allied troops relatively free of malaria. Chloroquine was discovered; vixax relapses prevented. More fundamentally, Shannon's approach to the study of drugs served as the base for a new pharmacology, emphasizing pharmacokinetics.

The conditions of wartime gave a certain stability to clinical investigation; because the problems were urgent, the full resources of the federal government could be used, and recruitment was easy. It was a short-lived stability, because the problems were solved so quickly. After the war, the team turned to other things for a while and then reassembled as the nucleus of the rapidly expanding NIH.

I had become interested in clinical pharmacology, had taken a three-year fellowship at Johns Hopkins, and later joined the faculty. I had duties both in medicine and pharmacology, and my general objective was to improve therapeutics using the new pharmacology. My laboratory was in Dr. E. K. Marshall's department. He had been a mainstay in the malaria drug development program and was well known for having worked out the pharmacology of sulfanilamide and its successors. His work on sulfaguanidine was a major factor in keeping the Japanese, who suffered terribly from dysentery, away from the southern coast of New Guinea and preventing access to Australia's northern ports. There was a tremendous backlog of new knowledge developed during the war. There were many young faculty members and fellows eager to get back into clinical research. So for five or six years there was stability in the life of a clinical investigator, a stability not so much dependent on good salaries as it was on the sheer excitement of the many opportunities. In bacterial chemotherapy, for example, many different penicillins were available for study, streptomycin and antituberculosis treatment were emerging, and the tetracyclines had been discovered. The same thing was happening in every field, and other marvelous new drugs appeared—nitrogen mustard, antifols, adrenocorticotropic hormone, cortisone.

Besides, NIH, having observed the effects of federal support of research for wartime emergencies, was undertaking a vast expansion of its research grants. This was done deliberately, I believe, to confer stability on careers in academic medicine including, of course, clinical research. This was a period that lasted some 20 years from about 1950 to 1970. I had little experience on the university side with this era of clinical research stability, because in 1954 I went to NIH.

NIH had been largely a laboratory-based effort until 1953 when the Clinical Center opened. My Baltimore colleagues kidded me about leaving clinical investigation to join the National Institute of Mouse Cancer. I became the first clinical director of NCI. I had had only the most general exposure to cancer research, so I guess I was recruited in order to bring my experience in chemotherapy of infectious diseases to the cancer problems. I am not going to recite the events of 20 years at NCI, but I do want to pay tribute to the team of clinical investigators in the early days of NCI, including James Holland, Roy Hertz, John Fahey, Jesse Steinfeld, Nathaniel Berlin, Alfred Ketcham, Emil Frei, Emil Freireich, Mortimer Lipsett, Philip Rubin, Herman Suit, and Paul Carbone. Moreover, because the military draft was still rigorously applied and because service in the Public Health Service qualified, NCI was able to recruit the top talent from the great medical schools and hospitals. Some of the clinical associates of the early days at NCI included Dick Silver, Tom Waldman, Sherm Weissman, Dan Nathans, Gerry Bodey, Evan Hersh, Bob Gallo, John Zeigler, Dane Boggs, Dave Nathan, Vincent De Vita, Bruce Chabner, Bob Young, Jim Belli, Don Morton, Marvin Romsdahl, Chuck Vogel, and Jim Pittman. Once tasting of NIH, with its unique depths in basic science, 500 research beds, full financial support from federal funds, and few teaching or patient care responsibilities, it is no wonder that many physicians found exciting careers in clinical investigation.

So this is another kind of stability—the stability of the free-standing research institute, free of the many demands placed on the physician in the university setting. Nevertheless, I had a yearning for one more stint of university life, particularly for a return to a large general hospital, so in 1974 I went to the University of Miami to take responsibility for its new cancer center. After 35 years in which I had spent almost all my time in one aspect or another of clinical investigation, I had trouble in identifying what I had come to recognize as clinical research. Of course there was a lot of cooperative group activity, but though this is an essential part of drug development, it did not to my mind present the opportunity for effective interchange of new ideas between basic science and clinical exploration.

One of the main problems for clinical research in a cancer center is that the model for cancer centers was developed for the free-standing research institute and then translated to the university setting. In the university cancer center there is little stability for the physician scientist, largely because salary sources are lacking. Except in a few institutions with large endowments, the salary of the physician-scientist must be pieced together from a half dozen sources and is heavily dependent on private practice income. Research grants, the so-called RO1s, which provide major funding toward salaries of basic scientists, are rarely available to the physician-scientist. This is mostly because peer review of clinical grants is carried out by basic scientists—a custom that reminds me of the Christian martyrs being thrown to the lions and tigers of the Roman circus. Center core grants provide almost nothing toward physicians' salaries because they have no RO1 grants. So the salary is put together from practice income, a few dollars from the university, contracts with industry, fund raising, and the Veterans Administration.

This is hardly a model that medical students want to follow. They see the financial instability of a career in clinical research, especially when they graduate with an average debt of $33,000. They see the elements making an academic career unattractive: the debts of medical students, the low salaries of fellowships, the drive toward family practice, the many duties of patient care, the difficulties in getting clinical grants, the revolution in health care services, and the regulatory obstacles to clinical research. According to one survey, the percentage of students considering a research career dropped from 49% in 1963 to 2% in 1976, so the pool of students from which the physician-scientists would be drawn has dried up.

But given an adequate salary, how much time can the academic physician spend at becoming a physician-scientist? The answer is precious little, because his or her day is more than full with patient care, teaching of house staff and students, committee service, paperwork for institutional review boards and cooperative groups, and more recently for the diagnosis-related group record keeping and other impositions of the revolution in providing health care. All the while in the laboratories of the basic scientists, new complex technologies appear almost daily. The technology has bypassed most physicians and is ever more rapidly disappearing in the distance.

Sunrise or sunset? I think the sun is setting for the physician-scientist as Gordon Gill has so eloquently described (Gill 1984). At least this seems inevitable for yesterday's image of the physician-scientist who has mastered all the laboratory technologies and can carry out his own research in patients. It must be said that there is belated recognition of his plight as NIH begins to support a few young clinical investigators. The great new foundations, such as the Howard Hughes Foundation imaginatively led by Don Fredrickson, recognize the need to rescue clinical investigation. These billion-dollar foundations are quite capable of pouring money into today's void. For example, the Hughes Foundation has recently announced a program to attract medical students to work at NIH. The physician-scientist may not completely disappear. Certainly at the NIH Clinical Center, with 500 of the country's 1,200 research beds, the physician-scientist will continue to exist. The same may well be true at a few other highly endowed research institutes and at Harvard, but I suspect they are a small brave band. It reminds me of another endangered species in Florida—the dusky seaside sparrow. There are only four elderly males still alive. As a last desperate step to preserve some of their genetic materials, crossbreeding with similar species is underway and preservation of their DNA in vitro is contemplated. So even if the sun sets on the physician-scientist, in the night to follow as in the monasteries of Iona in the Dark Ages, the unique resources of NIH intramural programs and the extraordinary resources efforts of the Hughes Foundation will preserve a few physician-scientists for tomorrow.

What happens to clinical investigation without physician-scientists? The vast array of new knowledge, which grows daily, in molecular genetics, in the cancer-causing viruses and their oncogenes, in immunology, in cell biology, seems to have the potential to solve some of the dark mysteries of human cancer. Who will do this in patients? Fuller Albright defined clinical investigation as "studies of sick people." Physicians must play a key role. But it is the laboratory scientist who sees how the arcane technology must be applied to sick people. The show cannot go on without the players from the laboratory. How can we get the Ph.D. from the seminars at Cold Spring Harbor onto the stage—the confusing and messy stage of clinical medicine—so that the drama can proceed? NIH can do it, as Bob Gallo daily demonstrates. Industry has done it. The Ph.D.s who have created such companies as Genentech are smart enough to find physicians who can work with them, and more and more these linkages will be forged in the research institutes. Perhaps these are the ways. What troubles me is that most of the physicians who are at the bedside are in the medical schools. These are the physicians who practice the superb medicine essential to clinical investigation. These are the physicians who define new problems arising in disease. These are the physicians who can design a valid clinical trial.

Academic medicine must look for new ways to bring together its physicians and scientists. We must think of ways to bring the scientist into an awareness of clinical disease; we must find a less harried life for the academic physician and free his time to work closely with his laboratory colleagues. This, of course, is happening in many ways. I need only point to the experience with acquired immune deficiency syndrome. The epidemic has frightened all of us into extraordinary efforts. Thrown together daily are clinicians, virologists, molecular biologists, epidemiologists, biostatisticians, hospital administrators, even cancer center directors, as they try to cope with the realities of a slow virus with exponential increase. It reminds me of the urgent research problems of World War II with their access to vast research funds and easy recruitment. Although crisis is not always the best model for everyday life, it contains a valuable lesson, and if we are wise we will use it to devise calmer linkages for all biomedical research.

In looking at this reddened sky, I have asked, with apologies to the poets, is this the sinking of that nebulous star we call the sun, or are these the rosy fingers of the dawn? As in so many things in life, one can turn to the wisdom of the Bible:

> The Pharisees and Sadducees came along, and as a test asked him to show them some sign in the sky. He gave them this reply: "In the evening you say, 'Red sky at night, the day will be bright'; but in the morning, 'Sky red and gloomy, the day will be stormy.'" (Matthew 16:2–3)

Children over the centuries have shortened this to "Red at night, sailors' delight; red in the morning, sailors take warning." Perhaps the red in the sky is both a sunrise and a sunset. It is sunset for the physician-scientist who could master an entire technology and follow a narrow interest in a few patients; the academic physician has returned to his older role—the superb care of patients and the teaching of the young. And it is a sunrise on a new day with its warning that we need to prepare for a stormy day of finding stability for the physicians in academia and in forging the linkages between these fine physicians and our incredible science.

References

Booth CC. 1979. The development of clinical science in Britain. *Br Med J* 1:1469–1473.

Booth CC. 1980. Clinical science in the 1980's. *Lancet* 2:904–907.

Feinstein AR, Koss N, Austin JHM. 1967. The changing emphasis in clinical research. I. Topics under investigation: An analysis of the submitted abstracts and selected programs at the annual "Atlantic City Meetings" during 1953 through 1965. *Ann Intern Med* 66:396–419.

Fredrickson DS. 1981. Biomedical research in 1980's. *N Engl J Med* 304:509–517.
Gill GN. 1984. The end of the physician-scientist? *American Scholar* 53:353–368.
Legato MJ. 1981. The disappearing doctors: Why are physicians leaving academic medicine? *The Sciences* 21:15, 18–19.
Oliver MF. 1977. The shrinking base of clinical science: Where are tomorrow's researchers? *J Clin Invest* 7:1–2.
Wyngaarden JB. 1979. The clinical investigator as an endangered species. *N Engl J Med* 301:1254–1259.

Contributors

Ervin Adam, M.D.
Professor
Departments of Virology and Epidemiology and of Obstetrics and Gynecology
Baylor College of Medicine
Houston, Texas

Ebrahim Ashayeri, M.D.
Associate Professor, Radiation Medicine
Howard University Hospital
Washington, D.C.

Kenneth D. Bagshawe, M.D.
Professor of Medical Oncology
Cancer Research Campaign Laboratories
Department of Medical Oncology
Charing Cross and Westminster Medical School
London, England

Samuel C. Ballon, M.D.
Professor and Director
Division of Gynecologic Oncology
Stanford University School of Medicine
Stanford, California

Bart Barlogie, M.D.
Professor of Medicine
Division of Medicine
and Head (ad interim)
Department of Hematology
The University of Texas M. D. Anderson Hospital and Tumor Institute at Houston
Houston, Texas

James M. Bowen, Ph.D.
Professor of Virology and
Vice President for Academic Affairs
The University of Texas M. D. Anderson Hospital and Tumor Institute at Houston
Houston, Texas

William M. Christopherson, M.D.
Professor of Pathology
Department of Pathology
University of Louisville School of Medicine
Health Sciences Center
Louisville, Kentucky

Larry J. Copeland, M.D.
Associate Professor
Department of Gynecology
The University of Texas M. D. Anderson Hospital and Tumor Institute at Houston
Houston, Texas

Peter M. Corry, Ph.D.
Professor
Department of Radiation Physics
The University of Texas M. D. Anderson Hospital and Tumor Institute at Houston
Houston, Texas

Catherine J. Cox, M.D.
Staff Pathologist
Falk Clinic Laboratory
Pittsburgh, Pennsylvania

Luis Delclos, M.D.
Professor of Radiotherapy
Department of Clinical Radiotherapy
The University of Texas M. D. Anderson Hospital and Tumor Institute at Houston
Houston, Texas

Gregorio Delgado, M.D.
Chief, Division of Gynecologic Oncology
Georgetown University Hospital
Washington, D.C.

Alon J. Dembo, M.B., F.R.C.P.(C)
Associate Professor
Department of Radiology
The University of Toronto
and Radiation Oncologist
The Princess Margaret Hospital
Toronto, Ontario
Canada

A. Dennis De Petrillo, M.D., F.R.C.S.(C)
Director, Division of Gynecologic Oncology
The University of Toronto
Chief, Department of Obstetrics and Gynecology
The Wellesley Hospital
and Professor
Department of Obstetrics and Gynecology
The University of Toronto
Toronto, Ontario
Canada

Creighton L. Edwards, M.D.
Professor and Ann Rife Cox Chair
Department of Gynecology
Experimental Gynecology Laboratory
The University of Texas M. D. Anderson Hospital and Tumor Institute at Houston
Houston, Texas

Clarence E. Ehrlich, M.D.
Professor and Chairman
Department of Obstetrics and Gynecology
Indiana University Medical Center
Indianapolis, Indiana

Arnold J. Eisenfeld, M.D.
Senior Research Scientist
Department of Obstetrics and Gynecology
Yale University School of Medicine
New Haven, Connecticut

Gilbert H. Fletcher, M.D.
Professor of Radiotherapy
Department of Clinical Radiotherapy
The University of Texas M. D. Anderson Hospital and Tumor Institute at Houston
Houston, Texas

Ralph S. Freedman, M.D., Ph.D.
Associate Professor
Department of Gynecology
The University of Texas M. D. Anderson Hospital and Tumor Institute at Houston
Houston, Texas

Herbert A. Fritsche, Ph.D.
Associate Biochemist, Associate Professor, and Chief of Clinical Chemistry
The University of Texas M. D. Anderson Hospital and Tumor Institute at Houston
Houston, Texas

H. Stephen Gallager, M.D.
Professor
Department of Pathology
The University of Texas M. D. Anderson Hospital and Tumor Institute at Houston
Houston, Texas

David M. Gershenson, M.D.
Associate Professor
Department of Gynecology
The University of Texas M. D. Anderson Hospital and Tumor Institute at Houston
Houston, Texas

Alfred L. Goldson, M.D.
Chairman, Radiation Medicine
Howard University Hospital
Washington, D.C.

Arthur D. Hamberger, M.D.
Clinical Associate Radiotherapist
The University of Texas M. D. Anderson Hospital and Tumor Institute at Houston
and Medical Director
Department of Radiotherapy
Memorial City General Hospital
Houston, Texas

Ronald B. Herberman, M.D.
Director, Pittsburgh Cancer Institute
and Professor of Medicine and Pathology
University of Pittsburgh
Pittsburgh, Pennsylvania

Richard B. Hochberg, Ph.D.
Professor of Obstetrics and Gynecology
Yale University School of Medicine
New Haven, Connecticut

John A. Holt, Ph.D.
Associate Professor
Department of Obstetrics and Gynecology
University of Chicago Hospitals and Clinics
Chicago, Illinois

Tod S. Johnson, Ph.D.
Associate Professor of Biophysics
Department of Hematology
Division of Medicine
The University of Texas M. D. Anderson Hospital and Tumor Institute at Houston
Houston, Texas

Lovell A. Jones, Ph.D.
Associate Professor
Department of Gynecology
Experimental Gynecology Laboratory
The University of Texas M. D. Anderson Hospital and Tumor Institute at Houston
Houston, Texas

Geri-Lynn Kasper, M.D.
Fellow, Gynecologic Oncology
Department of Gynecology
The University of Texas M. D. Anderson Hospital and Tumor Institute at Houston
Houston, Texas

Ruth L. Katz, M.D.
Chief, Section of Cytopathology
Department of Pathology
The University of Texas M. D. Anderson Hospital and Tumor Institute at Houston
Houston, Texas

Raymond H. Kaufman, M.D.
Ernst W. Bertner Chairman and Professor
Department of Obstetrics and Gynecology
and Professor, Department of Pathology
Baylor College of Medicine
Houston, Texas

John J. Kavanagh, M.D.
Departments of Gynecology and Chemotherapy Research
The University of Texas M. D. Anderson Hospital and Tumor Institute at Houston
Houston, Texas

Joseph S. Kong, M.D.
Assistant Professor
Department of Clinical Radiotherapy
The University of Texas M. D. Anderson Hospital and Tumor Institute at Houston
Houston, Texas

Alan J. Kunschner, M.D.
Associate Clinical Professor
Department of Obstetrics and Gynecology
University of Pittsburgh School of Medicine
Pittsburgh, Pennsylvania

Lamk M. Lamki, M.D.
Associate Professor
Department of Diagnostic Radiotherapy
Division of Diagnostic Imaging
The University of Texas M. D. Anderson Hospital and Tumor Institute at Houston
Houston, Texas

John S. Lazo, Ph.D.
Associate Professor of Pharmacology
Yale University School of Medicine
New Haven, Connecticut

Errol Lewis, M.D.
Associate Professor
Department of Diagnostic Radiology
Division of Diagnostic Imaging
The University of Texas M. D. Anderson Hospital and Tumor Institute at Houston
Houston, Texas

Frank J. Liu, M.D.
Assistant Pathologist
Assistant Professor of Laboratory Medicine
The University of Texas M. D. Anderson Hospital and Tumor Institute at Houston
Houston, Texas

Eva Lotzová, Ph.D.
Professor of Immunology
Department of General Surgery
The University of Texas M. D. Anderson Hospital and Tumor Institute at Houston
Houston, Texas

Neil J. MacLusky, Ph.D.
Associate Professor of Obstetrics and Gynecology
Yale University School of Medicine
New Haven, Connecticut

Maurie Markman, M.D.
Associate Chairman for Clinical Affairs
Department of Medicine
Memorial Sloan-Kettering Cancer Center
New York, New York

C. Paul Morrow, M.D.
Professor of Gynecology
University of Southern California School of Medicine
Los Angeles, California

Philip M. Mount, M.D.
Pathologist, U.S. Army Reserve Corps
Armed Forces Institute of Pathology
Washington, D.C.

Fredrick N. Naftolin, M.D.
Professor and Chairman
Department of Obstetrics and Gynecology
Yale University School of Medicine
New Haven, Connecticut

Henry J. Norris, M.D.
Chairman, Department of Gynecologic and Breast Pathology
Armed Forces Institute of Pathology
Washington, D.C.

Roland A. Pattillo, M.D.
Professor of Obstetrics and Gynecology
The Medical College of Wisconsin
Milwaukee, Wisconsin

Edmund S. Petrilli, M.D.
Associate Professor
Division of Gynecologic Oncology
Georgetown University Hospital
Washington, D.C.

M. Steven Piver, M.D.
Chief, Department of Gynecologic Oncology
Roswell Park Memorial Institute
Buffalo, New York

Michael F. Press, M.D., Ph.D.
Assistant Professor
Departments of Pathology and of Obstetrics and Gynecology
University of Chicago Hospitals and Clinics
Chicago, Illinois

Martin N. Raber, M.D.
Associate Professor of New Drug Studies
Department of Chemotherapy Research
Division of Medicine
The University of Texas M. D. Anderson Hospital and Tumor Institute at Houston
Houston, Texas

A. C. F. Ruckert
Research Technologist
Department of Gynecology and Obstetrics
The Medical College of Wisconsin
Milwaukee, Wisconsin

Felix N. Rutledge, M.D.
Professor and Chairman
Department of Gynecology
The University of Texas M. D. Anderson Hospital and Tumor Institute at Houston
Houston, Texas

Patton B. Saul, M.D.
Assistant Professor
Department of Gynecology
The University of Texas M. D. Anderson Hospital and Tumor Institute at Houston
Houston, Texas

Cherylyn A. Savary, Ph.D.
Project Investigator
Department of General Surgery
The University of Texas M. D. Anderson Hospital and Tumor Institute at Houston
Houston, Texas

Leslie R. Schover, Ph.D.
Assistant Professor of Urology (Psychology)
Section of Sexual Rehabilitation
Department of Urology
The University of Texas M. D. Anderson Hospital and Tumor Institute at Houston
Houston, Texas

Peter E. Schwartz, M.D.
Professor of Obstetrics and Gynecology
Director of Gynecologic Oncology
Yale University School of Medicine
New Haven, Connecticut

Henry F. Sears, M.D., F.A.C.S.
Associate Professor of Surgery
Harvard Medical School
New England Deaconess Hospital
Boston, Massachusetts

Jan C. Seski, M.D.
Assistant Clinical Professor
Department of Obstetrics and Gynecology
University of Pittsburgh School of Medicine
Pittsburgh, Pennsylvania

R. Michael Shier, B.S.C., M.D., F.R.C.S.(C)
Director, The Wellesley Hospital Colposcopy Unit
Deputy Chief, Department of Obstetrics and Gynecology
The Wellesley Hospital
and Assistant Professor
Department of Obstetrics and Gynecology
The University of Toronto
Toronto, Ontario
Canada

Elvio G. Silva, M.D.
Associate Professor
Department of Pathology
The University of Texas M. D. Anderson Hospital and Tumor Institute at Houston
Houston, Texas

C. Allen Stringer, M.D.
Assistant Professor
Department of Obstetrics, Gynecology, and Reproductive Sciences
The University of Texas Medical School at Houston
Houston, Texas

Sidney Wallace, M.D.
Professor of Radiology
Deputy Department Chairman
Department of Diagnostic Radiology
Division of Diagnostic Imaging
The University of Texas M. D. Anderson Hospital and Tumor Institute at Houston
Houston, Texas

J. Taylor Wharton, M.D.
Professor and Deputy Chairman
Department of Gynecology
The University of Texas M. D. Anderson Hospital and Tumor Institute at Houston
Houston, Texas

C. Gordon Zubrod, M.D.
Director, Papanicolaou Comprehensive Cancer Center
and Professor and Chairman
Department of Oncology
University of Miami School of Medicine
Miami, Florida

Index